MEDICAL
Terminology
&Anatomy
for CODING

Contents

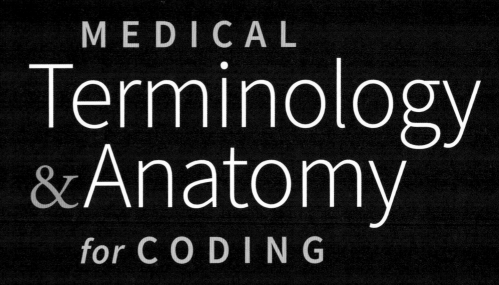

MEDICAL
Terminology
& Anatomy
for CODING

4TH EDITION

BETSY J. SHILAND

CCS, CPC, CPHQ, CTR, CHDA, CPB, EMT
AHIMA Approved ICD-10-CM/PCS Trainer
Former Assistant Professor
Allied Health Department
Community College of Philadelphia
Philadelphia, Pennsylvania

With 440 illustrations

ELSEVIER

Elsevier
3251 Riverport Lane
St. Louis, Missouri 63043

MEDICAL TERMINOLOGY & ANATOMY FOR CODING,
FOURTH EDITION

ISBN: 978-0-323-74957-2

Notices

Knowledge and best practice in this field are constantly changing. As new research and experience broaden our understanding, changes in research methods, professional practices, or medical treatment may become necessary.

Practitioners and researchers must always rely on their own experience and knowledge in evaluating and using any information, methods, compounds, or experiments described herein. In using such information or methods they should be mindful of their own safety and the safety of others, including parties for whom they have a professional responsibility.

With respect to any drug or pharmaceutical products identified, readers are advised to check the most current information provided (i) on procedures featured or (ii) by the manufacturer of each product to be administered, to verify the recommended dose or formula, the method and duration of administration, and contraindications. It is the responsibility of practitioners, relying on their own experience and knowledge of their patients, to make diagnoses, to determine dosages and the best treatment for each individual patient, and to take all appropriate safety precautions.

To the fullest extent of the law, neither the Publisher nor the authors, contributors, or editors, assume any liability for any injury and/or damage to persons or property as a matter of products liability, negligence or otherwise, or from any use or operation of any methods, products, instructions, or ideas contained in the material herein.

Previous editions copyrighted 2018, 2015, 2012.

Library of Congress Control Number: 2020938648

Publishing Director: Kristin Wilhelm
Senior Content Strategist: Linda Woodard
Senior Content Development Manager: Luke Held
Publishing Services Manager: Julie Eddy
Senior Project Manager: Abigail Bradberry
Designer: Brian Salisbury

Printed in India

Last digit is the print number: 9   8   7   6   5   4   3   2

Contributors

Erinn Kao, PharmD, RPh
Pharmacist
Rx Outreach, Inc.
St. Louis, MO

Previous Edition Reviewers

Bonnie Aspiazu, JD RHIA
Managing Director, School of Business and Health
  Sciences
ITT Educational Services, Inc.
Carmel, IN

Angela Campbell
Medical Insurance Manager, Eastern Illinois
  University
Charleston, IL
Assistant Professor, Northwestern College
Chicago, IL
Adjunct Faculty Member, The College of Health
  Care Professions
Houston, TX

Sandra Hertkorn
Director-Company Owner
Medical Information Systems, Physicians Billing
  Service
Sacramento-Carmichael, CA

Sue Manela, MBA
Assistant Professor of Office Administration
Northampton Community College
Bethlehem, PA

Cheryl Miller, MBA/HCM
Assistant Professor/Program Director
Westmoreland County Community College
Youngwood, PA

Terri Pizzano, BBA, MBA, CHTS IM, CHTS TR
Executive Health Care Consultant, HSM Consulting
Assistant Professor Health Care, IT, Business and
  General Education
Land O'Lakes, FL

Donna Reese, CPC, CPPM
Instructor
Northeast Technology Center-Kansas
Kansas, OK

Karen Smith, M.Ed., RHIA, CDIP, CPC
Assistant Professor
University of Arkansas for Medical Sciences,
  College of Health Professions
Little Rock, AR

Diana Wilson, CPC, CPMA, CPC-I
Adjunct Instructor, Course Writer
Ultimate Medical Academy
Tampa, FL

Preface

With ICD-11 on the horizon, the changes to ICD-10-CM/PCS just keep coming. Coders are constantly being required to raise their game in terms of knowledge of medical terminology, anatomy, and guidelines. Preparing for this edition had me using fistfuls of different colored sticky notes to remind me of the ICD-10-CM/PCS and CPT-4 changes on 93 pages with notes on 38 separate pages for extra research that needed to be done.

Our biggest change to this edition was the addition Appendix A, which serves to provide an introduction to ICD-10-CM Chapter 1: Certain Infectious and Parasitic Diseases. Historical context, an explanation of what the various organisms (and non-organisms) that cause the diseases and a new set of tables with word origins/definitions are included. The tables also include the cause of the disease for each disease, whether it be bacterial, viral, fungal, etc.

As always, it is important to remember that ICD-10 is a classification, a grouping of diseases and procedures. It is a collective best effort at this point in time as to how these diseases and procedures should be grouped. That's why we see constant changes in the classification, because our knowledge of medicine is always evolving. CPT-4 is also a nomenclature, literally a "calling of names." Billing for procedures for a provider requires a very specific designation of exactly what was done. For those coders who are amazed at the specificity of PCS, and are unfamiliar with CPT-4, a whole new way of organizing procedures is revealed (along with a significant amount of different terminology).

Medical Terminology and Anatomy for Coding prepares students for a coding, medical assisting, or health information management career with a focused delivery of content that allows them to recognize, recall, and apply their knowledge.

NEW TO THIS EDITION

The fourth edition continues the focus on ICD-10 terminology, with the following enhancements:

- New Basics of Infectious Disease appendix, which provides the basic information coders need to be able to understand infectious diseases and to code them correctly
- Additional and updated ICD-10 Guidelines and Notes provide connections between terminology and codes
- Updated CPT-4 anatomy and procedural coding alerts provide special information regarding coding in a physician office

UNIQUE FEATURES

- All the anatomy and physiology needed to correctly code using ICD-10-CM.
- Pathology terms organized by ICD-10 disease and disorder categories let you learn terms in the same order they are presented in the coding manual.
- Electronic health records allow students to view medical terminology in context.
- Oncology and Pharmacology appendices present the basics of these important subjects.
- Body Part Key provides a complete list of body parts and how they should be coded in ICD-10.

ORGANIZATION OF THE BOOK

Medical Terminology and Anatomy for Coding uses a scaffolding approach to carefully sequence learning from simple to complex. Students begin with an introduction to Greek and Latin word parts and rules for building terms. Next, they learn directional terminology, surface anatomy, and terms that are used to describe anatomical structures. The first body system discussed is the musculoskeletal system, which is key to understanding an enormous number of terms used in other body systems. A careful and thorough understanding of these first chapters is an investment that pays a substantial return on investment for the rest of the text. Students will find examples of word parts and terms covered in these first chapters that are used over and over again in the following chapters. A solid knowledge of word parts leads to an easier understanding of the location and function of anatomical terms. Word parts continue to play an important role in grasping the details of the pathologic terms for a particular body system and the procedural terms that diagnose and treat those diseases.

The internal structure of each chapter consists of small learning segments or "chunks." Concepts, terms, illustrations, and abbreviations for the anatomy and physiology, pathology, procedures, and pharmacology for a body system are covered and are then immediately followed by exercises that reinforce and assess your understanding and retention of the material. Special boxes alert you to terminology and coding pitfalls and electronic healthcare records provide practice of newly learned terminology.

FEATURES

Medical Terminology and Anatomy for Coding, fourth edition, is loaded with special features geared specifically to those who need to learn the terminology associated with ICD-10 and CPT.

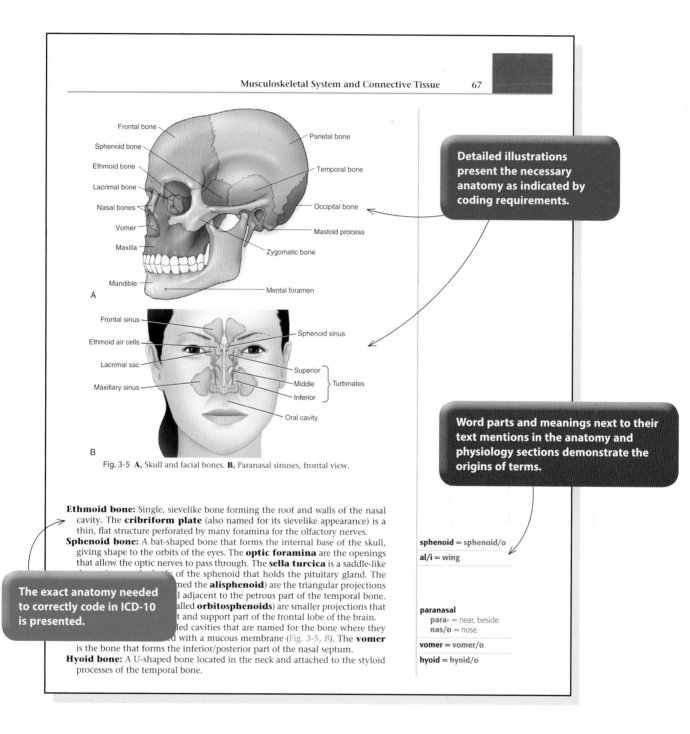

Musculoskeletal System and Connective Tissue   67

Frontal bone
Sphenoid bone
Ethmoid bone
Lacrimal bone
Nasal bones
Vomer
Maxilla
Mandible

Parietal bone
Temporal bone
Occipital bone
Mastoid process
Zygomatic bone
Mental foramen

A

Frontal sinus
Ethmoid air cells
Lacrimal sac
Maxillary sinus

Sphenoid sinus
Superior
Middle } Turbinates
Inferior
Oral cavity

B

Fig. 3-5 **A,** Skull and facial bones. **B,** Paranasal sinuses, frontal view.

Detailed illustrations present the necessary anatomy as indicated by coding requirements.

Word parts and meanings next to their text mentions in the anatomy and physiology sections demonstrate the origins of terms.

The exact anatomy needed to correctly code in ICD-10 is presented.

Ethmoid bone: Single, sievelike bone forming the roof and walls of the nasal cavity. The **cribriform plate** (also named for its sievelike appearance) is a thin, flat structure perforated by many foramina for the olfactory nerves.
Sphenoid bone: A bat-shaped bone that forms the internal base of the skull, giving shape to the orbits of the eyes. The **optic foramina** are the openings that allow the optic nerves to pass through. The **sella turcica** is a saddle-like ... of the sphenoid that holds the pituitary gland. The ...med the **alisphenoid**) are the triangular projections ... adjacent to the petrous part of the temporal bone. ...lled **orbitosphenoids**) are smaller projections that ... and support part of the frontal lobe of the brain. ...ed cavities that are named for the bone where they ... with a mucous membrane (Fig. 3-5, *B*). The **vomer** is the bone that forms the inferior/posterior part of the nasal septum.
Hyoid bone: A U-shaped bone located in the neck and attached to the styloid processes of the temporal bone.

sphenoid = sphenoid/o
al/i = wing

paranasal
para- = near, beside
nas/o = nose

vomer = vomer/o

hyoid = hyoid/o

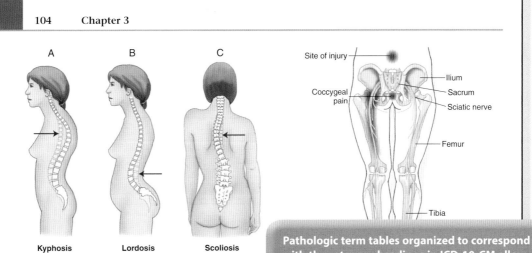

A   B   C

Kyphosis   Lordosis   Scoliosis

Fig. 3-17 **A,** Kyphosis. **B,** Lordosis. **C,** Scoliosis.

> Pathologic term tables organized to correspond with the category headings in ICD-10-CM allow students to begin to correlate terms with their location in the manual.

Terms Related to Systemic Connective Tissue Disorders (M30-M36) and Deforming Dorsopathies (M40-M54)—cont'd

Term	Word Origin	Definition
systemic lupus erythematosus (SLE)	*system/o* system *-ic* pertaining to *erythemat/o* red *-osus* noun ending	Chronic systemic inflammation of unknown etiology (cause). Characterized by distinctive and butterfly-like rash on nose and cheeks. Also called **disseminated lupus erythematosus (DLE)** (Fig. 3-20).
systemic scleroderma	*scler/o* hard *derm/o* skin *-a* noun ending	Disorder that causes hardening and thickening of the skin and connective tissues.

> Terminology specific to ICD-10, along with any synonyms, presents the exact terminology an ICD-10 coder might encounter while working with medical reports.

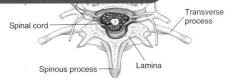

Fig. 3-19 Spinal stenosis. Bony overgrowth has narrowed the spinal canal and pinched the spinal nerves. Compare with normal vertebra in Fig. 3-6, *B*.

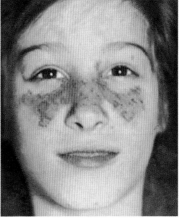

Fig. 3-20 The characteristic butterfly-like rash of SLE.

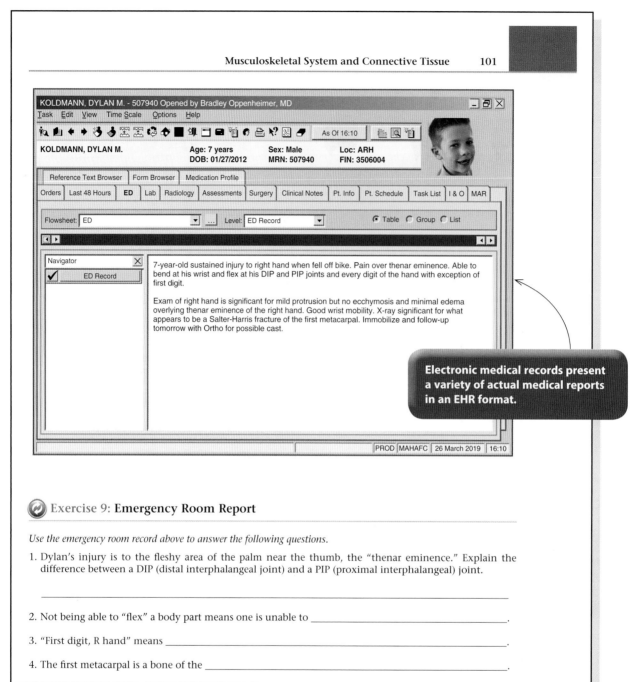

Musculoskeletal System and Connective Tissue   101

KOLDMANN, DYLAN M. - 507940 Opened by Bradley Oppenheimer, MD

Task   Edit   View   Time Scale   Options   Help

As Of 16:10

KOLDMANN, DYLAN M.

Age: 7 years   **Sex: Male**   **Loc: ARH**
DOB: 01/27/2012   **MRN: 507940**   **FIN: 3506004**

Reference Text Browser   Form Browser   Medication Profile

Orders | Last 48 Hours | **ED** | Lab | Radiology | Assessments | Surgery | Clinical Notes | Pt. Info | Pt. Schedule | Task List | I & O | MAR

Flowsheet: ED   Level: ED Record   ● Table ○ Group ○ List

Navigator

☑ ED Record

7-year-old sustained injury to right hand when fell off bike. Pain over thenar eminence. Able to bend at his wrist and flex at his DIP and PIP joints and every digit of the hand with exception of first digit.

Exam of right hand is significant for mild protrusion but no ecchymosis and minimal edema overlying thenar eminence of the right hand. Good wrist mobility. X-ray significant for what appears to be a Salter-Harris fracture of the first metacarpal. Immobilize and follow-up tomorrow with Ortho for possible cast.

> **Electronic medical records present a variety of actual medical reports in an EHR format.**

PROD | MAHAFC | 26 March 2019 | 16:10

Exercise 9: Emergency Room Report

Use the emergency room record above to answer the following questions.

1. Dylan's injury is to the fleshy area of the palm near the thumb, the "thenar eminence." Explain the difference between a DIP (distal interphalangeal joint) and a PIP (proximal interphalangeal) joint.

   _____

2. Not being able to "flex" a body part means one is unable to _____.

3. "First digit, R hand" means _____.

4. The first metacarpal is a bone of the _____.

tricuspid
 tri- = three
 cusp/o = point
 -id = pertaining to

semilunar
 semi- = half
 lun/o = moon
 -ar = pertaining to

bicuspid
 bi- = two
 cusp/o = point
 -id = pertaining to

annulus, ring = annul/o

papillary = papill/o

chordae = chord/o

upper body, whereas the lower body is drained by the **inferior vena cava.** Blood is squeezed from the **right atrium (RA)** to the **right ventricle (RV)** through the **tricuspid valve (TV).** Valves are considered to be competent (capable) if they open and close properly, letting through or holding back an expected amount of blood. Once in the right ventricle the blood is squeezed out through the pulmonary semilunar valve into the **pulmonary arteries (PA),** which carry deoxygenated blood to the lungs from the heart. These are the only arteries that carry deoxygenated blood. The main pulmonary artery (**pulmonary trunk**) divides into right and left arteries to supply each lung. The **conus arteriosus** is the cone-shaped extension of the right ventricle into the pulmonary trunk. In the capillaries of the lungs, the CO_2 is passed out of the blood and O_2 is taken in. The now-oxygenated blood continues its journey back from the lungs to the left side of the heart through the **pulmonary veins (PV).** These are the only veins that carry oxygenated blood. The blood then enters the heart through the **left atrium (LA)** and has to pass the **mitral valve (MV),** also termed the **bicuspid valve,** to enter the **left ventricle (LV).** When the left ventricle contracts, the blood finally pushes out through the aortic semilunar valve into the **aorta** (the largest artery in the body) and begins yet another cycle through the body. The first part of the aorta, the **ascending aorta,** rises toward the head, then bends into the aortic arch and continues downward through the chest as the descending thoracic aorta. Once it passes the diaphragm, it is termed the **abdominal aorta.**

Each valve has a fibrous ring at its base called the **annulus.** The bicuspid valve has two leaflets (cusps) that are attached to two nipple-like papillary muscles by the **chordae tendineae,** cordlike tendons. The **papillary muscles** open and close the heart valves. The **tricuspid valve** has three leaflets attached to three papillary muscles, connected again by chordae tendineae. When a writer refers to heartstrings being tugged at in sentimental situations, he/she is referring to the chordae tendineae.

 CPT Coding Alert!

CPT has several codes that reference the sinus of Valsalva, a cavity in the wall of the aorta that is at the beginning of the right or left coronary artery, or which has no natural outlet at all. The first two of these sinuses are referred to as coronary sinuses because of their outlet into coronary arteries, while the third is considered a noncoronary sinus. The sinus of Valsalva is important to recognize in regard to procedures because it may be the site of an aneurysm. Synonym: aortic sinus

CPT Coding Alerts notify students to physician-specific coding situations.

 CPT Coding Alert!

CPT references to the infundibulum of the heart refer to a conical structure in the anterosuperior portion of the right ventricle, at the entrance to the pulmonary trunk (arteries). Another name for the infundibulum of the heart is the conus arteriosus. The term *infundibulum* is from Latin for "funnel."

 Be Careful!   *Don't confuse **chordae** (tendineae) with **chordee**, a disorder of the male reproductive system.*

Be Careful! boxes remind students of potentially confusing look-alike or sound-alike word parts or terms.

The amount of blood expelled from the left ventricle is referred to as the **stroke volume,** while the percentage of blood expelled of the amount filling the ventricle is the **ejection fraction.** The ejection fraction is typically around 65%. Lower percentages occur in certain types of heart disease.

If a woman's heart rate is 80 beats per minute (BPM), that means her heart contracts almost 5000 times per hour and more than 100,000 times per day,

Match the lower appendicular combining forms with their meanings.

Combining Forms   **Lower Appendicula**
____ 11. patell/a   K. foot bone
____ 12. pub/o   L. lower portion of pe
____ 13. metatars/o   M. anklebone
____ 14. tibi/o   N. lower anterior pelvic bone
____ 15. ili/o   O. shinbone
____ 16. malleol/o   P. kneecap
____ 17. cox/o   Q. superior, widest bone of pelvis
____ 18. ischi/o   R. processes on distal tibia and fibula
____ 19. fibul/o, perone/o   S. thighbone
____ 20. femor/o   T. hip bone
____ 21. tars/o   U. lower lateral leg bone
____ 22. calcane/o   V. heel bone
____ 23. acetabul/o   W. great toe
____ 24. halluc/o   X. hip socket

Translate the terms.

25. interphalangeal _____

26. humeroulnar _____

27. infrapatellar _____

28. femoral _____

29. supraclavicular _____

To practice labeling the appendicular skeleton, click on **Label It.**

Joints

ICD-10-PCS classifies joints as being either upper or lower. As a coder, you will
need to recognize these joints and be able to categorize them appropriately. The
following introduction to the terminology of the joints is organized with the
PCS in mind.

PCS Guideline Alert

B2.1B Where the general body part values "upper" and "lower" are provided as an
option in the Upper Arteries, Lower Arteries, Upper Veins, Lower Veins, Muscles and
Tendons body systems, "upper" or "lower" specifies body parts located above or
below the diaphragm respectively.

Extensive intrachapter exercises and end-of-
chapter reviews offer many opportunities to
practice and review anatomy and terminology.

Frequent references to online games
and activities alert students to
opportunities for interactive learning.

ICD-10-CM and PCS Guideline Alert!
boxes are included to signal students
that ICD-10 guidelines are influenced
by medical terms being presented.

Shapes of Human Bones

Types	Examples
long bones	humerus (upper arm bone), femur (thighbone)
short bones	carpal (wristbone), tarsal (anklebone)
flat bones	sternum (breastbone), scapula (shoulder blade)
irregular bones	vertebra (backbone), stapes (a bone in the ear)
sesamoid	patella (kneecap)

> **Special ICD Note** boxes key students to ICD-10 features that affect their understanding of the terminology presented.

Note

Although the traditional method of explaining the organization of the skeleton is by dividing it into its axial and appendicular components, the ICD-10-PCS Medical Surgical section categorizes the skeleton into three different divisions (Fig. 3-3):

Head and facial bones: the skull, facial bones, and hyoid bone.

Upper bones: the left and right upper extremities (arm, hand, and finger bones); left and right glenoid cavity; scapula; clavicle; rib; and the sternum, as well as the cervical and thoracic vertebrae.

Lower bones: the left and right lower extremities (leg, foot, and toe bones), left and right pelvic bones (ilium, ischium, and pubis), acetabula, and the lumbar vertebrae, sacrum, and coccyx.

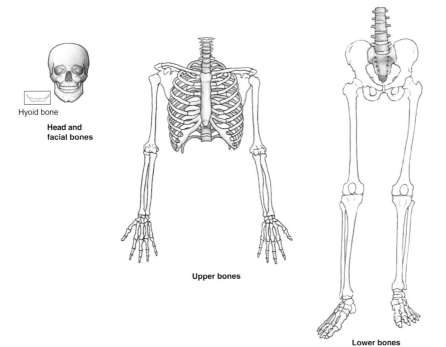

Hyoid bone

Head and facial bones

Upper bones

Lower bones

Fig. 3-3 Skeletal bones divided by ICD-10 PCS classifications.

PHARMACOLOGY

antibiotics: Treat bacterial infections. A commonly used oral agent to treat ear infections is amoxicillin (Amoxil). A topical example is ciprofloxacin with hydrocortisone (Cipro HC Otic).

ceruminolytics: Soften and break down earwax. An example is carbamide peroxide (Debrox).

decongestants: Relieve congestion associated with a cold, allergy, or sinus pressure. These drugs may be available as a nasal spray or an oral product. Examples include oxymetazoline (Kovanaze) and pseudoephedrine (Sudafed).

otics: Drugs applied directly to the external ear canal. These may be adminis tered in the form of solutions, suspensions, or ointments.

> Pharmacology in each body system chapter provides the most current medications and their usages.

RECOGNIZING SUFFIXES FOR PCS

Now that you've finished reading about the procedures for the ear, take at this review of the *suffixes* used in their terminology. Each of these suf associated with one or more root operations in the medical surgical sec one of the other categories in PCS.

> Summary tables of procedural suffixes and their corresponding root operations for each chapter show the correlation between suffixes and the 31 ICD-10 root operations.

Suffixes and Root Operations for the Ear

Suffix	Root Operation
-centesis	Drainage
-ectomy	Excision, resection
	Release
-plasty	Repair, replacement, supplement
-scopy	Inspection
-stomy	Drainage
-tomy	Drainage

> NEW! Infectious and Parasitic Disease Basics appendix provides the basic information coders need to be able to understand infectious diseases and to code them correctly.

Appendix A   Infectious and Parasitic Disease Basics

pathogen
path/o = disease
-gen = producing, produced by

The very first chapter of ICD-10, "Certain Infectious and Parasitic Diseases," presents a variety of concerns and questions for coders. Unlike the majority of chapters, it is not organized by body systems, but instead, is loosely organized around the **pathogens** that carry and transmit the ailments listed. The medi- cal terms for each of the diseases are often very different from the particular microbe that causes it, and each set of terms has its own naming conventions. Attempting to apply strict logic to neatly compartmentalize these diseases will be met with frustration, as the structure of the chapter has its roots in the 16th century with John Graunt's examination of the London Bills of Mortality (Fig. A-1). Over 400 years of medical science (including the use of naked eye and electron microscopy) has occurred in the interim, so some categories include only one type of pathogen, while others group together diseases by their mode

Appendix B   Oncology Basics

Coding charts with diagnoses from the **neoplasm** chapter of ICD-10-CM requires an understanding of the terminology describing the types of tumors, and the diagnostic and therapeutic procedures used to detect and treat each. Diagnostic coding guidelines determine how the tumor should be coded, depending on whether it is the original **cancer,** or one that has developed from it. Further detailed guidelines are given in regard to diagnoses that indicate admissions for treatments to either the original or subsequent formations. Coding the procedures used to diagnose and treat these various neoplasms necessitates an understanding of the terminology that is often used with cancer diagnosis and treatment, but is used less often with other pathologies.

Where there is life, there is cancer. Although the types of cancer and their incidence (the number of new cases diagnosed each year) may vary by geography, sex, race, age, and ethnicity, cancer exists in every population and has since ancient times. Archeologists have found evidence of cancer in dinosaur bones and human mummies. Written descriptions of cancer treatment have been discovered dating back to 1600 BC. The word *cancer* comes from the Greek word for *crab*. It was used by Hippocrates to describe the appearance of the most common type of cancer, carcinoma, as it invaded the tissue it inhabited.

neo- = new
-plasm = formation
cancer = carcin/o

Oncology Basics appendix introduces students to the concepts of cancer and neoplasms.

Pharmacy Basics appendix provides an easy-to-understand introduction to important pharmacological concepts and terms.

Appendix C   Pharmacology Basics

Simply stated, **pharmacology** is the study of drugs (also called *pharmaceuticals*). What is not so simple is the number of details that are involved with this field of study. Fortunately, many of the concepts and terms necessary to understand pharmacology are built from Greek and Latin word parts that will help you remember their definitions.

Pharmacists specialize in the preparation and dispensing of medications. Usually, these individuals work in a pharmacy—that is to say, a drugstore. They spend years studying the disciplines that make up pharmacology, such as **pharmacodynamics,** the action and effects of drugs on the tissues of the body; **pharmacokinetics,** the study of the movement of drugs through the body over time, and **pharmacotherapeutics,** the use of drugs in treating disease. See the table below for a breakdown of the word origins of these terms.

DRUG NAMES

Unlike diseases or procedures, each drug has at least three names. The **chemical name** is the scientific name that specifies the chemical composition of the drug. The **generic name** is its common name, often abbreviated from the chemical name. The copyrighted name that is given to the drug by its manufacturer is the **brand, trade, or proprietary name** and is accompanied by a symbol (an R

with a circle around it, meaning "registered," or TM, meaning "trademark") next to it. The TM abbreviation is used until the U.S. Patent and Trademark Office has registered the name, after which the symbol ® is used. Federal law protects the patent (an exclusive right to make and sell the drug) on a new drug. The manufacturer has several years to sell its uniquely formulated and named medication before another company may use the "recipe."

Acetylsalicylic acid, aspirin, and Ecotrin are the chemical, generic, and brand names of a common over-the-counter (OTC) medication used to treat pain and inflammation.

DRUG SOURCES

Medications are manufactured from a variety of sources. Animal, botanical, and mineral sources are common, along with synthetic and recombinant DNA technology. Willow bark, for example, is the source of aspirin, while the foxglove plant is used to extract digitalis to control heart arrhythmias. Fish are the source of oil to supplement diets with vitamins A, D, and omega-3 fatty acids. Calcium is the essential component in Tums and Rolaids, which soothe an upset stomach. Penicillin is an example of an organic synthetic drug, and Humulin is a form of insulin that has been developed through the use of recombinant DNA technology.

Appendix G   Normal Lab Values

Urine Reference Values*

Analyte	Conventional Units	SI Units
Acetone and acetoacetate, qualitative	Negative	Negative
Albumin		
Qualitative	Negative	Negative
Quantitative	10-100 mg/24 h	0.15-1.5 μmol/d
Amylase/creatinine clearance ratio	0.01-0.04	0.01-0.04
Bilirubin, qualitative	Negative	Negative
Creatinine	15-25 mg/kg/24 h	0.13-0.22 mmol/kg/d
Glucose (as reducing substance)	<250 mg/24 h	<250 mg/d
, qualitative	Negative	Negative
	4.6-8.0	4.6-8.0
	Negative	Negative
	10-150 mg/24 h	10-150 mg/d
Protein/creatinine ratio	<0.2	<0.2
Specific gravity		
Random specimen	1.003-1.030	1.003-1.030
24-hour collection	1.015-1.025	1.015-1.025
Urobilinogen	0.5-4.0 mg/24 h	0.6-6.9 μmol/d

*Values may vary depending on the method used.

> Normal Lab Values appendix provides a frame of reference when reading lab results.

Appendix H

> ICD-10 Body Part Index provides a complete list of body parts and how they should be coded.

Body Part Key

If You See This Body Part	Code to This Body
Abdominal aortic plexus	Abdominal Sympathetic Nerve
Abdominal esophagus	Esophagus, Lower
Abductor hallucis muscle	Foot Muscle, Right
	Foot Muscle, Left
Accessory cephalic vein	Cephalic Vein, Right
	Cephalic Vein, Left
Accessory obturator nerve	Lumbar Plexus
Accessory phrenic nerve	Phrenic Nerve
Accessory spleen	Spleen
Acetabulofemoral joint	Hip Joint, Right
	Hip Joint, Left

Student Resources

Electronic assets for students on Evolve include entertaining, interactive games and activities that have been designed to test specific areas of knowledge as you prepare for quizzes and exams. These games and activities are now gradable and scores will feed the instructor gradebook.

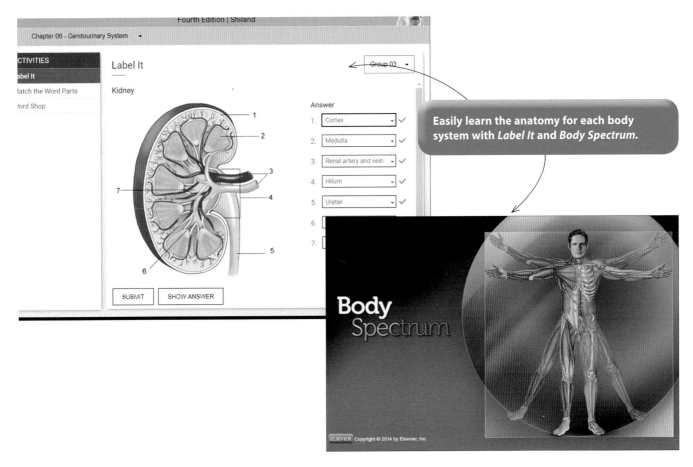

Easily learn the anatomy for each body system with *Label It* and *Body Spectrum*.

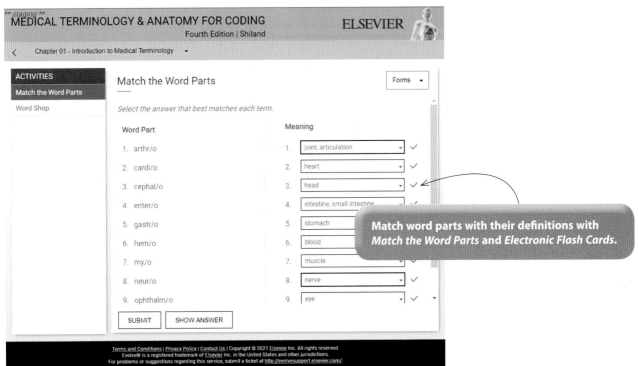

Match word parts with their definitions with *Match the Word Parts* and *Electronic Flash Cards*.

Build terms with *Word Shop*.

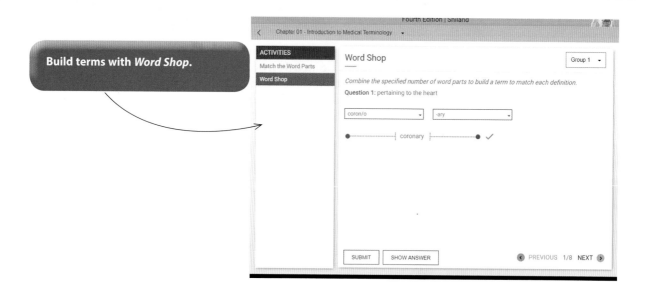

Become a *Medical Millionaire* by answering questions about pathology terms.

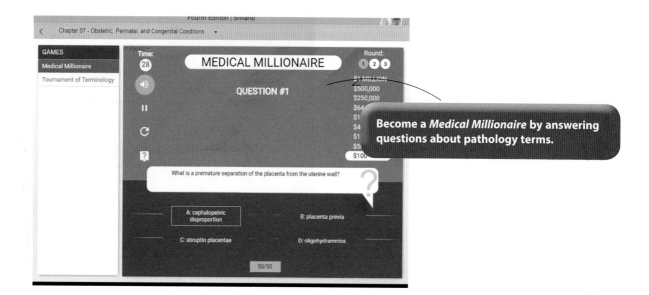

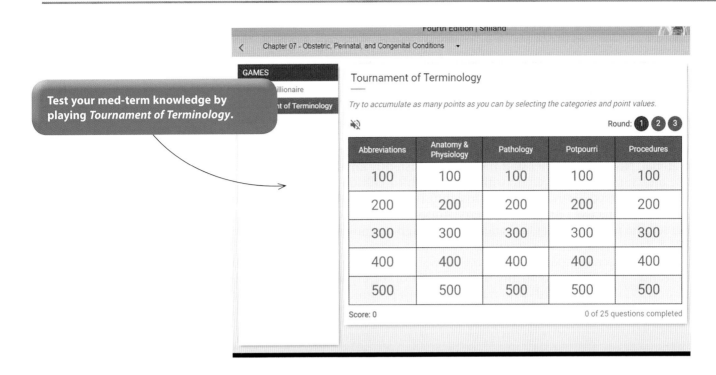

Test your med-term knowledge by playing *Tournament of Terminology.*

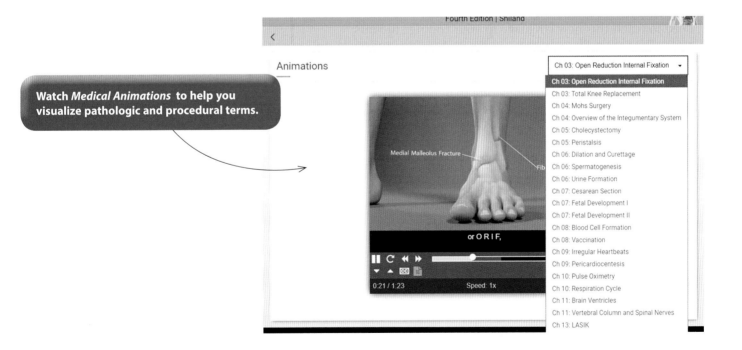

Watch *Medical Animations* to help you visualize pathologic and procedural terms.

WHY YOU NEED THIS BOOK

It is important to remember that all of us are affected by the codes that are generated by future coders. These codes are used to not only pay for care but will also determine future healthcare policy and influence medical research.

Learning the **specific** anatomy and terminology necessary for ICD-10 and CPT is the key to assigning codes correctly. Those who learn medical terminology and its direct connections to anatomy will **pass their coding tests** and learn to assign codes with more confidence and accuracy. This is the goal of Medical Terminology and Anatomy for Coding, *fourth edition.*

Betsy J. Shiland

Acknowledgments

As I worked on this fourth edition, I have been constantly aware of, and unendingly grateful to, the people who made this text possible. My first acknowledgements are to the instructors, students, and reviewers who provided feedback to guide the revision of this edition. I cannot adequately express my gratitude for feedback (positive and negative!) to help finely tune our presentation of this material. Next, the Elsevier staff has been consistently amazing with their expertise and support of the composition of the third edition. Brian Salisbury, our designer, worked his magic with an insightful plan that makes the content accessible and attractive. Abigail Bradberry, the senior production manager, shepherded the many changes and additions through the process with a deft, steady hand. Luke Held, senior content development manager, worked in a patient, behind-the scenes mode, to move the new arrangement and content from idea to reality. And where would any of this be, if not for my long-standing content strategist, Linda Woodard, who makes all things possible. Over the years, I realize how fortunate I am to have her as a strategist, ally, and friend.

TO THE INSTRUCTOR

You are the most important driving force behind your students' mastery of medical terminology. That's why we have provided you with all the resources you will need to teach this new language to your coding students:

- TEACH Lesson Plans help you prepare for class and make full use of the rich array of ancillaries and resources that come with your textbook. TEACH is short for "Total Education and Curriculum Help," which accurately describes how these lesson plans and lecture materials provide creative and innovative instructional strategies to both new and experienced instructors to the benefit of their students.

Each lesson plan contains:

- 50-minute lessons that correlates chapter objectives with content and teaching resources
- Convenient lists of key terms for each chapter
- Classroom activities and critical-thinking questions that engage and motivate students
- Assessment plans to help measure your students' knowledge base
- A PowerPoint presentation that includes over 1500 slides to make teaching a breeze. Slides are enhanced with additional images, and a 3-column format with word parts are included to help students make the connection between medical terms and the prefixes, suffixes, and combining forms used to make these terms. Each PPT includes copious notes for classroom instruction.
- A Test Bank that consists of over 4,500-questions. Multiple-choice, fill-in-the-blank, and true/false questions that can be sorted by subject, objective, and type of questions using ExamView. Many of the questions used for the games are also included in the Test Bank.
- Handouts that can be used for classroom quizzes or homework.

Visit http://evolve.elsevier.com/Shiland/coding for more information.

Contents

CHAPTER 1

Introduction to Healthcare Terminology

CHAPTER OUTLINE

OBJECTIVES

☐ State the derivation of most healthcare terms.

☐ Use the rules given to build and spell healthcare terms.

☐ Use the rules given to change singular terms to their plural forms.

☐ Recognize and recall an introductory word bank of prefixes, suffixes, and combining forms and their respective meanings.

ICD-10-CM Example from Tabular
R16 Hepatomegaly and splenomegaly, not elsewhere classified
   R16.0 Hepatomegaly, not elsewhere classified
     Hepatomegaly, not otherwise specified
   R16.1 Splenomegaly, not elsewhere classified
     Splenomegaly, not otherwise specified
   R16.2 Hepatomegaly with splenomegaly, not elsewhere classified
  Hepatosplenomegaly, not otherwise specified

ICD-10-PCS Example from Index
Hepatopancreatic ampulla
  – *see* Ampulla of Vater
Hepatopexy
  – *see* Repair, Hepatobiliary System and Pancreas **0FQ**
  – *see* Reposition, Hepatobiliary System and Pancreas **0FS**
Hepatorrhaphy
  – *see* Repair, Hepatobiliary System and Pancreas **0FQ**
Hepatotomy
  – *see* Drainage, Hepatobiliary System and Pancreas **0F9**

INTRODUCTION TO ICD-10 AND CPT-4

Technology is making our world feel smaller—and more complicated. The World Health Organization (WHO) has been publishing a listing of morbidity (disease) and mortality (death) data for more than 100 years. This listing is used to keep track of the rates of disease and death on much of our planet. Periodically, it is updated to reflect advances in medical science and new terminology. The use of the Internet to collect and publish statistics with this listing allows for faster dissemination of the information collected.

As of October 2015, the United States began using the International Classification of Diseases, 10th edition (ICD-10). The American adaptation of ICD-10 is titled ICD-10-CM (clinical modification); the CM represents a substantial expansion of the classification system to give more detailed information about diseases. Accompanying the ICD-10-CM volume is an ICD-10-PCS (Procedure Classification System), which has been developed to capture the vastly increased amount of information regarding the diagnostic and therapeutic techniques used to diagnose and treat disease. In the United States, both volumes of ICD serve to capture encoded disease and procedure information that may be used for billing, research, and public policy.

The American Medical Association produces a manual of *procedures* called CPT-4 (Current Procedural Terminology, 4th edition). The purpose of the manual is to help physicians and other healthcare professionals uniformly bill the specific services they perform. The terminology in CPT-4 is used to capture the details needed to describe the procedures performed. *It does not include diagnoses.* While many of the procedures are stated using the same terminology as ICD-10-PCS, CPT-4 includes codes for time, type of service (interpretation, technical services, supervision), and the level of difficulty in determining the services required. Sometimes the terminology differs from ICD-10 for anatomical structures or procedures. CPT-4 is a type of nomenclature, a detailing listing of individual *"names"* of procedures, while ICD-10-PCS is a classification, a *grouping* of procedures. **CPT Coding Alert!** boxes will highlight these differences throughout the text to assist you when coding.

Students who want to master the intricacies of coding and billing need to begin their study by learning the language of medical professionals and how that specific vocabulary is related to both ICD-10 and CPT-4 coding. This text will help you toward your goals by presenting the material in small, manageable segments with a variety of opportunities to test and reinforce the new material and concepts. **Guideline Alert!** and special **ICD-10 Note** boxes will notify you of special concerns for coders, while illustrations and tables will provide additional explanations.

DERIVATION OF HEALTHCARE TERMS

Healthcare terminology is a specialized vocabulary derived from Greek and Latin **word components (parts).** This terminology is used by professionals in the medical field to communicate with each other. By applying the process of "translating," or recognizing the word components and their meanings and using these to define the terms, anyone will be able to interpret literally thousands of medical terms.

The English language and healthcare terminology share many common origins. This proves to be an additional bonus for those who put forth the effort to learn hundreds of seemingly new word parts. Two excellent and highly relevant examples are the **combining forms** (the "subjects" of most terms) *gloss/o* and *lingu/o,* which mean "tongue" in Greek and Latin, respectively. Because the tongue is instrumental in articulating spoken language, Greek and Latin

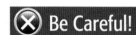

⊗ Be Careful!

ICD-10-CM is used for coding the diagnoses for both inpatient and outpatient procedures as well as for physician encounters. ICD-10-PCS is used to code inpatient procedures, while CPT-4 is used to code outpatient procedures and physician services.

equivalents appear, not surprisingly, in familiar English vocabulary. The table on this page illustrates the intersection of our everyday English language with the ancient languages of Greek and Latin and can help us to clearly see the connections. **Suffixes** (word parts that appear at the end of some terms) and **prefixes** (word parts that appear at the beginning of some terms) also are presented in this table.

Ancient Word Origins in Current English and Healthcare Terminology Usage		
Term	**Word Origins**	**Definition**
glossary	*gloss/o* tongue (Greek) *-ary* pertaining to	An English term meaning "an alphabetical list of terms with definitions."
glossitis	*gloss/o* tongue (Greek) *-itis* inflammation	A healthcare term meaning "inflammation of the tongue."
bilingual	*bi-* two *lingu/o* tongue (Latin) *-al* pertaining to	An English term meaning "pertaining to two languages."
sublingual	*sub-* under *lingu/o* tongue (Latin) *-al* pertaining to	A healthcare term meaning "pertaining to under the tongue."

Did you notice that these healthcare terms use the word origins literally, whereas English words are related to word origins but are not exactly the same? Fortunately, most healthcare terms may be assigned a simple definition through the use of their word parts.

TYPES OF HEALTHCARE TERMS

Translatable Terms

Translatable terms are those terms that can be broken into their Greek and Latin word parts and given a working definition based on the meanings of those word parts. Most medical terms are translatable, so learning word parts is important. The word parts are:
- **Combining form:** word root with its respective combining vowel.
  - **Word root:** word origin.
  - **Combining vowel:** a letter sometimes used to join word parts. Usually an "o" but occasionally an "e" or "i."
- **Suffix:** word part that appears at the end of a term. Suffixes are used to indicate whether the term is an anatomic, pathologic, or procedural term.
- **Prefix:** word part that sometimes appears at the beginning of a term. Prefixes are used to further define the absence, location, number, quantity, or state of the term.

In our first examples, *gloss/* and *lingu/* are word roots with an "o" as their combining vowel. *Gloss/o* and *lingu/o* are therefore combining forms; *-ary, -al,* and *-itis* are suffixes; and *bi-* and *sub-* are prefixes. Figs. 1-1 and 1-2 demonstrate the translation of the terms **glossitis** and **sublingual.**

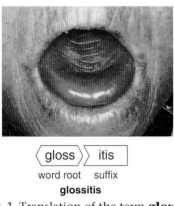

gloss | itis
word root | suffix
glossitis

Fig. 1-1 Translation of the term **glossitis.**

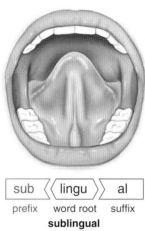

sub | lingu | al
prefix | word root | suffix
sublingual

Fig. 1-2 Translation of the term **sublingual.**

Nontranslatable Terms

Not all terms are composed of word parts that can be used to assemble a definition. These terms are referred to as nontranslatable **terms,** that is, words used in medicine whose definitions must be memorized without the benefit of Greek and Latin word parts. These terms will have a blank space in the word origin columns in the tables presented in the text or will include only a partial notation because the word origins either are not helpful or don't exist. Examples of these terms include the following:

- **Cataract:** From the Greek term meaning "waterfall." In healthcare language, this means "progressive loss of transparency of the lens."
- **Asthma:** From the Greek term meaning "panting." Although this word origin is understandable, the definition is "a respiratory disorder characterized by recurring episodes of paroxysmal dyspnea (difficulty breathing)."
- **Diagnosis:** The disease or condition that is identified after a healthcare professional evaluates a patient's signs, symptoms, and history. Although the term is built from word parts (*dia-,* meaning "through," "complete"; and *-gnosis,* meaning "state of knowledge"), using these word parts to form the definition of diagnosis, which is "a state of complete knowledge," really isn't very helpful.
- **Prognosis:** Similar to *diagnosis,* the term *prognosis* can be broken down into its word parts (*pro-,* meaning "before" or "in front of"; and *-gnosis,* meaning "state of knowledge"), but this does not give the true definition of the term, which is "a prediction of the probable outcome of a disease or disorder."
- **Sequela:** From the Latin meaning "to follow," a sequela is a condition that results from an injury or disease. It is also referred to in coding as a "late effect." When coding, the code for a sequela follows the code for its cause.

The following are examples of Guideline Alerts from the ICD-10-CM coding manual that use nontranslatable terms. CM and PCS Guideline Alerts are scattered throughout the text to help students understand the connection between choosing the most specific correct medical term and accurate, complete coding. Note the reference numbers that you can use to locate the actual guideline in your coding manual. All the guidelines in this book are from Section I.

CM Guideline Alert

I.B.10 SEQUELA (LATE EFFECTS)
A sequela is the residual effect (condition produced) after the acute phase of an illness or injury has terminated. There is no time limit on when a sequela code can be used. The residual may be apparent early, such as in cerebral infarction, or it may occur months or years later, such as that due to a previous injury. Examples of a sequela include: scar formation resulting from a burn, deviated septum due to a nasal fracture, and infertility due to tubal occlusion from old tuberculosis. Coding of sequela generally requires two codes sequenced in the following order: the condition or nature of the sequela is sequenced first. The sequela code is sequenced second.

- **Acute:** A term that describes an abrupt, severe onset to a disease *(acu-* means "sharp").
- **Chronic:** Developing slowly and lasting for a long time *(chron/o* means "time"). Diagnoses may be additionally described as being either acute or chronic.

 CM Guideline Alert

I.B.8 ACUTE AND CHRONIC CONDITION
If the same condition is described as both acute (subacute) and chronic, and separate subentries exist in the Alphabetic Index at the same indentation level, code both and sequence the acute (subacute) code first.

- **Sign:** An objective finding of a disease state (e.g., fever, high blood pressure, rash).
- **Symptom:** A subjective report of a disease (pain, itching).

- **Syndrome:** A group of signs and symptoms that consistently appear together.

 CM Guideline Alert

I.B.4 SIGNS AND SYMPTOMS
Codes that describe symptoms and signs, as opposed to diagnoses, are acceptable for reporting purposes when a related definitive diagnosis has not been established (confirmed) by the provider. Chapter 18 of ICD-10-CM—Symptoms, Signs, and Abnormal Clinical and Laboratory Findings, Not Elsewhere Classified (codesR00. 0R99)—contains many, but not all, codes for symptoms.

 CM Guideline Alert

I.B.15 SYNDROMES
Follow the Alphabetic Index guidance when coding syndromes. In the absence of Alphabetic Index guidance, assign codes for the documented manifestations of the syndrome. Additional codes for manifestations that are not an integral part of the disease process may also be assigned when the condition does not have a unique code.

- **Etiology:** Literally the "study of cause," although the term is used in coding to simply refer to the cause of a disease.
- **Manifestation:** An outward demonstration or perception. Signs and symptoms are manifestations of diseases.

 CM Guideline Alert

I.A.13 ETIOLOGY/MANIFESTATION CONVENTION ("CODE FIRST," "USE ADDITIONAL CODE," AND "IN DISEASES CLASSIFIED ELSEWHERE" NOTES)[1]

Certain conditions have both an underlying etiology and multiple body system manifestations due to the underlying etiology. For such conditions, the ICD-10-CM has a coding convention that requires the underlying condition be sequenced first, followed by the manifestation. Wherever such a combination exists, there is a "use additional code" note at the etiology code and a "code first" note at the manifestation code. These instructional notes indicate the proper sequencing order of the codes, etiology followed by manifestation.

In most cases the manifestation codes will have in the code title "in diseases classified elsewhere." Codes with this title are a component of the etiology/manifestation convention. The code title indicates that it is a manifestation code. "In diseases classified elsewhere" codes are never permitted to be used as first-listed or principal diagnosis codes. They must be used in conjunction with an underlying condition code, and they must be listed following the underlying condition.

[1]For more of this guideline, see ICD-10-CM Official Guidelines for Coding and Reporting.

Other types of terms that are not built from word parts include the following:
- **Eponyms:** Terms that are named after a person or place associated with the term. Examples include:
  - **Alzheimer's disease,** which is named after Alois Alzheimer, a German neurologist. The disease is a progressive mental deterioration.
  - **Achilles tendon,** a body part named after a figure in Greek mythology whose one weak spot was this area of his anatomy. Tendons are bands of tissue that attach muscles to bone. The Achilles tendon is the particular tendon that attaches the calf muscle to the heel bone *(calcaneus)*. Unlike some eponyms, this one does have a medical equivalent, the calcaneal tendon.
  - **Cesarean delivery,** the delivery of an infant through a surgical abdominal incision. Note that it is in PCS as an "extraction of products of conception" with body part, approach, device, and qualifier options. In CPT it is included under the heading "Cesarean delivery" with codes for delivery only, antepartum care, delivery and postpartum care, with hysterectomy, and with tubal ligation and delivery. The PCS body part, approach, device, and qualifier options are not part of the decision-making in choosing a CPT code.
  - **Portmanteau.** Sometimes medical terms are combinations of words that are not built from traditional Greek and Latin word parts. Portmanteaus (from an old French term for a suitcase) are terms that are a combination of two or more words. Botox, for example is a combination of the words *botulism* and *toxin*. Covid-19 is one of the newest medical terms, built from corona (co-) virus (vi-) + disease (d) and 19 (first discovered in 2019).

Abbreviations and Symbols

Abbreviations are terms that have been shortened to letters and/or numbers for the sake of convenience. Symbols are graphic representations of a term. Abbreviations and symbols are extremely common in written and spoken healthcare terminology but can pose problems for healthcare workers. The Joint Commission has published a "DO NOT USE" list of dangerously confusing abbreviations, symbols, and acronyms that should be avoided (see Appendix F). The Institute for Safe Medication Practices has provided a more extensive list. Each healthcare organization should have an official list, which includes the single meaning allowed for each abbreviation or symbol. Examples of acceptable abbreviations and symbols include the following:

- **Simple abbreviations:** A combination of letters (often, but not always, the first letters of significant word parts) and sometimes numbers
  - IM: abbreviation for "intramuscular" (pertaining to within the muscles)
  - C2: second cervical vertebra (second bone in neck)
- **Acronyms:** Abbreviations that are also pronounceable
  - CABG: coronary artery bypass graft (a detour around a blockage in an artery of the heart)
  - TURP: transurethral resection of the prostate (a surgical procedure that removes the prostate through the urethra)
- **Symbols:** Graphic representations of terms
  ♀ stands for *female*
  ♂ stands for *male*
  ↑ stands for *increased*
  ↓ stands for *decreased*
  + stands for *present*
  – stands for *absent*

 Exercise 1: **Derivation of Healthcare Terms and Nontranslatable Terms**

Match the following types of healthcare terms with their examples.

____ 1. symbol

____ 2. translatable term

____ 3. simple abbreviation

____ 4. eponym

____ 5. nontranslatable term

____ 6. acronym

A. CABG

B. Alzheimer's disease

C. ♀

D. glossitis

E. C2

F. asthma

Match the nontranslatable term to its definition.

____ 7. diagnosis

____ 8. prognosis

____ 9. acute

____ 10. chronic

____ 11. sign

____ 12. symptom

____ 13. syndrome

____ 14. etiology

____ 15. manifestation

____ 16. sequela

____ 17. portmanteau

A. outward demonstration or perception

B. a group of signs/symptoms that consistently appear together

C. a subjective report of a disease

D. cause of a disease

E. developing slowly and lasting a long time

F. objective finding of a disease

G. abrupt, severe onset to a disease

H. prediction of the probable outcome of a disease

I. a disease or condition that is determined by an evaluation

J. a condition that results from an injury or disease

K. combination of words not built from traditional word parts

TRANSLATING TERMS

Check, Assign, Reverse, Define (CARD) Method

Using Greek and Latin word components to decipher the meanings of healthcare terms requires a simple four-step process. You need to:
- **Check** for the word parts in a term.
- **Assign** meanings to the word parts.
- **Reverse** the meaning of the suffix to the front of your definition.
- **Define** the term.

Using Fig. 1-3, see how this process is applied to your first patient, Alex.

Most of the terms presented in this text appear in standardized tables. The term and its pronunciation appear in the first column, the word origin in the second, and a definition in the third. A table that introduces six healthcare terms that include six different combining forms and suffixes is provided on p. 9 (The use of prefixes will be introduced later.) Success in translating these terms depends on how well you remember the 12 word parts that are covered in the table. Once you master these 12 word parts, you will be able to recognize and define many other medical terms that use these same word parts—a perfect illustration of how learning a few word parts helps you learn many healthcare terms.

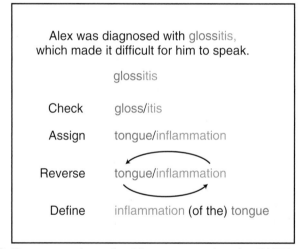

Fig. 1-3 How to translate a healthcare term using the **CARD** method.

The "wheels of terminology" included in Fig. 1-4 demonstrate how different suffixes can be added to a combining form to make a variety of terms.

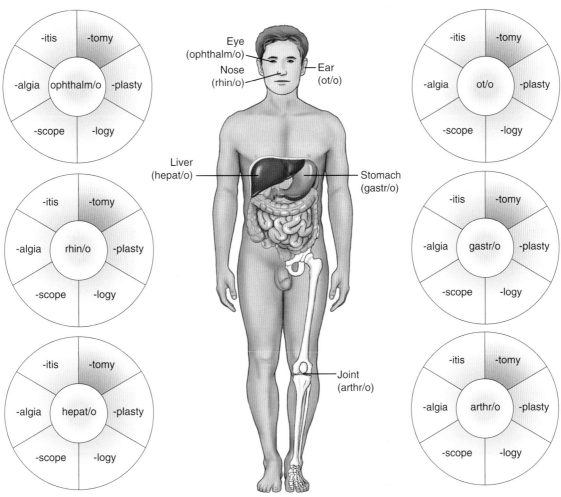

Fig. 1-4 Body parts and their combining forms. Surrounding the figure are "terminology wheels" that show how different suffixes can be added to a combining form to make a variety of terms.

Common Combining Forms and Suffixes

Combining Forms	Suffixes	Combining Forms	Suffixes
arthr/o = joint	-algia = pain	ot/o = ear	-logy = study of
gastr/o = stomach	-tomy = cutting	rhin/o = nose	-plasty = surgically forming
ophthalm/o = eye	-scope = instrument to view	hepat/o = liver	-itis = inflammation

The table below demonstrates how terms are presented in this book. Notice that the first column includes the term. The second column breaks the term down into word parts and their meanings. The third column includes the definition of the term and any synonyms.

Samples of Translatable Terms		
Term	Word Origins	Definition
arthralgia	*arthr/o* joint *-algia* pain of	Pain of a joint. Also called **arthrodynia**.
gastrotomy	*gastr/o* stomach *-tomy* cutting	Incision of the stomach.
hepatitis	*hepat/o* liver *-itis* inflammation	Inflammation of the liver.
ophthalmoscope	*ophthalm/o* eye *-scope* instrument to view	Instrument used to view the eye.
otology	*ot/o* ear *-logy* study of	Study of the ear.
rhinoplasty	*rhin/o* nose *-plasty* surgically forming	Surgically forming the nose.

Exercise 2: Combining Forms

Match the combining forms with their meaning

____ 1. ear
____ 2. stomach
____ 3. nose

____ 4. eye
____ 5. joint
____ 6. liver

A. rhin/o
B. arthr/o
C. ot/o

D. gastr/o
E. ophthalm/o
F. hepat/o

Exercise 3: Suffixes

Match the suffixes with their meanings.

____ 1. pain
____ 2. surgically forming
____ 3. instrument to view
____ 4. cutting
____ 5. study of

A. -tomy
B. -algia
C. -logy
D. -plasty
E. -scope

Exercise 4: Translating the Terms Using Check, Assign, Reverse, and Define

Using the method shown in Fig. 1-3 and the 12 word parts in the table on p. 8, translate and define these five NEW terms.

1. ophthalmology _____

2. otoplasty _____

3. gastralgia _____

4. arthroscope _____

5. rhinotomy _____

BUILDING TERMS

Now that you've seen how terms are translated, we will discuss how they are built. First, a few rules on how to spell healthcare terms correctly.

Spelling Rules

With a few exceptions, translatable healthcare terms follow five simple rules.

1. If the suffix starts with a vowel, a combining vowel is *not* needed to join the parts. For example, it is simple to combine the combining form **arthr/o** and suffix **-itis** to build the term **arthritis,** which means "an inflammation of the joints." The combining vowel "**o**" is not needed because the suffix starts with the vowel "**i.**"
2. If the suffix starts with a consonant, a combining vowel *is* needed to join the two word parts. For example, when building a term using **arthr/o** and **-plasty,** the combining vowel is retained and the resulting term is spelled **arthroplasty,** which refers to surgically forming a joint.
3. If a combining form ends with the same vowel that begins a suffix, one of the vowels is dropped. The term that means "inflammation of the inside of the heart" is built from the suffix **-itis** (inflammation), the prefix **endo-** (inside), and the combining form **cardi/o. Endo- + cardi/o + -itis** would result in *endocardiitis.* Instead, one of the i's is dropped, and the term is spelled **endo-carditis.**
4. If two or more combining forms are used in a term, the combining vowel is retained between the two, regardless of whether the second combining form begins with a vowel or a consonant. For example, joining **gastr/o** and **enter/o** (small intestine) with the suffix **-itis,** results in the term **gastroen-teritis.** Notice that the combining vowel is *kept* between the two combining forms (even though **enter/o** begins with the vowel "e"), and the combining vowel is *dropped* before the suffix **-itis.**
5. Sometimes when two or more combining forms are used to make a medical term, special notice must be paid to the order in which the combining forms are joined. For example, joining **esophag/o** (which means *esophagus),* **gastr/o** (which means *stomach),* and **duoden/o** (which means *duodenum,* the first part of the small intestines) with the suffix **-scopy** *(viewing)* produces

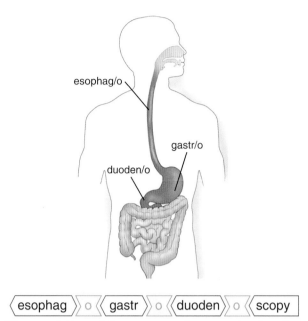

esophag/o

gastr/o

duoden/o

| esophag | o | gastr | o | duoden | o | scopy |

Fig. 1-5 The translation of the term **esophagogastroduodenoscopy.**

the term *esophagogastroduodenoscopy.* An **esophagogastroduodenoscopy** is a viewing of the esophagus, stomach, and duodenum. In this procedure, the examination takes place in a specific sequence, that is, esophagus first, stomach second, then the duodenum. Thus the term reflects the direction in which the scope travels through the body (Fig. 1-5).

Suffixes

The body systems chapters in this text (Chapters 3 through 15) include many combining forms that are used to build terms specific to each system. These combining forms will not be seen elsewhere, except as a sign or symptom of a particular disorder. **Suffixes,** however, are used over and over again throughout the text. Suffixes usually can be grouped according to their purposes. The following tables cover the major categories.

Noun-Ending Suffixes
Noun endings are used most often to describe anatomical terms. Noun endings such as *-icle, -ole,* and *-ule* describe a diminutive structure.

Adjective Suffixes
Adjective suffixes such as those listed below usually mean "pertaining to." For example, when the suffix *-ac* is added to the combining form *cardi/o,* the term *cardiac* is formed, which means "pertaining to the heart." Remember that when you see an adjective term, you need to see what it is describing. For example, cardiac pain is pain of the heart, and cardiac surgery is surgery done on the heart. An adjective tells only half of the story.

Noun-Ending Suffixes

Suffix	Meaning	Example	Word Origins	Definition
-icle	small, tiny	cuticle	*cut/o* skin *-icle* small	Small skin (surrounding the nail).
-is	structure, thing	hypodermis	*hypo-* under *derm/o* skin *-is* structure	Structure under the skin.
-ole	small, tiny	arteriole	*arteri/o* artery *-ole* small	Small artery.
-ule	small, tiny	venule	*ven/o* vein *-ule* small	Small vein.
-um	structure, thing, membrane	endocardium	*endo-* within *cardi/o* heart *-um* structure	Structure within the heart.
-y	condition, process of	polydactyly	*poly-* many, much, excessive, frequent *dactyl/o* digitus (finger, toe) *-y* condition, process of	Condition of excessive fingers or toes.

Adjective Suffixes

Suffix	Meaning	Example	Word Origins	Definition
-ac	pertaining to	cardiac	*cardi/o* heart *-ac* pertaining to	Pertaining to the heart.
-al	pertaining to	cervical	*cervic/o* neck *-al* pertaining to	Pertaining to the neck.
-ar	pertaining to	valvular	*valvul/o* valve *-ar* pertaining to	Pertaining to a valve.
-ary	pertaining to	coronary	*coron/o** heart, crown *-ary* pertaining to	Pertaining to the heart.
-eal	pertaining to	esophageal	*esophag/o* esophagus *-eal* pertaining to	Pertaining to the esophagus.
-ic	pertaining to	hypodermic	*hypo-* below *derm/o* skin *-ic* pertaining to	Pertaining to below the skin.
-ous	pertaining to	subcutaneous	*sub-* under *cutane/o* skin *-ous* pertaining to	Pertaining to under the skin.

*Coron/o literally means "crown," but is used most frequently to describe the arteries that supply blood to the heart, so the meaning "heart" has been added. The novel coronavirus (Covid-19) is our most recent addition to the medical lexicon. In this case, it refers to the crown-like appearance of the virus.

Pathology Suffixes
Pathology suffixes describe a disease process or a sign or symptom. The meanings vary according to the dysfunctions that they describe.

Pathology Suffixes				
Suffix	Meaning	Example	Word Origins	Definition
-algia	pain	cephalalgia	*cephal/o* head *-algia* pain	Pain in the head.
-cele	herniation	cystocele	*cyst/o* bladder, sac *-cele* herniation, protrusion	Herniation of the bladder.
-dynia	pain	cardiodynia	*cardi/o* heart *-dynia* pain	Pain in the heart.
-emia	blood condition	hyperlipidemia	*hyper-* excessive *lipid/o* fats *-emia* blood condition	Excessive fats in the blood.
-ia	condition	agastria	*a-* without *gastr/o* stomach *-ia* condition	Condition of having no stomach.
-itis	inflammation	gastroenteritis	*gastr/o* stomach *enter/o* small intestine *-itis* inflammation	Inflammation of the stomach and small intestine.
-malacia	softening	chondromalacia	*chondr/o* cartilage *-malacia* softening	Softening of the cartilage.
-megaly	enlargement	splenomegaly (Fig. 1-6)	*splen/o* spleen *-megaly* enlargement	Enlargement of the spleen.
-oma	tumor, mass	osteoma	*oste/o* bone *-oma* tumor, mass	Tumor of a bone.
-osis	abnormal condition	psychosis	*psych/o* mind *-osis* abnormal condition	Abnormal condition of the mind.
-pathy	disease process	gastropathy	*gastr/o* stomach *-pathy* disease process	Disease process of the stomach.
-ptosis	prolapse, drooping	hysteroptosis	*hyster/o* uterus *-ptosis* prolapse, drooping	Prolapse of the uterus.
-rrhage, -rrhagia	bursting forth	hemorrhage (Fig. 1-7)	*hem/o* blood *-rrhage* bursting forth	Bursting forth of blood.
-rrhea	discharge, flow	otorrhea	*ot/o* ear *-rrhea* discharge, flow	Discharge from the ear.

Continued

Pathology Suffixes—cont'd

Suffix	Meaning	Example	Word Origins	Definition
-rrhexis	rupture	cystorrhexis	*cyst/o* bladder, sac *-rrhexis* rupture	Rupture of the bladder.
-sclerosis	abnormal condition of hardening	arteriosclerosis	*arteri/o* artery *-sclerosis* abnormal condition of hardening	Abnormal condition of hardening of an artery
-spasm	spasm; sudden, involuntary contraction	bronchospasm	bronchus spasm	Spasm of a bronchus
-stenosis	abnormal condition of narrowing	tracheostenosis	*trache/o* trachea, windpipe *-stenosis* abnormal condition of narrowing	Abnormal condition of narrowing of the trachea or windpipe.

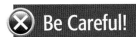 **Be Careful!** *Don't confuse* **-malacia,** *meaning softening, with* **-megaly,** *meaning enlargement.*

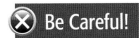 **Be Careful!** *Don't confuse* **-sclerosis,** *meaning hardening, with* **-stenosis,** *meaning narrowing.*

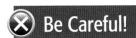 **Be Careful!** *Don't confuse* **-rrhage** *and* **-rrhagia,** *meaning bursting forth, with* **-rrhea,** *meaning discharge or flow.*

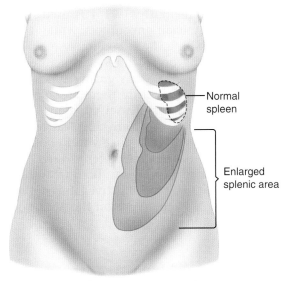

Fig. 1-6 Splenomegaly.

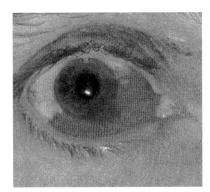

Fig. 1-7 Subconjunctival hemorrhage.

Exercise 5: Noun-Ending, Adjective, and Pathology Suffixes

Match the suffixes with their meanings.

____ 1. -icle, -ole, -ule	A. softening
____ 2. -megaly	B. abnormal condition of hardening
____ 3. -um	C. pain
____ 4. -ic, -al, -ous	D. prolapse
____ 5. -cele	E. small, tiny
____ 6. -malacia	F. blood condition
____ 7. -algia	G. enlargement
____ 8. -ptosis	H. abnormal condition of herniation, protrusion
____ 9. -emia	I. pertaining to
____ 10. -sclerosis	J. structure, thing, membrane

Using the method shown in Fig. 1-3 and the new word parts introduced in the preceding tables, translate and define these five NEW terms.

11. cardiomegaly _____

12. osteomalacia _____

13. valvulitis _____

14. cephalic _____

15. gastroptosis _____

Procedural Suffixes

So far, we have covered medical suffixes for nouns, adjectives, and terms that describe a variety of disease conditions. The next important category is procedural suffixes: what is done to diagnose (e.g., imaging, measurement, laboratory testing) or treat (e.g., removing, replacing, suturing) a patient with a given condition. It is very important that you recognize the difference between procedural suffixes and those that signify a condition.

The two sets of codes used to bill for these procedural services are CPT-4 and ICD-10-PCS. As mentioned previously, CPT-4 is used for reimbursement for outpatient procedures and physician encounters, while ICD-10-PCS is used by hospitals for their inpatient billing. Both coding systems use much of the same terminology, despite differing organizational structures. While CPT has more detail in particular procedures, PCS has greater specificity that includes approaches, devices, and qualifiers. Currently there are approximately 10,000 CPT codes and 80,000 PCS codes. CPT still uses eponyms (e.g., Whipple procedure, Cesarean section), while PCS uses only medical terminology, largely derived from word parts. This text will introduce you to both, along with synonyms, so that you are familiar with the various terms used by different physicians to describe the same or similar procedures. Both CPT and PCS (as well as CM) are updated annually. CPT updates are effective January 1 of each year. PCS updates take place each October 1. Keep an eye on the AMA and CDC websites to be aware of changes and additions.

CPT-4

CPT-4 is a 5-digit, multi-axial nomenclature. The axes are the type of service (evaluation and management, anesthesia, surgery, radiology, pathology and laboratory, and medicine) and, where appropriate, the body system, body part, and the specific procedure. Two-digit modifiers are appended to the CPT code to further define the service provided (e.g., bilateral procedures, repeat clinical diagnostic laboratory tests, and preventive services).

ICD-10-PCS

The PCS volume of ICD-10 is a multi-axial (meaning that it describes not just one, but several characteristics), 7-character classification system that replaces its predecessor, ICD-9-CM, volume 3. The overall structure of the classification begins with **Sections** (e.g., medical and surgical, obstetrics, imaging, measurement, and monitoring), broad categories that divide all of the procedures into one of 16 different types. The largest of the Sections, Medical and Surgical, is divided into **Body Systems,** which are a grouping of body parts, some of which appear as traditional body systems (e.g., endocrine system, respiratory system) and some as parts of body systems (e.g., heart and great vessels, upper arteries, lower arteries). Each of the body systems is then subdivided into 31 distinct Root Operations. A **Root Operation** is the goal of the procedure. Examples include a resection, which is defined as a "cutting out or off, without replacement, all of a body part," and an inspection, which is defined as "visually and/or manually exploring a body part." See the inside back cover of this text for a table of the root operations, their definitions, and possible suffixes. Each of these 31 Root Operations is then further coded for its specific Approach, Device, and Qualifer. An **Approach** is the method of access to the procedure site. A **Device** is the instrument that is used but is only specified when it remains after the procedure is completed. A **Qualifier** is any additional information particular to the procedure; it is a specified final character for the PCS. Just remember—the end goal of coding using PCS is to uniquely identify every procedure with one specific and exclusive code.

Examples of How Root Operations Relate to Suffixes

-centesis (surgical puncture) is a *drainage.*
-desis (binding) is a *fusion.*
-ectomy (cutting out) can be a *destruction,* a *resection,* an *excision,* or an *extirpation.*
-pexy (fixation, suspension) is a *repair* or *reposition.*
-plasty (surgically forming) can be an *alteration,* a *dilation,* a *repair,* a *supplement,* or a *replacement.*

-rrhaphy (suturing) is a *repair.*
-scopy (viewing) is an *inspection.*
-stomy (making a new opening) can be a *bypass* or a *drainage.*
-tomy (cutting) can be a *drainage* or *division.*
-tripsy (crushing) can be a *destruction,* *fragmentation,* or *occlusion.*

Procedure Suffixes

Suffix	Meaning	Example	Word Origins	Definition
-centesis	surgical puncture	amniocentesis	*amni/o* amnion, inner fetal sac *-centesis* surgical puncture	Surgical puncture of the inner fetal sac.*
-desis	binding	arthrodesis	*arthr/o* joint *-desis* binding	Binding of a joint.
-ectomy	cutting out	tonsillectomy	*tonsill/o* tonsil *-ectomy* cutting out	Cutting out the tonsils.

Pathology Suffixes—cont'd

Suffix	Meaning	Example	Word Origins	Definition
-graphy	recording	mammography	*mamm/o* breast *-graphy* recording	Recording the breast.
-metry	measuring	spirometry	*spir/o* breathing *-metry* measuring	Measuring breathing (Fig. 1-8).
-opsy	viewing	biopsy	*bi/o* living, life *-opsy* viewing	Viewing living tissue.
-pexy	suspension, fixation	patellapexy	*patell/a* kneecap, patella *-pexy* suspension, fixation	Suspension of the kneecap.
-plasty	surgically forming	rhinoplasty	*rhin/o* nose *-plasty* surgically forming	Surgically forming the nose.
-rrhaphy	suturing	splenorrhaphy	*splen/o* spleen *-rrhaphy* suturing	Suturing the spleen.
-scopy	viewing	esophagogastrodu-odenoscopy	*esophag/o* esophagus *gastr/o* stomach *duoden/o* duodenum *-scopy* viewing	Viewing the esophagus, stomach, and duodenum.
-stomy	making a new opening	colostomy	*col/o* colon, large intestine *-stomy* making a new opening	Making a new opening in the colon or large intestine (Fig. 1-9).
-tomy	cutting	osteotomy	*oste/o* bone *-tomy* cutting	Incision into the bone.
-tripsy	crushing	lithotripsy	*lith/o* stone *-tripsy* crushing	Crushing of stones.

*Please note that these simple definitions are used to demonstrate the value of learning the Greek and Latin word parts for translatable terms. The definitions in the body system chapters are more robust.

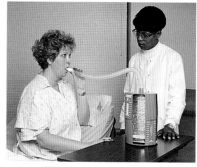

Fig. 1-8 Spirometry.

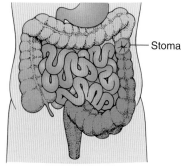

Stoma

Fig. 1-9 Colostomy.

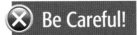 **Be Careful!** *Don't confuse* -**ectomy,** *meaning cutting out, with* -**stomy,** *meaning making a new opening, or* -**tomy,** *meaning cutting.*

Instrument Suffixes

Instruments are indicated by yet another set of suffixes. Note the obvious similarities to their procedural "cousins." For example, electrocardiography is a diagnostic procedure that is done to measure the electrical activity in the heart; an electrocardiograph is the instrument that is used to perform electrocardiography.

Instrument Suffixes

Suffix	Meaning	Example	Word Origins	Definition
-graph	instrument to record	electrocardiograph	*electr/o* electricity *cardi/o* heart *-graph* instrument to record	Instrument to record the electricity of the heart.
-meter	instrument to measure	thermometer	*therm/o* temperature, heat *-meter* instrument to measure	Instrument to measure temperature.
-scope	instrument to view	ophthalmoscope	*ophthalm/o* eye *-scope* instrument to view	Instrument to view the eye.
-tome	instrument to cut	osteotome	*oste/o* bone *-tome* instrument to cut	Instrument to cut bone (Fig. 1-10).
-tripter	machine to crush	lithotripter	*lith/o* stone *-tripter* machine to crush	Machine to crush stone.
-trite	instrument to crush	lithotrite	*lith/o* stone *-trite* instrument to crush	Instrument to crush stones (Fig. 1-11).

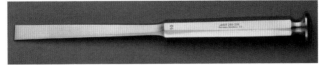

Fig. 1-10 Osteotome.

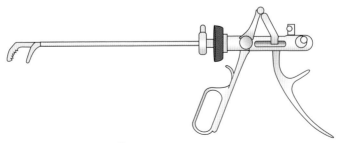

Fig. 1-11 Lithotrite.

Exercise 6: **Procedure and Instrument Suffixes**

Match the suffixes with their meanings.

____	1. -tome	A.	cutting out
____	2. -rrhaphy	B.	making a new opening
____	3. -graphy	C.	binding
____	4. -meter	D.	viewing
____	5. -plasty	E.	instrument to cut
____	6. -desis	F.	instrument to measure
____	7. -scopy	G.	cutting
____	8. -ectomy	H.	recording
____	9. -tomy	I.	suturing
____	10. -stomy	J.	surgically forming

Using the method shown in Fig. 1-3 and the new word parts introduced in the preceding tables, translate and define these five NEW terms.

11. arthrocentesis _____

12. spirometer _____

13. hysteroscopy _____

14. cystoscope _____

15. splenectomy _____

Prefixes

Prefixes modify a medical term by indicating a structure's or condition's:

- Absence
- Location
- Number or quantity
- State

Sometimes, as with other word parts, a prefix can have one or more meanings. For example, the prefix *hypo-* can mean "below" or "deficient."

To spell a term with the use of a prefix, simply add the prefix directly to the beginning of the term. No combining vowels are needed!

Prefixes

Prefix	Meaning	Example	Word Origins	Definition
a-	no, not, without	apneic	*a-* no, not, without *pne/o* breathing *-ic* pertaining to	Pertaining to without breathing.
an-	no, not, without	anophthalmia	*an-* without *ophthalm/o* eye *-ia* condition	Condition of without an eye.
ante-	forward, in front of, before	anteversion	*ante-* forward *vers/o* turning *-ion* process of	Process of turning forward.
anti-	against	antibacterial	*anti-* against *bacteri/o* bacteria *-al* pertaining to	Pertaining to against bacteria.
dys-	abnormal, difficult, bad, painful	dystrophy	*dys-* abnormal *-trophy* process of nourishment	Process of abnormal nourishment
endo-, end-	within	endoscopy	*endo-* within *-scopy* viewing	Viewing within.
epi-	above, upon	epigastric	*epi-* above *gastr/o* stomach *-ic* pertaining to	Pertaining to above the stomach.
hyper-	excessive, above	hyperglycemia	*hyper-* excessive, above *glyc/o* sugar, glucose *-emia* blood condition	Blood condition of excessive sugar.
hypo-	below, deficient	hypoglossal	*hypo-* below *gloss/o* tongue *-al* pertaining to	Pertaining to below the tongue.
inter-	between	intervertebral	*inter-* between *vertebr/o* vertebra, backbone *-al* pertaining to	Pertaining to between the backbones.
intra-	within	intramuscular	*intra-* within *muscul/o* muscle *-ar* pertaining to	Pertaining to within the muscle.

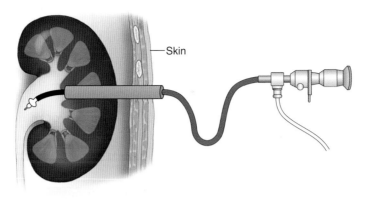

—Skin

Fig. 1-12 Percutaneous nephrolithotomy.

Prefixes—cont'd				
Prefix	**Meaning**	**Example**	**Word Origins**	**Definition**
neo-	new	neonatal	*neo-* new *nat/o* birth, born *-al* pertaining to	Pertaining to a newborn.
par-	near, beside	parotid	*par-* near *ot/o* ear *-id* pertaining to	Pertaining to near the ear.
para-	near, beside, abnormal	paraphilia	*para-* abnormal *phil/o* attraction *-ia* condition	Condition of abnormal attraction.
per-	through	percutaneous	*per-* through *cutane/o* skin *-ous* pertaining to	Pertaining to through the skin (Fig. 1-12).
peri-	surrounding, around	pericardium	*peri-* surrounding *cardi/o* heart *-um* structure	Structure surrounding the heart.
poly-	many, much, excessive, frequent	polyneuritis	*poly-* many, much, excessive, *neur/o* nerve *-itis* inflammation	Frequent inflammation of many nerves.
post-	after, behind	postnatal	*post-* after, behind *nat/o* birth, born *-al* pertaining to	Pertaining to after birth.
pre-	before, in front of	prenatal	*pre-* before *nat/o* birth, born *-al* pertaining to	Pertaining to before birth.
sub-	under, below	subhepatic	*sub-* under *hepat/o* liver *-ic* pertaining to	Pertaining to under the liver.
trans-	through, across	transurethral	*trans-* through *urethr/o* urethra *-al* pertaining to	Pertaining to through the urethra.

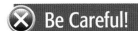 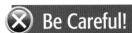 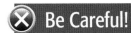 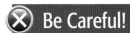

Don't confuse **inter-,** *meaning between, with* **intra-,** *meaning within.*

Don't confuse **ante-,** *meaning forward, with* **anti-,** *meaning against.*

Don't confuse **per-,** *meaning through, with* **peri-,** *meaning surrounding, and* **pre-,** *meaning before.*

Don't confuse **hyper-,** *meaning excessive, above, with* **hypo-,** *meaning below, deficient.*

Exercise 7: Prefixes

Match the prefixes with their meanings.

____ 1. anti-	A. under, below
____ 2. inter-	B. above, excessive
____ 3. poly-	C. against
____ 4. ante-	D. bad, difficult, painful
____ 5. hyper-	E. within
____ 6. dys-	F. many
____ 7. intra-	G. through
____ 8. peri-	H. between
____ 9. sub-	I. forward, in front of
____ 10. per-	J. around, surrounding

Using the method shown in Fig. 1-3 and the new word parts introduced in the preceding tables, translate and define these five terms.

11. subhepatic _____

12. pericardium _____

13. dyspneic _____

14. percutaneous _____

15. hypoglycemia _____

SINGULAR/PLURAL RULES

Because most healthcare terms end with Greek or Latin suffixes, making a healthcare term singular or plural is not always done the same way as it is in English. The following table gives the most common singular/plural endings and the rules for using them. Examples of unusual singular/plural endings and singular/plural exercises will be included throughout the text.

Rules for Using Singular and Plural Endings

If a Term Ends in:	Form the Plural by:	Singular Example	Plural Example	Plural Pronounced as:
-a	dropping the -a and adding -ae	vertebra (a bone in the spine)	vertebrae	Long a, e, or i, depending on the term
-is	dropping the -is and adding -es	arthrosis (an abnormal condition of a joint)	arthroses	seez
-ix or -ex	dropping the -ix or -ex and adding -ices	appendix	appendices	seez
-itis	dropping the -itis and adding -itides	arthritis (inflammation of a joint)	arthritides	deez
-nx	dropping the -nx and adding -nges	phalanx (a bone in the fingers or toes)	phalanges	ng (as in sing) and jeez
-um	dropping the -um and adding an -a	endocardium (the structure inside the heart)	endocardia	ah
-us	dropping the -us and adding an -i	digitus (a finger or toe)	digiti	eye
-y	dropping the -y and adding -ies	therapy (a treatment)	therapies	eez

http://evolve.elsevier.com/Shiland/coding
The Evolve website that comes with your book is loaded with entertaining interactive games and activities that will help you learn and review the material presented in each chapter. You can interactively:
- Study word parts
- Practice building terms
- Label anatomy
- Play games
- Watch animations
And much, much more!

Study on the go with these mobile-optimized assets:
- **Flash Cards**
- **Quick Quizzes**

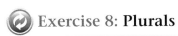 Exercise 8: **Plurals**

Change the singular terms to plural using the rules given in the preceding table.

1. esophag**us** (the tube joining the throat with the stomach) _____

2. lary**nx** (the voice box) _____

3. forn**ix** (an arched structure) _____

4. pleur**a** (the sac surrounding the lungs) _____

5. diagnos**is** _____

6. myocardi**um** _____

7. cardiomyopath**y** _____

8. hepat**itis** _____

Common Combining Forms

Combining Form	Meaning	Combining Form	Meaning
arteri/o	artery	lith/o	stone
arthr/o	joint	mamm/o	breast
bacteri/o	bacteria	muscul/o	muscle
bi/o	living, life	my/o	muscle
cardi/o	heart	nat/o	birth, born
cephal/o	head	neur/o	nerve
cervic/o	neck, cervix	ophthalm/o	eye
chondr/o	cartilage	oste/o	bone
col/o	large intestine, colon	ot/o	ear
coron/o	crown, heart	path/o	disease
cut/o	skin	ped/o	child
cutane/o	skin	phil/o	attraction
cyst/o	bladder, sac	pne/o	breathing
dent/i	tooth	psych/o	mind
derm/o	skin	rhin/o	nose
duoden/o	duodenum	somn/o	sleep
electr/o	electricity	spir/o	breathing
enter/o	small intestine	splen/o	spleen
esophag/o	esophagus	therm/o	heat, temperature
gastr/o	stomach	tonsill/o	tonsil
gloss/o	tongue	trache/o	trachea, windpipe
glyc/o	glucose, sugar	troph/o	nourishment, development
hem/o	blood	urethr/o	urethra
hepat/o	liver	valvul/o	valve
hyster/o	uterus	ven/o	vein
lingu/o	tongue	vers/o	turning
lipid/o	lipid, fat	vertebr/o	backbone, vertebra

Match the word parts to their definitions.

WORD PART DEFINITIONS

Prefixes		Definition
a-	1.	_____ between
anti-	2.	_____ through
dys-	3.	_____ near, beside
inter-	4.	_____ within
intra-	5.	_____ against
par-	6.	_____ no, not, without
para-	7.	_____ surrounding, around
per-	8.	_____ near, beside, abnormal
peri-	9.	_____ before, in front of
poly-	10.	_____ many, much, excessive, frequent
pre-	11.	_____ under, below
sub-	12.	_____ abnormal, difficult, painful, bad

Suffixes		Definition
-ar	13.	_____ pain
-dynia	14.	_____ discharge, flow
-ectomy	15.	_____ narrowing
-graphy	16.	_____ tumor, mass
-ia	17.	_____ machine to crush
-itis	18.	_____ inflammation
-metry	19.	_____ bursting forth
-oma	20.	_____ viewing
-osis	21.	_____ hardening
-pathy	22.	_____ cutting
-plasty	23.	_____ surgically forming
-rrhage	24.	_____ cutting out
-rrhaphy	25.	_____ recording
-rrhea	26.	_____ measuring
-sclerosis	27.	_____ suturing
-scopy	28.	_____ making a new opening
-stenosis	29.	_____ abnormal condition
-stomy	30.	_____ disease process
-tomy	31.	_____ pertaining to
-tripter	32.	_____ condition

WORDSHOP

Prefixes	Combining Forms	Suffixes
an-	cardi/o	-algia
endo-	cephal/o	-cele
hypo-	cervic/o	-ectomy
par-	col/o	-graphy
peri-	cyst/o	-ia
sub-	derm/o	-ic
	enter/o	-id
	gastr/o	-itis
	hepat/o	-megaly
	mamm/o	-scope
	ophthalm/o	-scopy
	ot/o	-stomy
	splen/o	-um
	tonsill/o	

Build the following terms by combining the above word parts. Some word parts may be used more than once. Some may not be used at all. The number in parentheses indicates the number of word parts needed.

Definition	Term
1. condition of without an eye (3)	
2. pertaining to near the ear (3)	
3. pertaining to under the liver (3)	
4. inflammation of the stomach and small intestines (3)	
5. instrument to view the eye (2)	
6. structure surrounding the heart (3)	
7. making a new opening of the colon (2)	
8. recording the breast (2)	
9. viewing within (2)	
10. cutting out the tonsils (2)	
11. herniation of the bladder (2)	
12. pertaining to the cervix (2)	
13. pain in the head (2)	
14. pertaining to below the skin (3)	
15. enlargement of the spleen (2)	

CHAPTER 2

Body Structure and Directional Terminology

ICD-10-CM Example from Tabular

S31.600 Unspecified open wound of abdominal wall, right upper quadrant with penetration into peritoneal cavity A

S31.601 Unspecified open wound of abdominal wall, left upper quadrant with penetration into peritoneal cavity A

S31.602 Unspecified open wound of abdominal wall, epigastric region with penetration into peritoneal cavity A

S31.603 Unspecified open wound of abdominal wall, right lower quadrant with penetration into peritoneal cavity A

S31.604 Unspecified open wound of abdominal wall, left lower quadrant with penetration into peritoneal cavity A

S31.605 Unspecified open wound of abdominal wall, periumbilic region with penetration into peritoneal cavity A

S31.609 Unspecified open wound of abdominal wall, unspecified quadrant with penetration into peritoneal cavity A

ICD-10-PCS Example

3 Administration
E Physiological Systems and Anatomical Regions
0 Introduction
Body System/Region:
    L Pleural Cavity
    M Peritoneal Cavity
    Q Cranial Cavity and Brain
    R Spinal Canal
    S Epidural Space
    U Joints
    Y Pericardial Cavity

CHAPTER OUTLINE

ORGANIZATION OF THE HUMAN BODY

ANATOMICAL POSITION AND SURFACE ANATOMY

POSITIONAL AND DIRECTIONAL TERMS

BODY CAVITIES

BODY REGIONS

PLANES OF THE BODY

ABBREVIATIONS

OBJECTIVES

☐ Recognize and use terms associated with the organization of the body.

☐ Recognize and use terms associated with positional and directional vocabulary.

☐ Recognize and use terms associated with the body cavities.

☐ Recognize and use terms associated with the abdominopelvic regions and quadrants.

☐ Recognize and use terms associated with planes of the body.

ORGANIZATION OF THE HUMAN BODY

The human body and its general state of health and disease may be understood by studying the various **body systems,** such as the digestive and respiratory systems. Each body system is composed of different **organs,** such as the stomach and lungs. These organs are made up of combinations of **tissues,** such as epithelial and muscular tissue, which in turn are composed of various **cells** that have very specialized functions.

All of these levels of organization are involved in a continual process of sensing and responding to conditions in the organism's environment. A negative change at one level of one system may cause a reaction throughout the entire body. **Homeostasis** is the normal dynamic process of balance needed to maintain a healthy body. When the body can no longer compensate for trauma or pathogens, disease, disorder, and dysfunction result.

organ = organ/o, viscer/o
tissue = hist/o
cell = cyt/o, cellul/o

homeostasis
   home/o = same
   -stasis = controlling

Cells

The smallest unit of the human body is the cell. Although there are a number of different types of cells, all of them share certain characteristics, one of them being **metabolism.** Metabolism is the act of converting energy by continually building up substances by **anabolism** and breaking down substances by **catabolism** for use by the body. Metabolism can be described as an equation:

$$\text{Metabolism} = \text{Anabolism} + \text{Catabolism}$$

See Fig. 2-1 for an illustration of a cell and the corresponding table below for a brief description of the pictured organelles and their functions.

metabolism
   meta- = change, beyond
   bol/o = throwing
   -ism = state of

anabolism
   ana- = up, apart
   bol/o = throwing
   -ism = state of

catabolism
   cata- = down
   bol/o = throwing
   -ism = state of

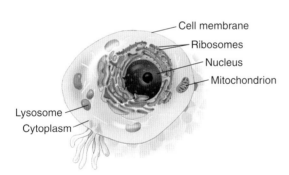

Fig. 2-1 The cell.

Cell Parts

Cell Part	Word Origin	Function
cytoplasm	**cyt/o** cell **-plasm** formation	Holds the organelles of the cell.
lysosome	**lys/o** dissolving **-some** body	Organelle that serves a digestive function for the cell.
ribosome	**rib/o** ribose **-some** body	Site of protein formation; contains RNA.
mitochondrion (pl. mitochondria)	**mitochondri/o** mitochondria **-on** structure	Converts nutrients to energy in the presence of oxygen.
nucleus (pl. nuclei)	**nucle/o** nucleus **-us** structure	Control center of cell; contains DNA, which carries genetic information.

To review the structure of a cell, click on **Body Spectrum.**

Tissues

There are four major categories of **tissues.** Within each type, the tissue either supports **(stromal** tissue) or does the actual work **(parenchymal** tissue) of the organ. For example, parenchymal nerve cells are the neurons that conduct the nervous impulse. Neuroglia are stromal nerve cells that enhance and support the functions of the nervous system. The four types of tissue include the following:

Epithelial: acts as an internal or external covering for organs, for example, the outer layer of the skin or the lining of the digestive tract. Note that the derivation of the term includes a combining form for the nipple *(thel/e)*. Originally the term *epithelium* was used to describe the membrane covering the nipple. Later, the usage was expanded to include all surface membranes, whether on the skin or mucosal membrane surfaces, that communicate with the outside of the body.

Connective: includes a variety of types, all of which have an internal structural network. Examples include bone, blood, cartilage, and fat.

Muscular: includes three types: heart muscle, skeletal muscle, and visceral muscle, all of which share the unique property of being able to contract and relax.

Nervous: includes cells that provide transmission of information to regulate a variety of functions, for example, neurons (nerve cells).

When tissue is destroyed by disease or trauma, the possibility of tissue replacement may be an option. **Autologous** tissue is that which is taken from one part of an individual's body and is transplanted to another location. *Auto-* means "self." An example would be a vein that is used to bypass a blocked coronary artery. If **nonautologous** tissue is used, it would mean that it is not from one's self, but from another human. A synonym for nonautologous is **allogeneic,** this time referring to being produced by a different human being. *All/o* means "different." **Zooplastic** tissue is that which is derived from an animal, for example, a cow or pig heart valve that is used to temporarily replace a structure until human donor tissue is available. *Zo/o* means "animal." If tissue is **syngeneic,** as in the case of identical twins, it refers to a genetically identical individual. *Syn-* means "together or joined," as in the sharing of the same DNA. Synonyms for the term *syngeneic* are **isoplastic, isogeneic,** and **isologous.** The combining form *is/o* means "equal." Note that the synonyms use all of the previous suffixes: *-plastic, -geneic, and -logous.*

Organs

Organs, also referred to as **viscera** *(sing.* viscus), are arrangements of various types of tissue that accomplish specific purposes. The heart, for example, is made up of muscle tissue, called **myocardium,** and it is lined with epithelial tissue known as **endocardium.** Organs are grouped within body systems but do have specific terms to describe their parts.

Parts of Organs

Organs can be divided into parts and have a set of terms that describe these various parts.

---

tissue = hist/o

stromal = strom/o

parenchymal
   par- = near
   en- = in
   chym/o = juice
   -al = pertaining to

epithelial
   epi- = upon
   thel/e = nipple
   -ial = pertaining to

muscle = my/o

fat = adip/o, lip/o

nervous = neur/o

organ = viscer/o, hist/o
myocardium
   myocardi/o = heart muscle
   -um = structure

endocardium
   endocardi/o = within the heart
   -um = structure

Parts of Organs

	Term	Combining Form	Definition
	apex	*apic/o*	The pointed extremity of a conical structure (*pl.* apices).
	body (corporis)	*corpor/o, som/o, somat/o*	The largest or most important part of an organ.
	cortex	*cortic/o*	The outer layer of an organ (*pl.* cortices).
	fornix	*fornic/o*	Any vaultlike or arched structure (*pl.* fornices).
	fundus	*fund/o*	The base or deepest part of a hollow organ that is farthest from the mouth of the organ (*pl.* fundi).
	hilum	*hil/o*	Recess, exit, or entrance of a duct into a gland, or of a nerve and vessels into an organ (*pl.* hila).
	lumen	*lumin/o*	The space within an artery, vein, intestine, or tube (*pl.* lumina).
	sinus	*sin/o, sinus/o*	A cavity or channel in bone, a dilated channel for blood, or a cavity that permits the escape of purulent (pus-filled) material (*pl.* sinuses). **Antrum** (*pl.* antra) and **sinus** are synonyms.
	vestibule	*vestibul/o*	A small space or cavity at the beginning of a canal.

Exercise 1: Intracellular Functions

Match each cell part with its function.

— 1. mitochondria   — 4. lysosomes   A. control center of cell
— 2. ribosomes   — 5. cytoplasm   B. holds organelles of cell
— 3. nucleus   C. digestive function
                                            D. responsible for energy production
                                            E. formation of proteins

Exercise 2: Types of Tissue

Match the characteristics of the tissue with its type.

— 1. contracts tissue   A. nervous
— 2. transmits information   B. epithelial
— 3. has an internal structural network   C. muscular
— 4. is an internal/external body covering D. connective

Exercise 3: Organ Parts

Match the combining forms with their meanings.

____ 1. fund/o   ____ 6. fornic/o
____ 2. lumin/o   ____ 7. hil/o
____ 3. sin/o   ____ 8. corpor/o
____ 4. apic/o   ____ 9. cortic/o
____ 5. vestibul/o

A. cavity/channel in bone/organ
B. pointed extremity of conical structure
C. archlike structure
D. base or deepest part of a hollow organ
E. entrance/exit/recess for ducts/vessels
F. space within an artery or tube
G. largest, most important part of organ, body
H. small space at beginning of a canal
I. outer layer of an organ

Exercise 4: Organ Parts

Fill in the blanks with the definitions of the following terms.

1. intraluminal_____

2. hilar_____

3. periapical_____

4. antral _____

5. vestibular_____

6. fundal_____

7. cortical_____

Fill in the blank with the correct organ part.

8. Fatty deposits may form in the _____ (space within) of the arteries, resulting in atherosclerosis.

9. Hector had a stone that was obstructing urine flow at the level of the _____ (exit/entrance) of the right kidney.

10. The x-rays showed a blunted _____ (tip) of the left lung.

11. The _____ (largest part) of the stomach was described as inflamed.

12. The paranasal _____ (cavities in bone) were completely blocked.

Body Systems

The organs of the body systems work together to perform certain defined functions. For example, movement is a function of the musculoskeletal system. Although each system has a number of functions, one must remember that the systems interact, and problems with one system can affect the function of other systems. For example, in the condition called *secondary hypertension,* disease in one body system (usually the lungs) causes a pathologic increase in blood pressure in the cardiovascular system. This hypertensive pressure is secondary to the primary cause (lung disease). Once the disorder of the initial system resolves, the hypertension disappears.

The following table lists each body system and its function.

> ⊗ **Be Careful!**
>
> *Do not confuse **my/o,** the combining form for* muscle, *with **myel/o,** the combining form for* spinal cord *or* bone marrow.

Body Systems

Body System	Functions
musculoskeletal	Support, movement, protection
integumentary	Cover and protection
gastrointestinal	Nutrition
urinary	Elimination of nitrogenous waste
reproductive	Reproduction
blood/lymphatic/ immune	Transportation of nutrients/waste, protection
cardiovascular	Transportation of blood
respiratory	Delivers oxygen to cells and removes carbon dioxide
nervous/behavioral	Receive/process information
special senses (eye and ear)	Information gathering, balance
endocrine	Effects changes through chemical messengers

Exercise 5: Body Systems and Functions

Matching.

____ 1. information gathering	A. integumentary
____ 2. delivers oxygen to cells and removes carbon dioxide	B. gastrointestinal
____ 3. reproduction	C. male and female reproductive
____ 4. cover and protection	D. musculoskeletal
____ 5. transportation of nutrients/waste, protection	E. endocrine
____ 6. effects changes through chemical messages	F. special senses
____ 7. receive/process information	G. blood, lymphatic, and immune
____ 8. nutrition	H. respiratory
____ 9. transportation of blood	I. nervous
____ 10. support, movement, protection	J. urinary
____ 11. elimination of nitrogenous waste	K. cardiovascular

Combining Forms for Body Organization

Meaning	Combining Form	Meaning	Combining Form
blood	hem/o, hemat/o	nerve	neur/o
bone	oste/o, osse/o	nipple	thel/e
break down, dissolve	lys/o	nucleus	kary/o, nucle/o
cell	cyt/o, cellul/o	organ, viscera	organ/o, viscer/o
epithelium	epitheli/o	same	home/o
fat	adip/o, lip/o	stroma	strom/o
heart	cardi/o	system	system/o
heart muscle	myocardi/o	to throw, throwing	bol/o
juice	chym/o	tissue	hist/o
muscle	my/o, muscul/o		

Prefixes for Body Organization

Prefix	Meaning
ana-	up, apart, away
cata-	down
en-	in
endo-	within
epi-	above, upon
meta-	beyond, change
para-	near, beside, abnormal

Suffixes for Body Organization

Suffix	Meaning
-al, -ous	pertaining to
-ia, -ism	condition, state of
-on	structure
-plasm	formation
-some	body
-stasis	controlling, stopping
-um	structure, thing, membrane
-us	structure

Specialties/Specialists and General Terms

The levels of organization of the body are accompanied by a number of specialties and their associated specialists.

Term	Word Origin	Definition
cytology	**cyt/o** cell **-logy** study of	The study of the cells. A cytologist specializes in the study of the cell. The suffix **-logist** means "one who specializes in the study of."
histology	**hist/o** tissue **-logy** study of	The study of tissues. A histologist specializes in the study of tissues.
anatomy	**ana-** up, apart, away **-tomy** cutting	To cut apart, the study of the structure of the body. An anatomist specializes in the structure of the body
physiology	**physi/o** growth **-logy** study of	The study of growth; the study of the function of the body. A physiologist specializes in the study of the function of the body.
pathology	**path/o** disease **-logy** study of	The study of disease. A pathologist specializes in the study of disease.
biopsy	**bi/o** life, living **-opsy** viewing	Process of viewing living tissue that has been removed for the purpose of diagnosis and/or treatment.
necropsy	**necr/o** death, dead **-opsy** viewing	Process of viewing dead tissue.
autopsy	**auto-** self **-opsy** viewing	Process of viewing by self; term commonly used to describe the examination of a dead body to determine cause(s) of death.

 Exercise 6: **Specialties/Specialists/General Terms**

Match the word parts to their definitions.

____ 1. physi/o
____ 2. necr/o
____ 3. ana-
____ 4. bi/o
____ 5. cyt/o
____ 6. auto-
____ 7. -opsy
____ 8. path/o
____ 9. -logy
____ 10. -logist

A. up, apart, away
B. disease
C. study of
D. cell
E. self

F. one who specializes in the study of
G. death, dead
H. process of viewing
I. life, living
J. growth

Exercise 7: Translating Terms

Write the meanings of the following terms.

1. cytology _____

2. pathologist _____

3. necropsy _____

4. histologist _____

5. biopsy _____

ANATOMICAL POSITION AND SURFACE ANATOMY

Now that you understand the levels of organization of the body, you need the terms that describe locations, positions, and directions on the body. A standard frame of reference, the **anatomical position,** is the position in which the body stands erect with face forward, arms at the sides, palms forward, with toes pointed forward. This position is used to describe the surface anatomy of the body, both front *(ventral)* and back *(dorsal)*. Fig. 2-2 shows the anatomical position, both front and back, and is labeled with all the surface anatomy labels you will encounter throughout this text.

Ventral Surface Anatomy Terms (Head and Neck)

Term	Word Origin	Definition
buccal	***bucc/o*** cheek ***-al*** pertaining to	Pertaining to the cheek.
cephalic	***cephal/o*** head ***-ic*** pertaining to	Pertaining to the head.
cervical	***cervic/o*** neck ***-al*** pertaining to	Pertaining to the neck. ***Collum*** is a term that refers to the entire neck.
cranial	***crani/o*** skull ***-al*** pertaining to	Pertaining to the skull.
facial	***faci/o*** face ***-al*** pertaining to	Pertaining to the face.
frontal	***front/o*** front ***-al*** pertaining to	Pertaining to the front, the forehead.
mental	***ment/o*** chin ***-al*** pertaining to	Pertaining to the chin. Because ment/o also refers to the mind, use context to help you chose the right definition.

Ventral Surface Anatomy Terms (Head and Neck)—Cont'd

Term	Word Origin	Definition
nasal	***nas/o*** nose ***-al*** pertaining to	Pertaining to the nose.
ocular	***ocul/o*** eye ***-ar*** pertaining to	Pertaining to the eye.
oral	***or/o*** mouth ***-al*** pertaining to	Pertaining to the mouth.
otic	***ot/o*** ear ***-ic*** pertaining to	Pertaining to the ear. Also called **auricular.**

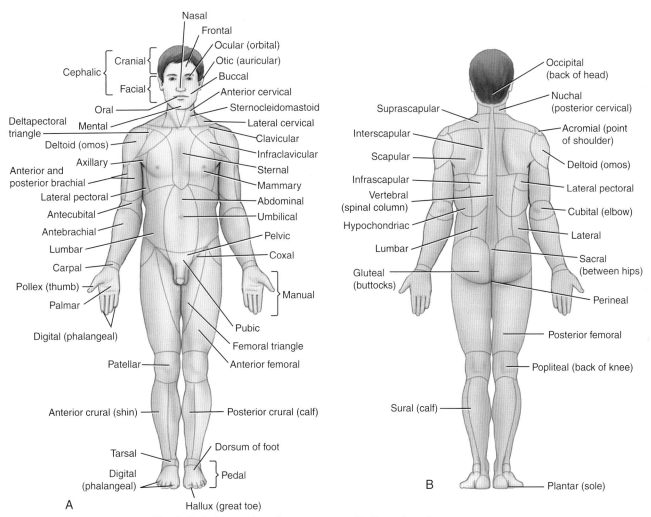

Fig. 2-2 **A,** Ventral surface anatomy. **B,** Dorsal surface anatomy.

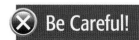 **Be Careful!**   The term **mental** means *pertaining to the chin* as well as *pertaining to the mind.*

Ventral Surface Anatomy (Trunk)

Term	Word Origin	Definition
abdominal	***abdomin/o*** abdomen ***-al*** pertaining to	Pertaining to the abdomen.
axillary	***axill/o*** axilla (armpit) ***-ary*** pertaining to	Pertaining to the armpit.
coxal	***cox/o*** hip ***-al*** pertaining to	Pertaining to the hip.
deltoid	***delt/o*** triangular ***-oid*** resembling	Pertaining to the deltoid muscle covering the shoulder. The combining form om/o is often used for the shoulder.
inguinal	***inguin/o*** groin ***-al*** pertaining to	Pertaining to the groin.
mammary	***mamm/o*** breast ***-ary*** pertaining to	Pertaining to the breast.
pelvic	***pelv/o, pelv/i*** pelvis ***-ic*** pertaining to	Pertaining to the pelvis.
pubic	***pub/o*** pubis ***-ic*** pertaining to	Pertaining to the pubis.
sternal	***stern/o*** sternum (breastbone) ***-al*** pertaining to	Pertaining to the breastbone.
thoracic	***thorac/o*** chest ***-ic*** pertaining to	Pertaining to the chest. Also called **pectoral.**
umbilical	***umbilic/o*** umbilicus (navel) ***-al*** pertaining to	Pertaining to the umbilicus.

Ventral Surface Anatomy (Arms and Legs)

Term	Word Origin	Definition
antecubital	***ante-*** forward, in front of, before ***cubit/o*** elbow ***-al*** pertaining to	Pertaining to the front of the elbow.
brachial	***brachi/o*** arm ***-al*** pertaining to	Pertaining to the arm. **Antebrachial** means pertaining to the forearm.
carpal	***carp/o*** wrist ***-al*** pertaining to	Pertaining to the wrist.

Ventral Surface Anatomy (Arms and Legs)—Cont'd

Term	Word Origin	Definition
crural	*crur/o* leg *-al* pertaining to	Pertaining to the leg.
digital	*digit/o* finger/toe *-al* pertaining to	Pertaining to the finger/toe. **Phalangeal** means pertaining to the bones in the fingers/toes.
femoral	*femor/o* thigh *-al* pertaining to	Pertaining to the thigh.
manual	*man/u* hand *-al* pertaining to	Pertaining to the hand.
palmar	*palm/o* palm *-ar* pertaining to	Pertaining to the palm. Also termed *volar.*
patellar	*patell/o, patell/a* kneecap *-ar* pertaining to	Pertaining to the kneecap.
pedal	*ped/o* foot *-al* pertaining to	Pertaining to the foot.
plantar	*plant/o* sole *-ar* pertaining to	Pertaining to the sole of the foot.
tarsal	*tars/o* ankle *-al* pertaining to	Pertaining to the ankle.

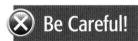 **Ped/o** means *foot* in the term *pedal,* but it can mean *child* or *children* in terms such as *pediatrics* and *pedodontics.*

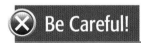 **Man/o** means *pressure* or *scanty* but **man/u** and **man/i** mean *hand.*

Dorsal Surface Anatomy Terms

Term	Word Origin	Definition
acromial	*acromi/o* acromion *-al* pertaining to	Pertaining to the acromion (highest point of shoulder).
dorsal	*dors/o* back *-al* pertaining to	Pertaining to the back.
gluteal	*glute/o* buttocks *-al* pertaining to	Pertaining to the buttocks.
lumbar	*lumb/o* lower back, loin *-ar* pertaining to	Pertaining to the lower back.

continued

Dorsal Surface Anatomy Terms—Cont'd

Term	Word Origin	Definition
nuchal	***nuch/o*** neck ***-al*** pertaining to	Pertaining to the neck, especially the back of the neck.
olecranal	***olecran/o*** elbow ***-al*** pertaining to	Pertaining to the elbow.
perineal	***perine/o*** perineum ***-al*** pertaining to	Pertaining to the perineum. The perineum is the space between the external genitalia and the anus.
popliteal	***poplite/o*** back of knee ***-eal*** pertaining to	Pertaining to the back of the knee.
sacral	***sacr/o*** sacrum ***-al*** pertaining to	Pertaining to the sacrum.
scapular	***scapul/o*** scapula, shoulder blade ***-ar*** pertaining to	Pertaining to the scapula.
sural	***sur/o*** calf ***-al*** pertaining to	Pertaining to the calf.
vertebral	***vertebr/o*** vertebra, spine ***-al*** pertaining to	Pertaining to the spine.

Exercise 8: Surface Anatomy Terms

Match the word parts with their definitions.

____ 1. cephal/o

____ 2. cervic/o

____ 3. brachi/o

____ 4. crur/o

____ 5. ped/o

____ 6. axill/o

____ 7. thorac/o

____ 8. mamm/o

____ 9. digit/o

____ 10. carp/o

____ 11. glute/o

____ 12. vertebr/o

____ 13. ot/o

____ 14. or/o

____ 15. crani/o

____ 16. man/u

____ 17. cubit/o

____ 18. plant/o

____ 19. bucc/o

____ 20. tars/o

A. armpit

B. wrist

C. mouth

D. breast

E. elbow

F. buttocks

G. head

H. cheek

I. backbones

J. arm

K. leg

L. ankle

M. neck

N. hand

O. sole

P. chest

Q. ear

R. foot

S. skull

T. fingers/toes

To practice labeling surface anatomy, click on **Label It.**

POSITIONAL AND DIRECTIONAL TERMS

Positional and directional terms are used in healthcare terminology to describe up and down, middle and side, and front and back. Because people may be lying down, raising their arms, and so on, standard English terms cannot be used to describe direction. The following table lists directional and positional terms as opposite pairs, with their respective combining forms or prefixes and illustrations. For example, x-rays may be taken from the front of the body to the back —an **anteroposterior (AP)** view—or from the back to the front—a **postero-anterior (PA)** view (Figs. 2-3 and 2-4). *Note that the terms are built from the perspective of the technician taking the x-ray.* The midline of the body is an imaginary line drawn from the crown of the head down between the eyes, through the chest, and separating the legs.

anteroposterior
  anter/o = front
  poster/o = back
  -ior = pertaining to

posteroanterior
  poster/o = back
  anter/o = front
  -ior = pertaining to

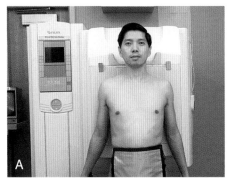
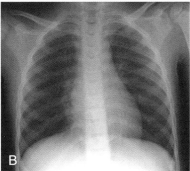

Fig. 2-3 **A,** Patient positioned for anteroposterior (AP) x-ray of the chest. **B,** AP chest x-ray.

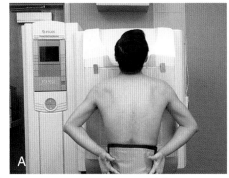
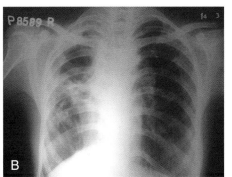

Fig. 2-4 **A,** Patient positioned for posteroanterior (PA) x-ray of the chest. **B,** PA chest x-ray.

Positional and Directional Terms

	Term	Word Origin	Definition
	anterior (ant)	**anter/o** front **-ior** pertaining to	Pertaining to the front.
	ventral	**ventr/o** belly **-al** pertaining to	Pertaining to the belly side.
	posterior (pos)	**poster/o** back **-ior** pertaining to	Pertaining to the back.
	dorsal	**dors/o** back **-al** pertaining to	Pertaining to the back of the body.
	superior (sup)	**super/o** upward **-ior** pertaining to	Pertaining to upward.
	cephalad	**cephal/o** head **-ad** toward	Toward the head.
	inferior (inf)	**infer/o** downward **-ior** pertaining to	Pertaining to downward.
	caudad	**caud/o** tail **-ad** toward	Toward the tail.
	medial	**medi/o** middle **-al** pertaining to	Pertaining to the middle (midline).
	lateral (lat)	**later/o** side **-al** pertaining to	Pertaining to the side.
	ipsilateral	**ipsi-** same **later/o** side **-al** pertaining to	Pertaining to the same side.

Positional and Directional Terms—Cont'd

	Term	Word Origin	Definition
	contralateral	***contra-*** opposite ***later/o*** side ***-al*** pertaining to	Pertaining to the opposite side.
	unilateral	***uni-*** one ***later/o*** side ***-al*** pertaining to	Pertaining to one side.
	bilateral	***bi-*** two ***later/o*** side ***-al*** pertaining to	Pertaining to two sides.
	superficial (external)		On the surface of the body.
	deep (internal)		Away from the surface of the body.
	proximal	***proxim/o*** near ***-al*** pertaining to	Pertaining to near the origin.
	distal	***dist/o*** far ***-al*** pertaining to	Pertaining to far from the origin.
	dextrad*	***dextr/o*** right ***-ad*** toward	Toward the right.

continued

Positional and Directional Terms—Cont'd

	Term	Word Origin	Definition
	sinistrad*	**sinistr/o** left **-ad** toward	Toward the left.
	afferent	**af-** toward **fer/o** to carry **-ent** pertaining to	Pertaining to carrying toward a structure.
	efferent	**ef-** away from **fer/o** to carry **-ent** pertaining to	Pertaining to carrying away from a structure.
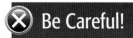	**supine**		Lying on one's back.
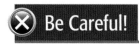	**prone**		Lying on one's belly.

*This is the *patient's,* not the reader's, right and left.

⚠ CM Guideline Alert

B.12 REPORTING SAME DIAGNOSIS CODE MORE THAN ONCE
Each unique ICD-10-CM diagnosis code may be reported only once for an encounter. This applies to bilateral conditions when there are no distinct codes identifying laterality or two different conditions classified to the same ICD-10-CM diagnosis code.

B.13 LATERALITY
Some ICD-10-CM codes indicate laterality, specifying whether the condition occurs on the left, right, or is bilateral. If no bilateral code is provided and the condition is bilateral, assign separate codes for both the left and right side. If the side is not identified in the medical record, assign the code for the unspecified side.

    When a patient has a bilateral condition and each side is treated during separate encounters, assign the "bilateral" code (as the condition still exists on both sides), including for the encounter to treat the first side. For the second encounter for treatment after one side has previously been treated and the condition no longer exists on that side, assign the appropriate unilateral code for the side where the condition still exists (e.g., cataract surgery performed on each eye in separate encounters). The bilateral code would not be assigned for the subsequent encounter, as the patient no longer has the condition in the previously treated site. If the treatment on the first side did not completely resolve the condition, then the bilateral code would still be appropriate.

⊗ Be Careful!
Do not confuse **anter/o,** meaning *front,* with **antr/o,** meaning *a cavity.*

⊗ Be Careful!
Do not confuse **bi-,** meaning *two,* with **bi/o,** meaning *life.*

Exercise 9: Word Parts for Positional and Directional Terms

Match the word parts with their definitions.

_____ 1. bi-	A. same
_____ 2. infer/o	B. side
_____ 3. anter/o	C. toward (suffix)
_____ 4. ef-	D. upward
_____ 5. medi/o	E. right
_____ 6. proxim/o	F. opposite
_____ 7. uni-	G. left
_____ 8. later/o	H. pertaining to
_____ 9. poster/o	I. two
_____ 10. contra-	J. near
_____ 11. super/o	K. back
_____ 12. af-	L. away from
_____ 13. sinistr/o	M. middle
_____ 14. ipsi-	N. front
_____ 15. dist/o	O. toward
_____ 16. dextr/o	P. downward
_____ 17. -ad	Q. far
_____ 18. -ior	R. one

Exercise 10: Positional and Directional Terms

Match the terms with their correct definitions.

_____ 1. medial	A. pertaining to downward
_____ 2. inferior	B. pertaining to carrying away from a structure
_____ 3. distal	C. pertaining to the middle
_____ 4. anterior	D. pertaining to the opposite side
_____ 5. dorsal	E. away from the surface of the body
_____ 6. supine	F. pertaining to far from the origin
_____ 7. prone	G. pertaining to carrying toward a structure
_____ 8. deep	H. pertaining to the same side
_____ 9. contralateral	I. pertaining to the back of the body
_____ 10. ipsilateral	J. lying on one's back
_____ 11. afferent	K. pertaining to the front
_____ 12. efferent	L. lying on one's belly

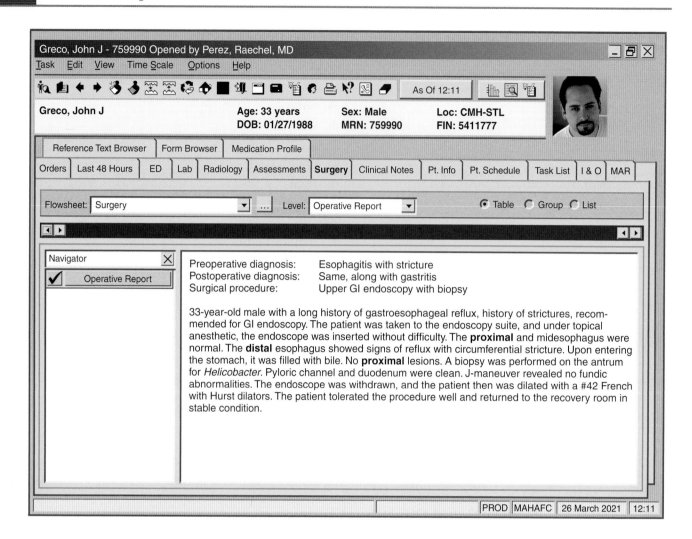

Greco, John J - 759990 Opened by Perez, Raechel, MD

Task   Edit   View   Time Scale   Options   Help

Greco, John J

Age: 33 years   Sex: Male   Loc: CMH-STL
DOB: 01/27/1988   MRN: 759990   FIN: 5411777

Reference Text Browser   Form Browser   Medication Profile

Orders   Last 48 Hours   ED   Lab   Radiology   Assessments   **Surgery**   Clinical Notes   Pt. Info   Pt. Schedule   Task List   I & O   MAR

Flowsheet: Surgery   Level: Operative Report   ⦿ Table   ○ Group   ○ List

Navigator
✓   Operative Report

Preoperative diagnosis: Esophagitis with stricture
Postoperative diagnosis: Same, along with gastritis
Surgical procedure: Upper GI endoscopy with biopsy

33-year-old male with a long history of gastroesophageal reflux, history of strictures, recommended for GI endoscopy. The patient was taken to the endoscopy suite, and under topical
anesthetic, the endoscope was inserted without difficulty. The **proximal** and midesophagus were
normal. The **distal** esophagus showed signs of reflux with circumferential stricture. Upon entering
the stomach, it was filled with bile. No **proximal** lesions. A biopsy was performed on the antrum
for *Helicobacter*. Pyloric channel and duodenum were clean. J-maneuver revealed no fundic
abnormalities. The endoscope was withdrawn, and the patient then was dilated with a #42 French
with Hurst dilators. The patient tolerated the procedure well and returned to the recovery room in
stable condition.

PROD MAHAFC   26 March 2021   12:11

Exercise 11: Operative Report

Using the operative report above, answer the following questions.

1. Which organ was described as inflamed before the operation?_____

2. After the operation, which organ/organs were described as inflamed?_____

3. Translate "The proximal and midesophagus were normal."_____

4. Which end of the esophagus was farthest from the point of origin? Circle one. *(proximal esophagus, mid-esophagus, distal esophagus)*

BODY CAVITIES

dorsal = dors/o

ventral = ventr/o

The body is divided into five cavities (Fig. 2-5). Two of these five cavities are in the back of the body and are called the **dorsal cavities.** The other three cavities are in the front of the body and are called the **ventral cavities.** Most of the body's organs are in one of these five body cavities.

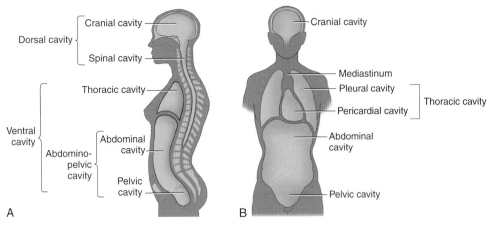

Fig. 2-5 Body cavities.

Dorsal Cavities

The **cranial cavity** contains the brain and is surrounded and protected by the cranium, or skull. The **spinal cavity** contains the spinal cord and is surrounded and protected by the bones of the spine, or vertebrae.

Ventral Cavities

The **thoracic** cavity contains the heart, lungs, esophagus, and trachea (windpipe) and is protected by the ribs, the **sternum** (breastbone), and the **vertebrae** (backbones). This chest cavity is further divided into the two **pleural cavities** that contain the lungs; the **mediastinum,** the space between the lungs; and the **pericardial cavity,** which holds the heart.

The pleura is a double-folded serous (watery) membrane that provides a small amount of lubrication that allows the lungs to contract and expand with minimal friction. The side of the membrane that is closest to the lung is called the visceral pleura, whereas the side that is closest to the body wall is the parietal pleura.

The pericardial cavity shares a similar structure to the pleural cavity, again having a double-folded serous membrane designed to avoid friction on the organ that it encloses. This time the inner membrane is termed the visceral pericardium, whereas the outer membrane is the parietal pericardium.

The **abdominopelvic cavity** is composed of two cavities (abdominal and pelvic) that are not separated by any physical structure. Because nothing physically separates the abdominal and pelvic cavities, they are often collectively referred to as the abdominopelvic cavity.

The **abdominal cavity** contains the stomach, liver, gallbladder, pancreas, spleen, and intestines, whereas the pelvic cavity contains the bladder and reproductive organs. The only anterior protections for the abdominal cavity are the skin and muscles covering it, and in the back, just the vertebrae. It is separated from the thoracic cavity by a broad dome-shaped muscle called the **diaphragm.**

The **pelvic cavity** contains the bladder and reproductive organs. These organs are cradled on the sides and in the back by the pelvic bones.

The entire abdominopelvic cavity is lined with yet another serous membrane called the **peritoneum.** The **parietal** layer of the peritoneum lines the abdominopelvic cavity, whereas the visceral layer surrounds its organs. The term parietal is derived from a Latin term for "the wall"; hence this layer is always the one closest to the body wall. The visceral layer of the peritoneum (or pericardium) is the one that is closest to the organ or organs that it encloses. The greater and

---

cranial = **crani/o**

spinal = **spin/o**

thoracic = **thorac/o**

sternum = **stern/o**

vertebrae = **vertebr/o**

mediastinum = **mediastin/o**

pleural = **pleur/o**

abdominopelvic
   abdomin/o = abdomen
   pelv/o = pelvis
   -ic = pertaining to

abdomen = abdomin/o, celi/o, lapar/o

diaphragm = **diaphragmat/o, diaphragm/o, phren/o**

pelvis = **pelv/o, pelv/i**

wall = **pariet/o**

peritoneum = **peritone/o**

retroperitoneum
  retro- = behind
  peritone/o =
  peritoneum
  -um = structure

lesser **omenta** are extensions of the visceral peritoneum that hold and support the cavity's organs. The fold of the peritoneum that joins the parietal and visceral layers and attaches it to the posterior wall of the abdominal cavity is called the **mesentery.** The **retroperitoneum** is the space behind the peritoneum that contains the kidneys, aorta, ureters, duodenum, and pancreas.

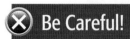 **Be Careful!** *The term* **abdomen** *refers to a region, whereas the* **stomach** *is an organ.*

Exercise 12: Body Cavities

Match the organ with the appropriate body cavity.

___ 1. cranial   ___ 4. spinal   A. spinal cord   D. brain
___ 2. abdominal   ___ 5. thoracic   B. bladder   E. heart
___ 3. pelvic   C. stomach

BODY REGIONS

In ICD-10-PCS, knowledge of the organization of the body is essential to accurate coding. At times, coders will not be able to assign a procedure to a specific part of a body system. In these cases, *general anatomical regions* are used (character 2 of the code). The choices can include a body part *(ex.* head); a body cavity *(ex.* pelvic cavity); or a tract *(ex.* respiratory tract).

 PCS Guideline Alert

B2. BODY SYSTEM
General guidelines
    B2.1a The procedure codes in the general anatomical regions body systems can only be used when the procedure is performed on an anatomical region rather than a specific body part (e.g., root operations Control and Detachment, Drainage of a body cavity) or, on the rare occasion when no information is available to support assignment of a code, to a specific body part. *Example:* Control of postoperative hemorrhage is coded to the root operation Control found in the general anatomical regions body systems.

umbilical = umbilic/o,
  omphal/o

lumbar = lumb/o

hypochondriac
  hypo- = under
  chondr/o = cartilage
  -iac = pertaining to

epigastric
  epi- = upon, above
  gastr/o = stomach
  -ic = pertaining to

hypogastric
  hypo- = under
  gastr/o = stomach
  -ic = pertaining to

iliac = ili/o

inguinal = inguin/o

Abdominopelvic Regions

The **abdominopelvic regions** are the nine regions that lie over the abdominopelvic cavity (Fig. 2-6). The area in the center of the abdominopelvic region is called the **umbilical** area. Laterally, to the left and right of this area, are the **lumbar** regions. They are called the lumbar regions because they are bound by the lumbar vertebrae. Superior to the lumbar regions, and below the ribs, are the **hypochondriac** regions. Medial to the hypochondriac regions, and superior to the umbilical region, is the **epigastric** region. Inferior to the umbilical region is the **hypogastric** region, and lateral to the sides of the hypogastric region are, respectively, the right and left **iliac** regions, sometimes referred to as the **inguinal** regions.

Abdominopelvic Quadrants

A simpler method of naming a location in the abdominopelvic area is to divide the area into quadrants, using the navel as the intersection. These quadrants are referred to as either right or left, upper or lower (Fig. 2-7). In the right upper

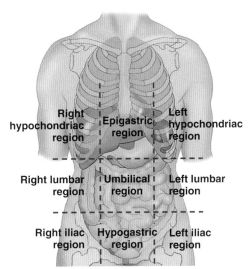

Fig. 2-6 Abdominopelvic regions. *Left and right are from the patient's perspective, not yours.*

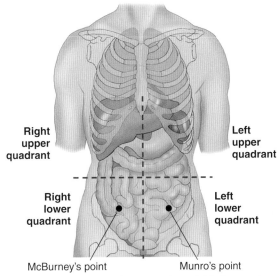

Fig. 2-7 Abdominopelvic quadrants with Munro's and McBurney's points. *Left and right are from the patient's perspective, not yours.*

Be Careful!

Do not confuse **hypo,** meaning *under* or *deficient,* with **hyper-,** meaning *above* or *excessive.*

Be Careful!

Do not confuse **ile/o,** meaning *ileum* (part of the intestine), with **ili/o,** meaning *ilium* (part of the hip).

quadrant (RUQ) lies the liver. In the left upper quadrant (LUQ) lie the stomach and the spleen. The appendix is in the right lower quadrant (RLQ). If a patient complains of pain in the area of **McBurney's point,** the area that is approximately two thirds of the distance between the navel and the hip bone in the RLQ, appendicitis is suspected. Except for the appendix, the left lower quadrant (LLQ) contains organs similar to the lower right. In the LLQ, halfway between the navel and the hip bone, is **Munro's point.** This is a standard site of entrance for surgeons who perform laparoscopic surgery.

PLANES OF THE BODY

Another way of describing the body is by dividing it into planes, or flat surfaces, that are imaginary cuts or sections through the body. The use of plane terminology is common when imaging of internal body parts by computed tomography (CT) scans, magnetic resonance imaging (MRI), positron emission tomography (PET) scans, or other imaging techniques is described. Figs. 2-8 to 2-10 show the three body planes and corresponding views of the brain.

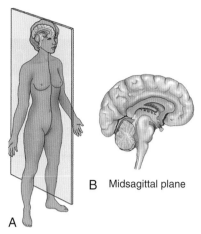

B Midsagittal plane

Fig. 2-8 A, Midsagittal plane. **B,** Midsagittal section of the brain.

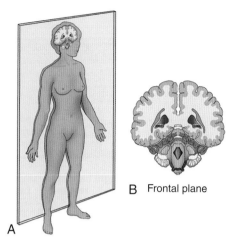

B Frontal plane

Fig. 2-9 A, Frontal plane. **B,** Frontal section of the brain.

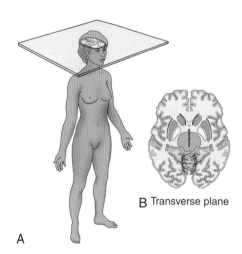

B Transverse plane

Fig. 2-10 A, Transverse plane. **B,** Transverse section of the brain.

sagittal = sagitt/o
mid- = middle

frontal = front/o

Sagittal planes are vertical planes that separate the sides from each other (see Fig. 2-8). A **midsagittal plane,** also termed the median plane, separates the body into equal right and left halves. The **frontal** (or **coronal)** plane divides the body into front and back portions (see Fig. 2-9). The **transverse** plane (also called **cross-sectional)** divides the body horizontally into an upper part and a lower part (see Fig. 2-10) . And finally, the **oblique** plane, not as commonly used as the first three, divides the body at a slanted angle.

Combining Forms for Body Cavities, Abdominopelvic Quadrants and Regions, and Planes

Meaning	Combining Form	Meaning	Combining Form
abdomen	abdomin/o, celi/o, lapar/o	diaphragm	diaphragmat/o, diaphragm/o, phren/o
back	dors/o	front, bellyside	front/o, ventr/o
cartilage	chondr/o	groin	inguin/o
cranium (skull)	crani/o		

Combining Forms for Body Cavities, Abdominopelvic Quadrants and Regions, and Planes—Cont'd

Meaning	Combining Form	Meaning	Combining Form
ilium	ili/o	spine	spin/o
		sternum	stern/o
lower back, loin	lumb/o	stomach	gastr/o
mediastinum	mediastin/o	thorax (chest)	thorac/o
organ	viscer/o, organ/o	umbilicus (navel)	umbilic/o, omphal/o
pelvis	pelv/i, pelv/o	vertebra	vertebr/o
peritoneum	peritone/o	wall	pariet/o
pleura	pleur/o		

Prefixes for Body Cavities, Abdominopelvic Quadrants and Regions, and Planes

Prefix	Meaning
epi-	above, upon
hyper-	excessive, above
hypo-	deficient, below, under
mid-	middle
trans-	through, across
retro-	behind, backward

Exercise 13: Abdominopelvic Regions

Using your knowledge of directional terms and the nine abdominopelvic regions, answer the following questions.

1. Superior to the umbilical region is the _____ region.

2. Lateral to the umbilical region are the left and right _____ regions.

3. Medial to the left and right inguinal regions is the _____ region.

4. Inferior to the lumbar regions are the left and right _____ regions.

5. Lateral to the epigastric region are the right and left _____ regions.

To practice labeling the abdominopelvic regions, click on **Label It.**

Exercise 14: Planes of the Body

1. Which plane divides the body into superior and inferior portions? _____

2. Which plane divides the body into equal left and right sections? _____

3. Which plane divides the body into anterior and posterior sections? _____

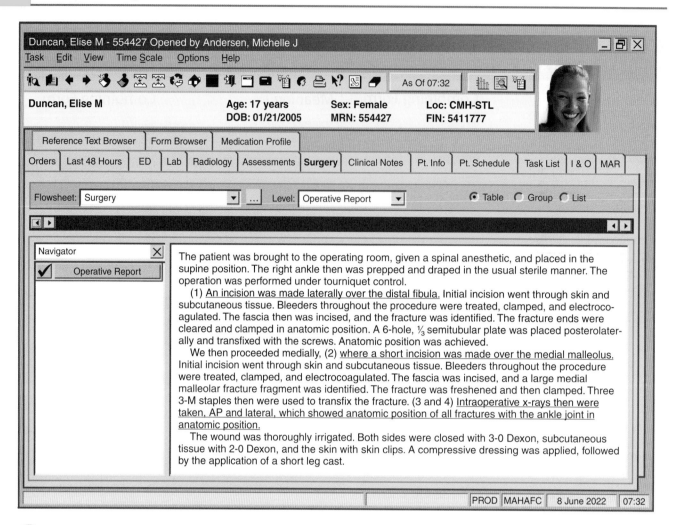

 Exercise 15: **Operative Report**

Refer to the operative report above to answer the following questions.

1. "An incision was made laterally over the distal fibula." If you know that the fibula is one of the lower lateral leg bones, the distal end is *closer to the* _____ .

2. The malleoli are processes at the distal ends of the fibula and tibia. The medial malleolus is on the _____ *surface* of the leg.

3. The "intraoperative x-rays" were taken _____ the operation.

4. The AP view of the ankle joint fracture was taken from _____.

Abbreviations

Abbreviation	Definition	Abbreviation	Definition
ant	anterior	MRI	magnetic resonance imaging
AP	anteroposterior	PA	posteroanterior
CT	computed tomography	PET	positron emission tomography
inf	inferior	pos	posterior
lat	lateral	RLQ	right lower quadrant
LLQ	left lower quadrant	RUQ	right upper quadrant
LUQ	left upper quadrant	sup	superior

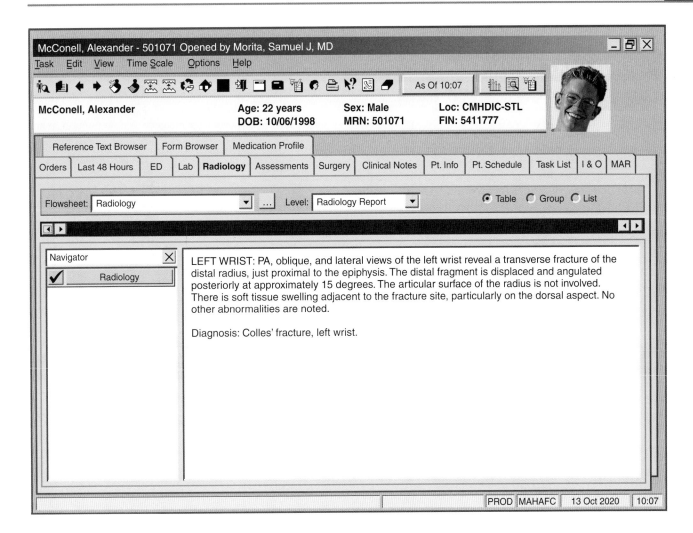

Exercise 16: **Radiology Report**

Refer to the radiology report above to answer the following questions.

1. Which end of the radius was fractured? The end closest to the wrist or the end nearest the elbow?

_____

2. Was the bone displaced backward or forward?_____

3. What does *dorsal* mean?_____

4. A PA view means_____.

Go to the Evolve website to interactively build terms, label images, memorize word parts, and practice using directional and positional terms in context.

Match the word parts to their definitions.

WORD PART DEFINITIONS

Prefixes	Definition
af-	1. _____above, upon
ante-	2. _____forward, in front of, before
bi-	3. _____one
contra-	4. _____within
ef-	5. _____two
endo-	6. _____toward
epi-	7. _____same
ipsi-	8. _____opposite
meta-	9. _____away from
uni-	10. _____change, beyond

Combining Forms	Definition
anter/o	11. _____organ
axill/o	12. _____downward
brachi/o	13. _____front
caud/o	14. _____far
cephal/o	15. _____middle
cervic/o	16. _____armpit
corpor/o	17. _____upward
crani/o	18. _____near
crur/o	19. _____left
cyt/o	20. _____arm
dextr/o	21. _____tail
dist/o	22. _____leg
hist/o	23. _____side
infer/o	24. _____right
inguin/o	25. _____back
lapar/o	26. _____tissue
later/o	27. _____body
medi/o	28. _____head
poster/o	29. _____skull
proxim/o	30. _____cell
sinistr/o	31. _____groin
super/o	32. _____neck
thorac/o	33. _____chest
viscer/o	34. _____abdomen

WORDSHOP

Prefixes	Combining Forms	Suffixes
bi-	abdomin/o	-ad
contra-	anter/o	-al
hyper-	crani/o	-ar
hypo-	cyt/o	-ic
in-	dextr/o	-ia
inter-	gastr/o	-ior
intra-	hist/o	-logy
ipsi-	inguin/o	-oid
mid-	later/o	-plasm
	lumb/o	
	pelv/i	
	poster/o	
	sagitt/o	
	super/o	
	thorac/o	

Build body structure and directional terms by combining the word parts above. Some word parts may be used more than once. Some may not be used at all. The number in parentheses indicates the number of word parts needed.

Definition	Term
1. pertaining to the middle of the sagittal plane (3)	
2. pertaining to two sides (3)	
3. toward the right (2)	
4. pertaining to back to front (3)	
5. pertaining to the chest (2)	
6. pertaining to the abdomen and pelvis (3)	
7. pertaining to the lower back (2)	
8. pertaining to the opposite side (3)	
9. formation of cells (2)	
10. pertaining to upward (2)	
11. pertaining to the groin (2)	
12. the study of tissue (2)	
13. pertaining to under the stomach (3)	
14. pertaining to the same side (3)	
15. pertaining to within the skull (3)	

Sort the terms below into the correct categories.

TERM SORTING

Organization of the Body	Positional and Directional Terms	Body Cavities and Planes	Abdominal Regions and Quadrants

afferent	iliac	sinus
anterior	inguinal	spinal
apex	lateral	stroma
coronal	lumbar	superior
cranial	lumen	supine
cytoplasm	midsagittal	system
distal	nucleus	thoracic
efferent	organ	transverse
epigastric	pleural	umbilical
hilum	posterior	pelvic
hypochondriac	prone	vestibule
hypogastric	sagittal	

Replace the highlighted text with the correct terms.

TRANSLATIONS

1. Susie was being treated for a cut on the **pertaining to the sole of the foot** surface of her foot and a wart on the **pertaining to the palm** surface of her hand.	
2. Maureen located a vein in the **pertaining to the front of the elbow** space of the patient's left arm for a blood draw.	
3. The patient described her leg pain as **pertaining to two sides,** although occasionally it seemed to be only on the right.	
4. Sam had canker sores on his **pertaining to the cheek** membrane.	
5. The patient had a **process of viewing living tissue that has been removed for the purpose of diagnosis** of a mole that had recently increased in size.	
6. The **space within an artery, vein, intestine, or tube** of one of the patient's coronary arteries was completely blocked.	
7. The paralyzed patient had fractured one of the bones in his **pertaining to the chest** spine.	
8. Nora had a fracture of the **pertaining to far from the origin** phalanx of her right index finger.	
9. A tumor growing in the patient's **the space between the lungs** pressed on his esophagus.	
10. The patient's right hemispheric stroke affected the **pertaining to the opposite** side of her body.	
11. The patient was in a **lying on one's back** position so that the physician could examine her abdomen.	
12. Jeremy complained of pain resulting from a/an **lateral to the sides of the hypogastric region** hernia.	
13. The man had **pertaining to the chest** and **pertaining to the hip** contusions.	
14. Mr. Jones had **pertaining to above the stomach** pain.	

Musculoskeletal System and Connective Tissue

ICD-10-CM Example from Tabular

M43.1 Spondylolisthesis

Excludes 1 acute traumatic of lumbosacral region (S33.1)

acute traumatic of sites other than lumbosacral—code to feature vertebra, by region

congenital spondylolisthesis (Q76.2)

M43.10 Spondylolisthesis, site unspecified

M43.11 Spondylolisthesis, occipito-atlanto-axial region

M43.12 Spondylolisthesis, cervical region

M43.13 Spondylolisthesis, cervicothoracic region

M43.14 Spondylolisthesis, thoracic region

M43.15 Spondylolisthesis, thoracolumbar region

M43.16 Spondylolisthesis, lumbar region

M43.17 Spondylolisthesis, lumbosacral region

M43.18 Spondylolisthesis, sacral and sacrococcygeal region

M43.19 Spondylolisthesis, multiple sites in spine

ICD-10-PCS Example from Index

Bursectomy
- *See* Excision, Bursae and Ligaments ØMB
- *See* Resection, Bursae and Ligaments ØMT

Bursocentesis
- *See* Drainage, Bursae and Ligaments ØM9

Bursography
- *See* Plain Radiography, Non-Axial Upper Bones BPØ
- *See* Plain Radiography, Non-Axial Lower Bones BQØ

Bursotomy
- *See* Division, Bursae and Ligaments ØM8
- *See* Drainage, Bursae and Ligaments ØM9

CHAPTER OUTLINE

OBJECTIVES

☐ Recognize and use terms related to the anatomy and physiology of the musculoskeletal system.

☐ Recognize and use terms related to the pathology of the musculoskeletal system.

☐ Recognize and use terms related to the procedures for the musculoskeletal system.

Learning terminology of the musculoskeletal system (MS) (Fig. 3-1) is best done sequentially. Studying the names and locations of the bones and bone markings will help you recognize the names and locations of the joints and ligaments. Learning the names of the bones and muscle actions will be reinforced in the names of the muscles and tendons. Remembering the terms for surface anatomy and directional terms studied in the second chapter will help you with the terms for many of the structures in this body system.

New terminology will include Greek and Latin terms for shapes and sizes. Some of the word parts may help you remember the locations and characteristics of anatomical structures by visualizing their Greek or Latin meanings. Remember that linking what you already know to new material, using repetition, and putting that new knowledge into use are all ways to make the new material stick.

A quick note: Some of these terms will reappear in other chapters, so keep an eye on the margins for terms that are "recyclable" and have uses in other body

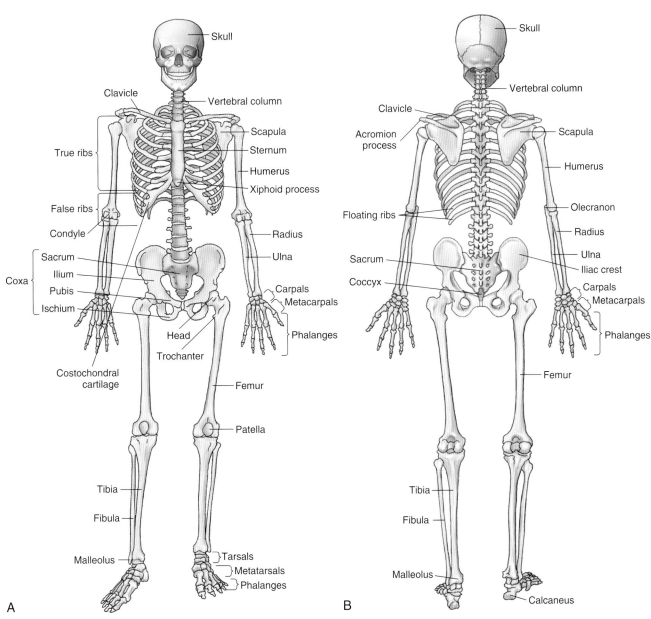

A   B

Fig. 3-1 Axial and appendicular skeleton.

systems. Being aware of this ahead of time will keep you from being confused with word parts that appear in more than one body system.

FUNCTIONS OF THE MUSCULOSKELETAL SYSTEM AND CONNECTIVE TISSUE

The musculoskeletal system is composed of three interrelated parts: the **bones, joints** (articulations), and **muscles.** Bones are connected to one another by fibrous bands of tissue called **ligaments.** Muscles are attached to the bone by bands of tissue called **tendons.** The tough fibrous covering of the muscles (and some nerves and blood vessels) is called the **fascia.**[1] These structures:
1. act as a framework for the organ systems
2. protect many of the body's organs
3. provide the organism with the ability to move
4. provide formation of blood cells
5. act as storage for mineral salts (calcium and phosphorus) and fat cells

ANATOMY AND PHYSIOLOGY

Skeletal System

The skeletal system is composed of two types of connective tissue: cartilage and bone. Both are composed of a structural protein termed **collagen.** Note that the derivation of *coll/a* (glue) is related to the nature of the substance formed when connective tissue is boiled, not any function of the protein itself.

This chapter includes all the anatomy necessary to assign ICD-10 musculoskeletal system codes, including detail on annular ligaments, the cribriform plate and the gemellus muscles. See Appendix H for a complete list of body parts and how they should be coded.

Cartilage

Cartilage is composed of collagen fibers and cartilage cells **(chondrocytes).** Together, these substances form its internal structure, termed a **matrix.**

Three varieties of cartilage (elastic cartilage, fibrocartilage, and hyaline cartilage) form flexible tissues in different locations in the body.
- **Elastic cartilage,** with its stretchy elastin fibers, forms parts of the ears and nose, along with the temporary bones in the fetal skeleton. This elastic cartilage is later replaced by bone in a process termed **endochondral ossification.**
- **Fibrocartilage,** named for the bundles of collagen fibers in it, is found in the discs between the backbones (vertebrae) and pubic bones in the pelvis.
- **Hyaline cartilage** (also termed **glassy cartilage** for its appearance) that covers the ends of the long bones and serves to cushion and protect the joints is called **articular cartilage.** Hyaline cartilage also forms the attachments of the ribs to the breastbone (costochondral cartilage) and parts of the voice box, windpipe, and bronchi.

The covering of the elastic and hyaline cartilage (with the exception of the articular cartilage) is called the **perichondrium,** which is instrumental in supplying the tissue with nutrients. Cartilage lacks a nerve supply, which means

---

[1]ICD-10 has reclassified disorders of the fascia to the chapter on the skin. For purposes of continuity, the fascia and its associated disorders will be addressed in this chapter.

---

musculoskeletal
  muscul/o = muscle
  skelet/o = skeleton
  -al = pertaining to

bone = oste/o, oss/i, osse/o

joint = arthr/o, articul/o

muscle = muscul/o, my/o, myos/o

ligament = ligament/o, syndesm/o

tendon = tendin/o, tendon/o, ten/o

fascia = fasci/o

cartilage = chondr/o, cartilag/o

costochondral
  cost/o = rib
  chondr/o = cartilage
  -al = pertaining to

perichondrium
  peri- = surrounding, around
  chondr/o = cartilage
  -ium = structure

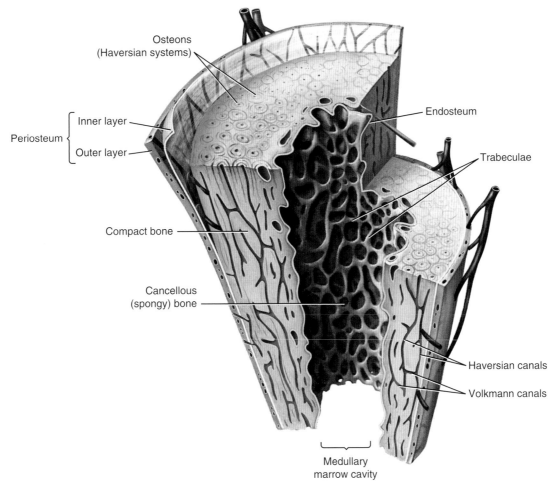

Fig. 3-2 Compact and cancellous bone.

that wear-and-tear joint disease is not sensed until pain is registered by the bones. Also, because cartilage is avascular (meaning that it does not have a blood supply), disorders of the cartilage are often slow to heal.

 CPT Coding Alert!

CPT has a specific code for an introduction of autologous chondrocyte implantation (ACI) into the knee. The procedure uses the body's own hyaline cartilage cells to replace the missing articular cartilage.

Bone

As opposed to cartilage, bones (osseous tissue) are inflexible structures. There are two types of osseous tissue: **cortical** (also called **compact**) and **cancellous** (also called **spongy** or **trabecular**) bone (Fig. 3-2). The cortical bone is the dense, stronger, outer segment of bones, whereas cancellous bone is the more open, weaker part.

Bone Formation

Once formed, bones are continually engaged in the process of renewing themselves. During the process of **osteogenesis** (also called **ossification**), connective tissue cells are turned into **osteoblasts.** Osteoblasts are immature cells that build bone.

bone = oste/o, oss/i, osse/o

osteogenesis
  oste/o = bone
  -genesis = production, origin

osteoblast
    oste/o = bone
    -blast = embryonic

osteocyte
    oste/o = bone
    -cyte = cell

osteoclast
    oste/o = bone
    -clast = breaking down

trabecula = trabecul/o

hematopoiesis
    hemat/o = blood
    -poiesis = formation

axial = axi/o

appendicular =
    appendicul/o

Osteocytes are mature bone cells, and **osteoclasts** are cells that break down bone to release the calcium salts as needed by the body.

A bone's matrix is formed by a fibrous protein substance that provides a framework in which the mineral salts (calcium, phosphate, and hydroxide) are deposited. This chemical compound is termed **hydroxyapatite** (also spelled *hydroxylapatite* and *apatite*), and it is this substance that gives bone its latticelike structure. Hydroxyapatite is also a major component of teeth.

Osteons (also called the **Haversian systems**) are the cylindrical units within the harder] outer cortical bone that are built up in layers by this deposition process with a mature osteoblast, now called an **osteocyte,** in its middle. The surrounding layers are called **lamellae,** a term meaning "little plates." It might help to note the relationship to the word *lamination,* with its similar meaning of a composition of layers. The bodies of the osteocytes occupy the spaces (**lacunae**) in the calcified matrix. Their cytoplasmic processes extend into the tiny canals (termed **canaliculi**) that join the lacunae to each other. Unlike cartilage, osseous tissue is vascular, with its required blood supply furnished through a series of passageways. These passageways are both the Haversian and Volkman canals. The **Haversian canals** are located longitudinally to the long axis of the bone, whereas the **Volkman canals** join each of the Haversian canals in a horizontal fashion. Cancellous bone is composed of **trabeculae** ("little beams"—as in tiny construction girders) in a much less dense, open network that allows space for the storage of fat cells and the formation of blood (hematopoiesis).

Skeleton

The Greeks named the skeleton for the dried-up remains of a withered corpse. Today we recognize the term *skeleton* to represent the bones of the body without any of the muscles, ligaments, bursae, or tendons that accompany the musculoskeletal system, regardless of their state of hydration.

A normal skeleton is composed of 206 bones (slight variation occurs in the tailbone, feet, hands, and knee bones), many of which are paired with a mirrored left or right likeness. For the purposes of assigning accurate codes, it is necessary to learn the names of each of these 206 bones, categorize them as to their location, and note when a disease or condition affects either the right, left, or bilateral locations (e.g., right, left, or both knee joints).

The skeleton itself can be divided into two parts: the **axial skeleton,** which is the skull, vertebrae (back bones), and rib cage, and the **appendicular skeleton,** which is the shoulder and pelvic girdles, and the upper and lower extremities (Fig. 3-1). The **shoulder girdle** connects the arms to the axial skeleton with the shoulder blades (scapulae) and collarbones (clavicles). The **pelvic girdle** provides attachment for the legs with its two pelvic (coxal) bones.

Bone Shapes

Bones can be divided by their shapes: long, short, flat, irregular, and sesamoid. Although the shape is often important to their supportive or protective functions (long—mostly those of the arms, legs, fingers and toes; short—boxy, cube-shaped like those of the wrist or ankle; flat—like the sternum, scapulae, and most of the skull bones; irregular—the vertebrae and hip bones; and sesamoid—the kneecap), the structure of these shapes is of particular importance to understanding the terminology needed for ICD-10. Long bones, for example, the upper arm bone, help to explain the different types of osseous tissue and the composition of bone at a microscopic and macroscopic level.

Shapes of Human Bones

Types	Examples
long bones	humerus (upper arm bone), femur (thighbone)
short bones	carpal (wristbone), tarsal (anklebone)
flat bones	sternum (breastbone), scapula (shoulder blade)
irregular bones	vertebra (backbone), stapes (a bone in the ear)
sesamoid	patella (kneecap)

ICD Note

Although the traditional method of explaining the organization of the skeleton is by dividing it into its axial and appendicular components, the ICD-10-PCS Medical Surgical section categorizes the skeleton into three different divisions (Fig. 3-3):

- Head and facial bones: the skull, facial bones, and hyoid bone.
- Upper bones: the left and right upper extremities (arm, hand, and finger bones); left and right glenoid cavity; scapula; clavicle; rib; and the sternum, as well as the cervical and thoracic vertebrae.
- Lower bones: the left and right lower extremities (leg, foot, and toe bones), left and right pelvic bones (ilium, ischium, and pubis), acetabula, and the lumbar vertebrae, sacrum, and coccyx.

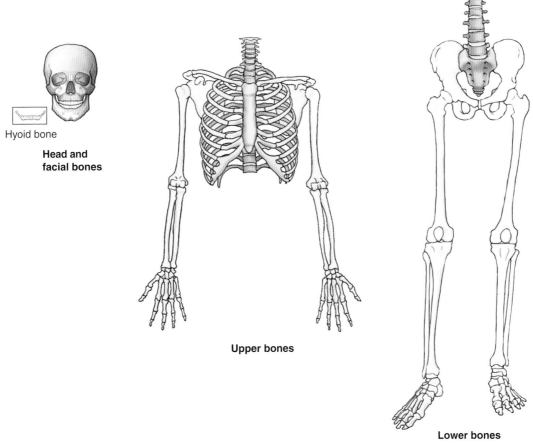

Hyoid bone

**Head and
facial bones**

Upper bones

Lower bones

Fig. 3-3 Skeletal bones divided by ICD-10 PCS classifications.

diaphysis
    dia- = through
    -physis = growth, nature

epiphysis
    epi- = above
    -physis = growth, nature

periosteum
    peri- = surrounding
    oste/o = bone
    -um = structure

endosteum
    endo- = within
    oste/o = bone
    -um = structure

bone marrow = **myel/o**

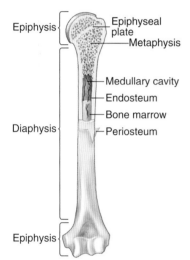

Fig. 3-4 Long bone.

Bone Structure

The shaft of a long bone (Fig. 3-4) is termed the **diaphysis,** whereas the ends are called the **epiphyses** (*sing.* **epiphysis**). The end that is closer to the trunk is termed the **proximal epiphysis,** whereas the end that is farther away is called the **distal epiphysis.** The growth plate (also called the **epiphyseal plate** or the **physis**) is the site of growth for bone lengthening. This plate is "sealed" when growth stops, typically around the ages of 18-20 in most people.

The tissue that surrounds the bones is called the **periosteum,** which has specialized cells called **nociceptors** to provide the sensation of pain when damage occurs.

The inner lining of the center of the bones is called the **endosteum.** The **medullary** (medull/o) **cavity** is the center of the bone within the endosteum. There are two types of **bone marrow** in the medullary cavities. Red bone marrow produces blood cells, whereas yellow bone marrow stores fat. The yellow bone marrow is stored in the center of the cortical (compact) bone, whereas the red marrow is located in the spongy bone of long bones as well as the flat bones of the body. Red bone marrow gives rise to the stem cells that differentiate into red blood cells, platelets, and most of the white blood cells.

Bone Markings

Each bone has characteristic protrusions and/or indentations that function as attachments for ligaments and muscles and access for blood vessels and nerves. These bone markings are called **processes** (the protrusions) and **depressions** (the indentations). By taking the time to study their names and characteristics, learning the names of muscles, ligaments, and joints will be much easier. A table of the most common bone depressions and processes is provided below.

Bone Depressions

Depression	Combining Form	Meaning/Function	Example
fissure	fissur/o	Fairly deep cleft or groove	Sphenoidal fissure
foramen	foramin/o	Opening or hole	Foramen magnum, mental foramina
fossa	foss/o	Hollow or depression, especially on the surface of the end of a bone	Olecranal fossa
fovea		Small pit or depression	Fovea capitis of humerus
sinus/antrum	sinus/o, sin/o, antr/o	Cavity or channel lined with a membrane	Paranasal sinuses
sulcus	sulc/o	General term that refers to a groove or depression in an anatomical structure, not as deep as a fissure	Intertubercular sulcus of humerus

Bone Processes

Process	Combining Form	Meaning/Function	Example
condyle	condyl/o	Rounded projection at the end of a bone that anchors the ligaments and articulates with adjacent bones	Medial condyle of the femur
crest		Narrow elongated elevation	Iliac crest
epicondyle	epicondyl/o	Projection on the surface of the bone above the condyle	Lateral epicondyle of the humerus
facet		Small smooth, flat articular surface	Vertebral facets
head (capitis)		Rounded, usually proximal portion of some long bones	Femoral head, humeral head
neck		Narrowed area distal to a bone head	Femoral neck
ramus		Branchlike extension	Mandibular ramus
spine	spin/o	Thornlike projection	Spinous process of vertebra
trochanter	trochanter/o	One of two bony projections on the proximal ends of the femurs that serve as points of attachment for muscles	Greater trochanter
tubercle	tubercul/o	Nodule or small raised area	Costal tubercle
tuberosity		Elevation or protuberance; larger than a tubercle	Ischial tuberosity

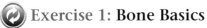 **Exercise 1: Bone Basics**

Match the bone word parts with their meanings.

____ 1. myel/o	A. bone
____ 2. -physis	B. foramen, hole
____ 3. peri-	C. above, upon
____ 4. condyl/o	D. cell
____ 5. spin/o	E. bone marrow
____ 6. sin/o	F. surrounding, around
____ 7. foramin/o	G. embryonic
____ 8. -um	H. spine
____ 9. -blast	I. breaking down
____ 10. epi-	J. growth, nature
____ 11. foss/o	K. hollow, depression
____ 12. endo-	L. condyle, knob
____ 13. oste/o	M. within
____ 14. -cyte	N. sinus, cavity
____ 15. -clast	O. structure

Fill in the blank.

16. Osteoblasts _____ bone, whereas osteoclasts _____ bone.

17. The shaft of a long bone is called the _____; the ends of a long bone are called _____(plural!).

18. The outer covering of bone is the _____, whereas the inner lining
    is the _____.

19. A foramen, a sinus, and a fossa are examples of bone _____. A condyle, a
    trochanter, and a tuberosity are examples of bone _____.

20. A synonym for a sinus is a/an _____.

21. What are the five bone shapes? _____.

22. The axial skeleton comprises _____.

23. The appendicular skeleton comprises _____.

24. The ICD-10-PCS divides the entire skeleton into three categories. What are they?

    _____.

25. Describe the difference between cortical and cancellous bone. _____.

To practice labeling the bones of the musculoskeletal system, click on **Label It.**

skull, cranium = crani/o
face = faci/o

frontal = front/o

parietal = pariet/o
occipital = occipit/o

temporal = tempor/o
mastoid = mastoid/o

styloid = styl/o
ethmoid = ethmoid/o

Axial Skeleton

The axial skeleton includes the skull, spine, and rib cage (see Fig. 3-1).

Skull

The skull is made up of two parts: the **cranium,** which encloses and protects the
brain, and the **facial bones** (Fig. 3-5).

Cranium

Frontal bone: Forms the anterior part of the skull and the forehead. The zygomatic process is the section of the frontal bone that extends toward the cheek.

Parietal bones: Paired bones that form the sides of the cranium.

Occipital bone: Forms the posteroinferior portion of the skull. Notable is a
   large hole at the ventral surface in this bone, the foramen magnum (magnum means *large*), which allows brain communication with the spinal
   cord.

Temporal bones: Paired bones that form the inferior two sides of the cranium.
   The **mastoid process** is the small, rounded protruding bone posterior to the
   ear. The petrous part of the temporal bone is the hard, stonelike portion of the
   temporal bone that protectively houses the external auditory canal and middle and inner ear. The tympanic portion is the lower area that encircles the
   eardrum. The **zygomatic process** is the anterior projection that forms the
   inferior portion of the cheek. The **styloid process** is a thin, pointed projection at the base of the temporal bone that serves as a point of attachment for
   ligaments and muscles.

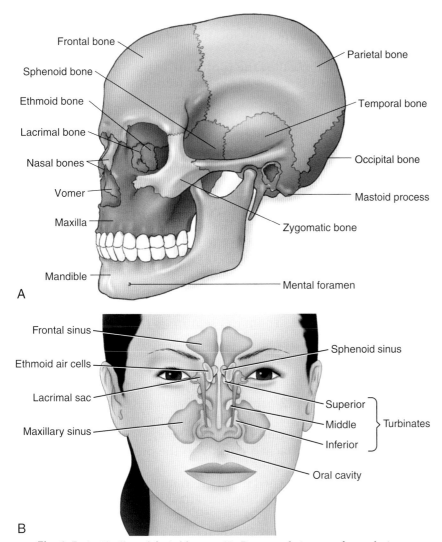

Fig. 3-5 A, Skull and facial bones. **B,** Paranasal sinuses, frontal view.

Ethmoid bone: Single, sievelike bone forming the roof and walls of the nasal cavity. The **cribriform plate** (also named for its sievelike appearance) is a thin, flat structure perforated by many foramina for the olfactory nerves.

Sphenoid bone: A bat-shaped bone that forms the internal base of the skull, giving shape to the orbits of the eyes. The **optic foramina** are the openings that allow the optic nerves to pass through. The **sella turcica** is a saddle-like depression on the body of the sphenoid that holds the pituitary gland. The **greater wings** (also termed the **alisphenoid**) are the triangular projections that form the cranial wall adjacent to the petrous part of the temporal bone. The **lesser wings** (also called **orbitosphenoids**) are smaller projections that form the back of the orbit and support part of the frontal lobe of the brain.

Paranasal sinuses: Air-filled cavities that are named for the bone where they are located. Each is lined with a mucous membrane (Fig. 3-5, *B*). The **vomer** is the bone that forms the inferior/posterior part of the nasal septum.

Hyoid bone: A U-shaped bone located in the neck and attached to the styloid processes of the temporal bone.

sphenoid = sphenoid/o

al/i = wing

paranasal
 para- = near, beside
 nas/o = nose

vomer = vomer/o

hyoid = hyoid/o

zygoma = zygom/o, zygomat/o	
lacrimal = lacrim/o	
maxilla = maxill/o	
jaw = gnath/o	
mandible = mandibul/o	
palatine = palat/o	
nasal = nas/o	

Facial Bones

Use Fig. 3-5 to locate the names and locations of the majority of the following facial bones:

Zygoma: Cheekbone. Also called the **malar or zygomatic bone.**

Lacrimal bones: Paired bones at the corner (canthus) of each eye that cradle the tear ducts.

Orbit: The bony socket of the eyeball. It is composed of the ethmoid, frontal, lacrimal, maxilla, palatine, sphenoid, and zygomatic bones.

Maxilla: Upper jawbone. Also called the **maxillary bone.** The maxillary alveolar processes are the cavities that hold the teeth in.

Mandible: Lower jawbone. Also called the **mandibular bone.** The **mental foramina** are the holes in the central part (body) of the mandible. The rami are posterior vertical projections. The **condyloid process** is a posterior projection of the ramus that articulates with the temporal bone. The **coronoid process** is the anterior projection of the ramus. The mandibular notch is the depression between the coronoid and condylar processes.

Palatine bones: Structures that make up part of the roof of the mouth.

Nasal bones: Pair of small bones that make up the bridge of the nose. The **vomer** is the bone that forms the posterior/inferior part of the **nasal septum** between the nostrils. The nasal septum is the wall that separates the nostrils.

rib = cost/o	
costochondral **cost/o** = rib **chondr/o** = cartilage **-al** = pertaining to	

Rib Cage

The **ribs** (costae) consist of 12 pairs of thin, flat bones attached to the thoracic vertebrae in the back. The head and neck of the ribs are closest to the vertebrae. The three types of ribs can be categorized as follows:

- **True ribs:** Seven pairs attached directly to the breastbone (sternum) in the front of the body
- **False ribs:** Three pairs attached to the sternum by cartilage
- **Floating ribs:** Two pairs of ribs not attached in the front of the body at all

In addition to ribs, the rib cage includes the **sternum,** also known as the breastbone. The sharp point at the most inferior aspect of the sternum is called the **xiphoid process.** The combining form *xiph/o* is derived from the Greek word for sword, which the xiphoid resembles.

sternum = stern/o	
xiphoid = xiph/o	
body = corpor/o	

The **corporis** (body) of the sternum is the main central portion. The **manubrium** is the upper section that articulates with the collarbones. *Manubri/o* means "handle," a reference to the swordlike **xiphoid process.** The **suprasternal notch** (also called the **jugular notch** and **fossa jugularis sternalis**) is the small indentation in the superior edge of the manubrium.

spine = spin/o	
vertebra = vertebr/o	

Spine

The **spinal** or **vertebral column** is divided into five regions from the neck to the tailbone. It is composed of 26 bones called the **vertebrae** (see Fig. 3-6). The following table lists the bones in the spine.

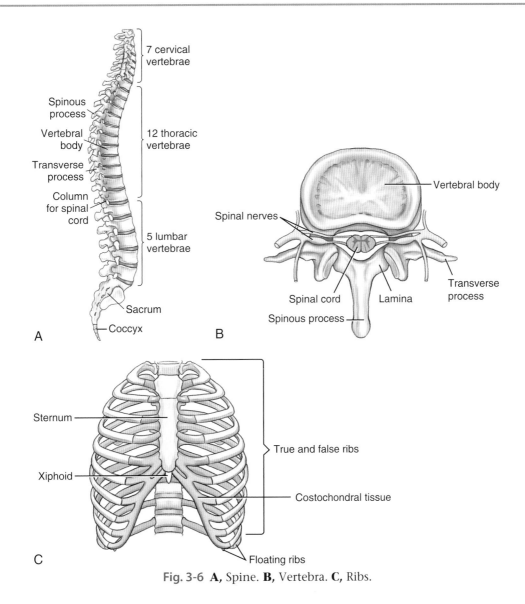

Fig. 3-6 **A**, Spine. **B**, Vertebra. **C**, Ribs.

Bones of the Spine

Region	Type and Abbreviation
cervical	neck bones (C1-C7)
thoracic	upper back (T1-T12)
lumbar	lower back (L1-L5)
sacral	sacrum (S1-S5) (5 bones fused as one)
coccygeal (tailbone)	coccyx or tailbone

cervical = cervic/o

thoracic = thorac/o

lumbar = lumb/o

sacral = sacr/o

coccygeal = coccyg/o

C1 is called the atlas, named for the Greek god who held up the heavens. C2 is called the axis for its role in permitting rotation of the head. Unique to C2 is the dens (also termed the odontoid process), which is a small toothlike projection for the first cervical vertebra to rotate around.

The **vertebral foramen** is the opening in the center of each vertebra where the spinal cord passes. The **vertebral arch** (also called the **neural arch**) is the posterior part of the bone. It consists of two laminae, the spinous process, the

lamina = lamin/o

articular = articul/o

vertebral pedicles, and the facets. **Laminae** are thin, platelike structures that form parts of the arch on either side of the spinous process. The **spinous process** is the thornlike projection on the back of a vertebra. **Vertebral pedicles** connect the laminae to the vertebral body. **Facets** are small, rounded processes that articulate between vertebrae. Also called **articular processes,** they are either inferior or superior.

 ## Exercise 2: Axial Skeletal Combining Forms

Match each axial skeletal term with its correct combining form.

____ 1. cervic/o	A. lower jawbone
____ 2. lamin/o	B. rib
____ 3. ethmoid/o	C. backbone
____ 4. chondr/o	D. lower back
____ 5. thorac/o	E. cheekbone
____ 6. crani/o	F. roof and walls of nasal cavity
____ 7. occipit/o	G. cartilage
____ 8. cost/o	H. roof of mouth
____ 9. zygomat/o	I. neck
____ 10. lumb/o	J. skull
____ 11. mandibul/o	K. lamina of vertebra
____ 12. coccyg/o	L. upper jawbone
____ 13. vertebr/o	M. back of skull
____ 14. palat/o	N. chest
____ 15. maxill/o	O. tailbone
____ 16. stern/o	P. breastbone

Translate the following terms below using your knowledge of word parts.

17. submandibular _____

18. costochondral _____

19. lumbosacral _____

20. thoracic _____

21. substernal _____

To practice labeling the axial skeleton, click on **Label It.**

Appendicular Skeleton

The appendicular skeleton is divided into the **upper appendicular** and **lower appendicular** skeletons.

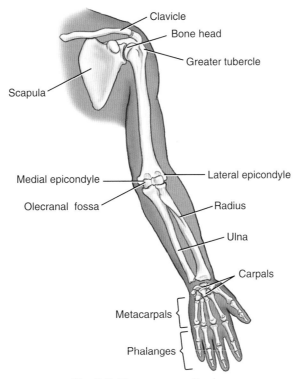

Fig. 3-7 Upper appendicular.

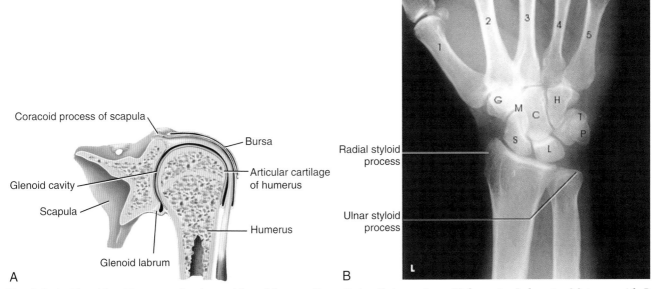

A   B

Fig. 3-8 **A,** Shoulder; **B,** x-ray of wrist and hand bones; *C*, capitate; *G*, trapezium; *H*, hamate; *L*, lunate; *M*, trapezoid; *P*, pisiform; *S*, scaphoid; *T*, triquetrum. (*S, L, P, T* = proximal bones; *G, M, C, H* = distal bones)

Upper Appendicular Skeleton

The upper appendicular skeleton (Fig. 3-7) includes the shoulder girdle (scapula, clavicle, upper humerus) and the arm bones. Refer to Fig. 3-8, *A* for a closer look at the shoulder.

Scapula: The scapulae, or shoulder blades, are flat bones that help to support the arms. The **acromion process** is the lateral protrusion of the scapula that forms the highest point of the shoulder. The **glenoid cavity** (the arm socket)

scapula = scapul/o

acromion process = acromi/o

glenoid = glen/o

**clavicle = clavicul/o,
cleid/o**

humerus = humer/o

radius = radi/o

ulna = uln/o

olecranon = olecran/o

wrist = carp/o

**metacarpus =
metacarp/o**

phalanx = phalang/o

interphalangeal
  inter- = between
  phalang/o = phalanx
  -eal = pertaining to

digitus = digit/o, dactyl/o

is the depression in the scapula that is the seat of the head of the humerus (syn. glenoid fossa). The **coracoid process** is the beaklike process of the scapula that serves as a point of attachment for muscles and ligaments in the shoulder.

Clavicle: The clavicle, or collarbone, is one of a pair of long, curved horizontal bones that attach to the upper sternum at one end and the acromion process of the scapula at the other. These bones help to stabilize the shoulder anteriorly. A "wishbone" is composed of the fused clavicles of a bird.

Humerus: Upper arm bone. The bone head (caput) is the proximal enlarged round end that articulates with the glenoid cavity. The anatomical neck is immediately below the humeral head, whereas the surgical neck is below the tuberosities distal to the anatomical neck. The greater tubercle is the larger of two protuberances, whereas the adjacent lesser tubercle is obviously the other. Both function as points of attachment for muscles. The long, narrow part of the humerus shaft is capped by the medial and lateral epicondyles at the distal end.

Radius: Lower lateral arm bone parallel to the ulna. The distal end articulates with the thumb side of the hand. The **ulnar notch** is the small cavity that articulates with the ulna at the distal end of the radius. It is also called the **sigmoid cavity.** Sigmoid just means "s" shaped. You'll see this adjective again describing a section of the large intestine.

Ulna: Lower medial arm bone. The distal end articulates with the little finger side of the hand. The radial notch is the cavity that articulates with the radius at its proximal end. The **radial notch** is also termed the **lesser sigmoid cavity.** The **olecranon** is a proximal projection of the ulna that forms the tip of the elbow. Commonly known as the **funny bone,** this structure is actually a process.

Carpus: The eight bones of the carpus (wrist) are each named for a shape and are in two rows. The distal row (closest to the palm) has the scaphoid, lunate, triquetrum and pisiform, while the proximal row (closest to the forearm) has the trapezium, trapezoid, capitate and hamate. They are listed from lateral to medial using anatomical position with the palms forward. (see Fig. 3-8, *B* for a radiograph of the carpus and metacarpus bones).

Metacarpus: One of the five bones that form the middle part of the hand.

Phalanx: One of the 14 bones that constitute the fingers of the hand, two in the thumb and three in each of the other four fingers (pl. phalanges). The three bones in each of the four fingers are differentiated as proximal, medial/middle, and distal. The joints between these are referred to as proximal and distal interphalangeal (PIP, DIP) joints. When one is referring to a whole finger (or toe), the term **digitus** is used. The thumb is called the **pollex.** Additional tiny sesamoid bones can be found in the hand between some of the interphalangeal and metacarpophalangeal joints. These bones help to change the direction of tendons and relieve friction on a joint.

 PCS Guideline Alert

B4.7 If a body system does not contain a separate body part value for fingers, procedures performed on the fingers are coded to the body part value of the hand. If a body system does not contain a separate body part value for toes, procedures performed on the toes are coded to the body part value for the foot.
   Example: Excision of a finger muscle is coded to one of the hand muscle body part values in the Muscles body system.

 CPT Coding Alert!

CPT codes amputation by the body part removed. In regard to fingers or toes, the amputation is named at the level of the phalanx (or metacarpal/tarsal). ICD-10 uses rays (phalanges and metacarpal/tarsal) or partial rays to describe amputations.

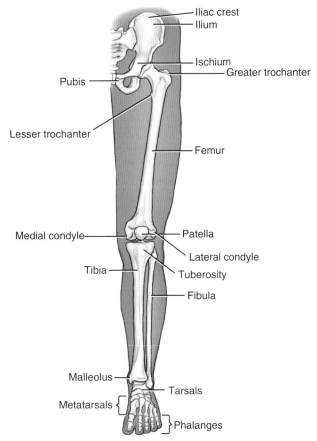

Fig. 3-9 Lower appendicular.

 CPT Coding Alert!

CPT has a specific code for pollicization (creation of a thumb from another finger). ICD-10-PCS groups transfers of index fingers together, specifying right or left only.

Lower Appendicular Skeleton

The lower half of the appendicular skeleton can be divided into the pelvic girdle (the **bony pelvis, sacrum,** and **coccyx**) and the leg bones (Fig. 3-9). The pelvis is composed of two **coxal** (hip) bones that are connected in the front at the pubic symphysis and in the back at the sacrum. Each coxa is composed of three fused bones that together form the hip socket, the **acetabulum,** for the head of the thighbone. The three fused bones are the:

Ilium: The superior and widest bone of the pelvis. The iliac crest is the upper edge of the bone.

Ischium: The lower, posterior portion of the pelvic bone.

Pubis or pubic bone: The lower anterior part of the pelvic bone. The obturator foramina are the two openings between the ischium and pubis on both sides of the pelvic bone. The term *obturate* means to "stop up" or "block," and was used to name this opening because on dissection it was found to be filled with muscles and nerves.

The leg is composed of the:

Femur: Thighbone, upper leg bone. The femoral head articulates with the hip bone at the acetabulum. The femoral neck connects the head to the shaft where two protuberances, the greater and lesser trochanters, serve as sites of

pelvis = pelv/i, pelv/o	
sacrum = sacr/o	
coccyx = coccyg/o	
hip = cox/o	
acetabulum = acetabul/o	
ilium = ili/o	
ischium = ischi/o	
pubis = pub/o	
femur = femor/o	

patella = patell/o, patell/a	
tibia = tibi/o	
fibula = fibul/o, perone/o	
malleolus = malleol/o	
tarsus = tars/o	
calcaneus = calcane/o	
cuboid = cuboid/o	
cuneiforms = cune/o	
talus = tal/o	
navicular = navicul/o	
metatarsus = metatars/o	
phalanx = phalang/o	
hallux = halluc/o	

muscle attachment. At the distal end of the shaft are medial and lateral condyles that articulate with the condyles of the tibia. Slightly above those are the medial and lateral epicondyles.

Patella: Kneecap, a sesamoid bone that is encased in the quadriceps femoris tendon and helps to protect the knee joint.

Tibia: Shinbone, lower medial leg bone. The proximal end of the tibia has both medial and lateral condyles, whereas the distal end has a medial malleolus, a process that extends inward.

Fibula: Smaller, lower lateral leg bone. The head of the fibula is at its proximal end, where it articulates with the lateral condyle of the tibia. The body (shaft) of the fibula has a diamond-like appearance, with each of the four surfaces named for the direction it faces: anteromedial, anterolateral, posteromedial and posterolateral. The lateral **malleolus** is the process that extends outward at the distal end of the bone.

Tarsus: One of the seven bones of the ankle including the **calcaneus** (heel bone), **cuboid** (box-shaped), **cuneiforms** (medial, lateral, and intermediate wedge-shaped bones), **navicular** (boat-shaped), and **talus** (the second-largest tarsal bone). The talus is named from the Latin for its shape like a die (singular of dice), as it was used as a game piece in ancient times.

Metatarsus: One of the five small, long bones in the foot between the tarsals and the phalanges.

Phalanx: One of 14 toe bones, 2 in the great toe and 3 in each of the other four toes. The term for the great toe is the **hallux.** As in the hands, sesamoid bones are also present in the feet where the first metatarsal bone joins the great toe.

Note

When coding fingers or toes, be aware of the term "ray." It refers to all of the phalanges as well as the corresponding metacarpals or metatarsals. For example, a complete detachment (amputation) of the 5th ray of the foot is a removal of the fifth metatarsal as well as the three corresponding phalanges (proximal, middle/middle, and distal). This is also the case in CPT.

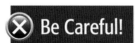 **Be Careful!**   *Do not confuse* **perone/o,** *meaning* fibula, *with* **peritone/o,** *meaning* the lining of the abdomen.

 Exercise 3: The Appendicular Skeleton

Match the upper appendicular combining forms with their meanings.

Combining Forms
_____ 1. humer/o
_____ 2. scapul/o
_____ 3. uln/o
_____ 4. olecran/o
_____ 5. clavicul/o, cleid/o
_____ 6. metacarp/o
_____ 7. digit/o
_____ 8. phalang/o
_____ 9. radi/o
_____ 10. carp/o

Upper Appendicular Bones
A. collarbone, clavicle
B. wristbone
C. finger, toe
D. one of the finger or toe bones
E. lower lateral arm bone
F. upper arm bone
G. lower medial arm bone
H. elbow
I. shoulder blade
J. hand bone

Match the lower appendicular combining forms with their meanings.

Combining Forms

____ 11. patell/a
____ 12. pub/o
____ 13. metatars/o
____ 14. tibi/o
____ 15. ili/o
____ 16. malleol/o
____ 17. cox/o
____ 18. ischi/o
____ 19. fibul/o, perone/o
____ 20. femor/o
____ 21. tars/o
____ 22. calcane/o
____ 23. acetabul/o
____ 24. halluc/o

Lower Appendicular Bones

K. foot bone
L. lower portion of pelvis
M. anklebone
N. lower anterior pelvic bone
O. shinbone
P. kneecap
Q. superior, widest bone of pelvis
R. processes on distal tibia and fibula
S. thighbone
T. hip bone
U. lower lateral leg bone
V. heel bone
W. great toe
X. hip socket

Translate the terms.

25. interphalangeal _____

26. humeroulnar _____

27. infrapatellar _____

28. femoral _____

29. supraclavicular _____

To practice labeling the appendicular skeleton, click on **Label It.**

Joints

ICD-10-PCS classifies joints as being either upper or lower. As a coder, you will need to recognize these joints and be able to categorize them appropriately. The following introduction to the terminology of the joints is organized with the PCS in mind.

 PCS Guideline Alert

B2.1B Where the general body part values "upper" and "lower" are provided as an option in the Upper Arteries, Lower Arteries, Upper Veins, Lower Veins, Muscles and Tendons body systems, "upper" or "lower" specifies body parts located above or below the diaphragm respectively.

PCS Guideline Alert

B4.5 Procedures performed on tendons, ligaments, bursae, and fascia supporting a joint are coded to the body part in the respective body system that is the focus of the procedure. Procedures performed on joint structures themselves are coded to the body part in the joint body systems.

Example: Repair of the anterior cruciate ligament of the knee is coded to the knee bursae and ligament body part in the bursae and ligaments body system. Knee arthroscopy with shaving of articular cartilage is coded to the knee joint body part in the Lower Joints body system.

PCS Guideline Alert

B4.6. If a procedure is performed on the skin, subcutaneous tissue, or fascia overlying a joint, the procedure is coded to the following body part:
- Shoulder is coded to Upper Arm
- Elbow is coded to Lower Arm
- Wrist is coded to Lower Arm
- Hip is coded to Upper Leg
- Knee is coded to Lower Leg
- Ankle is coded to Foot

joint = articul/o, arthr/o

synarthrosis
  syn- = together
  arthr/o = joint
  -sis = condition

amphiarthrosis
  amphi- = both
  arthr/o = joint
  -sis = condition

diarthrosis
  dia- = through
  arthr/o = joint
  -sis = condition

synovial = synovi/o

bursa = burs/o

meniscus = menisc/o

Joints, or **articulations** as they are sometimes called, are the parts of the body where two or more bones of the skeleton join. Examples of joints include the knee, which joins the tibia and the femur, and the elbow, which joins the humerus with the radius and ulna. Joints provide **range of motion (ROM)**, the range through which a joint can be extended and flexed. Different joints have different ROMs, ranging from no movement at all to full range of movement. Categorized by ROM, they are as follows:

No ROM: Most **synarthroses** are immovable joints held together by fibrous cartilaginous tissue. The suture lines of the skull are examples of synarthroses.
Limited ROM: Amphiarthroses are joints joined together by cartilage that are slightly movable, such as the vertebrae of the spine or the pubic bones.
Full ROM: Diarthroses are joints that have free movement. The most commonly known are ball-and-socket joints (such as the hip) and hinge joints (such as the knees). Other examples of diarthroses include the elbows, wrists, shoulders, and ankles. See Fig. 3-12 for an illustration of a knee joint that shows the bones, muscles, tendons, bursae, synovial membrane, and cavity in the knee.

Diarthroses, or **synovial joints,** as they are frequently called, are the most complex of the joints. Because these joints help a person move around for a lifetime, they are designed to efficiently cushion the jarring of the bones and to minimize friction between the surfaces of the bones. Many of the synovial joints have **bursae** (*sing.* bursa), which are sacs of fluid that are located between the bones of the joint and the tendons that hold the muscles in place. Bursae help cushion the joints when they move. Synovial joints also have joint capsules that enclose the ends of the bones, a synovial membrane that lines the joint capsules and secretes fluid to lubricate the joint, and articular cartilage that covers and protects the bone. The **menisci** (*sing.* meniscus) consist of crescent-shaped cartilage in the knee joint that additionally cushions the joint.

Upper Joints

Head Joints

temporomandibular joint	Articulation between the temporal (tempor/o) and the lower jawbone (mandibul/o).

Upper Spine Joints

occipital-cervical joint	The first joint between the base of the skull (occipit/o) and first cervical vertebra (the atlas).
cervical vertebral joint atlantoaxial joint cervical facet joint cervical vertebral joint cervical vertebral disc	One of the articulations between the seven cervical vertebrae (C1-C7). Articulation between C1 (atlant/o) and C2 (axi/o). Articulation between the adjoining facets of the vertebrae of the neck (cervic/o). Articulation between two or more of the cervical vertebrae. The cartilaginous pad between the vertebrae of the neck.
cervicothoracic vertebral joint cervicothoracic facet joint cervicothoracic vertebral disc	Articulation between the last cervical vertebra (C7) and the first thoracic (thorac/o) vertebra (T1). Articulation of the facet joints between C7 and T1. Intervertebral disk between C7 and T1.
thoracic vertebral joint (T2-7) costotransverse joint costovertebral joints thoracic facet joints thoracic vertebral joints thoracic vertebral disc	Any of the articulations between the second (T2) and seventh (T7) thoracic vertebrae. Articulation between the posterior end of the six ribs (cost/o) and T2-T7 vertebrae. Any of the articulations between the ribs (cost/o) and the thoracic vertebrae, including the floating and false ribs. Any of the articulations between the facet processes of the thoracic vertebrae. Any of the articulations between the eighth (T8) and twelfth (T12) vertebrae. The intervertebral disc between any of the thoracic vertebral joints.
thoracolumbar joint* thoracolumbar facet joints thoracolumbar disc	Articulation between the final thoracic vertebra (T12) and the first lumbar (lumb/o) vertebra (L1). Articulations between the facet processes of T12 and L1. Intervertebral disc between T12 and L1.

*This is the last of the upper joints of the spine.

Upper Extremity Joints

sternoclavicular joint	Articulation between the manubrium of the breastbone (stern/o) and the medial end of the collarbone (clavicul/o).
acromioclavicular joint	Articulation between the acromion process (acromi/o) of the scapula and the lateral end of the collarbone.
humeroulnar joint (Fig. 3-10)	Articulation between the upper arm bone (humer/o) and the lower medial arm bone (uln/o).
humeroradial joint (Fig. 3-10)	Articulation between the upper arm bone and the lower lateral arm bone (radi/o).
proximal radioulnar joint (Fig. 3-10)	Articulation between the lower arm bones nearest to the humerus.
carpal joints	Articulations between the individual carpal bones (**intercarpal joints**) and between the proximal row (scaphoid, lunate, and triquetral) and the distal row (trapezium, trapezoid, capitate, and hamate) termed the **midcarpal joint.**

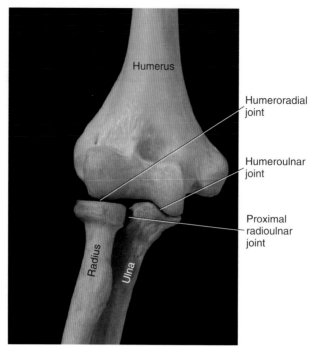

Fig. 3-10 Right elbow joints.

Upper Extremity Joints–cont'd

wrist joints	Articulations between the distal end of the lower lateral arm bone and the carpal bones **(radiocarpal joint)** and between the distal ends of both lower arm bones **(distal radioulnar joint).**
metacarpal joints	Joints between the distal row of the carpal bones and the five metacarpal bones are **metacarpocarpal/carpometacarpal joints.** The carpo-metacarpal joint of the thumb, also known as the **trapeziometacarpal joint,** connects the trapezium to the first metacarpal bone.
metacarpophalangeal joints	Articulations between the metacarpals (metacarp/o) and the proximal finger bones (phalang/o).
finger phalangeal joints	Articulations between either the far two bones **(distal interphalangeal [DIP])** or near two bones **(proximal interphalangeal [PIP]).**

Exercise 4: Upper Joints

Match the joint to its definition.

____ 1. humeroulnar joint

____ 2. cervicothoracic joint

____ 3. radioulnar joint

____ 4. interphalangeal joint

____ 5. sternoclavicular joint

____ 6. humeroradial joint

____ 7. occipital-cervical joint

____ 8. atlantoaxial joint

____ 9. costovertebral joint

____ 10. acromioclavicular joint

A. between the proximal ends of the two lower arm bones

B. between the breastbone and the collarbone

C. between the base of the skull and the first neck bone

D. between the ribs and the vertebrae

E. between a process on the scapula and the collarbone

F. between the ends of the finger bones

G. between the upper arm bone and the lower lateral arm bone

H. between the upper arm bone and the lower medial arm bone

I. between C7 and T1

J. between the first and second cervical vertebrae

Lower Joints

Lower Spine Joints

lumbar vertebral joint lumbar facet joint lumbar vertebral disc	Articulation between two lumbar (lumb/o) vertebrae. Articulation between superior and inferior lumbar facets. The cartilaginous pad between the lumbar vertebrae.
lumbosacral joint lumbosacral disc	Articulation between lumbar vertebrae and the sacrum (sacr/o). The cartilaginous pad between the fifth lumbar vertebra and the first sacral vertebra.
sacrococcygeal joint	Articulation between the sacrum and the coccyx (coccyg/o). Synonym is the coccygeal joint.
sacroiliac joint	Articulation between the sacrum and the ilium (ili/o) of the pelvic bone.

Lower Extremity Joints

hip joint	Articulation between the acetabulum of the hip and the femur.
knee joint femoropatellar joint femorotibial joint lateral meniscus medial meniscus inferior tibiofibular joint (ankle joint)	Articulations between the thighbone and the shinbone, and the thighbone and the kneecap. The articulation between the femur (femor/o) and the patella (patell/a). The articulation between the femur and the tibia (tibi/o). A crescent-shaped pad of cartilage that cushions the knee joint to the side. A crescent-shaped pad of cartilage that cushions the knee joint in the middle. Articulation between the lower end of the tibia and fibula (fibul/o).
tarsal joint calcaneocuboid joint cuboidonavicular joint cuneonavicular joint intercuneiform joint subtalar (talocalcaneal) joint talocalcaneonavicular joint	One of the many articulations between the seven tarsal bones. Articulation between the calcaneus (calcane/o) and the cuboid (cuboid/o). Articulation between the cuboid and the navicular (navicul/o). Articulation between the cuneiform (cune/o) bones and the navicular. Articulation between the three cuneiform bones. Articulation between the talus (tal/o) and the calcaneus. Articulation between the talus, calcaneus, and navicular bones.
metatarsal-tarsal joint	Articulation between a metatarsal and one of the tarsal (tars/o) bones.
metatarsal-phalangeal joint	Articulation between one of the metatarsals (metatars/o) and a proximal phalanx (phalang/o).
toe phalangeal joint (Fig. 3-11) PIP (proximal interphalangeal joint) DIP (distal interphalangeal joint)	One of the articulations between the phalanges of the toes. Articulation between the proximal and medial phalanges. Articulation between the distal and medial phalanges.

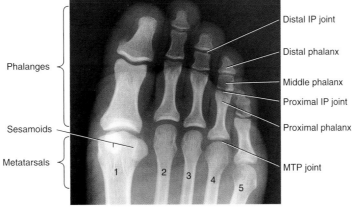

Fig. 3-11 Phalangeal joints of the toes.

Exercise 5: Lower Joints

Match the joint to its definition:

____ 1. interphalangeal joint
____ 2. hip joint
____ 3. lumbar joint
____ 4. talocalcaneal joint
____ 5. sacrococcygeal joint
____ 6. intercuneiform joint
____ 7. medial meniscus
____ 8. femoropatellar joint
____ 9. sacroiliac joint
____ 10. femorotibial joint

A. between the lower backbones
B. between the talus and heel bone
C. between the sacrum and tailbone
D. between the thighbone and the shinbone
E. cartilage on the inner edges of the knee joint
F. between the thighbone and the hip bone
G. between the wedge-shaped bones of the foot
H. between the bones of the toes
I. between the upper hip bone and the fused vertebrae of the spine
J. between the thighbone and the kneecap

ligament = ligament/o, syndesm/o

bursa = burs/o

synovial = synovi/o

Ligaments and Bursae

Ligaments are strong bands of white fibrous connective tissue that connect one bone to another at the joints.

Bursae are the sacs that appear in some synovial joints with the function of providing additional cushioning. The sacs are lined with a **synovial membrane** and filled with **synovial fluid,** a clear, viscous lubricating liquid. The term *synovial* is derived from its similar appearance to egg white.

The names of the bursae and ligaments echo the names of their associated bones and joints. If you have been working in sequence, the combining forms should help you recognize the location of many of these structures.

 ## PCS Guideline Alert

B4.3 Bilateral body part values are available for a limited number of body parts. If the identical procedure is performed on the contralateral body parts, and a bilateral body part value exists for that body part, a single procedure is coded using the bilateral body part value. If no bilateral body part value exists, code each procedure separately using the appropriate body part value.

Head and Neck Ligaments

alar ligament of axis	The winglike (al/i) ligament that connects the skull to the second cervical vertebra.
cervical interspinous ligament	The ligaments that connect the spinous processes of the cervical (cervic/o) vertebrae.
cervical intertransverse ligament	The ligaments that connect the cervical vertebrae between the transverse processes.
cervical ligamentum flavum	The yellow bandlike ligaments that connect the laminae of the vertebrae of the neck.
lateral temporomandibular ligament	The ligament that attaches the temporal (tempor/o) and mandibular (mandibul/o) bones.
sphenomandibular ligament	The ligament that attaches the sphenoid bone (sphen/o) to the mandible.
stylomandibular ligament	The ligament that connects the styloid (styl/o) process of the temporal bone to the mandible.
transverse ligament of atlas	The transverse ligament of the atlas is instrumental in holding the dens of the second cervical vertebrae against the anterior arch for the purpose of stabilizing the neck.

Shoulder Ligaments and Bursa

acromioclavicular ligament	The ligament that joins the acromion process (acromi/o) to the collarbones (clavicul/o).
coracoacromial ligament	The ligament that connects the coracoid process (corac/o) to the acromion process.
coracoclavicular ligament	The ligament that connects the coracoid process to the collarbone.
coracohumeral ligament	The ligament that joins the coracoid process with the humerus (humer/o).
glenohumeral ligament	The ligament that joins the glenoid cavity (glen/o) to the humerus.
glenoid ligament (labrum)	The ligament within the glenoid cavity. Also termed the **glenoid labrum.**
interclavicular ligament	The ligament between the collarbones.
sternoclavicular ligament	The ligament joining the sternum (stern/o) to the clavicles.
subacromial bursa	The subacromial bursa is located between the head of the humerus and under (sub-) the acromion process.
transverse humeral ligament	The transverse humeral ligament is between the greater and lesser tubercles (tuberosities) of the humerus.

Elbow Ligaments and Bursa

annular ligament	The annular ligament is a ringlike structure that encircles the head of the radius.
olecranon bursa	The olecranon bursa cushions the elbow joint.
radial collateral ligament	The radial collateral ligament connects the humerus to the radius.
ulnar collateral ligament (UCL)	The ulnar collateral ligament has an anterior and posterior portion, both connecting the humerus to the ulna.

Wrist Ligaments

palmar ulnocarpal ligament	Connects the ulnar (uln/o) styloid process to carpal (carp/o) (the lunate, capitate, and triquetral) bones.
radial collateral carpal ligament	Connects the styloid process of the radius to the wrist bones.
radiocarpal ligament	Connects the radius (radi/o) to the wrist bones. Also termed the **volar radiocarpal.** Volar means pertaining to the palm of the hand or the sole of the foot.
radioulnar ligament	Connects the radius and the ulna.
ulnar collateral carpal ligament	Connects the ulna to the wrist bones.

Hand Ligaments

carpometacarpal ligament	Connects the wrist bones to the metacarpals (metacarp/o).
intercarpal ligament	Connects the carpal bones.
interphalangeal ligament	Connects the bones of the fingers (phalang/o) to each other.
lunotriquetral ligament	Connects the lunate and the triquetral bones.
metacarpal ligament	Connects the metacarpals.
metacarpophalangeal ligament	Connects the metacarpals to the phalanges.
pisohamate ligament	Connects the pisiform and hamate bones.
pisometacarpal ligament	Connects the pisiform and metacarpal bones.
scapholunate ligament	Connects the scaphoid (scaphoid/o) to the lunate bone.
scaphotrapezium ligament	Connects the scaphoid to the trapezium.

Trunk Ligaments

iliolumbar ligament	Connects the ilium (ili/o) to the lumbar (lumb/o) vertebrae.
interspinous ligament	Connects the spinous processes of the vertebrae.
intertransverse ligament	Connects the transverse processes to each other.
ligamentum flavum	Broad yellow ligament that connects the laminae of the vertebrae.
pubic ligament	Connects the pubic bones.
sacrococcygeal ligament	Connects the sacrum (sacr/o) and the coccyx (coccyg/o).
sacroiliac ligament	Connects the sacrum (sacr/o) to the ilium.
sacrospinous ligament	Connects the sacrum (sacr/o) to the spinous processes of the ischial spine.
sacrotuberous ligament	Connects the sacrum (sacr/o) to the tuberosity of the ischium.
supraspinous ligament	Connects the tops (supra-) of the spinous processes.

Thorax Ligaments

costotransverse ligament	Connects the back of the neck of a rib (cost/o) to the adjacent transverse process of the corresponding vertebra.
costoxiphoid ligament	Connects the ribs (cost/o) and the xiphoid process of the sternum.
sternocostal ligament	Connects the sternum (stern/o) and the ribs.

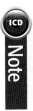

ICD Note Although most ligaments connect bones around a joint, some ligaments are not the expected fibrous bands of connective tissue. Instead, they are folds of peritoneal tissue (the lining of the abdominopelvic cavity) that hold the abdominopelvic cavity viscera (organs) in place. These are not considered organs of the musculoskeletal system, but are referenced in the digestive and urogenital systems.

Hip Ligaments and Bursa

iliofemoral ligament	Connects the ilium and the femur (femor/o).
ischiofemoral ligament	Connects the ischium (ischi/o) and the femur.
pubofemoral ligament	Connects the pubis (pub/o) and the femur.
transverse acetabular ligament	Ligament that is part of the acetabular labrum and serves to keep the femoral head in place.
trochanteric bursa	Cushions the hip joint.

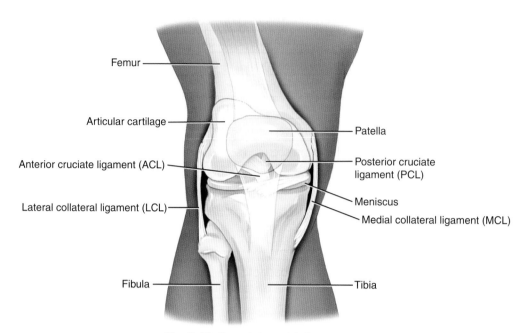

Fig. 3-12 Knee joint with ligaments.

Knee Ligaments and Bursa (Fig. 3-12)

anterior cruciate ligament (ACL)	Connects the femur and tibia by crossing the front of the knee.
lateral collateral ligament (LCL)	Connects the femur and fibula on the outer (lateral) side of the knee.
ligament of head of fibula	Connects the fibula to the tibia over the patella (patell/a).
medial collateral ligament (MCL)	Connects the femur and tibia at the inner (medial) part of the knee.
patellar ligament	Connects the kneecap to the tibia.
popliteal ligament	Connects the femur to the tibia in the back of the knee.
posterior cruciate ligament (PCL)	Connects the femur to the tibia by crossing in the back of the knee.
prepatellar bursa	Largest bursa in knee joint. Cushions the knee in front (pre-) of the patellar ligament.

Ankle Ligaments

calcaneofibular ligament	Connects the heel bone (calcane/o) and the fibula (fibul/o).
deltoid ligament	Triangular-shaped ligament that connects the medial malleolus of the tibia to the navicular, calcaneus, and talus bones.
ligament of the lateral malleolus	Connects the lateral malleolus of the fibula to the bones of the foot. May be the calcaneofibular ligament, or the anterior or posterior talofibular ligaments.
talofibular ligament	Connects the talus (tal/o) to the fibula with anterior and posterior segments.

Foot Ligaments

calcaneocuboid ligament	Connects the heel bone to the cuboid bone.
cuneonavicular ligament	Connects the cuneiform (cune/o) bones to the navicular bone.
intercuneiform ligament	Connects the cuneiform bones to each other.
interphalangeal ligament	Connects the phalanges to each other.
metatarsal ligament	Connects the metatarsals to each other.
metatarsophalangeal ligament	Connects the metatarsals (metatars/o) to the phalanges.
subtalar ligament	Connects the talus to the calcaneus.
talocalcaneonavicular ligament	Connects the talus to the heel bone and the navicular (navicul/o) bone.
tarsometatarsal ligament	Connects the tarsals (tars/o) to the metatarsals.

Exercise 6: Ligaments and Bursae

Match the ligaments and bursae to their definitions.

_____ 1. costoxiphoid ligament
_____ 2. ischiofemoral ligament
_____ 3. talocalcaneonavicular ligament
_____ 4. popliteal ligament
_____ 5. acromioclavicular
_____ 6. coracohumeral ligament
_____ 7. olecranon bursa
_____ 8. carpometacarpal ligament
_____ 9. trochanteric bursa
_____ 10. temporomandibular ligament
_____ 11. interphalangeal ligament
_____ 12. iliolumbar ligament
_____ 13. prepatellar bursa
_____ 14. subtalar ligament
_____ 15. glenohumeral ligament

A. cushions the elbow joint
B. joins the coracoid process with the humerus
C. connects the ischium and the femur
D. attaches the temporal and lower jawbones
E. connects the bones of the fingers to each other
F. connects the ilium to the lower back vertebrae
G. connects the ribs and the xiphoid process of the sternum
H. cushions the hip joint
 I. connects the talus to the heel bone and navicular bone
J. joins the glenoid cavity to the upper arm
K. cushions the knee in front of the patellar ligament
L. connects the talus to the calcaneus
M. connects the femur to the tibia in the back of the knee
N. connects the wrist bones to the metacarpals.
O. joins the acromion process to the collarbones

Muscles

Muscle is a tissue that is composed of cells with the ability to contract and relax. Because of those two specialized actions, the body is able to move. The muscles in the human body are further specialized into three different functions:
- **Skeletal muscle** that allows the skeleton to move voluntarily
- **Smooth muscle** that is responsible for involuntary movement of the organs
- **Heart muscle** that pumps blood to the circulatory system.

Fig. 3-13 shows posterior and anterior views of the major skeletal muscles of the body. ICD-10-PCS requires knowledge of all of the muscles and knowledge of where they are in the body. The muscles will be presented with their locations and word part meanings, as well as grouped as they are in the classification.

muscle = muscul/o, my/o, myos/o

skeletal muscle = rhabdomy/o

smooth muscle = leiomy/o

heart muscle = myocardi/o

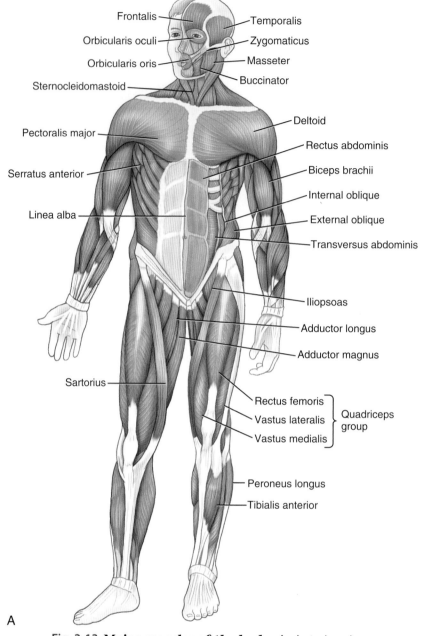

Fig. 3-13 **Major muscles of the body. A,** Anterior view.

tendon = tendin/o, ten/o, tend/o

Muscles are attached to bones by strong fibrous bands of connective tissue called **tendons.** The bone that is at the end of the attachment that does not move and is also nearest to the trunk is called the **origin (O);** the bone that is at the end that does move and is farthest from the trunk is termed the **insertion (I).** The function of a muscle is its **action (A).** For example, to close your mouth (A), you would need to use the masseter muscle, which has its origin in the maxilla (upper jaw) and its insertion in the mandible (lower jaw). Note that the upper jaw does not move, but the lower jaw does, raising that bone upward. Tables and illustrations of the variety of muscle actions are included to familiarize you with the terms and types of movements you will encounter in your work.

Muscles can be categorized into three main types: **prime mover muscles, synergistic muscles,** and **antagonist muscles.** The prime movers (also

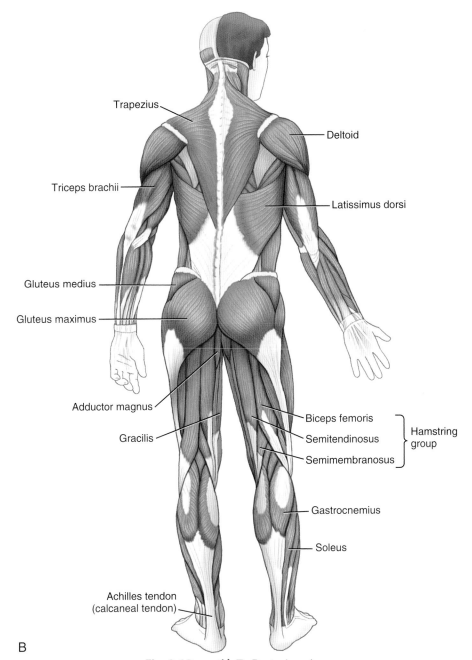

Fig. 3-13 cont'd B, Posterior view.

B

called **agonist muscles**) are those that are responsible for the main muscle movement. **Synergist muscles** (*syn-* meaning "together" and *erg/o* meaning "work") assist in carrying out the main movement or "work" of the muscle by either stabilizing a joint or helping the actual movement to happen. **Antagonist muscles** have an opposite function to the prime mover. A good example is again the biceps brachii. When it flexes (contracts) and functions as a prime mover, several other muscles (pectoral, deltoid, latissimus dorsi) assist in their role as synergist muscles. The triceps brachii on the back of the arm extends and acts as an antagonist.

  Fascia is a structure of connective tissue that surrounds muscles, groups of muscles, blood vessels, and nerves, binding some structures together while permitting others to slide smoothly over each other. Fascia is composed of dense connective tissue that contains closely packed bundles of fibers oriented in a wavy pattern parallel to the direction of pull.

Muscle Actions

	Action	Word Origin	Description
	extension	*ex-* out *tens/o* stretching *-ion* process of	Process of stretching out; increasing the angle of a joint.
	flexion	*flex/o* bending *-ion* process of	Process of decreasing the angle of a joint.
	abduction	*ab-* away from *duct/o* carrying *-ion* process of	Process of carrying away from the midline.
	adduction	*ad-* toward *duct/o* carrying *-ion* process of	Process of carrying toward the midline.
	supination		Turning the palm or medial side of the foot upward.
	pronation		Turning the palm or medial edge of foot downward.
	dorsiflexion	*dors/i* back *flex/o* bending *-ion* process of	Process of bending back.
	plantar flexion	*plant/o* sole *-ar* pertaining to *flex/o* bending *-ion* process of	Lowering the foot; pointing the toes away from the shin.

Continued

Muscle Actions—cont'd

	Action	Word Origin	Description
	eversion	*e-* out *vers/o* turning *-ion* process of	Process of turning out.
	inversion	*in-* in *vers/o* turning *-ion* process of	Process of turning in.
	protraction	*pro-* forward *tract/o* pulling *-ion* process of	Process of pulling forward; the forward movement of a muscle.
	retraction	*re-* backward *tract/o* pulling *-ion* process of	Process of backward pulling; the backward movement of a muscle.
	rotation	*rot/o* wheel *-ation* process of	Process of a bone turning on its axis (like a wheel).
	circumduction	*circum-* around *duct/o* carrying *-ion* process of	Process of carrying around; the circular movement of the distal end of a limb around its point of attachment.

Exercise 7: Muscle Actions

Match the muscle action with the correct definition.

____	1. plantar flexion	A. process of turning in
____	2. circumduction	B. process of bending
____	3. pronation	C. process of bone turning on its axis
____	4. inversion	D. process of bending back
____	5. adduction	E. process of pulling backward
____	6. extension	F. turning the palm downward
____	7. protraction	G. process of carrying away from (the midline)
____	8. rotation	H. turning the palm upward
____	9. supination	I. process of turning out
____	10. eversion	J. process of pulling forward
____	11. dorsiflexion	K. process of stretching out
____	12. abduction	L. process of carrying around
____	13. flexion	M. process of carrying toward (the midline)
____	14. retraction	N. lowering the foot

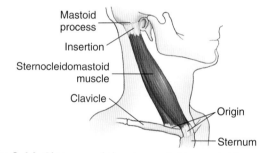

Fig. 3-14 Close-up of the sternocleidomastoid muscle.

sternocleidomastoid
  stern/o = sternum
  cleid/o = clavicle
  mastoid/o = mastoid

Muscle Naming Conventions

There are some general muscle naming conventions that will help you. Refer to the table below for examples of how muscles are named by their location, number of insertions, size, shape, and muscle action. The final type of naming convention that appears in the table is by its origins and insertion. For example, the sternocleidomastoid muscle (Fig. 3-14) originates in the sternum and collarbone and inserts on the mastoid process.

Muscle Naming Conventions

Naming Device	Name of Muscle	Word Origin	Definition
location	zygomaticus	*zygomatic/o* zygoma *-us* noun ending	Cheek muscle.
number of insertions	biceps brachii	*bi-* two ***ceps** heads *brachi/o* arm *-i* noun ending	Muscle that flexes upper arm.
size	gluteus maximus	*glute/o* buttock *-us* noun ending *maxim/o* large *-us* noun ending	Large buttock muscle.
shape	deltoid	*delt/o* triangle *-oid* like	Triangular muscle in shoulder.
muscle action	adductor longus	*ad-* toward *duct/o* carrying *-or* one who *long/o* long *-us* noun ending	Upper leg muscle that carries the leg back to the midline.
origin/insertion	sternocleidomastoid	*stern/o* breastbone *cleid/o* collarbone *mastoid/o* mastoid process	Muscle that originates in the sternum and collarbone and inserts on the mastoid process (see Fig. 3-14).

ceps* is a variation of **cephal/o, the combining form for head. These word parts are used for "the head" or the beginning of a structure and also are used for bones (bone heads), as well as muscle heads.

Additionally, the naming themes use synonyms and antonyms. Here are some shortcut opposites with their meanings:
- Brevis is short and longus is long.
- Minimus is small and maximus, magnus, and vastus are large.
- Lateralis is to the side and medialis is to the middle.
- Adductors pull *toward* the midline, whereas abductors pull *away* from the midline.
- Extensors straighten out, whereas flexors bend.
- Levators raise, whereas depressors lower.

Head Muscles

auricularis muscle	Moves the ears (auricul/o).
masseter muscle	Closes the jaw.
pterygoid muscle	Winglike muscle that raises, lowers, and allows side-to-side movement of the mandible.
splenius capitis muscle	Bandlike muscle that holds the head upright; located in back of neck.
temporalis muscle	Raises the lower jaw.
temporoparietalis muscle	Paired scalp muscles over the temporal and parietal regions.

Head Muscles—cont'd

facial muscles	A group of muscles of the face.
buccinator muscles	Cheek (bucc/o) muscles; compress cheek against teeth.
corrugator supercilii muscle	Wrinkles forehead (above eyelids). Cili/o refers to the small hairs in the eyelids, or eyelashes. The term *supercilious*, meaning "haughty," is derived from one arching his/her eyebrows disdainfully. Corrug/o means "wrinkled," as in corrugated cardboard.
depressor anguli oris muscle	Lowers corners of mouth (or/o).
depressor labii inferioris muscle	Lowers lower lip (labi/o).
depressor septi nasi muscle	Lowers wall in nose (nas/o).
depressor supercilii muscle	Lowers eyebrows.
levator anguli oris muscle	Raises corners of mouth.
levator labii superioris alaeque nasi muscle	Raises upper lip and nostrils (wings) of nose.
levator labii superioris muscle	Raises upper lip.
mentalis muscle	Wrinkles chin (ment/o), protrudes lower lip.
nasalis muscle	Raises corners of nostrils.
occipitofrontalis muscle	Also called **epicranius muscle** for its location on top of the skull. Composed of two muscles that are joined by a broad, flat tendon, the galea aponeurotica.
orbicularis oris muscle	Encircles mouth and serves to pucker lips. The "kissing" muscle.
procerus muscle	Draws eyebrows together and down (as in frowning).
risorius muscle	Pulls the angles of the mouth backward. The "smiling" muscle.
zygomaticus muscle	Raises angle of mouth up and to the side.

Neck Muscles

anterior vertebral muscle	Group of muscles (longi colli and capitis, recti capitis anterior and lateralis) located in the front of the backbones that help the head and neck bend. Note that coll/o means "neck," as in the word collar.
arytenoid muscle	Moves vocal cords together (adduction).
cricothyroid muscle	Lengthens and tenses vocal cords.
infrahyoid muscle	A group of four muscles (omohyoid, thyrohyoid, sternohyoid, and sternothyroid) under the hyoid bone that move the hyoid and larynx downward while speaking. The thyr/o reference is due to the proximity of these muscles to the thyroid gland.
levator scapulae muscle	Raises the shoulder blades.
platysma muscle	Broad, flat muscle that tenses the lower face and neck.
scalene muscle	Raises the ribs and flexes the neck.
splenius cervicis muscle	Bandlike muscle that bends and extends the neck.
sternocleidomastoid muscle	Rotates and tilts head to opposite side.
suprahyoid muscle	Group of muscles (geniohyoid, mylohyoid, digastric and stylohyoid) that raise the tongue and widen the esophagus.
thyroarytenoid muscle	Thickens the vocal cords.

Tongue, Palate, and Pharynx Muscles

chondroglossus muscle	Lowers the tongue (gloss/o).
genioglossus muscle	Lowers and protrudes the tongue.
hypoglossus muscle	Lowers and pulls tongue backward.
inferior longitudinal muscle	Located under and extending the length of the tongue; changes shape of tongue for chewing and swallowing.
levator veli palatini muscle	Raises the soft palate while swallowing.
palatoglossal muscle	Raises tongue.
palatopharyngeal muscle	Aids in swallowing.
pharyngeal constrictor muscle	Narrows throat (pharyng/o) for swallowing.
salpingopharyngeus muscle	Raises nasopharynx (part of the throat behind nasal cavity).
styloglossus muscle	Raises and retracts tongue for swallowing.
stylopharyngeus muscle	Raises voice box and nasopharynx; used in swallowing.
superior longitudinal muscle	Located on dorsum of tongue; changes shape of tongue for chewing and swallowing.
tensor veli palatini muscle	Controls tension of the soft palate.

Shoulder Muscles

deltoid muscle	Triangular muscle that flexes, abducts, and extends the arm.
infraspinatus muscle	Laterally rotates arm. Named for its origin in the infraspinous fossa of the scapula.
subscapularis muscle	Adducts and medially rotates arm. Located under the scapula.
supraspinatus muscle	Assists deltoid at the shoulder. Named for its origin in the supraspinous fossa of the scapula.
teres major muscle	Large round muscle that extends arm and medially rotates shoulder.
teres minor muscle	Smaller round muscle that laterally rotates arm.

The rotator cuff is composed of the infraspinatus, the subscapularis, the supraspinatus, and the teres minor muscles.

Medial rotation is also called **internal rotation.** Lateral rotation is also called **external rotation.**

Upper Arm Muscles

biceps brachii muscle	"Two-headed" arm (brachi/o) muscle that flexes and supinates forearm at elbow.
brachialis muscle	Flexes forearm at elbow.
coracobrachialis muscle	Flexes and medially rotates arm at shoulder.
triceps brachii muscle	"Three-headed" muscle that extends forearm at elbow.

Lower Arm Muscles

anatomical snuffbox	Also called the **radial fossa,** this is a triangular depression on the radial side of the back of the hand. Named for its sometime use in earlier times as a place to put powdered tobacco for sniffing.
brachioradialis muscle	Flexes forearm at elbow.
extensor carpi radialis muscle	Extends and abducts hand at the wrist.
extensor carpi ulnaris muscle	Extends and adducts hand at the wrist.
flexor carpi radialis muscle	Flexes and abducts hand at the wrist.
flexor carpi ulnaris muscle	Flexes and adducts hand at the wrist.
palmaris longus muscle	Flexes wrist.
pronator quadratus muscle	Pronates forearm. Named for its four sides (two insertions and two origins).
pronator teres muscle	Round muscle that pronates forearm and flexes the elbow.

Hand Muscles

hypothenar eminence	Group of muscles (abductor, adductor, and opponens digiti minimi) that move the little finger.
palmar interosseous muscle	Also called the **interossei volares,** with *volar* meaning "pertaining to the palm of the hand or sole of the foot." Located between the bones of the palm of the hand, these serve to flex the fingers at the metacarpophalangeal joints and extend the interphalangeal joints.
thenar muscle	Group of muscles (abductor, flexor, and opponens pollicis brevis, with pollic/o referring to the pollex, the thumb) that move the thumb.

Trunk Muscles

coccygeus muscle	Pulls the tailbone forward ("tucking the tail") and supports the organs of the pelvis.
erector spinae muscle	Extends and bends the spine and head to the side.
interspinalis muscle	Extends the spine. Located between the spinous processes of the backbones.
intertransversarius muscle	Located between the transverse processes of the backbones, this muscle serves to flex the trunk sideways.
latissimus dorsi muscle	Adducts, extends, and medially rotates the humerus.
levator ani muscle	Helps to raise the pelvic floor around the anus.
quadratus lumborum muscle	Extends and flexes the vertebral column to the side. Named for its insertion on four of the lumbar vertebrae.
rhomboid major muscle	Pulls the shoulder blade back and rotates to lower the glenoid cavity.
rhomboid minor muscle	A smaller version of rhomboid major, rhomboid minor also pulls the shoulder blade back and rotates to lower the glenoid cavity.

Continued

Trunk Muscles—cont'd

serratus posterior muscle	A notched appearance in the back of the body, these muscles raise the ribs.
transversospinalis muscle	Located between the transverse and spinous processes of the backbones, they act as rotators of the spine.
trapezius muscle	A broad, table-like muscle, this one raises, rotates, and pulls the shoulder blades backward.

Thorax Muscles

intercostal muscle	Located between (inter-) the ribs (cost/o), they assist in inhalation.
levatores costarum muscle	12 small muscles that attach the ribs to the backbones; help to raise the ribs in respiration.
pectoralis major muscle	Large chest (pector/o) muscle that flexes, adducts, and medially rotates the arm at the shoulder.
pectoralis minor muscle	Smaller chest muscle that raises and lowers the shoulder blades.
serratus anterior muscle	Notched muscle in the front of the body that rotates the shoulder blades upward.
subclavius muscle	Muscle located under (sub-) the collarbone (clav/o) that pulls it downward.
subcostal muscle	Muscles that pull the ribs (cost/o) down (sub-) in respiration.
transverse thoracis muscle	Chest muscles that pull the ribs and costal cartilage downward. Named for their location crossing the chest from the breastbone to the ribs.

Abdomen Muscles

external oblique muscle	The outer diagonal muscles that flex and rotate the torso.
internal oblique muscle	The inner diagonal muscles that support and compress the abdomen as well as rotate the vertebral column.
pyramidalis muscle	Tenses the linea alba, the "white line" that is a tendon located in the midline of the abdominal muscles.
rectus abdominis muscle	Straight abdominal muscles that compress the internal abdominal organs and flex the trunk.
transverse abdominis muscle	Crosswise abdominal muscles that compress and support internal abdominal organs.

Perineum Muscles

bulbospongiosus muscle	Contracts the vagina in females and empties the urethra in males.
cremaster muscle	Raises and lowers the scrotum in males.
deep transverse perineal muscle	Provides support for the perineum.
ischiocavernosus muscle	Assists the bulbospongiosus muscle.
superficial transverse perineal muscle	Helps resist increased intrapelvic pressure.

Hip Muscles

gemellus muscle	The two forms, superior and inferior, of this muscle laterally rotate and extend the thigh from the hip. Also allows for abduction of the flexed thigh at the hip. Its name is derived from its Latin meaning of "little twin."
gluteus maximus muscle	Extends the thigh at the hip and rotates the thigh laterally. Glute/o is the combining form for buttocks.
gluteus medius muscle	Abducts and medially rotates the thigh at the hip.
gluteus minimus muscle	Abducts and medially rotates the thigh at the hip.
iliacus muscle	Flexes hips and stabilizes the hip joint. Named for its attachment to the ilium.
obturator muscles	Rotate and abduct the thigh. Named for their location in the obturator foramen.
piriformis muscle	Pear-shaped muscle that rotates the thigh.
psoas muscle	One of two muscles (major and minor) that flex the hip, trunk, and vertebral column. *Psoa* means "loin."
quadratus femoris muscle	Rotates the thigh laterally at the hip.
tensor fasciae latae muscle	Tensors are muscles that tighten a structure; fasciae is the plural form of the bandlike covering of muscles, and latae is the plural form meaning "broad." These muscles abduct, medially rotate, and flex the thigh at the hip.

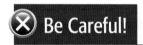 **Be Careful!** The pisiform bone is in the wrist, while the piriformis muscle is in the hip.

Upper Leg Muscles

adductor brevis muscle	This is the shorter muscle that carries the thigh toward the midline.
adductor longus muscle	This is the longer muscle that carries the thigh toward the midline and also rotates the thigh medially at the hip.
adductor magnus muscle	Large muscle that adducts the thigh at the hip.
biceps femoris muscle	"Two-headed" muscle that flexes the leg at the knee, rotates it laterally, and extends the thigh at the hip. One of the three "hamstrings," muscles in the back of the thigh.
gracilis muscle	Slender muscle that adducts the thigh at the hip.
pectineus muscle	Adducts and flexes the thigh at the hip.
quadriceps muscle	Also called the **quadriceps,** this is a "four-headed" group of thigh muscles. The muscles are the three vastus muscles (intermediate, lateral, and medial) and the rectus muscle. They extend the lower leg at the knee joint.
rectus femoris muscle	Straight muscle in the thigh. One of the muscles in the quadriceps.
sartorius muscle	*Sartorius* refers to a tailor in the sense that this is the muscle extended when one sits in a cross-legged position.
semimembranosus muscle	Extends thigh at hip. Flexes and rotates leg medially. One of the three "hamstrings," muscles in the back of the thigh.
semitendinosus muscle	Extends thigh at hip. Flexes and medially rotates leg at knee. One of the three "hamstrings," muscles in the back of the thigh.
vastus intermedius muscle	One of the quadriceps. Extends the lower leg at the knee.
vastus lateralis muscle	One of the quadriceps. Extends the lower leg at the knee.
vastus medialis muscle	One of the quadriceps. Extends the lower leg at the knee.

Lower Leg Muscles

extensor digitorum longus muscle	Extends lateral four digits and dorsiflexes the foot at the ankle.
extensor hallucis longus muscle	Extends the great toe and dorsiflexes the foot at the ankle.
fibularis brevis muscle	Everts the foot.
fibularis longus muscle	Everts the foot.
flexor digitorum longus muscle	Flexes the lateral four digits and plantar flexes the foot at the ankle.
flexor hallucis longus muscle	Flexes the great toe and plantar flexes the foot at the ankle.
gastrocnemius muscle	Plantar flexes the foot at the ankle, raises the heel during walking, and flexes the leg at the knee joint.
peroneus brevis muscle	Same as fibularis brevis (perone/o = fibula).
peroneus longus muscle	Same as the fibularis longus.
popliteus muscle	Flexes the leg at the knee. Named for its location in the space behind the knee.
soleus muscle	Plantar flexes the foot at the ankle. (*Soleus* is named for the shape of the fish of the same name and is another muscle of the calf of the leg.)
tibialis anterior muscle	Muscle in the front of the shinbone that dorsiflexes the foot at the ankle and inverts the foot. If you need to remember that it inverts the foot, remember that the tibia is the inner of the two lower leg bones.
tibialis posterior muscle	Muscle in the back of the shinbone that plantar flexes the foot at the ankle and inverts the foot.

Foot Muscles

abductor hallucis muscle	Abducts and flexes the great toe (halluc/o).
adductor hallucis muscle	Adducts the great toe.
extensor digitorum brevis muscle	Extends the lateral digits (2-4). Located on the upper surface of the foot.
extensor hallucis brevis muscle	Flexes the proximal phalanx of the great toe.
flexor digitorum brevis muscle	Flexes the lateral four digits and their interphalangeal joints.
flexor hallucis brevis muscle	The short great toe muscle that allows it to bend.
quadratus plantae muscle	The four (quadra-) muscles on the sole of the foot (plant/o) that assist in flexing the lateral four digits.

Exercise 8: **Muscles**

Match the muscle to its definition.

____ 1. mentalis	A. draws eyebrows together
____ 2. risorius	B. flexes forearm at elbow
____ 3. procerus	C. raises tongue
____ 4. palatoglossal	D. assist in inhalation
____ 5. deltoid	E. wrinkles chin, protrudes lower lip
____ 6. brachialis	F. helps raise pelvic floor around the anus
____ 7. pronator teres	G. rotates the thigh
____ 8. levator ani	H. "the smiling muscle"
____ 9. intercostals	I. pronates forearm and flexes elbow
____ 10. piriformis	J. flexes, abducts, and extends arm

Match the muscle to its definition.

____ 11. quadriceps	K. slender muscle that adducts the thigh at the hip
____ 12. gracilis	L. flexes wrist
____ 13. soleus	M. large round muscle that extends arm and medially rotates shoulder
____ 14. interspinalis	N. plantar flexes the foot at the ankle
____ 15. adductor hallucis	O. closes the jaw
____ 16. masseter	P. raises the ribs and flexes the neck
____ 17. scalene	Q. group of four muscles that extend the lower leg at the knee
____ 18. teres major	R. raises, rotates, and pulls shoulder blades backward
____ 19. palmaris longus	S. adducts the great toe
____ 20. trapezius	T. extends the spine

To practice labeling some of the major muscles, click on **Label It.**

Tendons

Tendons are strong bands of fibrous connective tissue that connect muscles to bone. Because this type of tissue has a poor blood supply, it is slow to heal when injured.

A strong, broad, flat sheet of fibrous connective tissue that serves as a tendon is called an **aponeurosis.** Aponeuroses often merge with other tendons to attach muscles to bone. Tendon sheaths have a characteristic membranous lining and are the covering of certain tendons. **Fascia** is the tough outer covering of both the muscles and the tendons.

Tendons are categorized in ICD-10-CM as either upper body or lower body, meaning above or below the diaphragm. The only two specific tendons listed are the patellar tendon of the knee and the **Achilles tendon,** also called the **calcaneal tendon** in the lower leg.

Achilles tendon =
achill/o

Combining Forms for the Anatomy of the Musculoskeletal System

Meaning	Combining Form	Meaning	Combining Form
acromion	acromi/o	metatarsus (foot bone)	metatars/o
bone marrow	myel/o	muscle (heart)	myocardi/o, cardiomy/o
bone	oste/o, osse/o, oss/i	muscle (smooth)	leiomy/o
bursa	burs/o	muscle (skeletal)	rhabdomy/o
calcaneus (heel bone)	calcane/o	muscle	my/o, myos/o, muscul/o
carpus (wrist)	carp/o	neck	cervic/o
cartilage	chondr/o, cartilag/o	occiput	occipit/o
chin	ment/o, geni/o	olecranon	olecran/o
clavicle (collarbone)	clavicul/o, cleid/o	palatine bone	palat/o
coccyx (tailbone)	coccyg/o	parietal bone	pariet/o
condyle	condyl/o	patella (kneecap)	patell/o, patell/a
elbow (olecranon)	olecran/o	pelvis	pelv/i, pelv/o
epicondyle	epicondyl/o	phalanx (one of the bones of the fingers or toes)	phalang/o
ethmoid	ethmoid/o		
femur (thighbone)	femor/o		
fibula (lower lateral leg bone)	fibul/o, perone/o	pubis (pubic bone)	pub/o
		radius (lower lateral arm bone)	radi/o
finger, toe (whole), digitus	dactyl/o, digit/o	rib (costa)	cost/o
foramen	foramin/o	sacrum	sacr/o
frontal bone	front/o	scapula (shoulder blade)	scapul/o
glenoid	glen/o		
hallux	halluc/o	sinus	sin/o, sinus/o, antr/o
humerus (upper arm bone)	humer/o	skeleton	skelet/o
		skull (cranium)	crani/o
ilium	ili/o	sphenoid	sphenoid/o
ischium	ischi/o	spinal column, spine	spin/o, rachi/o, vertebr/o
jaw (entire)	gnath/o	sternum, breastbone	stern/o
joint (articulation)	arthr/o, articul/o	tarsus (anklebone)	tars/o
lacrima	lacrim/o	temporal bone	tempor/o
lamina	lamin/o	tendon	tendin/o, tendon/o, ten/o, tend/o
ligament	ligament/o, syndesm/o		
lower back	lumb/o	thorax (chest)	thorac/o
mandible (lower jawbone)	mandibul/o	tibia (shinbone)	tibi/o
		ulna	uln/o
maxilla (upper jawbone)	maxill/o	vertebra (backbone)	vertebr/o, spondyl/o
		vomer	vomer/o
meniscus	menisc/o	xiphoid process	xiph/o
metacarpus (hand bone)	metacarp/o	zygoma (cheekbone)	zygomat/o

Prefixes for the Anatomy of the Musculoskeletal System

Prefix	Meaning	Prefix	Meaning
ab-	away from	ex-, e-	out
ad-	toward	in-	in
amphi-	both	inter-	between
bi-	two	intra-	within
circum-	around	peri-	surrounding, around
dia-	through, complete	pro-	forward
endo-, end-	within	re-	back
epi-	above, upon	syn-	together, joined

Suffixes for the Anatomy of the Musculoskeletal System

Suffix	Meaning	Suffix	Meaning
-ar, -al, -ic, -ous, -eal	pertaining to	-physis	growth
		-poiesis	formation
-blast	embryonic	-sis	condition
-clast	breaking down	-um	structure
-cyte	cell		
-genesis	production, origin		
-oid	resembling, like		

You can review the anatomy of the musculoskeletal system by clicking on **Body Spectrum,** then **Muscular** and **Skeletal.**

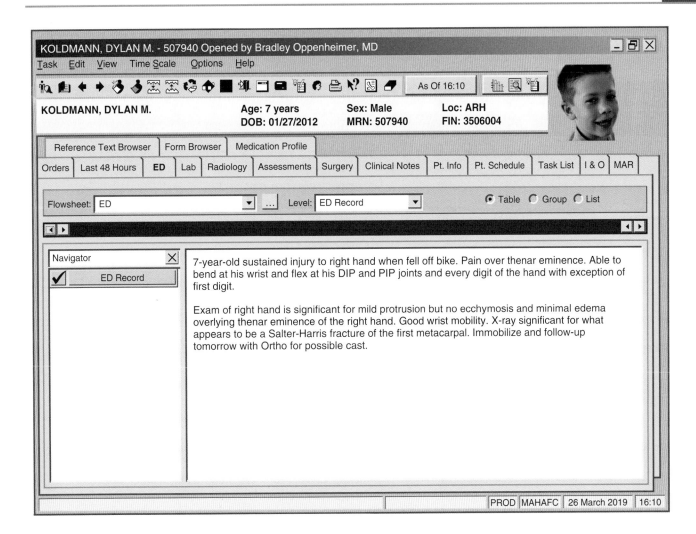

Within the ED Record screen:

7-year-old sustained injury to right hand when fell off bike. Pain over thenar eminence. Able to bend at his wrist and flex at his DIP and PIP joints and every digit of the hand with exception of first digit.

Exam of right hand is significant for mild protrusion but no ecchymosis and minimal edema overlying thenar eminence of the right hand. Good wrist mobility. X-ray significant for what appears to be a Salter-Harris fracture of the first metacarpal. Immobilize and follow-up tomorrow with Ortho for possible cast.

 Exercise 9: **Emergency Room Report**

Use the emergency room record above to answer the following questions.

1. Dylan's injury is to the fleshy area of the palm near the thumb, the "thenar eminence." Explain the difference between a DIP (distal interphalangeal joint) and a PIP (proximal interphalangeal) joint.

_____

2. Not being able to "flex" a body part means one is unable to _____.

3. "First digit, R hand" means _____.

4. The first metacarpal is a bone of the _____.

PATHOLOGY

Terms Related to Arthropathies (MØØ-M25) and Dentofacial Anomalies (M26-M27)

Term	Word Origin	Definition
arthrosis	*arthr/o* joint *-osis* abnormal condition	Abnormal condition of a joint; may be hemarthrosis, hydrarthrosis, or pyarthrosis (blood, fluid, or pus, respectively, in a joint cavity).
bunion	*bunion/o* bunion	Fairly common painful enlargement and inflammation of the first metatarsophalangeal joint (the base of the great toe). Also called **hallux valgus.**
contracture	*con-* together *tract/o* pulling *-ure* condition	Chronic fixation of a joint in flexion (such as a finger) caused by atrophy and shortening of muscle fibers after a long period of disuse.
crepitus	*crepit/o* crackling *-us* thing	Crackling sound heard in joints.
gout		Type of arthritis due to excessive uric acid that causes crystals to form. The joints then become swollen and inflamed.
osteoarthritis (OA)	*oste/o* bone *arthr/o* joint *-itis* inflammation	Joint disease characterized by degenerative articular cartilage and a wearing down of the bones' edges at a joint; considered a "wear and tear" disorder. Also called **degenerative joint disease** (DJD) (Fig. 3-15).
osteophytosis	*oste/o* bone *phyt/o* growth, nature *-osis* abnormal condition	Abnormal bone growth in a joint. Bouchard nodes are osteophytes of the proximal interphalangeal joints in rheumatoid arthritis (Fig. 3-16).

Continued

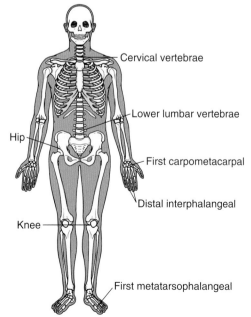

Cervical vertebrae

Lower lumbar vertebrae

Hip

First carpometacarpal

Distal interphalangeal

Knee

First metatarsophalangeal

Fig. 3-15 Joints most frequently involved in osteoarthritis.

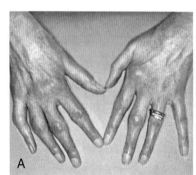
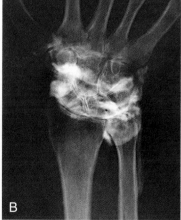

Fig. 3-16 **A,** Bouchard nodes seen in rheumatoid arthritis of the hands. Moderate involvement. **B,** Arthrogram of wrist showing RA and resultant osteophytosis.

Terms Related to Arthropathies (MØØ-M25) and Dentofacial Anomalies (M26-M27)—cont'd

Term	Word Origin	Definition
rheumatoid arthritis (RA)	*rheumat/o* watery flow *-oid* resembling, like *arthr/o* joint *-itis* inflammation	Chronic inflammatory joint disease affecting the lining of the joints that is thought to be autoimmune in nature. Usually occurs after age 40 and is more common in women (see Fig. 3-16). Diagnosed with blood tests for an elevated erythrocyte sedimentation rate (ESR), a rheumatoid factor test, and anticyclic citullinated peptide (anti-CCP) antibodies.
temporomandibular joint disorder (TMJ)	*tempor/o* temporal bone *mandibul/o* lower jaw *-ar* pertaining to	Dysfunctional temporomandibular joint, accompanied by gnathalgia (jaw pain).

Terms Related to Systemic Connective Tissue Disorders (M3Ø-M36) and Deforming Dorsopathies (M4Ø-M54)

Term	Word Origin	Definition
ankylosing spondylitis	*ankyl/o* stiffening *spondyl/o* vertebra *-itis* inflammation	Chronic inflammatory disease of idiopathic origin, which causes a fusion of the spine.
herniated intervertebral disk	*inter-* between *vertebr/o* vertebra *-al* pertaining to	Protrusion of the central part of the disk that lies between the vertebrae, resulting in compression of the nerve root and pain.
kyphosis	*kyph/o* round back *-osis* abnormal condition	Extreme posterior curvature of the thoracic area of the spine (Fig. 3-17, *A*).
lordosis	*lord/o* swayback *-osis* abnormal condition	Swayback; exaggerated anterior curve of the lumbar vertebrae (lower back) (Fig. 3-17, *B*).
polymyositis	*poly-* many *myos/o* muscle *-itis* inflammation	Chronic idiopathic inflammation of a number of voluntary muscles.
sciatica		Inflammation of the sciatic nerve. Symptoms include pain and tenderness along the path of the nerve through the thigh and leg (Fig. 3-18).
scoliosis	*scoli/o* curvature *-osis* abnormal condition	Lateral S curve of the spine that can cause an individual to lose inches in height (Fig. 3-17, *C*).
spinal stenosis	*spin/o* spine *-al* pertaining to *stenosis* abnormal condition of narrowing	Abnormal condition of narrowing of the spinal canal with attendant pain, sometimes caused by osteoarthritis or spondylolisthesis (Fig. 3-19).
spondylolisthesis	*spondyl/o* vertebra *-listhesis* slipping	Condition resulting from the partial forward dislocation of one vertebra over the one beneath it.
spondylosis	*spondyl/o* vertebra *-osis* abnormal condition	An abnormal condition characterized by stiffening of the vertebral joints.

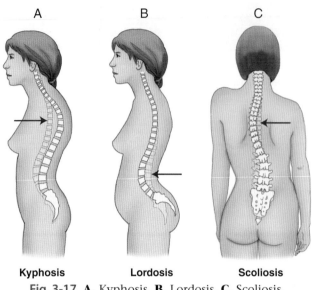

A   B   C

Kyphosis   **Lordosis**   **Scoliosis**

Fig. 3-17 **A,** Kyphosis. **B,** Lordosis. **C,** Scoliosis.

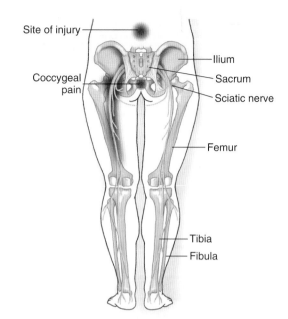

Fig. 3-18 Sciatica.

Terms Related to Systemic Connective Tissue Disorders (M3Ø-M36) and Deforming Dorsopathies (M4Ø-M54)—cont'd

Term	Word Origin	Definition
systemic lupus erythematosus (SLE)	*system/o* system *-ic* pertaining to *erythemat/o* red *-osus* noun ending	Chronic systemic inflammation of unknown etiology (cause). Characterized by distinctive and butterfly-like rash on nose and cheeks. Also called **disseminated lupus erythematosus (DLE)** (Fig. 3-20).
systemic scleroderma	*scler/o* hard *derm/o* skin *-a* noun ending	Disorder that causes hardening and thickening of the skin and connective tissues.

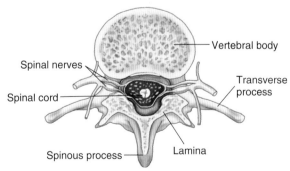

Fig. 3-19 Spinal stenosis. Bony overgrowth has narrowed the spinal canal and pinched the spinal nerves. Compare with normal vertebra in Fig. 3-6, *B.*

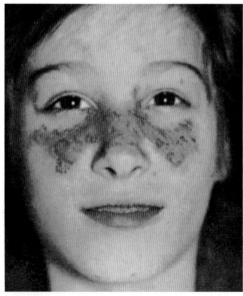

Fig. 3-20 The characteristic butterfly-like rash of SLE.

Exercise 10: Arthropathies and Dentofacial Anomalies; Systemic Connective Tissue Disorders and Dorsopathies

Fill in the blanks using the terms from the list below.

rheumatoid arthritis	**ankylosing spondylitis**	**arthrosis**
crepitus	**spinal stenosis**	**sciatica**
bunion	**herniated intervertebral disk**	**SLE**
TMJ	**contracture**	**scleroderma**
osteophytosis	**lordosis**	**gout**

1. An abnormal condition of a joint is called _____.

2. A painful enlargement and inflammation of the joint at the base of the great toe is _____.

3. Chronic fixation of a joint in flexion is called _____.

4. _____ is a crackling sound heard in joints.

5. A type of arthritis due to excessive uric acid that causes crystals to form is _____.

6. Abnormal bone growth in a joint is called _____.

7. _____ is an autoimmune inflammatory joint disease.

8. _____ is a dysfunctional temporomandibular joint, accompanied by gnathalgia.

9. A chronic inflammatory disease that causes fusion of the spine is _____.

10. A protrusion of the central part of the disk that lies between the vertebrae is called _____.

11. Another word for swayback is _____.

12. Inflammation of the sciatic nerve causes _____.

13. An abnormal, painful narrowing of the spinal canal is called _____.

14. _____ is a chronic systemic inflammation characterized by a butterfly-like rash on the nose and cheeks.

15. A disorder that causes hardening and thickening of the skin and connective tissue is _____.

Build the terms.

16. inflammation of a bone and joint _____

17. inflammation of many muscles _____

18. condition of slipping of the vertebrae _____

19. abnormal condition of vertebra _____

20. abnormal condition of curvature _____

21. abnormal condition of round back _____

Terms Related to Soft Tissue Disorders (M60-M79)

Term	Word Origin	Definition
Baker's cyst	*cyst/o* sac, bladder	Cyst of synovial fluid in the popliteal area of leg; often associated with rheumatoid arthritis.
bursitis	*burs/o* bursa *-itis* inflammation	Inflammation of a bursa.
fibromyalgia	*fibr/o* fiber *my/o* muscle *-algia* pain	Disorder characterized by musculoskeletal pain, fatigue, muscle stiffness and spasms, and sleep disturbances.
lateral epicondylitis	*epi-* above, upon *condyl/o* condyle *-itis* inflammation	Inflammation of the tendon on the outer side of the elbow accompanied by pain and tenderness. Also called **tennis elbow.**
plantar fasciitis	*plant/o* sole *-ar* pertaining to *fasci/o* fascia *-itis* inflammation	Inflammation of the fascia on the sole of the foot.
rhabdomyolysis	*rhabdomy/o* striated muscle *-lysis* breakdown, destruction	Breakdown of striated/skeletal muscle.
tendinitis	*tendin/o* tendon *-itis* inflammation	Inflammation of a tendon.

Terms Related to Osteopathies and Chondropathies (M8Ø-M94)

Term	Word Origin	Definition
chondromalacia	*chondr/o* cartilage *-malacia* softening	Softening of the cartilage.
costochondritis	*cost/o* rib *chondr/o* cartilage *-itis* inflammation	Inflammation of the cartilage of the ribs.
osteitis deformans	*oste/o* bone *-itis* inflammation *deformans* misshapen	Misshaped bone resulting from inflammation. Also known as **Paget's disease of the bone.**
osteomalacia	*oste/o* bone *-malacia* softening	Softening of bone caused by loss of minerals from the bony matrix as a result of vitamin D deficiency. When osteomalacia occurs in childhood, it is called **rickets.**
osteomyelitis	*oste/o* bone *myel/o* bone marrow *-itis* inflammation	Inflammation of the bone and bone marrow.
osteoporosis	*oste/o* bone *por/o* passage *-osis* abnormal condition	Loss of bone mass, which results in the bones being fragile and at risk for fractures (Fig. 3-21). Osteopenia refers to a less severe bone mass loss.

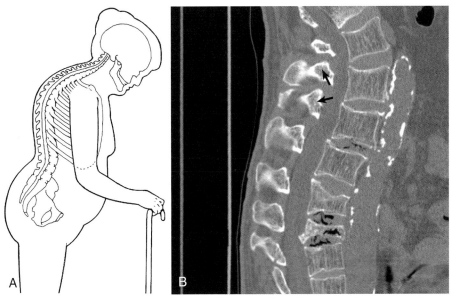

Fig. 3-21 **A,** The hallmark of osteoporosis: the dowager hump. Affected persons lose height, have a bent spine, and appear to sink into their hips. **B,** X-ray demonstrating a compression fracture of T12 and L1 subsequent to osteoporosis.

Exercise 11: Soft Tissue Disorders; Osteopathies and Chondropathies

Fill in the blanks using the terms from the list below.

Baker's cyst	**plantar fasciitis**	**osteitis deformans**
bursitis	**rhabdomyolysis**	**osteomalacia**
lateral epicondylitis	**costochondritis**	**osteomyelitis**

1. Inflammation of the cartilage of the ribs is called _____.

2. A synovial fluid cyst behind the back of the knee is called _____.

3. Inflammation of a bursa is called _____.

4. Paget's disease of the bone is also known as _____.

5. Inflammation of the fascia on the sole of the foot is called _____.

6. _____ is a condition in which the striated or skeletal muscle breaks down.

7. Softening of the bone is called _____.

8. Tennis elbow is also known as _____.

9. Inflammation of the bone and bone marrow is called _____.

Translate the terms.

10. chondromalacia _____

11. osteoporosis _____

12. tendinitis _____

13. fibromyalgia _____

Trauma

Fractures

Put simply, a fracture (fx, #) is a broken bone. However, there are a number of types of breaks, each with its own name. Most fractures occur as a result of trauma, but some can result from an underlying disease, such as osteoporosis or cancer; these **pathologic fractures** are also sometimes called **spontaneous fractures.** All fractures may be classified into simple (closed) or compound (open) fractures. Fractures are additionally characterized as **nondisplaced fractures,** meaning that the broken bones are still in alignment, or **displaced fractures,** meaning that the ends of the fractured bones are not in alignment (Fig. 3-22). The break in a simple fracture does not rupture the skin, but a compound fracture splits open the skin, which allows more opportunity for infection to take place. See the table on the next page.

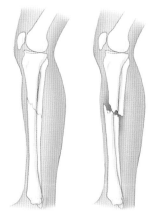

Nondisplaced   Displaced
fracture   fracture

Fig. 3-22 Nondisplaced and displaced fractures.

Sprain/Strain and Dislocation/Subluxation

A **sprain** is a traumatic injury to a joint involving the ligaments. Swelling, pain, and discoloration of the skin may be present. The severity of a sprain is measured in grades. Grade I sprain is an overstretching, Grade II is a partial tear, and Grade III is a complete tear. **A strain** is a lesser injury, usually described as overuse or overstretching of a muscle or tendon.

A bone that is completely out of its place in a joint is called a **dislocation.** If the bone is partially out of the joint, it is considered to be a **subluxation.** This can be a congenital or an acquired condition.

Compartment Syndrome

Compartment syndrome is a potentially serious medical condition that is a result of swelling within the fascia. The increased pressure limits the blood supply, which in turn may lead to nerve and muscle damage. Treatment involves an incision of the fascia to release the pressure (fasciotomy).

 CM Guideline Alert

19.a APPLICATION OF 7th CHARACTERS IN CHAPTER 19

Most categories in Chapter 19 have a 7th character requirement for each applicable code. Most categories in this chapter have three 7th character values (with the exception of fractures): A, initial encounter; D, subsequent encounter; and S, sequela. Categories for traumatic fractures have additional 7th character values. While the patient may be seen by a new or different provider over the course of treatment for an injury, assignment of the 7th character is based on whether the patient is undergoing active treatment and not whether the provider is seeing the patient for the first time.

For complication codes, active treatment refers to treatment for the condition described by the code, even though it may be related to an earlier precipitating problem. For example, code T84.50XA, infection and inflammatory reaction due to unspecified internal joint prosthesis, initial encounter, is used when active treatment is provided for the infection, even though the condition relates to the prosthetic device, implant or graft that was placed at a previous encounter.

7th character "A," initial encounter, is used for each encounter where the patient is receiving active treatment for the condition.

7th character "D," subsequent encounter, is used for encounters after the patient has completed active treatment of the condition and is receiving routine care for the condition during the healing or recovery phase.

The aftercare Z codes should not be used for aftercare for conditions such as injuries or poisonings, where 7th characters are provided to identify subsequent care. For example, for aftercare of an injury, assign the acute injury code with the 7th character "D" (subsequent encounter).

7th character "S," sequela, is for use for complications or conditions that are as a direct result of a condition, such as scar formation after a burn. The scars are sequelae of the burn. When using 7th character "S," it is necessary to use both the injury code that precipitated the sequela and the code for the sequela itself. The "S" is added only to the injury code, not the sequela code. The 7th character "S" identifies the injury responsible for the sequela. The specific type of sequela (e.g., scar) is sequenced first, followed by the injury code.

CM Guideline Alert

19.C. CODING OF TRAUMATIC FRACTURES
The principles of multiple coding of injuries should be followed in coding fractures. Fractures of specified sites . . . are coded individually by site in accordance with both the provisions within specific categories and the level of detail furnished by medical record content.

A fracture not indicated as open or closed should be coded to closed. A fracture not indicated as displaced or not displaced should be coded to displaced.

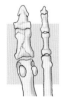

Comminuted   Compression

Note **ICD** The Gustilo classification for open fractures is used to give more information about the type of wound caused by the break. It includes information about the size of the wound, presence or absence of contamination, and additional complications.

Colles'   Complicated

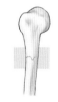

Impacted   Hairline

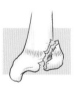

Greenstick   Salter-Harris

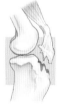

Avulsion fracture
Fig. 3-23 Fractures.

Terms Related to Injury, Poisoning, and Certain Other Consequences of External Causes (SØØ-T88)

Type	Definition
FRACTURES (Fig. 3-23)	
avulsion	Part of the bone is pulled away by a tendon or ligament.
Colles'	Fracture at distal end of the radius at the epiphysis. Often occurs when patient has attempted to break his/her fall.
comminuted	Bone is crushed and/or shattered into multiple pieces.
complicated	Bone is broken and pierces an internal organ.
compression	Fractured area of bone collapses on itself.
greenstick	Partially bent and partially broken. Relatively common in children.
hairline	Minor fracture appearing as a thin line on x-ray. May not extend through bone.
impacted	Broken bones with ends driven into each other.
Salter-Harris	Fracture of epiphyseal plate in children.
torus	Compression injury in children in which the bone does not break, but buckles because of its pliable nature. Also called a buckle fracture.

Terms Related to Injury, Poisoning, and Certain Other Consequences of External Causes (SØØ-T88)—cont'd

Type	Definition
Other Trauma (Figs. 3-24 and 3-25)	
dislocation	Bone that is completely out of its joint socket.
subluxation	Partial dislocation.
sprain	Traumatic injury to ligaments of a joint, including tearing of a ligament.
strain	Overstretching of muscle or a tendon.

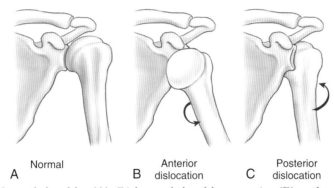

A Normal   B Anterior dislocation   C Posterior dislocation

Fig. 3-24 Normal shoulder **(A)**. Dislocated shoulder, anterior **(B)** and posterior **(C)**.

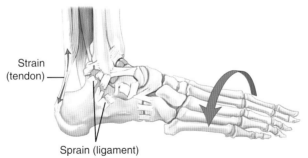

Strain (tendon)

Sprain (ligament)

Fig. 3-25 Strain vs. sprain.

Exercise 12: **Fractures**

Match the fractures with their definitions.

____ 1. complicated
____ 2. greenstick
____ 3. Colles'
____ 4. impacted
____ 5. comminuted
____ 6. simple/closed
____ 7. compound/open
____ 8. hairline
____ 9. pathologic

A. broken bone pierces internal organ
B. broken bone pierces skin
C. spontaneous fracture as a result of disease
D. bone is partially bent and partially broken
E. bone is broken, skin is closed
F. distal end of radius is broken
G. ends of broken bone are driven into each other
H. fracture appears as a line on the bone and fracture may not be completely through bone
I. bone is crushed

 Exercise 13: **Other Trauma**

1. A partial displacement of a bone at a joint is a _____; full displacement

   is a _____.

2. An injury that can be described in grades and involves the soft tissue of a joint is a _____

   _____.

3. An overstretching of a muscle is a _____.

4. Swelling within the confines of a muscle fascia can lead to _____.

Terms Related to Benign Neoplasms Except Benign Neuroendocrine Tumors (D1Ø-D36)		
Term	**Word Origin**	**Definition**
chondroma	*chondr/o* cartilage *-oma* tumor, mass	Benign tumor of the cartilage, usually occurring in children and adolescents.
exostosis	*ex-* out *oste/o* bone *-osis* abnormal condition	Abnormal condition of bony growth. Also called **hyperostosis** and **osteochondroma.**
leiomyoma	*leiomy/o* smooth muscle *-oma* tumor, mass	Benign tumor of smooth muscle. The most common leiomyoma is in the uterus and is termed a **fibroid.**
osteoma	*oste/o* bone *-oma* tumor, mass	Benign bone tumor, usually of compact bone.
rhabdomyoma	*rhabdomy/o* skeletal muscle *-oma* tumor, mass	Benign tumor of striated/voluntary/skeletal muscle.

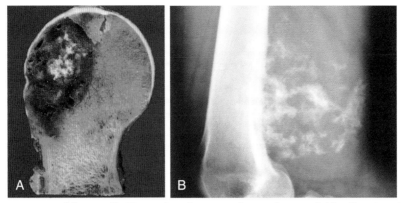

Fig. 3-26 **A,** Chondrosarcoma of femur. **B,** X-ray showing prominent dense calcification in a large neoplastic mass.

Terms Related to Malignant Neoplasms (C4Ø-C49)		
Term	**Word Origin**	**Definition**
chondrosarcoma	*chondr/o* cartilage *-sarcoma* connective tissue cancer	Malignant tumor of the cartilage. Occurs most frequently in adults (Fig. 3-26).
leiomyosarcoma	*leiomy/o* smooth muscle *-sarcoma* connective tissue cancer	Malignant tumor of smooth muscle. Most commonly appearing in the uterus.
osteosarcoma	*oste/o* bone *-sarcoma* connective tissue cancer	Malignant tumor of bone. Also called **Ewing's sarcoma.** Most common children's bone cancer.
rhabdomyosarcoma	*rhabdomy/o* skeletal muscle *-sarcoma* connective tissue cancer	Highly malignant tumor of skeletal muscle. Also called **rhabdosarcoma** or **rhabdomyoblastoma.**

Exercise 14: Neoplasms

Match the neoplasms with their definitions.

_____ 1. rhabdomyosarcoma
_____ 2. osteosarcoma
_____ 3. leiomyosarcoma
_____ 4. chondrosarcoma

A. connective tissue cancer of bone
B. connective tissue cancer of cartilage
C. connective tissue cancer of skeletal muscle
D. connective tissue cancer of smooth muscle

Build the term.

5. Benign tumor of skeletal muscle _____

6. Benign bone tumor _____

7. Benign tumor of smooth muscle _____

8. Benign tumor of cartilage _____

9. An abnormal condition of out(growth) of bone _____

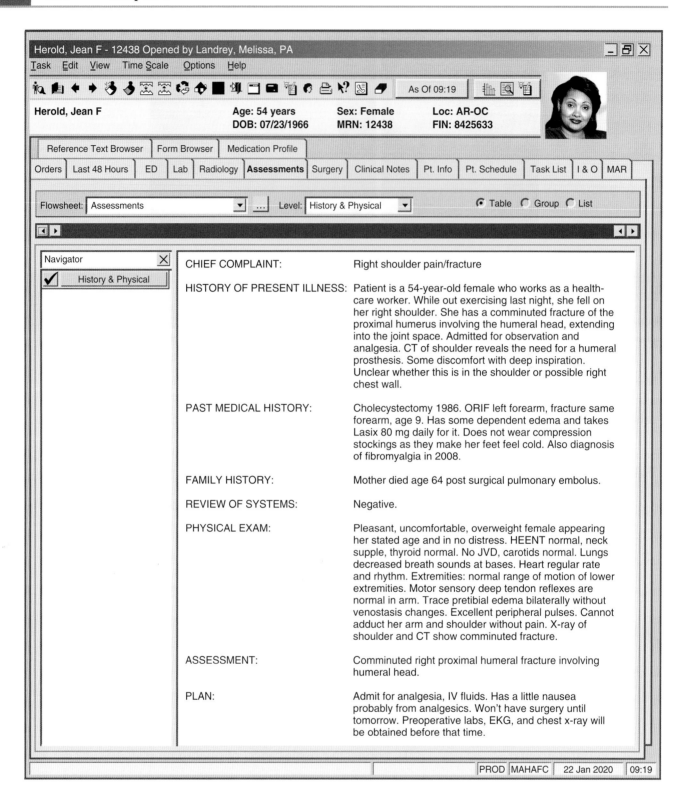

Herold, Jean F - 12438 Opened by Landrey, Melissa, PA

Task   Edit   View   Time Scale   Options   Help

Herold, Jean F

| Age: 54 years | Sex: Female | Loc: AR-OC |
| DOB: 07/23/1966 | MRN: 12438 | FIN: 8425633 |

Reference Text Browser | Form Browser | Medication Profile

Orders | Last 48 Hours | ED | Lab | Radiology | **Assessments** | Surgery | Clinical Notes | Pt. Info | Pt. Schedule | Task List | I & O | MAR

Flowsheet: Assessments   Level: History & Physical   ● Table ○ Group ○ List

Navigator

✓ History & Physical

CHIEF COMPLAINT: Right shoulder pain/fracture

HISTORY OF PRESENT ILLNESS: Patient is a 54-year-old female who works as a health-care worker. While out exercising last night, she fell on her right shoulder. She has a comminuted fracture of the proximal humerus involving the humeral head, extending into the joint space. Admitted for observation and analgesia. CT of shoulder reveals the need for a humeral prosthesis. Some discomfort with deep inspiration. Unclear whether this is in the shoulder or possible right chest wall.

PAST MEDICAL HISTORY: Cholecystectomy 1986. ORIF left forearm, fracture same forearm, age 9. Has some dependent edema and takes Lasix 80 mg daily for it. Does not wear compression stockings as they make her feet feel cold. Also diagnosis of fibromyalgia in 2008.

FAMILY HISTORY: Mother died age 64 post surgical pulmonary embolus.

REVIEW OF SYSTEMS: Negative.

PHYSICAL EXAM: Pleasant, uncomfortable, overweight female appearing her stated age and in no distress. HEENT normal, neck supple, thyroid normal. No JVD, carotids normal. Lungs decreased breath sounds at bases. Heart regular rate and rhythm. Extremities: normal range of motion of lower extremities. Motor sensory deep tendon reflexes are normal in arm. Trace pretibial edema bilaterally without venostasis changes. Excellent peripheral pulses. Cannot adduct her arm and shoulder without pain. X-ray of shoulder and CT show comminuted fracture.

ASSESSMENT: Comminuted right proximal humeral fracture involving humeral head.

PLAN: Admit for analgesia, IV fluids. Has a little nausea probably from analgesics. Won't have surgery until tomorrow. Preoperative labs, EKG, and chest x-ray will be obtained before that time.

PROD | MAHAFC | 22 Jan 2020 | 09:19

Exercise 15: **Admission Record**

Using the admission record on the previous page, answer the following questions:

1. Which bone did she break while exercising? Give the medical and English names. _____

2. Did she fracture the area closest to her shoulder or farther from her shoulder? Circle one.

3. Describe the type of fracture sustained. _____

4. What other MS disorder does she currently have? _____

5. What does "cannot adduct her arm and shoulder without pain" mean? _____

PROCEDURES

 Be aware that many of the musculoskeletal procedural codes depend on the correct identification of a left or right anatomical term. A little common sense (certainly there are left and right kneecaps, but only one sacrum) and knowledge of the anatomy of that particular system will help when checking one's work.

 PCS Guideline Alert

B2.1b Where the general body part values "upper" and "lower" are provided as an option in the Upper Arteries, Lower Arteries, Upper Veins, Lower Veins, Muscles and Tendons body systems, "upper" or "lower" specifies body parts located above or below the diaphragm, respectively.

 PCS Guideline Alert

B4.1b If the prefix "peri-" is combined with a body part to identify the site of the procedure and the site of the procedure is not further specified, then the procedure is coded to the body part named. This guideline applies only when a more specific body part value is not available.

This is where you reap the benefits of learning the bone processes, because they are used within the procedural part of coding to address specific parts of bones and name many muscles, ligaments, and tendons. With the general terms for the bones, you'll need to decide whether it's a procedure on the head and facial bones, upper bones, or lower bones. With the more specific terms, you'll need to think back to where the bone is in the skeleton and how it would be categorized.

 Be Careful!   **Geni/o** *means* chin, *whereas* **-gen** *means* producing *and* **gen/u** *means* knee.

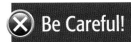 **Be Careful!**   **Ment/o** *means both* chin *and* mind.

Terms Related to Bone Procedures

Term	Word Origin	Definition
acetabuloplasty	*acetabul/o* acetabulum *-plasty* surgically forming	Reconstruction of the acetabulum to correct hip dysplasia, remove metastatic lesions, or as part of hip replacement surgery.
alveoloplasty	*alveol/o* small cavity *-plasty* surgically forming	Surgically shaping the alveolus of the jaw in preparation for dentures.
amputation		Removal of a limb when there are no feasible options to save it.
bunionectomy	*bunion/o* bunion *-ectomy* cutting out	Cutting off a bunion (Fig. 3-27).
carpectomy	*carp/o* carpus, wristbone *-ectomy* cutting out	Cutting off part or all of a wristbone. A **proximal row carpectomy** is done to reduce pain but maintain ROM.
chondrectomy	*chondr/o* cartilage *-ectomy* cutting out	Surgically cutting off part or all of a damaged cartilage.
claviculectomy	*clavicul/o* collarbone, clavicle *-ectomy* cutting out	Cutting off part or all of a collarbone. A **partial** (or distal) **claviculectomy** is performed to reduce pain in the acromioclavicular (AC) joint due to osteoarthritis.
condylotomy	*condyl/o* condyle *-tomy* cutting	Cutting a condyle (e.g., to treat TMJ).
costectomy	*cost/o* rib *-ectomy* cutting out	Cutting out part or all of a rib. May be done as part of a procedure to treat scoliosis.
densitometry	*densit/o* density *-metry* measuring	Process of measuring bone density. An example is **dual energy x-ray absorptiometry (DEXA)** (Fig. 3-28).
discography	*disc/o* disc *-graphy* recording	X-ray recording of an intervertebral disc using a contrast medium to establish a diagnosis for herniated discs.
genioplasty	*geni/o* chin *-plasty* surgically forming	Surgical formation to augment or reduce the size of the chin. Also called **mentoplasty**.

Continued

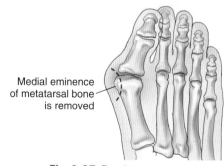

Medial eminence of metatarsal bone is removed

Fig. 3-27 Bunionectomy.

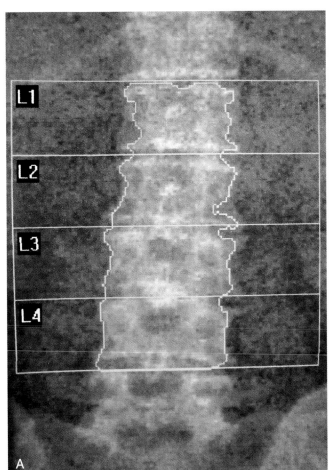

A

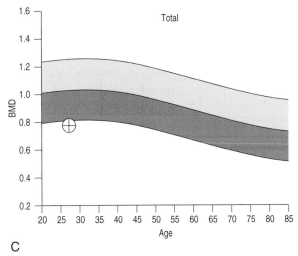

DXA Results Summary:

Region	Area (cm²)	BMC (g)	BMD (g/cm²)	T – Score	PR (%)	Z – Score	AM (%)
L1	9.38	6.66	0.711	–1.9	77	–1.9	77
L2	10.49	7.73	0.737	–2.6	72	–2.6	72
L3	12.07	10.16	0.842	–2.2	78	–2.2	78
L4	13.15	10.65	0.810	–2.8	73	–2.7	73
Total	45.08	35.20	0.781	–2.4	75	–2.4	75

B

C

Fig. 3-28 DEXA scan of the spine showing osteoporosis.

Terms Related to Bone Procedures—cont'd

Term	Word Origin	Definition
kyphoplasty	*kyph/o* round back *-plasty* surgically forming	Minimally invasive procedure designed to address the pain of fractured vertebrae resulting from osteoporosis or cancer. A balloon is used to inflate the area of fracture before a cement-like substance is injected. The substance hardens rapidly, and pain relief is immediate in most patients (Fig. 3-29).
mandibulectomy	*mandibul/o* mandible, lower jaw *-ectomy* cutting out	Cutting off part or all of the lower jaw. May be done to treat cancer of the jaw.
metatarsectomy	*metatars/o* metatarsus, foot bone *-ectomy* cutting out	Cutting off part or all of a foot bone to surgically treat intractable metatarsal pain.
osteoclasis	*oste/o* bone *-clasis* breaking	Surgical fracture of a bone to correct a malformation.

Terms Related to Bone Procedures—cont'd

Term	Word Origin	Definition
patellapexy	*patell/a* kneecap, patella *-pexy* fixation	Fixing the kneecap to the femur to stabilize the joint.
sacrectomy	*sacr/o* sacrum *-ectomy* cutting out	Cutting off part or all of the sacrum, usually to remove an attached tumor.
scapulopexy	*scapul/o* shoulder blade, scapula *-pexy* fixation	Fixing the shoulder blade in place to treat a protruding shoulder blade.
sequestrectomy	*sequestr/o* sequestrum *-ectomy* cutting out	Cutting out a necrosed (dead) bone fragment to prevent or correct possible complications (Fig. 3-30).
spondylosyndesis	*spondyl/o* vertebra *syn-* joined, together *-desis* binding	Binding the vertebrae together to stabilize the spine. Also called **spinal fusion** and **spondylodesis** (Fig. 3-31).
sternotomy	*stern/o* breastbone, sternum *-tomy* cutting	Cutting the sternum to allow access to the heart and thoracic cavity.
tarsectomy	*tars/o* tarsus, anklebone *-ectomy* cutting out	Cutting out one of the tarsal bones. May be done to correct an abnormally high arch of the foot.

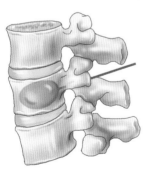

Fig. 3-29 Kyphoplasty.

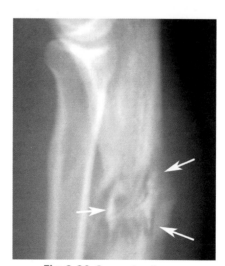

Fig. 3-30 Sequestrectomy.

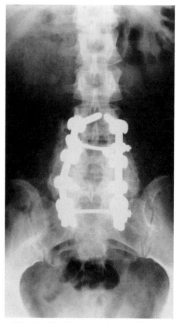

Fig. 3-31 Spondylosyndesis.

Setting Fractures

Broken bones must be "set"—that is, aligned and immobilized. The most common method is with a plaster cast. If a bone does not mend and realign correctly, it is said to be a **malunion.** If no healing takes place, it is **a nonunion.** A piece of bone that does not have a renewed blood supply will die; this tissue then is called **a sequestrum.** Removal of dirt, damaged tissue, or foreign objects from a wound is one of the first steps in repairing an open fracture. This removal of debris is called **débridement.** Methods of fixation and alignment are described as follows:

External fixation (EF): Noninvasive reposition and stabilization of broken bones in which no opening is made in the skin; instead, the stabilization takes place mainly through devices external to the body that offer traction (Fig. 3-32, *A*).

Internal fixation (IF): Reposition and stabilization of broken bones in their correct position, using devices such as pins, screws, plates, and so on, which are fastened to the bones to maintain correct alignment (Fig. 3-32, *B*).

Reduction: Alignment and immobilization of the ends of a broken bone. Also called **manipulation.** *Open reduction* (OR) requires incision of the skin; *closed reduction* (CR) does not require incision. An *open reduction internal fixation (ORIF)* is commonly performed to repair serious fractures with plates and screws.

A **spica cast** is a type of immobilization used to hold a limb close to the trunk (usually for the shoulder or hip).

A **Minerva cast** is used to immobilize the head and neck.

A **gauntlet cast** is one that extends from below the elbow to the palm of the hand.

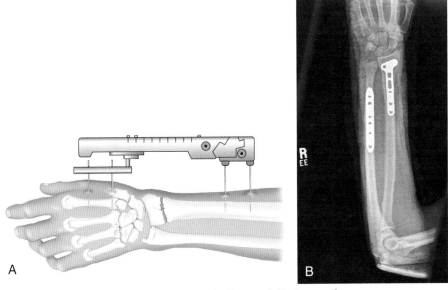

Fig. 3-32 Fixation. **A,** External. **B,** Internal.

CPT Coding Alert!

CPT lists a number of different casts and casting methods as treatments including immobilization. PCS groups all casting into a single digit, whereas CPT names the specific type under the particular body part. For example, types of casts for the body and upper extremity include the shoulder spica, Minerva type, and gauntlet casts.

Click on **Animations** to see a demonstration of an open reduction internal fixation (ORIF) procedure.

  ## Exercise 16: Bone Procedures

Match the procedure to its definition.

____ 1. spondylosyndesis	A. cutting out an anklebone
____ 2. tarsectomy	B. cutting out a rib
____ 3. scapulopexy	C. cutting the breastbone
____ 4. sternotomy	D. fixing a shoulder blade
____ 5. osteoclasis	E. binding the vertebrae together
____ 6. costectomy	F. surgical fracture of a bone to correct a malformation
____ 7. débridement	G. surgically forming a small cavity
____ 8. amputation	H. removal of a limb
____ 9. alveoloplasty	I. removal of debris

Build the terms.

10. cutting out dead bone _____

11. fixation of a kneecap _____

12. measuring density _____

13. cutting out cartilage _____

14. surgically forming a chin _____

15. breaking a bone _____

16. recording a disc _____

Terms Related to Joint, Muscle, and Fascia Procedures

Term	Word Origin	Definition
achillorrhaphy	*achill/o* Achilles tendon *-rrhaphy* suturing	Suturing a ruptured Achilles/calcaneal tendon.
acromioplasty	*acromi/o* acromion *-plasty* surgically forming	Forming the acromion process to correct a defect as in rotator cuff surgery.
arthrocentesis	*arthr/o* joint *-centesis* surgical puncture	Surgical puncture of a joint to remove fluid, pus, or blood.
arthrodesis	*arthr/o* joint *-desis* binding	Binding a joint in order to stabilize it.
arthrography	*arthr/o* joint *-graphy* recording	X-ray recording of a joint.
arthroplasty	*arthr/o* joint *-plasty* surgically forming	Surgically forming a joint. Examples include **total knee replacement (TKR)** and total **hip replacement (THR)** (Fig. 3-33).

Continued

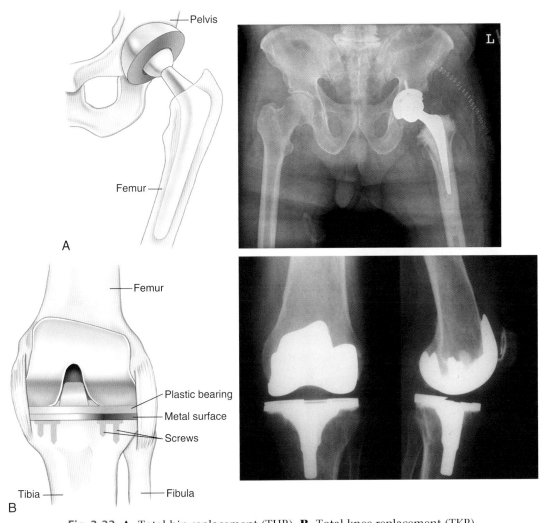

Fig. 3-33 A, Total hip replacement (THR). **B,** Total knee replacement (TKR).

Click on Animations to view a demonstration of a total knee replacement (TKR).

Terms Related to Joint, Muscle, and Fascia Procedures—cont'd

Term	Word Origin	Definition
arthroscopy	*arthr/o* joint *-scopy* viewing	Internal viewing of a joint, especially the shoulder and knees, to aid in the diagnosis of ligament tears and injuries (Fig. 3-34).
arthrotomy	*arthr/o* joint *-tomy* cutting	An incision of a joint, usually as a means of access for a surgical procedure, such as a joint replacement. It may also be performed to provide drainage for infection.
bursectomy	*burs/o* bursa *-ectomy* cutting out	Cutting out part or all of a bursa.
bursocentesis	*burs/o* bursa *-centesis* surgical puncture	Surgical puncture of a bursa to remove excess fluid.
discectomy	*disc/o* disc *-ectomy* cutting out	Removal of an intervertebral disc. Also called **diskectomy**.

Continued

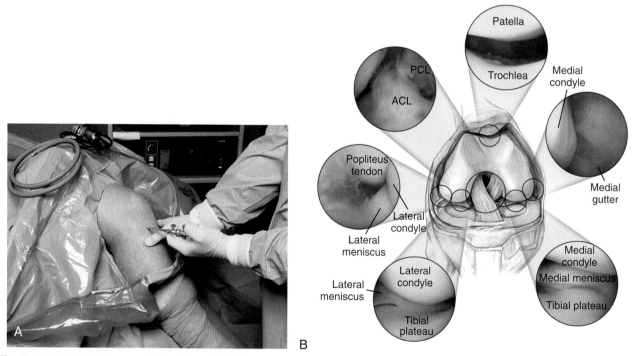

Fig. 3-34 A, Arthroscopy of the knee. **B,** Knee structures that can be seen during arthroscopy at six different points (circles).

Terms Related to Joint, Muscle, and Fascia Procedures—cont'd

Term	Word Origin	Definition
electromyography (EMG)	*electr/o* electricity *my/o* muscle *-graphy* recording	Recording the electrical activity of skeletal muscles. May be used to diagnose low back pain (Fig. 3-35).
fasciotomy	*fasci/o* fascia *-tomy* cutting	Incision of the fascia; used to treat acute compartment syndrome.
laminectomy	*lamin/o* lamina, thin plate *-ectomy* cutting out	Cutting out one of the vertebral laminae to treat spinal stenosis (Fig. 3-36).
meniscectomy	*menisc/o* meniscus *-ectomy* cutting out	Cutting out a meniscus to treat a tear of the meniscus.
myopexy	*my/o* muscle *-pexy* fixation	Fixing a muscle in place. Used to treat a visual defect of eye muscles.
synovectomy	*synov/o* synovial membrane *-ectomy* cutting out	Cutting out a synovial membrane to treat severe rheumatoid arthritis or hemarthrosis.
tendolysis	*tend/o* tendon *-lysis* release, destruction	Releasing a tendon from adhesions to improve flexion. Also called **tenolysis.**
tenomyoplasty	*ten/o* tendon *my/o* muscle *-plasty* surgically forming	Surgical repair of a muscle and a tendon.

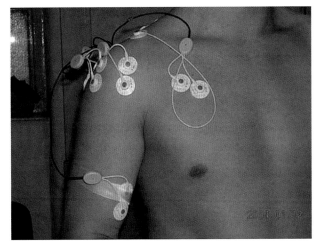

Fig. 3-35 Placement of the electrodes in electromyography (EMG).

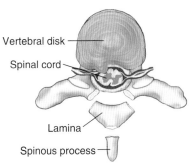

Vertebral disk

Spinal cord

Lamina

Spinous process

Fig. 3-36 Laminectomy.

Exercise 17: Joint, Muscle, and Fascia Procedures

Match the procedure to its definition.

____ 1. achillorrhaphy	A. releasing a tendon
____ 2. arthroscopy	B. recording a joint
____ 3. acromioplasty	C. surgically forming the acromion process
____ 4. bursectomy	D. surgical puncture of a bursa
____ 5. tendolysis	E. incision of the fascia
____ 6. bursocentesis	F. cutting out a vertebral lamina
____ 7. arthrography	G. cutting out a bursa
____ 8. fasciotomy	H. viewing a joint
____ 9. laminectomy	I. suturing the tendon of the heel

Translate the term.

10. arthrocentesis _____

11. arthrodesis _____

12. myopexy _____

13. electromyography _____

14. tenomyoplasty _____

PHARMACOLOGY

analgesics: Reduce pain. Examples include hydromorphone (Dilaudid), oxycodone (Oxycontin), acetaminophen (Tylenol), and NSAIDs such as naproxen (Anaprox).

antigout agents or antihyperuricemic agents: Treat gout by reducing the buildup of uric acid in joints. Examples include allopurinol (Zyloprim), colchicine (Colcrys), and lesinurad (Zurampic).

anti-inflammatories: Reduce inflammation. Examples include steroidal and nonsteroidal anti-inflammatory drugs (NSAIDs). Methylprednisolone (Medrol) is an example of a steroid; ibuprofen (Advil) and celecoxib (Celebrex) are examples of NSAIDs.

bisphosphonates: Inhibit bone loss to treat diseases such as osteoporosis, Paget's disease, or bone cancer. Examples include alendronate (Fosamax) and zoledronic acid (Zometa).

disease-modifying antirheumatic drugs (DMARDs): Slow progression of rheumatoid arthritis while also reducing signs and symptoms. Examples include leflunomide (Arava), etanercept (Enbrel), and infliximab (Remicade).

muscle relaxants: Relieve pain caused by muscle spasms by relaxing the skeletal muscles. Examples include cyclobenzaprine (Flexeril) and carisoprodol (Soma).

Exercise 18: Pharmacology

1. What class of drugs may prevent osteoporosis? _____.

2. Rheumatoid arthritis progression may be treated with _____.

3. NSAIDs are used to treat what kinds of symptoms? _____

4. _____ are used to treat muscle spasms.

RECOGNIZING SUFFIXES FOR PCS

Now that you've finished reading about the procedures for the musculoskeletal system, take a look at this review of the **suffixes** used in their terminology. Each of these suffixes is associated with one or more root operations in the medical surgical section or one of the other categories in PCS.

Suffixes and Root Operations for the Musculoskeletal System

Suffix	Root Operation
-clasis	Division
-desis	Fusion
-ectomy	Excision, resection, extirpation
-pexy	Repair, reposition
-plasty	Repair, replacement, supplement, alteration
-tomy	Release, division, drainage

Abbreviations

Abbreviation	Meaning	Abbreviation	Meaning
A	action	MS	musculoskeletal
ACL	anterior cruciate ligament	O	origin
C1-C7	first cervical through seventh cervical vertebrae	OA	osteoarthritis
CR	closed reduction	OR	open reduction
CREF	closed reduction external fixation	ORIF	open reduction internal fixation
DEXA, DXA	dual energy x-ray absorptiometry	PIP	proximal interphalangeal joint
DIP	distal interphalangeal joint	PCL	posterior cruciate ligament
DJD	degenerative joint disease	RA	rheumatoid arthritis
DLE	disseminated lupus erythematosus	ROM	range of motion
EF	external fixation	S1-S5	first sacral through fifth sacral segments
EMG	electromyography	SLE	systemic lupus erythematosus
Fx, #	fracture	T1-T12	first thoracic through twelfth thoracic vertebrae
I	insertion	THR	total hip replacement
IF	internal fixation	TKR	total knee replacement
L1-L5	first lumbar through fifth lumbar vertebrae	TMJ	temporomandibular joint disorder
LCL	lateral collateral ligament	UCL	ulnar collateral ligament
MCL	medial collateral ligament		

Go to the Evolve website to interactively build terms, label images, memorize word parts and practice using musculoskeletal terms in context.

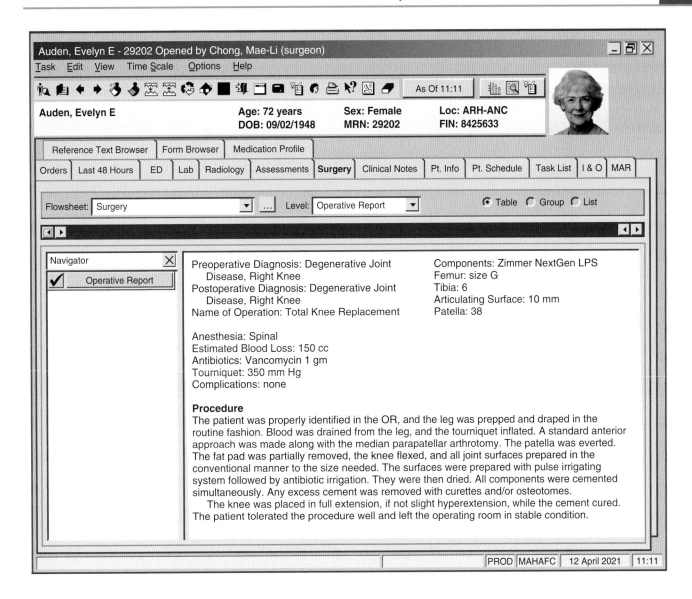

Auden, Evelyn E - 29202 Opened by Chong, Mae-Li (surgeon)

Task Edit View Time Scale Options Help

Auden, Evelyn E

Age: 72 years
DOB: 09/02/1948

Sex: Female
MRN: 29202

Loc: ARH-ANC
FIN: 8425633

Reference Text Browser | Form Browser | Medication Profile

Orders | Last 48 Hours | ED | Lab | Radiology | Assessments | **Surgery** | Clinical Notes | Pt. Info | Pt. Schedule | Task List | I & O | MAR

Flowsheet: Surgery   Level: Operative Report   ● Table ○ Group ○ List

Navigator   ✕

✓ Operative Report

Preoperative Diagnosis: Degenerative Joint
    Disease, Right Knee
Postoperative Diagnosis: Degenerative Joint
    Disease, Right Knee
Name of Operation: Total Knee Replacement

Anesthesia: Spinal
Estimated Blood Loss: 150 cc
Antibiotics: Vancomycin 1 gm
Tourniquet: 350 mm Hg
Complications: none

Components: Zimmer NextGen LPS
Femur: size G
Tibia: 6
Articulating Surface: 10 mm
Patella: 38

Procedure
The patient was properly identified in the OR, and the leg was prepped and draped in the routine fashion. Blood was drained from the leg, and the tourniquet inflated. A standard anterior approach was made along with the median parapatellar arthrotomy. The patella was everted. The fat pad was partially removed, the knee flexed, and all joint surfaces prepared in the conventional manner to the size needed. The surfaces were prepared with pulse irrigating system followed by antibiotic irrigation. They were then dried. All components were cemented simultaneously. Any excess cement was removed with curettes and/or osteotomes.
    The knee was placed in full extension, if not slight hyperextension, while the cement cured. The patient tolerated the procedure well and left the operating room in stable condition.

PROD MAHAFC   12 April 2021   11:11

Exercise 19: Healthcare Report

Using the operative report above, answer the following questions.

1. A synonym for the preoperative diagnosis of degenerative joint disease is _____.

2. An "anterior approach" to the knee would be through which part of the knee?

_____

3. What is the patella? _____

4. To what does the term *parapatellar* refer? _____

5. What is an arthrotomy? _____

6. If the patella was everted, how would it be placed? _____

7. What is an osteotome? _____

8. What would hyperextension be? _____

Match the word parts to their definitions.

WORD PART DEFINITIONS

Prefix/Suffix
-algia
-centesis
-clasis
-desis
-listhesis
-malacia
-osis
peri-
-physis
-sarcoma

Combining Form
arthr/o
carp/o
cervic/o
chondr/o
cleid/o
coccyg/o
cost/o
dactyl/o
femor/o
gnath/o
humer/o
mandibul/o
my/o
myel/o
olecran/o
oste/o
patell/a
phalang/o
rhabdomy/o
scapul/o
spondyl/o
zygomat/o

Definition

1. _____ binding
2. _____ pain
3. _____ surgical puncture
4. _____ connective tissue cancer
5. _____ softening
6. _____ slipping
7. _____ surrounding, around
8. _____ intentional breaking
9. _____ growth
10. _____ abnormal condition

Definition

11. _____ collarbone
12. _____ bone
13. _____ jaw (entire)
14. _____ skeletal muscle
15. _____ upper arm bone
16. _____ wrist
17. _____ cheekbone
18. _____ thighbone
19. _____ neck
20. _____ vertebra
21. _____ cartilage
22. _____ bone marrow
23. _____ finger/toe (whole)
24. _____ finger/toe bone
25. _____ rib
26. _____ muscle
27. _____ elbow
28. _____ tailbone
29. _____ kneecap
30. _____ joint
31. _____ lower jaw
32. _____ shoulder blade

WORDSHOP

Prefixes	Combining Forms	Suffixes
an-	arthr/o	-al
inter-	chondr/o	-desis
peri-	disc/o	-ectomy
poly-	geni/o	-graphy
	leiomy/o	-itis
	myel/o	-lysis
	myos/o	-malacia
	my/o	-oma
	oste/o	-osis
	phyt/o	-pexy
	rhabdomy/o	-sarcoma
	spondyl/o	-um
	vertebr/o	

Build musculoskeletal terms by combining the word parts above. Some word parts may be used more than once. Some may not be used at all. The number in parentheses indicates the number of word parts needed.

Definition	Term
1. structure surrounding bone (3)	
2. inflammation of many muscles (3)	
3. pertaining to between vertebrae (3)	
4. softening of cartilage (2)	
5. connective tissue cancer of bone (2)	
6. breakdown or destruction of skeletal muscle (2)	
7. abnormal condition of bone growth (3)	
8. binding of a joint (2)	
9. fixation of a muscle (2)	
10. cutting out of cartilage	
11. recording a disc (2)	
12. binding together of vertebrae (3)	
13. surgical puncture of a bursa (2)	
14. tumor of smooth muscle (2)	
15. surgical repair of the chin (2)	

Sort the terms into the correct categories.

TERM SORTING

Anatomy and Physiology	Pathology	Procedures

amputation	diaphysis	osteosarcoma
arthrocentesis	digitus	patellapexy
arthrodesis	EMG	perichondrium
arthrography	endosteum	radius
arthrosis	fibromyalgia	rhabdomyoma
arthrotomy	genioplasty	sacrectomy
articulation	humerus	scapula
bunion	lamellae	scapulopexy
bursitis	laminectomy	sciatica
carpectomy	ligament	SLE
cartilage	meniscectomy	spondylolisthesis
chondromalacia	osteoclasis	sternum
contracture	osteogenesis	tendinitis
costa	osteomyelitis	TMJ
densitometry	osteoporosis	ulna

Replace the underlined text with the correct terms.

TRANSLATIONS

1. Ms. Alston was diagnosed with **softening of the cartilage** of her knee and a **cyst of synovial fluid in the popliteal area of her leg.**	
2. The patient had **surgical puncture of a joint** to treat his **abnormal condition of blood in the joint** of the left knee.	
3. Dr. Matthews performed **an alignment and immobilization** of the right **collarbone** of 5-year-old Caitlin, who had fallen while jumping on her bed.	
4. Sarah Henderson had **abnormal bone growths** in the **joints between the bones of her fingers**.	
5. The patient had **an extreme posterior curvature of the thoracic area of the spine** that was a result of her **loss of bone mass.**	
6. The patient was admitted for **an inflammation of the bone and bone marrow** of his **lower lateral arm bone.**	
7. The patient complained of **inflammation of the fascia on the sole of the foot** and **inflammation of a tendon.**	
8. **A procedure that records the electrical activity of muscles** was used to confirm Mr. Travis' **chronic, idiopathic inflammation of many muscles.**	
9. An x-ray revealed a **partially bent and partially broken** fracture of the child's right **upper arm bone.**	
10. The patient sustained two broken bones: a **fracture at the distal end of her radius at the epiphysis on her right arm** and a **minor fracture appearing as a thin line on x-ray** of her left thumb.	
11. Mrs. Anderhub had **a removal of a bunion** to correct her **painful enlargement and inflammation of the first metatarsophalangeal joint.**	
12. The patient underwent a **removal of an intervertebral disc** to treat his **protrusion of the central part of vertebral disk.**	
13. The high jumper was admitted for **suturing of a ruptured calcaneal tendon** that was complicated by a **severe traumatic injury to the ligaments of a joint.**	

ICD-10-CM Example from Tabular
L21 Seborrheic dermatitis
  Excludes 2 infective dermatitis (**L30.3**)
    seborrheic keratosis (**L82.-**)
  L21.0 Seborrhea capitis
    Cradle cap
  L21.1 Seborrheic infantile dermatitis
  L21.8 Other seborrheic dermatitis
  L21.9 Seborrheic dermatitis, unspecified
    Seborrhea, NOS

ICD-10-PCS Example from Index
  Onychectomy
  see Excision, Skin and Breast **ØHB**
  see Resection, Skin and Breast **ØHT**
  Onychoplasty
  see Repair, Skin and Breast **ØHQ**
  see Replacement, Skin and Breast **ØHR**
  Onychotomy
  see Drainage, Skin and Breast **ØH9**

CHAPTER OUTLINE

FUNCTIONS OF THE SKIN AND SUBCUTANEOUS TISSUE

ANATOMY AND PHYSIOLOGY

PATHOLOGY

PROCEDURES

PHARMACOLOGY

RECOGNIZING SUFFIXES FOR PCS

ABBREVIATIONS

OBJECTIVES

☐ Recognize and use terms related to the anatomy and physiology of the skin and subcutaneous tissue

☐ Recognize and use terms related to the pathology of the skin and subcutaneous tissue

☐ Recognize and use terms related to the procedures for the skin and subcutaneous tissue

FUNCTIONS OF THE SKIN AND SUBCUTANEOUS TISSUE

The most important function of the **skin** (integument) is that it acts as the first line of defense in protecting the body from disease by providing an external barrier. It also helps regulate the temperature of the body, provides information about the environment through the sense of touch, assists in the synthesis of vitamin D (essential for the normal formation of bones and teeth), and helps eliminate waste products from the body. It is the largest organ of the body and accomplishes its diverse functions with assistance from its accessory structures, which include the **hair, nails,** and two types of **glands: sebaceous** (oil) and **sudoriferous** (sweat). Any impairment of the skin has the potential to lessen its ability to carry out these functions, which can lead to disease. It is important to note that the subcutaneous tissue also serves as an attachment to the muscles and bones beneath it.

ANATOMY AND PHYSIOLOGY

Skin

The skin is composed of two layers: the **epidermis,** which forms the outermost layer, and the **dermis** or **corium,** the inner layer (Fig. 4-1). The dermis is attached to a layer of connective tissue called the **hypodermis** or the **subcutaneous layer,** which is mainly composed of fat (adipose tissue).

This chapter includes all the anatomy necessary to assign ICD-10 skin and subcutaneous tissue codes, including detail on sebaceous glands, sweat glands, and the dermis. See Appendix H for a complete list of body parts and how they should be coded.

Go to Evolve to watch an animation on the anatomy of the integumentary system.

skin = derm/o, dermat/o, cut/o, cutane/o	
hair = trich/o, pil/o	
nail = onych/o, ungu/o	
oil, sebum = seb/o, sebac/o	
sweat = hidr/o, sudor/i	

epidermis
  epi- = above
  derm/o = skin
  -is = structure

hypodermis
  hypo- = below
  derm/o = skin
  -is = structure

subcutaneous
  sub- = under
  cutane/o = skin
  -ous = pertaining to

fat = adip/o, lip/o

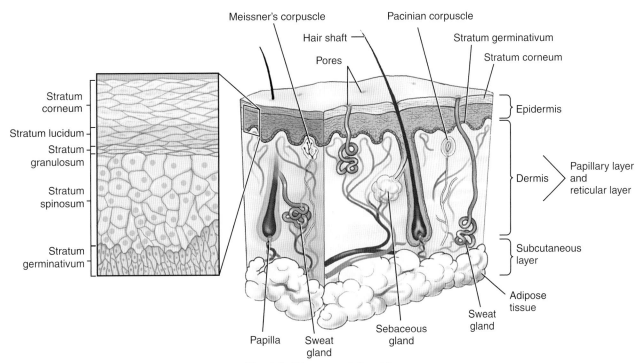

Fig. 4-1 Diagram of the skin.

scaly, squamous =
   squam/o

---

avascular
   a- = without
   vascul/o = vessel
   -ar = pertaining to

---

basal = bas/o

---

melanocyte
   melan/o = black
   -cyte = cell

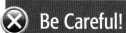 **Be Careful!**

Don't confuse **strata,** *meaning* layers, *with* **striae,** *meaning* stretch marks.

---

keratin
   kerat/o = hard, horny
   -in = substance

---

sudoriferous
   sudor/i = sweat
   -ferous = pertaining to
      carrying

---

sebaceous
   sebac/o = oil
   -ous = pertaining to

---

sweat gland =
   hidraden/o

---

sweat = hidr/o, sudor/i

---

eccrine
   ec- = out, outward
   -crine = to secrete

Epidermis

The epidermis is composed of several different layers, or strata, of epithelial tissue. Epithelial tissue covers many of the external and internal surfaces of the body. Because the type of epithelial tissue that covers the body has a microscopic layered, scaly appearance, it is referred to as **stratified squamous epithelium.**

Although there is a limited blood supply to the epidermis (it is **avascular**—that is, it contains no blood vessels), constant activity is taking place. New skin cells are formed in the basal (bottom) layer of the epidermis, the **stratum germinativum** (also called the **stratum basale**). The term **germinativum** is derived from *germ/i,* meaning "sprout," and *nat/o,* meaning "birth." So this is where the skin cells "sprout" and are "born," that is to say, where they develop, or germinate. This layer is also the site where **melanin** (a black pigment) is produced by **melanocytes.** When the skin is exposed to ultraviolet light, the melanocytes secrete more melanin. Birthmarks, age spots, and freckles result from the clumping of melanocytes in the basal layer of the skin. Individuals have different skin colors because of varying numbers of melanocytes. **Merkel cells,** also located in the basal layer of the skin, are thought to have a function in tactile perception. The most common site of these cells is in the finger tips. Along with melanocytes, Merkel cells are notable because of the rare possibility of their becoming cancerous.

The new cells move outward toward the next layer, the **stratum spinosum,** composed of flattened **keratinocytes,** then the **stratum granulosum.** The stratum granulosum is the layer in which the cells become filled with granules, which eventually transform to become the hardened protective cells in the stratum corneum. The next layer, the **stratum lucidum,** which is present only in thickened skin (e.g., soles of the feet), is made up of a few rows of clear, flattened keratinocytes. The outermost layer, the **stratum corneum,** has many rows of cells that are completely cornified (characterized by a hardened, horny nature) and that shed regularly.

During the transition from the lowest layer to the outer layer, these cells are called keratinocytes because they are filled with **keratin,** which is a hard protein material. The hardness of the keratin adds to the protective nature of the skin, giving it a waterproof property that helps retain moisture within the body. Note that *kerat/o* and *corne/o* both refer to the property of hardness. These combining forms will be encountered again in the anatomy of the eye, where they both refer to the cornea, the hard outer layer of the eye.

Dermis

The dermis, or **corium,** is the thick, underlying layer of the skin that is composed of vascular connective tissue arranged in two layers. The papillary layer is the thin upper layer composed of fibers made from protein and collagen that regulates blood flow through its extensive vascular supply. The reticular layer is the lower, thicker layer, which also is composed of collagen fibers. This layer holds the hair follicles, sudoriferous and sebaceous glands, and the sensory receptors. **Meissner's corpuscles** provide sensitivity to light touch, while **Pacinian corpuscles** sense pressure. Specialized heat and cold receptors relay information to the brain for regulating body temperature (thermoregulation).

Subcutaneous Tissue

The subcutaneous layer, a passageway for nerves and blood vessels, is connective tissue composed of lipocytes (fat cells). Aside from its role as a means of attachment to the muscles and bones beneath it, it also provides insulation from the cold, a protective cushion for bones and organs, and an energy reserve.

Accessory Structures
Glands

The sudoriferous, or sweat, glands are located in the dermis and provide one means of thermoregulation for the body. **Eccrine glands,** most densely in the hands, feet, and forehead, secrete sweat through tiny openings in the surface of the skin called **pores.** Eccrine glands are principally responsible for cooling the body. **Apocrine glands,** located in the armpits and groin, begin secretion after puberty and, aside from discharging sweat through the hair follicles, may be responsible for an individual's unpleasant body odor. Eccrine glands are named for secreting their sweat directly to the outside *(ec-)* of the body. Apocrine glands are named for a separation *(apo-)* of part of the secreting cell that enters the gland before it is discharged to the surface of the body. The secretion of sweat is called **perspiration.**

The **sebaceous glands** secrete an oily, acidic substance called **sebum,** which helps to lubricate hair and the surface of the skin. The acidic nature of sebum is key in inhibiting the growth of bacteria.

Hair

Hair has its roots in the dermis; these roots, together with their coverings, are called **hair follicles.** The visible part is called the **hair shaft.** Underneath the follicle is a nipple-shaped structure that encloses the capillaries called the **papilla.** Epithelial cells on top of the papilla are responsible for the formation of the hair shaft. When these cells die, hair can no longer regenerate, and hair loss occurs. Like skin, hair is colored by melanin, but in hair, there are two types. Eumelanin gives hair a black or brown color, while pheomelanin results in red or blond hair. Individuals who have very little melanin will have gray hair, while those with no melanin have white hair.

The main function of hair is to assist in thermoregulation by holding heat near the body. When cold, hair stands on end (piloerection), holding a layer of air as insulation near the body.

Nails

Nails cover and thus protect the dorsal surfaces of the distal bones of the fingers and toes. The part that is visible is the **nail body** (also called the **nail plate**), whereas the **nail root** (matrix) is in a groove under a small fold of skin at the base of the nail. The **nail bed** is the highly vascular tissue under the nail that appears pink when the blood is oxygenated or blue/purple when it is oxygen deficient (Fig. 4-2). The moonlike white area in the base of the nail is called the **lunula** (meaning little moon), behind which new growth occurs. The small fold of skin above the lower part of the nail is called the **cuticle**, or **eponychium**. The **paronychium** is the fold of skin that is near the sides of the nail. The **hyponychium** is the skin distal to the nail bed under the free edge of the nail plate. It is also referred to as the onychodermal band.

apocrine	
apo- = separate, away from	
-crine = to secrete	

sebum, oil = seb/o, sebac/o	

hair = trich/o, pil/o	
follicle = follicul/o	
papilla, nipple = papill/o	
eu- = healthy, normal	
phe/o = dark	
nail = onych/o, ungu/o	

eponychium
  epi- = above
  onych/o = nail
  -ium = structure

paronychium
  par- = near
  onych/o = nail
  -ium = structure

hyponychium
  hypo = under, below
  onych/o = nail
  -ium = structure

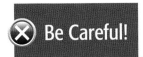 **Be Careful!** *Don't confuse* **papill/o,** *meaning* papilla *or* nipple, *describing a shape, with* **papul/o,** *which means* pimple, *and* **pupill/o,** *meaning* the pupil of the eye.

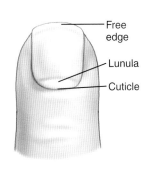

CPT Coding Alert!

CPT specifies a biopsy of a "nail unit" to include the hyponychium as well as the nail bed, plate, matrix, and proximal and lateral folds.

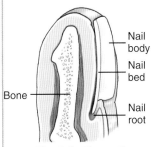

Fig. 4-2 The nail.

Exercise 1: Anatomy and Physiology

Match the integumentary term to its word part.

____	1. follicle	A.	squam/o
____	2. fat	B.	follicul/o
____	3. black	C.	pil/o, trich/o
____	4. scaly	D.	apo-
____	5. sweat	E.	sudor/i, hidr/o
____	6. hard, horny	F.	derm/o, dermat/o, cutane/o
____	7. skin	G.	ec-
____	8. oil, sebum	H.	kerat/o
____	9. hair	I.	adip/o
____	10. nail	J.	sebac/o, seb/o
____	11. away from	K.	onych/o, ungu/o
____	12. out	L.	-crine
____	13. to secrete	M.	melan/o
____	14. blood vessel	N.	vascul/o
____	15. nipple-like	O.	papill/o
____	16. dark	P.	phe/o
____	17. healthy, normal	Q.	eu-

To practice labeling the structure of the skin, click on **Label It.**

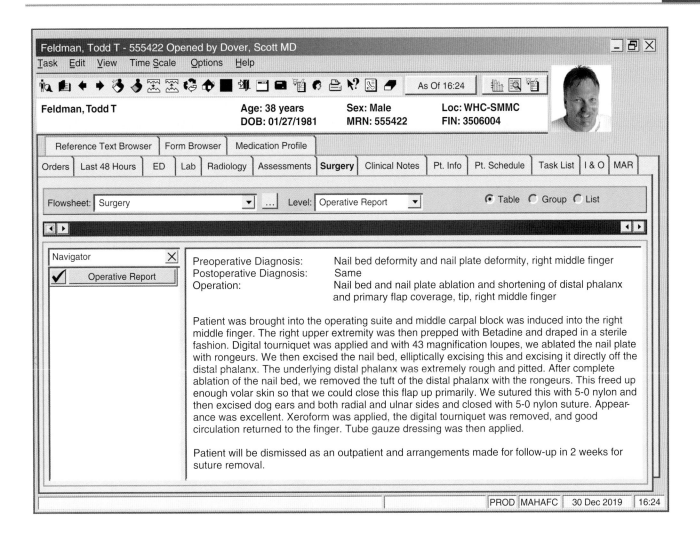

Feldman, Todd T - 555422 Opened by Dover, Scott MD

Task   Edit   View   Time Scale   Options   Help

Feldman, Todd T | Age: 38 years | Sex: Male | Loc: WHC-SMMC
| DOB: 01/27/1981 | MRN: 555422 | FIN: 3506004

Reference Text Browser | Form Browser | Medication Profile

Orders | Last 48 Hours | ED | Lab | Radiology | Assessments | **Surgery** | Clinical Notes | Pt. Info | Pt. Schedule | Task List | I & O | MAR

Flowsheet: Surgery   Level: Operative Report   • Table ○ Group ○ List

Navigator   ×
✓ Operative Report

Preoperative Diagnosis: Nail bed deformity and nail plate deformity, right middle finger
Postoperative Diagnosis: Same
Operation: Nail bed and nail plate ablation and shortening of distal phalanx and primary flap coverage, tip, right middle finger

Patient was brought into the operating suite and middle carpal block was induced into the right middle finger. The right upper extremity was then prepped with Betadine and draped in a sterile fashion. Digital tourniquet was applied and with 43 magnification loupes, we ablated the nail plate with rongeurs. We then excised the nail bed, elliptically excising this and excising it directly off the distal phalanx. The underlying distal phalanx was extremely rough and pitted. After complete ablation of the nail bed, we removed the tuft of the distal phalanx with the rongeurs. This freed up enough volar skin so that we could close this flap up primarily. We sutured this with 5-0 nylon and then excised dog ears and both radial and ulnar sides and closed with 5-0 nylon suture. Appearance was excellent. Xeroform was applied, the digital tourniquet was removed, and good circulation returned to the finger. Tube gauze dressing was then applied.

Patient will be dismissed as an outpatient and arrangements made for follow-up in 2 weeks for suture removal.

PROD | MAHAFC | 30 Dec 2019 | 16:24

 Exercise 2: **Operative Report**

Using the operative report above, answer the following questions:

1. What are the nail bed and nail plate?

_____

2. Where is the "volar skin" located? (Refer to Chapter 2 if you've forgotten.) _____

3. What is a "digital tourniquet," and why do you think it was used?

4. From your knowledge of the anatomy of a nail, what, if any, parts of the nail do you think remain?

_____

Combining Forms for the Anatomy of the Integumentary System

Meaning	Combining Form	Meaning	Combining Form
base, bottom	bas/o	papilla, nipple	papill/o
black, dark	melan/o, phe/o	scaly	squam/o
fat	adip/o, lip/o	sebum, oil	seb/o, sebac/o
follicle	follicul/o	skin	derm/o, dermat/o, cut/o, cutane/o
hair	trich/o, pil/o	sweat	hidr/o, sudor/i
hard, horny	kerat/o, corne/o	sweat gland	hidraden/o
nail	onych/o, ungu/o	vessel	vascul/o

Prefixes for the Anatomy of the Integumentary System

Prefix	Meaning
a-	no, not, without
apo-	separate, away from
ec-	out, outward
epi-	above
eu-	healthy, normal
hypo-, sub-	under, below
par-	near

Suffixes for the Anatomy of the Integumentary System

Suffix	Meaning
-al, -ar, -ous, -ic	pertaining to
-crine	to secrete
-cyte	cell
-ferous	pertaining to carrying
-ium	structure

You can review the anatomy of the integumentary system by clicking on **Body Spectrum,** then **Integumentary.**

PATHOLOGY

Skin Lesions

A skin l**esion** is any visible, localized abnormality of skin tissue. It can be described as either primary or secondary. **Primary lesions** (Fig. 4-3) are early skin changes that have not yet undergone natural evolution or change caused by manipulation. **Secondary lesions** (Fig. 4-4) are the result of natural evolution or manipulation of a primary lesion.

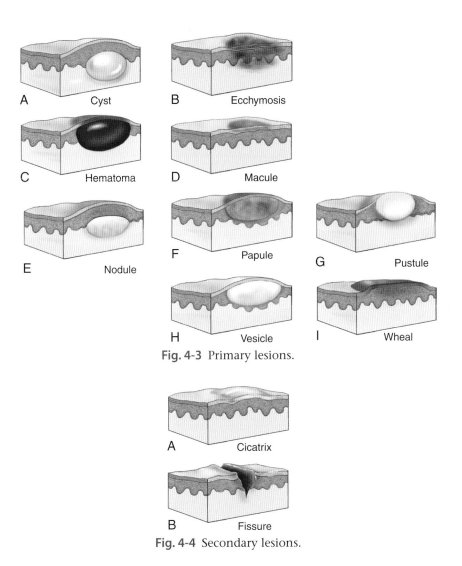

A   Cyst

B   Ecchymosis

C   Hematoma

D   Macule

E   Nodule

F   Papule

G   Pustule

H   Vesicle

I   Wheal

Fig. 4-3 Primary lesions.

A   Cicatrix

B   Fissure

Fig. 4-4 Secondary lesions.

Terms Related to Primary Skin Lesions

Term	Word Origin	Definition
cyst	*cyst/o* sac, bladder	Nodule filled with a semisolid material, such as a keratinous or sebaceous cyst (see Fig. 4-3, *A*).
ecchymosis (pl. ecchymoses)	*ec-* out *chym/o* juice *-osis* abnormal condition	Hemorrhage or extravasation (leaking) of blood into the subcutaneous tissue. The resultant darkening is commonly described as a bruise (see Fig. 4-3, *B*).
hematoma	*hemat/o* blood *-oma* mass, tumor	Collection of extravasated blood trapped in the tissues and palpable to the examiner, such as on the ear (see Fig. 4-3, *C*).
macule	*macul/o* spot *-ule* small	Flat blemish or discoloration less than 1 cm, such as a freckle, port-wine stain, or tattoo (see Fig. 4-3, *D*).
nodule	*nod/o* knot *-ule* small	Palpable, solid lesion less than 2 cm, such as a very small lipoma (fatty tumor) (see Fig. 4-3, *E*).
papule	*papul/o* pimple *-ule* small	Raised, solid skin lesion raised less than 1 cm, such as a pimple (see Fig. 4-3, *F*).
patch		Large, flat nonpalpable macule, larger than 1 cm.
petechia (pl. petechiae)		Tiny ecchymosis within the dermal layer.
plaque		Raised, plateaulike papule greater than 1 cm, such as a psoriatic lesion or seborrheic keratosis.
purpura	*purpur/o* purple *-a* noun ending	Massive hemorrhage into the tissues under the skin.
pustule	*pustul/o* pustule *-ule* small	Superficial, elevated lesion containing pus that may be the result of an infection, such as acne (see Fig. 4-3, *G*).
telangiectasia	*tel/e* far *angi/o* vessel *-ectasia* dilation	Permanent dilation of groups of superficial capillaries and venules.
tumor		Nodule more than 2 cm; any mass or swelling, including neoplasms.
vesicle	*vesicul/o* blister or small sac	Circumscribed, elevated lesion containing fluid and smaller than ½ cm, such as an insect bite. If larger than ½ cm, it is termed a **bulla**. Commonly called a **blister** (see Fig. 4-3, *H*).
wheal		Circumscribed, elevated papule caused by localized edema, which can result from a bug bite (see Fig. 4-3, *I*).

Terms Related to Secondary Skin Lesions

Term	Word Origin	Definition
atrophy	*a-* no, not, without *-trophy* process of nourishment	Paper-thin, wasted skin often occurring in the aged or as stretch marks (**striae**) from rapid weight gain.
cicatrix (pl. cicatrices)		A scar—an area of fibrous tissue that replaces normal skin after destruction of some of the dermis (see Fig. 4-4, *A*).
eschar	*eschar/o* scab	Dried serum, blood, and/or pus. May occur in inflammatory and infectious diseases, such as impetigo, or as the result of a burn. Also called a **scab**.
fissure		Cracklike lesion of the skin, such as an anal fissure (see Fig. 4-4, *B*).
keloid		Type of scar that is an overgrowth of tissue at the site of injury in excess of the amount of tissue necessary to repair the wound. The extra tissue is partially due to an accumulation of collagen at the site (Fig. 4-5).
ulcer		Circumscribed, craterlike lesion of the skin or mucous membrane resulting from **necrosis**, or tissue death, that can accompany an inflammatory, infectious, or malignant process. An example is a **pressure ulcer** seen sometimes in bedridden patients (see Fig. 4-14).

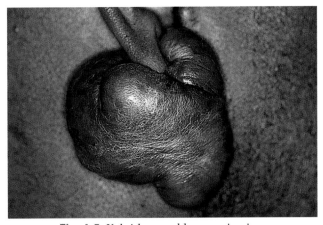

Fig. 4-5 Keloid caused by ear piercing.

Exercise 3: Skin Lesions

Match the primary lesions with their definitions.

____ 1. vesicle
____ 2. papule
____ 3. wheal
____ 4. ecchymosis
____ 5. macule
____ 6. pustule

A. extravasated blood into subcutaneous tissue caused by trauma
B. flat blemish or discoloration
C. circumscribed, raised papule
D. superficial, elevated lesion containing pus
E. circumscribed, raised lesion containing fluid
F. solid, raised skin lesion

Match the smaller version of a primary skin lesion with the larger version.

____ 7. petechia
____ 8. vesicle
____ 9. papule
____ 10. macule
____ 11. nodule

A. plaque
B. tumor
C. ecchymosis
D. bulla
E. patch

Match the secondary lesions with their definitions.

____ 12. ulcer
____ 13. cicatrix
____ 14. fissure
____ 15. atrophy
____ 16. eschar

A. paper-thin, wasted skin
B. scab
C. cracklike lesion
D. circumscribed, craterlike lesion
E. scar

Terms Related to Infections of the Skin and Subcutaneous Tissue (LØØ-LØ8) and Bullous Disorders (L1Ø-L14)

Term	Word Origin	Definition
abscess		A collection of pus in any part of the body, formed by a localized infection.
cellulitis	*cellul/o* cell *-itis* inflammation	Diffuse, spreading, acute inflammation within solid tissues. The most common cause is a *Streptococcus pyogenes* infection (Fig. 4-6).
furuncle		Localized, suppurative staphylococcal skin infection originating in a gland or hair follicle and characterized by pain, redness, and swelling (Fig. 4-7). If two or more furuncles are connected by subcutaneous pockets, it is termed a **carbuncle.**
impetigo		Superficial vesiculopustular skin infection, normally seen in children, but possible in adults (Fig. 4-8).
omphalitis	*omphal/o* navel *-itis* inflammation	Inflammation of the navel.
onychia	*onych/o* nail *-ia* condition	Inflammation of the fingernail. Also called **onychitis.**
paronychia	*par-* beside, near *onych/o* nail *-ia* condition	Infection of the skin beside the nail.
pemphigus		Autoimmune disorder characterized by large blisters of the skin and mucous membranes.
pilonidal cyst	*pil/o* hair *nid/o* nest *-al* pertaining to	Growth of hair in a cyst in the sacral region.
pyoderma	*py/o* pus *-derma* skin condition	A purulent (containing pus) bacterial skin disease.

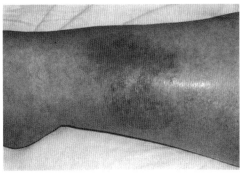

Fig. 4-6 Cellulitis of the lower leg.

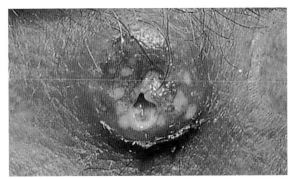

Fig. 4-7 Furuncle.

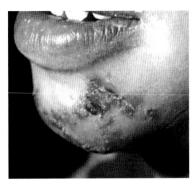

Fig. 4-8 Impetigo.

Terms Related to Dermatitis and Eczema (L20-L30)

Term	Word Origin	Definition
atopic dermatitis	*a-* no, not, without *top/o* place, location *-ic* pertaining to *dermat/o* skin *-itis* inflammation	Chronic, pruritic (itchy), superficial inflammation of the skin usually associated with a family history of allergic disorders.
contact dermatitis	*dermat/o* skin *-itis* inflammation	Irritated or allergic response of the skin that can lead to an acute or chronic inflammation (Fig. 4-9).
eczema		Superficial inflammation of the skin, characterized by vesicles, weeping, and pruritus. Also called **dermatitis.**
pruritus	*prurit/o* itching *-us* noun ending	Itching. May be described as occurring in a specific body area (e.g., ani, scroti, vulvae).
seborrheic dermatitis	*seb/o* sebum *-rrheic* pertaining to discharge *dermat/o* skin *-itis* inflammation	Inflammatory scaling disease of the scalp and face. In newborns, this is known as **cradle cap** or **seborrheic capitis.**

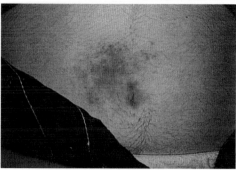

Fig. 4-9 Contact dermatitis caused by allergy to metal snap on pants.

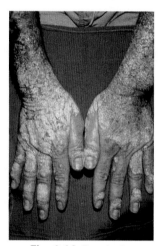

Fig. 4-10 Psoriasis.

Terms Related to Papulosquamous (L40-L45) Urticaria and Erythema (L49-L54) and Radiation-Related Disorders of the Skin and Subcutaneous Tissue (L55-L59)

Term	Word Origin	Definition
actinic keratosis	*act/i* rays *-in* substance *-ic* pertaining to *kerat/o* hard, horny *-osis* abnormal condition	Skin lesions caused by prolonged sun exposure.
psoriasis		Common chronic skin disorder characterized by circumscribed, salmon-red patches covered by thick, dry, silvery scales that are the result of excessive development of epithelial cells (Fig. 4-10).
urticaria		Skin condition characterized by wheals. May be caused by allergies, insect bites, drugs, or stress. Also called **hives**.

Exercise 4: Various Skin Diseases and Disorders

Fill in the blanks with the correct terms from the list below.

cellulitis	**pemphigus**	**contact dermatitis**	**psoriasis**
furuncle	**pilonidal cyst**	**seborrheic dermatitis**	**urticaria**
impetigo	**atopic dermatitis**	**pruritus**	**actinic keratosis**

1. Autoimmune skin disorder characterized by large blisters_____

2. An irritated or allergic response of the skin that can lead to an acute or chronic inflammation

    _____

3. Diffuse spreading inflammation within solid tissues_____

4. Inflammatory scaling disease of the scalp and face_____

5. Term that means itching_____

6. Chronic skin disorder characterized by circumscribed salmon-red patches_____

7. Growth of hair in a cyst in the sacral region of the skin_____

8. A superficial vesiculopustular skin infection normally seen in children_____

9. Skin lesion caused by prolonged sun exposure_____

10. Skin condition characterized by wheals_____

11. Localized, suppurative staphylococcal skin infection in a gland or hair follicle _____

12. Chronic, pruritic superficial inflammation of the skin, usually associated with a family history of
    allergic disorders_____

Build the terms.

13. inflammation of the navel_____

14. pertaining to a hair nest_____

15. condition of nail_____

16. condition beside the nail_____

Terms Related to Disorders of Skin Appendages (L60-L75)

Term	Word Origin	Definition
acne vulgaris	*vulgar/o* common *-is* noun ending	Inflammatory disease of the sebaceous glands characterized by papules, pustules, inflamed nodules, and **comedones** (*sing.* **comedo**), which are plugs of sebum that partially or completely block a pore. Blackheads are open comedones, and whiteheads are closed comedones.
alopecia		Hair loss, resulting from genetic factors, aging, or disease (Fig. 4-11).
anhidrosis	*an-* no, not, without *hidr/o* sweat *-osis* abnormal condition	A condition in which a person produces little or no sweat.
bromhidrosis	*brom/o* odor, stench *hidr/o* sweat *-osis* abnormal condition	Disorder of the apocrine sweat glands; a condition of abnormal body odor. Note that the combining vowel o is dropped in this term.
folliculitis	*follicul/o* follicle *-itis* inflammation	Inflammation of the hair follicles, which may be superficial or deep, acute or chronic.
hidradenitis suppurativa	*hidraden/o* sweat gland *-itis* inflammation	Inflammation of the sweat glands (Fig. 4-12).
hyperhidrosis	*hyper-* excessive *hidr/o* sweat *-osis* abnormal condition	Excessive perspiration caused by heat, strong emotion, menopause, hyperthyroidism, or infection.
hypertrichosis	*hyper-* excessive *trich/o* hair *-osis* abnormal condition	Abnormal condition of excessive hair; also known as **hirsutism.**

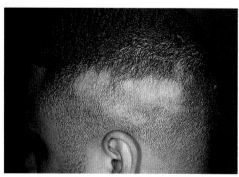

Fig. 4-11 Alopecia.

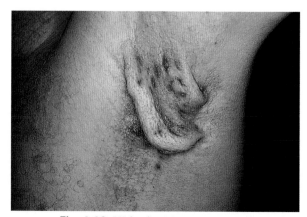

Fig. 4-12 Hidradenitis suppurativa.

Terms Related to Disorders of Skin Appendages (L60-L75)—cont'd

Term	Word Origin	Definition
keratinous cyst	*kerat/o* hard, horny *-in* substance *-ous* pertaining to	Benign cavity lined by keratinizing epithelium and filled with sebum and epithelial debris. Also called a **sebaceous cyst.**
milia		Tiny, superficial keratinous cysts caused by clogged oil ducts.
miliaria		Minute vesicles and papules, often with surrounding erythema (redness), caused by occlusion of sweat ducts during times of exposure to heat and high humidity.
onychocryptosis	*onych/o* nail *crypt-* hidden *-osis* abnormal condition	Abnormal condition of hidden (ingrown) nail.
onychodystrophy	*onych/o* nail *dys-* abnormal *-trophy* nourishment, development	Abnormally developed fingernails or toenails.
onychogryphosis	*onych/o* nail *gryph/o* curved *-osis* abnormal condition	Abnormally thickened and curved fingernails or toenails.
onycholysis	*onych/o* nail *-lysis* loosening	Separation of the nail plate from the nail bed (Fig. 4-13).
onychomalacia	*onych/o* nail *-malacia* softening	Softening of the nails.
poliosis	*poli/o* gray *-osis* abnormal condition	Localized patch of gray or white hair due to lack of melanin caused by disease.

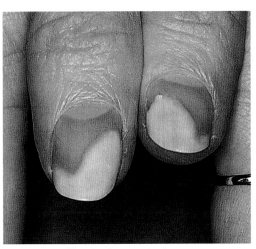

Fig. 4-13 Onycholysis.

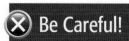 **Be Careful!**   **Paronychium** *is the structure that surrounds the nail.*
Paronychia *is an infection of the nail.*

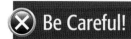 **Be Careful!**   *Don't confuse* **milia,** *a condition resulting from oil-filled ducts,*
with **miliaria,** *a condition resulting from sweat-filled ducts.*

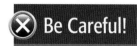 **Be Careful!**   **Hidr/o** *with an* **i** *means sweat;* **hydr/o** *with a* **y** *means water.*
Both are pronounced HYE droh.

Exercise 5: **Disorders of Skin Appendages**

Build the terms.

1. abnormal condition of curved nail _____

2. softening of the nail _____

3. abnormal condition of hidden nail _____

4. abnormal condition of excessive hair _____

5. inflammation of a hair follicle _____

6. abnormal condition of gray _____

7. abnormal condition of no sweating _____

8. abnormal condition of sweat odor _____

9. inflammation of a sweat gland _____

10. abnormal nail development _____

Terms Related to Other Disorders of the Skin and Subcutaneous Tissue (L80-L99)

Term	Word Origin	Definition
callus		Common, painless thickening of the stratum corneum at locations of external pressure or friction.
chloasma		Increased pigmentation on face, often during pregnancy. Also called **melasma** and "mask of pregnancy."
corn		Horny mass of condensed epithelial cells overlying a bony prominence as the result of pressure or friction; also referred to as a **clavus**.
discoid lupus erythematosus (DLE)	*disc/o* disc *-oid* like *lupus* *erythemat/o* red *-osus* pertaining to	Chronic inflammatory autoimmune condition that is limited to the skin. Characterized by red round-shaped lesions. Also referred to as **discoid erythematosus**.
dyschromia	*dys-* abnormal *chrom/o* color *-ia* condition	Abnormality of skin pigmentation. **Hyperchromia** is abnormally increased pigmentation. **Hypochromia** is abnormally decreased pigmentation.
ichthyosis	*ichthy/o* fish *-osis* abnormal condition	Category of dry skin that has the scaly appearance of a fish. It ranges from mild to severe. The mild form is known as **xeroderma**.
lentigo		Darkened macules usually caused by sun exposure. Also called **age spots** (*pl.* lentigines).
leukoderma	*leuk/o* white *-derma* skin condition	Loss of skin pigmentation.
pressure ulcer		Inflammation, ulcer, or sore in the skin over a bony prominence, such as an elbow, ankle, hip, or heel. Most often seen in aged, debilitated, cachectic (wasted), or immobilized patients; pressure sores or ulcers are graded by stages of severity. Also known as a **bedsore, decubitus ulcer, or pressure sore** (Fig. 4-14). **Stage 1** pressure ulcers are characterized by inflammation in the epidermis and/or dermis with focal (localized) edema and redness. **Stage 2** pressure ulcers have partial thickness (epidermis and dermis) involvement with a break in the surface of the skin. The shallow ulcer that results may be accompanied by blisters and a serous (watery) discharge. **Stage 3** pressure ulcers have full-thickness (epidermis, dermis, and subcutaneous tissue) involvement with skin loss, redness, and a purulent (pus-filled) discharge. **Stage 4** pressure ulcers have full-thickness skin loss with necrosis that descends through to the muscles, tendons, and bone.

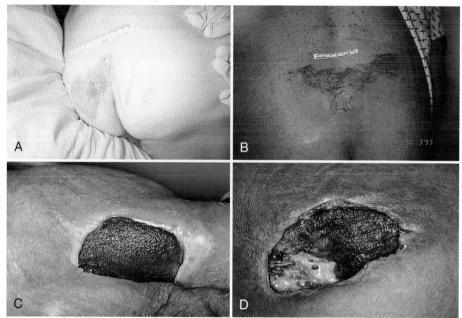

Fig. 4-14 A, Stage 1 pressure ulcer. **B,** Stage 2 pressure ulcer. **C,** Stage 3 pressure ulcer. **D,** Stage 4 pressure ulcer.

Terms Related to Other Disorders of the Skin and Subcutaneous Tissue (L80-L99)—cont'd

Term	Word Origin	Definition
seborrheic keratosis	*seb/o* sebum *-rrheic* pertaining to discharge *kerat/o* hard, horny *-osis* abnormal condition	Benign circumscribed, pigmented, superficial warty skin lesion.
skin tags		Small soft, pedunculated (with a stalk) lesions that are harmless outgrowths of epidermal and dermal tissue, usually occurring on the neck, eyelids, armpits, and groin; usually occur in multiples. Also known as **acrochordons** (Fig. 4-15).
vitiligo		Benign acquired disease of unknown origin, consisting of irregular patches of various sizes lacking in pigment (Fig. 4-16).
xerosis cutis	*xer/o* dry *-osis* abnormal condition *cut/o* skin *-is* noun ending	Dry skin

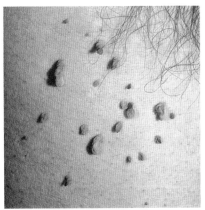

Fig. 4-15 Skin tags (acrochordons).

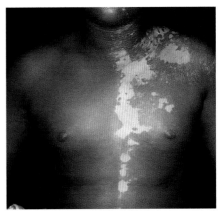

Fig. 4-16 Vitiligo.

CM Guideline Alert

C12.a1. PRESSURE ULCER STAGE CODES
1) Pressure Ulcer Stages
Codes from category L89, Pressure ulcer, are combination codes that identify the site of the pressure ulcer as well as the stage of the ulcer.

The ICD-10-CM classifies pressure ulcer stages based on severity, which is designated by stages 1-4, unspecified stage, and unstageable.

Assign as many codes from category L89 as needed to identify all the pressure ulcers the patient has, if applicable.

CPT Coding Alert!

CPT codes the removal of skin tags by the *number* removed, with one code for up to 15 removed and a separate add-on code for each additional 10.

Exercise 6: Other Disorders of the Skin and Subcutaneous Tissue

Match the terms to their definitions.

_____ 1. callus
_____ 2. pressure ulcer
_____ 3. corn
_____ 4. leukoderma
_____ 5. discoid lupus erythematosus
_____ 6. chloasma
_____ 7. dyschromia
_____ 8. ichthyosis
_____ 9. vitiligo
_____ 10. lentigo

A. dry, scaly skin
B. age spot
C. "mask of pregnancy"
D. irregular patches of loss of pigment
E. abnormality of skin pigmentation
F. common thickening of stratum corneum
G. clavus, mass of cells over a bony prominence
H. bedsore
I. loss of skin pigmentation
J. autoimmune skin disorder

Terms Related to Viral Infections Characterized by Skin and Mucous Membrane Lesions (B00-B09)

Term	Word Origin	Definition
exanthematous diseases	*exanthemat/o* rash *-ous* pertaining to	Generally, viral diseases characterized by a specific type of rash **(exanthem)**. The main ones are measles, rubella, fifth disease, roseola, and chicken pox.
herpes simplex virus (HSV)		Viral infection characterized by clusters of small vesicles filled with clear fluid on raised inflammatory bases on the skin or mucosa. HSV-1 causes fever blisters **(herpetic stomatitis)** and **keratitis,** an inflammation of the cornea. HSV-2 is more commonly known as **genital herpes**.
herpes zoster		Acute, painful rash caused by reactivation of the latent varicella-zoster virus. Also known as **shingles** (Fig. 4-17).
verruca *(pl.* verrucae)		Common contagious epithelial growths usually appearing on the skin of the hands, feet, legs, and face; can be caused by any of 60 types of the human papillomavirus (HPV) (Fig. 4-18). Also called **warts.**

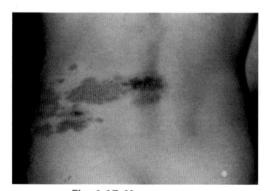

Fig. 4-17 Herpes zoster.

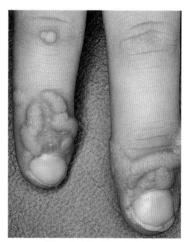

Fig. 4-18 Verruca.

Terms Related to Mycoses (B35-B49)

Term	Word Origin	Definition
candidiasis		Yeast infection in moist, occluded areas of the skin (armpits, inner thighs, underneath pendulous breasts) and mucous membranes. Also called **moniliasis.**
dermatomycosis	*dermat/o* skin *myc/o* fungus *-osis* abnormal condition	Fungal infection of the skin. Also called **dermatophytosis.**
onychomycosis	*onych/o* nail *myc/o* fungus *-osis* abnormal condition	Abnormal condition of nail fungus. Also called **tinea unguium** (Fig. 4-19).
tinea capitis	*capit/o* head *-is* structure	Fungal infection of the scalp; also known as **scalp ringworm.**
tinea corporis	*corpor/o* body *-is* structure	Ringworm of the body, manifested by pink to red papulosquamous annular (ringlike) plaques with raised borders; also known as **ringworm** (Fig. 4-20).
tinea cruris	*crur/o* leg *-is* structure	A fungal infection that occurs mainly on external genitalia and upper legs in males, particularly in warm weather; also known as **jock itch.**
tinea pedis	*ped/o* foot *-is* structure	Fungal infection of the foot; also known as **athlete's foot.**

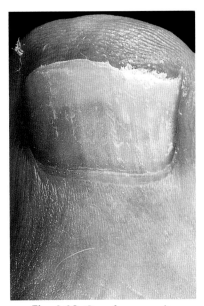

Fig. 4-19 Onychomycosis.

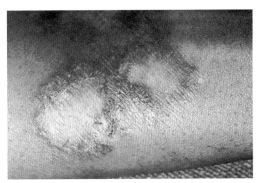

Fig. 4-20 Tinea corporis.

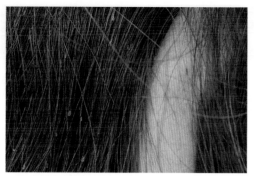

Fig. 4-21 Pediculosis.

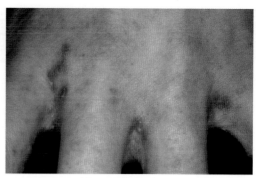

Fig. 4-22 Scabies.

Terms Related to Pediculosis, Acariasis, and Other Infestations (B85-B89)		
Term	Word Origin	Definition
pediculosis	*pedicul/i* lice *-osis* abnormal condition	Parasitic infestation with lice, involving the head, body, or genital area (Fig. 4-21).
scabies		Parasitic infestation caused by mites; characterized by pruritic papular rash (Fig. 4-22).

Exercise 7: Viral Infections, Mycoses, and Infestations

Match these fungal or yeast infections with their definitions or synonyms.

____ 1. athlete's foot

____ 2. ringworm of scalp

____ 3. moniliasis

____ 4. jock itch

____ 5. rash

____ 6. ringworm of body

____ 7. shingles

____ 8. warts

A. tinea corporis

B. tinea cruris

C. tinea capitis

D. tinea pedis

E. verrucae

F. candidiasis

G. herpes zoster

H. exanthem

Build the healthcare term.

9. infestation with lice

_____

10. virus causing herpetic stomatitis

_____

11. infestation with mites

_____

12. fungal infection of the skin

_____

CM Guideline Alert

C19.d. Coding of Burns and Corrosions
The ICD-10-CM makes a distinction between burns and corrosions. The burn codes are for thermal burns, except sunburns, that come from a heat source, such as a fire or hot appliance. The burn codes are also for burns resulting from electricity and radiation. Corrosions are burns due to chemicals. The guidelines are the same for burns and corrosions.

Current burns (T20-T25) are classified by depth, extent, and by agent (X code). Burns are classified by depth as first degree (erythema), second degree (blistering), and third degree (full-thickness involvement). Burns of the eye and internal organs (T26-T28) are classified by site, but not by degree.

 CM Guideline Alert

19a. Code Extensions
Most categories in Chapter 19 have 7th character extensions that are required for each applicable code. Most categories in this chapter have three extensions (with the exception of fractures): A, initial encounter, D, subsequent encounter, and S, sequela.*

*See Chapter 3, page 109, for the rest of this guideline.

Burns

Burns are injuries to tissues that result from exposure to thermal, chemical, electrical, or radioactive agents (covered in the Injury, Poisoning and Certain Other Consequences of External Causes). They may be classified into four different degrees of severity, depending on the layers of the skin that are damaged. Coders must categorize burns higher than second degree according to the "rule of nines" (Fig. 4-23) that divides the body into percentages that are, for the most part, multiples of nine: the head and neck equal 9%, each upper limb 9%, each lower limb 18%, the front and back of the torso 36%, and the genital area 1%. Fig. 4-24 is an illustration of the different degrees of burns.
- **Superficial burn:** Burn in which only the first layer of the skin, the epidermis, is damaged; also known as a **first-degree burn.** Characterized by redness (erythema), tenderness, and hyperesthesia (extreme sensitivity), with no scar development. (See Fig. 4-25, *A*.)

hyperesthesia
hyper- = excessive
esthesi/o = feeling, sensation
-ia = condition

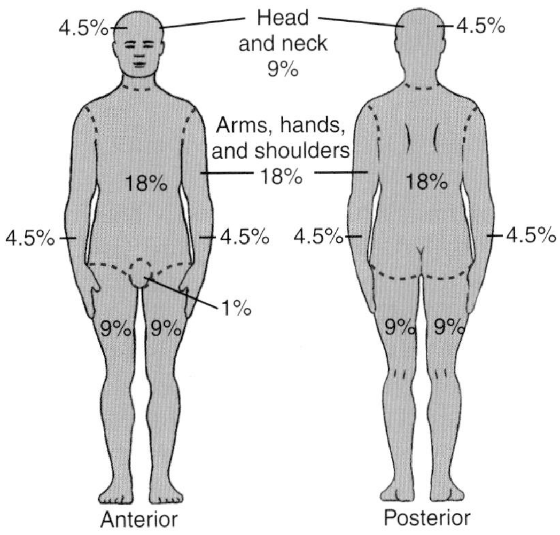

Fig. 4-23 Rule of nines for estimating extent of burns.

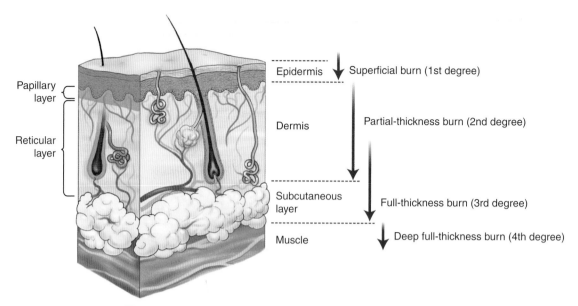

Fig. 4-24 Degrees of burns and depth of tissue involvement.

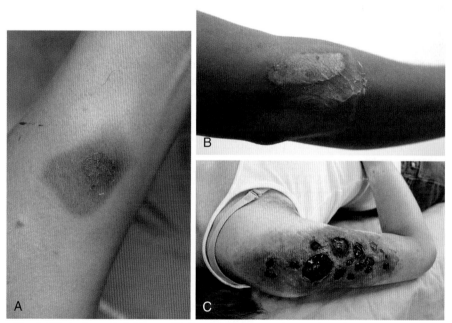

Fig. 4-25 A, Superficial burn. **B,** Partial-thickness burn. **C,** Full-thickness burn.

- **Partial-thickness burn:** Burn in which only the first and second layers of the skin (epidermis and part of the dermis) are affected; sometimes called a **second-degree burn.** If the burn extends to the papillary level, it is classified as a **superficial partial-thickness burn.** If it extends farther, to the reticular layer, it is classified as a **deep partial-thickness burn.** Characterized by redness, blisters, and pain, with possible scar development. (See Fig. 4-25, *B.*)
- **Full-thickness burn:** Burn that damages the epidermis, dermis, and subcutaneous tissue; also known as a **third-degree burn.** Pain is not present because the nerve endings in the skin have been destroyed. Skin appearance may be deep red, pale gray, brown, or black. Scar formation is likely. (See Fig. 4-25, *C.*)

- **Deep full-thickness burn:** Although not a universally accepted category, some burn specialists use this category to describe a rare burn that extends beyond the subcutaneous tissue into the muscle and bone. Also called a **fourth-degree burn.**

 Exercise 8: Burns

Match the characteristics of the burns listed with their degree.

____ 1. superficial
____ 2. partial thickness
____ 3. full thickness
____ 4. deep full thickness

A. Ironing a blouse for work, Rhonda burned her hand, resulting in blisters and erythema.
B. John suffered burns over two thirds of his body with many areas of tissue burned to the bone.
C. Because Kristin forgot to reapply her sunblock, she sustained a sunburn that resulted in painful, reddened skin.
D. Smoking in bed resulted in burns that destroyed the epidermis and dermis and extended through the hypodermis on the victim's chest and shoulders.

Terms Related to Benign Skin Growths (D10-D36)

Term	Word Origin	Definition
angioma	*angi/o* vessel *-oma* tumor, mass	Localized vascular lesion that includes **hemangiomas** (Fig. 4-26), **vascular nevi**, and **lymphangiomas**.
dermatofibroma	*dermat/o* skin *fibr/o* fiber *-oma* tumor, mass	Fibrous tumor of the skin that is painless, round, firm, and usually found on the extremities.
dysplastic nevus (*pl.* nevi)	*dys-* abnormal *plast/o* formation *-ic* pertaining to *nev/o* birthmark *-us* structure, thing	A nevus is a pigmented lesion often present at birth. It is also called a **mole.** Various abnormal changes of a pigmented congenital skin blemish give rise to concern for progression to malignancy. Changes of concern are categorized as ABCDE. **A**symmetry **B**orders, irregular **C**olors, changes or uneven pigmentation **Di**ameter, increasing size or >6 mm **E**volution, refers to change over recent weeks or months
lipoma	*lip/o* fat *-oma* tumor, mass	Fatty tumor that is a soft, movable subcutaneous nodule (Fig. 4-27).

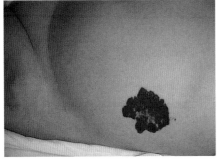

Fig. 4-26 Hemangioma.

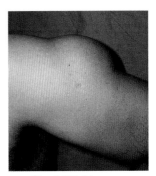

Fig. 4-27 Lipoma.

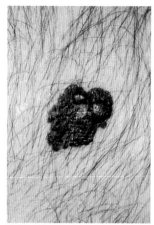

Fig. 4-28 Malignant melanoma on arm.

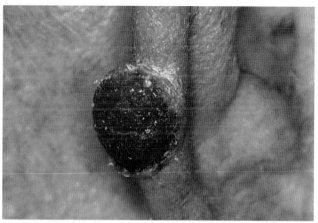

Fig. 4-29 Squamous cell carcinoma on the ear.

Terms Related to Malignant Neoplasms (C00-C96)

Term	Word Origin	Definition
basal cell carcinoma (BCC)	*bas/o* base *-al* pertaining to *carcinoma* cancer of epithelial origin	The most common form of skin cancer, it originates in the stratum germinativum of the epidermis. It usually occurs on the face as a result of sun exposure and rarely metastasizes (spreads to distant sites).
Kaposi's sarcoma (KS)	*sarcoma* connective tissue cancer	A rare form of skin cancer that takes the form of red/blue/brown/purple nodules, usually on the extremities. One form appears most often in patients with deficient immune systems.
malignant melanoma	*melan/o* black, dark *-oma* tumor, mass	This cancerous tumor arises from mutated melanocytes. This particular cancer is the leading cause of death from all skin diseases (Fig. 4-28).
Merkel cell carcinoma		A rare cancer of Merkel cells that may occur as the result of sun exposure or a weakened immune system.
squamous cell carcinoma (SCC)	*squam/o* scaly *-ous* pertaining to *carcinoma* cancer of epithelial origin	The second most common type of skin cancer, also caused by sun exposure, but developing from squamous cells (Fig. 4-29).

Exercise 9: Benign Skin Growths and Malignant Neoplasms

Match the malignant neoplasms to their definitions.

____ 1. squamous cell carcinoma

____ 2. Kaposi's sarcoma

____ 3. basal cell carcinoma

____ 4. malignant melanoma

A. most common type of skin cancer, derived from basal level of epidermis; rarely metastasizes

B. cancer arising from mutated pigment cells

C. malignancy of squamous skin cells

D. rare form of skin cancer that appears most often in patients with deficient immune systems

Translate the terms.

5. dermatofibroma _____

6. angioma _____

7. lipoma _____

PROCEDURES

Biopsy procedures are coded using the root operations Excision, Extraction, or Drainage and the qualifier Diagnostic.

 PCS Guideline Alert

B4.3 Bilateral body part values are available for a limited number of body parts. If the identical procedure is performed on the contralateral body parts and a bilateral body part value exists for that body part, a single procedure is coded using the bilateral body part value. If no bilateral body part value exists, code each procedure separately using the appropriate body part value.

 PCS Guideline Alert

B4.6 If a procedure is performed on the skin, subcutaneous tissue, or fascia overlying a joint, the procedure is coded to the following body part:
• Shoulder is coded to Upper Arm
• Elbow is coded to Lower Arm
• Wrist is coded to Lower Arm
• Hip is coded to Upper Leg
• Knee is coded to Lower Leg
• Ankle is coded to Foot

 PCS Guideline Alert

B3.4 If a diagnostic Excision, Extraction, or Drainage procedure (biopsy) is followed by a more definitive procedure, such as Destruction, Excision, or Resection at the same procedure site, both the biopsy and the more definitive treatment are coded.

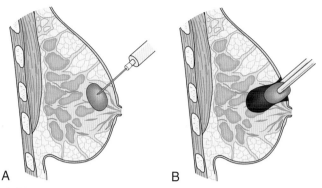

A,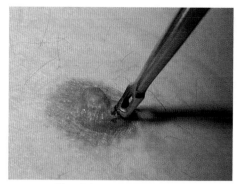

Fig. 4-30 **A,** Fine needle aspiration of the breast, **B,** Excisional biopsy of the breast.

Fig. 4-31 Punch biopsy.

Terms Related to Biopsies

Term	Word Origin	Definition
core biopsy		Sampling of tissue with a needle to withdraw tissue from the epidermis and dermis for diagnostic purposes. Samples from core needle biopsies collect tissue to be sent to the lab to determine its histology, while fine needle aspiration collects cells to be sent to cytology to determine cellular abnormalities.
excisional biopsy		Biopsy (bx) in which the entire tumor may be removed with borders as a means of diagnosis and treatment.
exfoliation		Scraping or shaving off samples of friable (easily crushed) lesions for a laboratory examination called **exfoliative cytology.**
fine needle aspiration (FNA)		Aspiration of fluid from lesions to obtain samples of fluid and cells for culture and examination using a thin needle. Coders must note if imaging guidance is used and if so, which type (ultrasound, fluoroscopic, CT, or MRI). (Fig. 4-30).
incisional biopsy		Biopsy in which large tissue samples may be obtained by excising a wedge of tissue and suturing the incision.
punch biopsy		Biopsy in which a tubular punch is inserted through to the subcutaneous tissue, and the tissue is cut off at the base (Fig. 4-31).

Terms Related to Laboratory Tests

Term	Word Origin	Definition
bacterial analyses		Culture and serology of lesions to help diagnose such disorders as impetigo.
fungal tests		Cultures of scrapings of lesions used to identify fungal infections, such as tinea pedis, tinea capitis, and tinea cruris.
sweat tests		Laboratory test for abnormally high levels of sodium and chloride present in the perspiration of persons with cystic fibrosis.
tuberculosis (TB) skin tests		Intradermal test (e.g., **Mantoux test**) using purified protein derivative (PPD) to test for either dormant or active tuberculosis; much more accurate test than the multiple puncture tine test, which had been used for screening purposes (Fig. 4-32).
Tzanck test		Microscopic examination of lesions for the purpose of diagnosing herpes zoster and herpes simplex.
viral culture		Sampling of vesicular fluid for the purpose of identifying viruses.

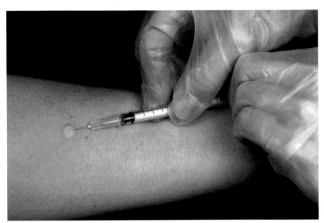

Fig. 4-32 Mantoux test. The technician is in the process of correctly placing a Mantoux tuberculin skin test in the recipient's forearm, which will cause a 6- to 10-mm wheal (i.e., a raised area of skin surface) to form at the injection site.

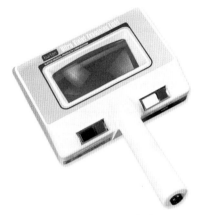

Fig. 4-33 Wood's light.

Terms Related to Laboratory Tests—cont'd		
Term	Word Origin	Definition
Wood's light examination		Method used to identify a variety of skin infections through the use of a Wood's light, which produces ultraviolet light; tinea capitis and *Pseudomonas* infections in burns are two of the disorders it can reveal (Fig. 4-33).
wound and abscess cultures		Lab samplings that can identify pathogens in wounds, such as diabetic or decubitus ulcers, postoperative wounds, or abscesses.

Exercise 10: Biopsies and Laboratory Tests

Fill in the blanks with the correct terms from the list below.

excisional   **incisional**   **punch**

exfoliation   **needle aspiration**

1. An entire tumor is removed in a/an _____ biopsy.

2. Fluid from a lesion is aspirated to obtain samples for culture in a/an _____ biopsy.

3. A wedge of tissue is removed and the incision is sutured in a/an _____ biopsy.

4. Samples of friable lesions are scraped or shaved off in _____.

5. A cylindrical punch is inserted into the subcutaneous tissue layer, and the tissue is cut off at the base in a/an _____ biopsy.

Match the following disorders with the tests that may be used to diagnose them.

_____ 6. ringworm
_____ 7. impetigo
_____ 8. cystic fibrosis
_____ 9. tuberculosis
_____ 10. herpes zoster simplex
_____ 11. *Pseudomonas*
_____ 12. bedsore, infection

A. Wood's light examination
B. Mantoux test
C. bacterial analysis
D. wound and abscess culture
E. sweat test
F. fungal test
G. Tzanck test

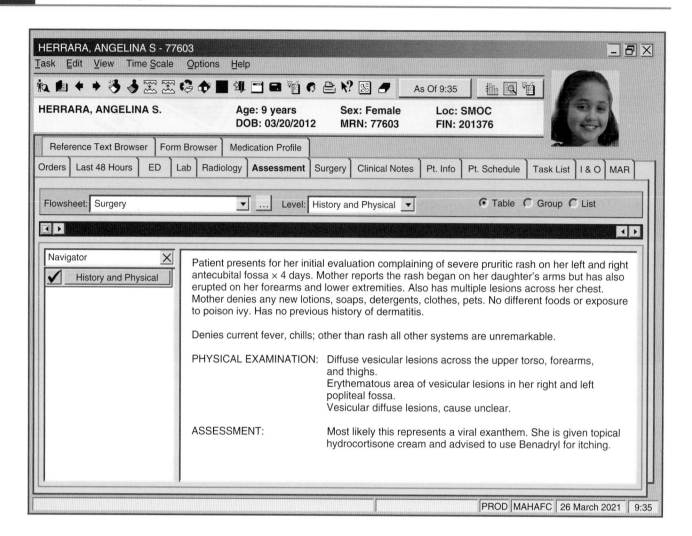

HERRARA, ANGELINA S - 77603

Task   Edit   View   Time Scale   Options   Help

HERRARA, ANGELINA S.

Age: 9 years   Sex: Female   Loc: SMOC
DOB: 03/20/2012   MRN: 77603   FIN: 201376

As Of 9:35

Reference Text Browser | Form Browser | Medication Profile

Orders | Last 48 Hours | ED | Lab | Radiology | **Assessment** | Surgery | Clinical Notes | Pt. Info | Pt. Schedule | Task List | I & O | MAR

Flowsheet: Surgery   Level: History and Physical   ◉ Table ○ Group ○ List

Navigator

✔ History and Physical

Patient presents for her initial evaluation complaining of severe pruritic rash on her left and right antecubital fossa × 4 days. Mother reports the rash began on her daughter's arms but has also erupted on her forearms and lower extremities. Also has multiple lesions across her chest. Mother denies any new lotions, soaps, detergents, clothes, pets. No different foods or exposure to poison ivy. Has no previous history of dermatitis.

Denies current fever, chills; other than rash all other systems are unremarkable.

PHYSICAL EXAMINATION: Diffuse vesicular lesions across the upper torso, forearms, and thighs.
Erythematous area of vesicular lesions in her right and left popliteal fossa.
Vesicular diffuse lesions, cause unclear.

ASSESSMENT: Most likely this represents a viral exanthem. She is given topical hydrocortisone cream and advised to use Benadryl for itching.

PROD | MAHAFC | 26 March 2021 | 9:35

 Exercise 11: **Progress Note**

Review the progress note above and answer the following questions.

1. How do we know that her rash is itchy?

_____

2. What phrase tells us that she has had no skin inflammations diagnosed in the past?

_____

3. What characteristic would "vesicular" lesions have?

_____

4. "Exanthem" is a medical term for what?

_____

The work of replacing skin can be a complicated procedure including several separate activities. Two types of surgical replacement can include grafts and flaps. The use of a flap as replacement tissue means that it has an intact blood supply (because it comes from the patient's own body). Grafts, however, do not have an intact blood supply. They can be from an identical twin (isograft), another person (allograft), another species (xenograft), or, again, the patient herself (autograft).

Terms Related to Grafting Techniques and Other Therapies

Term	Word Origin	Definition
allograft	*allo-* other	Harvest of skin from another human donor for temporary transplant until an autograft is available. Also called a **homograft.**
autograft	*auto-* self	Harvest of the patient's own skin for transplant (Fig. 4-34).
dermatome	*dermat/o* skin *-tome* instrument to cut	Instrument used to remove split-skin grafts (Fig. 4-35).
flap		Section of skin transferred from one location to an immediately adjacent one. Also called a **skin graft.**
laser therapy		Procedure to repair or destroy tissue, particularly in the removal of tattoos, warts, port-wine stains, and psoriatic lesions.
occlusive therapy	*occlus/o* to close *-ive* pertaining to	Use of a nonporous, occlusive dressing to cover a treated area to enhance the absorption and effectiveness of a medication; used to treat psoriasis, lupus erythematosus, and chronic hand dermatitis.
psoralen plus ultraviolet A (PUVA) therapy		Directing a type of ultraviolet light (UV) onto psoriatic lesions.

Continued

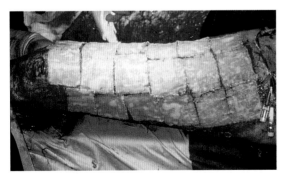

Fig. 4-34 Epithelial autografts. Thin sheets of skin are attached to gauze backing.

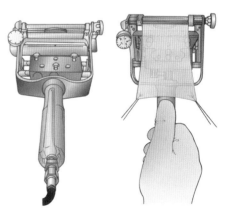

Fig. 4-35 Dermatome.

Procedures on skin and breast glands and ducts are coded to the body system Skin and Breast. Diagnoses of the breast glands, however, are classified to the Genitourinary body system in ICD-10-CM.

Terms Related to Grafting Techniques and Other Therapies—cont'd

Term	Word Origin	Definition
skin grafting (SG)		Skin transplant performed when normal skin cover has been lost as a result of burns, ulcers, or operations to remove cancerous tissue
full-thickness graft		Free skin graft in which full portions of both the epidermis and the dermis are used.
split-thickness skin graft (STSG)		Skin graft in which the epidermis and parts of the dermis are used
xenograft	*xen/o* foreign	Temporary skin graft from another species, often a pig, used until an autograft is available. Also called a **heterograft.**

CPT Coding Alert!

Adjacent tissue repairs in CPT specify the location and size, while skin replacement surgery includes the source of the grafts used.

Terms Related to Tissue Removal and Other Procedures

Term	Word Origin	Definition
cauterization	*cauter/i* burn *-zation* process of	Destruction of tissue by burning with heat.
cryosurgery	*cry/o* extreme cold	Destruction of tissue through the use of extreme cold, usually liquid nitrogen.
curettage		Scraping of material from the wall of a cavity or other surface to obtain tissue for microscopic examination; this is done with an instrument called a **curette** (Fig. 4-36).
débridement		First step in wound treatment, involving removal of dirt, foreign bodies (FB), damaged tissue, and cellular debris from the wound or burn to prevent infection and to promote healing.

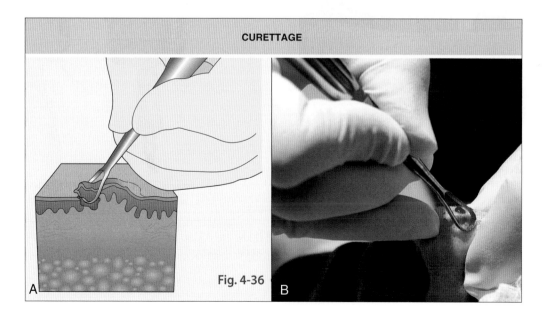

CURETTAGE

Fig. 4-36

Maps of tumor

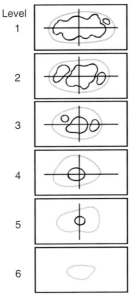

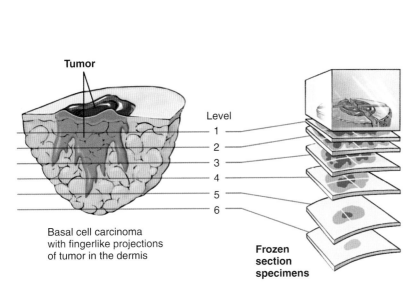

Tumor

Basal cell carcinoma
with fingerlike projections
of tumor in the dermis

Level
1
2
3
4
5
6

Frozen
section
specimens

Level
1
2
3
4
5
6

Maps
of tumor
location
drawn
from frozen
section
specimens,
indicating
areas of
remaining
tumor that
must be
removed

Fig. 4-37 Mohs surgery.

 Click on **Animations** to watch a demonstration of Mohs surgery.

Terms Related to Tissue Removal and Other Procedures—cont'd

Term	Word Origin	Definition
escharotomy	*eschar/o* scab *-tomy* cutting	Surgical incision into necrotic tissue resulting from a severe burn. This may be necessary to prevent edema leading to ischemia (loss of blood flow) in underlying tissue.
incision and drainage (I&D)		Cutting open and removing the contents of a wound, cyst, or other lesion.
Mohs surgery		Repeated removal and microscopic examination of layers of a tumor until no cancerous cells are present (Fig. 4-37).
onychectomy	*onych/o* nail *-ectomy* cutting out	Removal of nail usually to treat trauma. The procedure allows the nail to regrow normally.
onychoplasty	*onych/o* nail *-plasty* surgically forming	Surgical treatment usually including removal of the nail matrix to treat ingrown toenails.
onychotomy	*onych/o* nail *-tomy* cutting	Cutting the nail to drain the subungual hematoma.
shaving (paring)		Slicing off thin sheets of tissue to remove lesions.

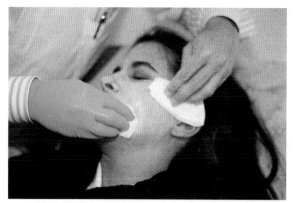

Fig. 4-38 Application of a chemical peel.

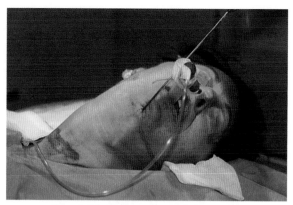

Fig. 4-39 Liposuction of the neck.

Terms Related to Cosmetic Procedures

Term	Word Origin	Definition
blepharoplasty	*blephar/o* eyelid *-plasty* surgically forming	Surgical repair of the eyelid.
chemical peel		Use of a mild acid to produce a superficial burn; normally done to remove wrinkles (Fig. 4-38).
dermabrasion	*derm/o* skin *-abrasion* scraping	Surgical procedure to resurface the skin; used to remove acne scars, nevi, wrinkles, and tattoos.
dermatoplasty	*dermat/o* skin *-plasty* surgically forming	Transplant of living skin to correct effects of injury, operation, or disease.
lipectomy	*lip/o* fat *-ectomy* cutting out	Removal of fatty tissue.
liposuction	*lip/o* fat	Technique for removing adipose tissue with a suction pump device (Fig. 4-39).
rhytidectomy	*rhytid/o* wrinkle *-ectomy* cutting out	Surgical operation to remove wrinkles. Commonly known as a "face-lift."

Exercise 12: Grafting, Tissue Removal, Cosmetic, and Other Procedures

1. Explain the differences among the following:

   A. autograft_____

   B. allograft_____

   C. xenograft_____

2. Which type of graft includes the epidermis and the dermis?_____

3. What instrument is used to cut skin for grafting?_____

Fill in the blanks with the correct terms from the list below.

cauterization	**débridement**	**occlusive therapy**
cryosurgery	**incision and drainage**	**shaving**
curettage	**laser therapy**	**Mohs surgery**

4. _____is used to destroy tattoos.

5. Removing dirt, foreign bodies, damaged tissue, and cellular debris from a wound is called _____.

6. The destruction of tissue by burning with heat is called_____.

7. The destruction of tissue through the use of extreme cold is called_____.

8. Scraping of material from the wall of a cavity is called_____.

9. I&D is_____.

10. Another term for paring is_____.

11. Covering an area to enhance absorption of medicine is called_____.

12. Removal of a tumor by layers is called_____.

Build the terms.

13. cutting out wrinkles_____

14. cutting out fat_____

15. surgically forming the eyelid_____

16. scraping of skin_____

17. surgically forming the skin_____

18. surgically forming a nail_____

PHARMACOLOGY

anesthetic agents: Cause loss of sensation; topically applied anesthetic agents act locally on affected area. Examples include lidocaine (Xylocaine) and benzocaine (Orajel).

antibacterials: Prevent and treat bacterial growth. Topical agents such as erythromycin (Erygel) and clindamycin (Benzaclin) are used to treat acne. Triple antibiotic ointment containing bacitracin, polymixin B, neomycin (Neosporin), silver sulfadiazine (Silvadene), and mupirocin (Bactroban) are used to prevent and treat skin or wound infections. Oral agents for the treatment of acne include erythromycin (Ery-Tab), tetracycline (Sumycin), and minocycline (Minocin).

antifungals: Treat fungal infections. Topical agents include nystatin (Nystop), butenafine (Lotrimin Ultra), ciclopirox (Loprox), and econazole (Ecoza).

antihistamines: Suppress the allergic response to reduce itching, redness, and swelling. Diphenhydramine (Benadryl) is available in oral and topical formulations. Other oral agents include chlorpheniramine (Chlor-Trimeton), cetirizine (Zyrtec), and loratadine (Claritin).

antiinflammatories: Reduce inflammation. Oral agents include prednisone and NSAIDs such as aspirin; topical agents include hydrocortisone (Cortizone), fluocinonide (Vanos), and triamcinolone (Kenalog).

antipsoriatics: Treat psoriasis. Examples include anthralin (Drithocreme) and calcipotriene (Dovonex).

antiseptics: Prevent infection by destroying microbials on skin or tissue surface with topical application of agent. Examples include iodine and chlorhexidine (Hibistat).

antivirals: Reduce the effect of viruses. Examples include valacyclovir (Valtrex) and acyclovir (Zovirax) for the treatment of herpes simplex virus (cold sores or genital herpes) and herpes zoster (shingles).

emollients: Soften and moisturize the skin; applied topically. Emollients come in the form of lotions, creams, ointments, and bath additives. A couple of well-known nonprescription products containing emollients are Aveeno and Eucerin.

immunomodulators or **immunosuppressants:** Agents that suppress the body's immune system. Topical agents such as pimecrolimus (Elidel) and tacrolimus (Protopic) are used to treat atopic dermatitis and eczema.

keratolytics: Break down hardened skin and shed the top layer of dead skin to treat warts, calluses, corns, acne, rosacea, or psoriasis; applied topically. Examples include salicylic acid (Compound W), podofilox (Condylox), and the alternative medicine cantharidin.

pediculicides: Destroy lice; applied topically. Examples include malathion (Ovide), lindane (Kwell), and permethrin (Nix).

protectives or **protectants:** Protect the skin against sunlight with sun protection factors (SPFs); applied topically. Common SPF active ingredients include oxybenzone and avobenzone.

psoralens: Absorb UVA (ultraviolet A) light to treat skin conditions such as eczema and psoriasis. One example is methoxsalen (Uvadex).

retinoids: Alter the growth of the top layer of skin and may be used to treat acne, reduce wrinkles, and treat psoriasis. Retinoids are derived from vitamin A. Examples include tretinoin (Retin-A), isotretinoin (Claravis), and tazarotene (Tazorac).

scabicides: Destroy mites and scabies. Examples include permethrin (Elimite) and crotamiton (Eurax).

Exercise 13: Pharmacology

Match the following pharmaceutical agents with their actions.

____ 1. softens the skin
____ 2. alters the growth of the outer layer of skin
____ 3. lessens itching
____ 4. prevents infection
____ 5. treats viral infection
____ 6. treats lice
____ 7. suppresses the immune system

A. antihistamine
B. antiseptic
C. retinoid
D. emollient
E. antiviral
F. immunomodulator
G. pediculicide

RECOGNIZING SUFFIXES FOR PCS

Now that you've finished reading about the procedures for the skin and subcutaneous tissue, take a look at this review of the *suffixes* used in their terminology. Each of these suffixes is associated with one or more root operations in the medical surgical section or one of the other categories in PCS.

Suffixes and Root Operations for the Skin and Subcutaneous Tissue

Suffix	Root Operation
-abrasion	Extraction
-ectomy	Excision, resection, alteration
-graft	Repair
-plasty	Repair, replacement, reposition, supplement
-tomy	Drainage

Abbreviations

Abbreviation	Meaning	Abbreviation	Meaning
BCC	basal cell carcinoma	KS	Kaposi's sarcoma
bx	biopsy	PPD	purified protein derivative
DLE	discoid lupus erythematosus	PUVA	psoralen plus ultraviolet A
FB	foreign body	SCC	squamous cell carcinoma
FNA	fine needle aspiration	SG	skin graft
HPV	human papillomavirus	STSG	split-thickness skin graft
HSV-1	herpes simplex virus 1	TB	tuberculosis
HSV-2	herpes simplex virus 2		
I&D	incision and drainage		

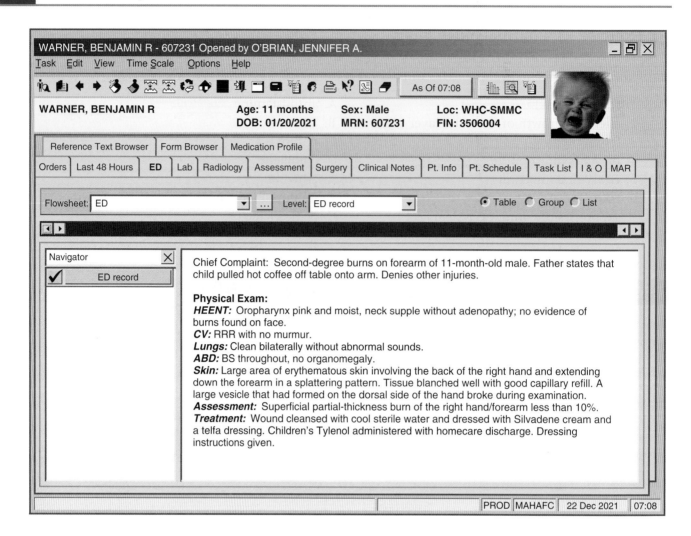

WARNER, BENJAMIN R - 607231 Opened by O'BRIAN, JENNIFER A.

Task Edit View Time Scale Options Help

WARNER, BENJAMIN R

| Age: 11 months | Sex: Male | Loc: WHC-SMMC |
| DOB: 01/20/2021 | MRN: 607231 | FIN: 3506004 |

Reference Text Browser | Form Browser | Medication Profile

Orders | Last 48 Hours | **ED** | Lab | Radiology | Assessment | Surgery | Clinical Notes | Pt. Info | Pt. Schedule | Task List | I & O | MAR

Flowsheet: ED   Level: ED record   ⦿ Table ○ Group ○ List

Navigator

✓   ED record

Chief Complaint: Second-degree burns on forearm of 11-month-old male. Father states that child pulled hot coffee off table onto arm. Denies other injuries.

Physical Exam:
HEENT: Oropharynx pink and moist, neck supple without adenopathy; no evidence of burns found on face.
CV: RRR with no murmur.
Lungs: Clean bilaterally without abnormal sounds.
ABD: BS throughout, no organomegaly.
Skin: Large area of erythematous skin involving the back of the right hand and extending down the forearm in a splattering pattern. Tissue blanched well with good capillary refill. A large vesicle that had formed on the dorsal side of the hand broke during examination.
Assessment: Superficial partial-thickness burn of the right hand/forearm less than 10%.
Treatment: Wound cleansed with cool sterile water and dressed with Silvadene cream and a telfa dressing. Children's Tylenol administered with homecare discharge. Dressing instructions given.

| PROD | MAHAFC | 22 Dec 2021 | 07:08 |

 Exercise 14: ED Record

Using the ED record above, answer the questions below.

1. Describe a superficial partial-thickness burn._____

_____

2. What are the characteristics that make this a second-degree burn?

_____

3. What is a vesicle?

_____

Go to the Evolve website to interactively build terms, label images, memorize word parts and practice using integumentary terms in context.

Match the word parts to their definitions.

WORD PART DEFINITIONS

Prefix/Suffix
crypt-
-derma
hyper-
-itis
-lysis
-oma
-osis
par-
-trophy
-ule

	Definition
1. _____	excessive
2. _____	abnormal condition
3. _____	loosening
4. _____	tumor, mass
5. _____	small
6. _____	hidden
7. _____	skin condition
8. _____	inflammation
9. _____	beside, near
10. _____	development, nourishment

Combining Form
adip/o
chrom/o
cutane/o
eschar/o
follicul/o
hidr/o
hidraden/o
kerat/o
macul/o
melan/o
myc/o
onych/o
papul/o
pedicul/i
pil/o
rhytid/o
seb/o
squam/o
ungu/o
vascul/o
vesicul/o
xer/o

	Definition
11. _____	sweat
12. _____	black, dark
13. _____	nail
14. _____	color
15. _____	wrinkle
16. _____	follicle
17. _____	vessel
18. _____	pimple
19. _____	spot
20. _____	vesicle
21. _____	dry
22. _____	nail
23. _____	hard, horny
24. _____	sweat gland
25. _____	skin
26. _____	lice
27. _____	sebum, oil
28. _____	scab
29. _____	scaly
30. _____	hair
31. _____	fat
32. _____	fungus

WORDSHOP

Prefixes	Combining Forms	Suffixes
a-	blephar/o	-ectomy
an-	chrom/o	-ia
crypt-	cutane/o	-ic
dys-	dermat/o	-itis
hyper-	fibr/o	-lysis
par-	follicul/o	-malacia
sub-	hidr/o	-oma
	melan/o	-osis
	myc/o	-ous
	onych/o	-plasty
	rhytid/o	-rrheic
	seb/o	-stomy
	trich/o	-trophy

Build skin terms by combining the word parts above. Some word parts may be used more than once. Some may not be used at all. The number in parentheses indicates the number of word parts needed.

Definition	Term
1. abnormal condition of excessive hair (3)	
2. process of no nourishment (2)	
3. cutting out wrinkles (2)	
4. pertaining to discharge of oil (2)	
5. condition of near the nail (3)	
6. abnormal condition of no sweat (3)	
7. surgically forming the eyelid (2)	
8. softening of the nail (2)	
9. inflammation of a follicle (2)	
10. condition of abnormal color (3)	
11. pertaining to under the skin (3)	
12. abnormal condition of fungus of the skin (3)	
13. tumor of skin fiber (3)	
14. loosening of the nail (2)	
15. abnormal condition of hidden nail (3)	

Sort the terms into the correct categories.

TERM SORTING

Anatomy and Physiology	Pathology	Procedures

allograft

alopecia

angioma

atrophy

blepharoplasty

corium

curettage

cuticle

cryosurgery

débridement

dermatomycosis

dermatoplasty

dermis

dyschromia

eczema

epidermis

eponychium

escharotomy

excisional bx

follicle

furuncle

hyperhidrosis

keratin

liposuction

lunula

Mantoux test

melanocyte

onychectomy

onychomycosis

papilla

paronychia

paronychium

perspiration

plaque

rhytidectomy

sebaceous gland

sebum

tinea pedis

Tzanck test

urticaria

verruca

vesicle

Wood's light

xenograft

Replace the underlined text with the correct terms.

TRANSLATIONS

1. John was treated for **athlete's foot** after a positive fungal test.

2. The patient visited her dermatologist because of **itching** due to hives.

3. Melanie said she had **an abnormal condition of excessive sweat** as the reason for her appointment with her physician.

4. Stephanie went to see her podiatrist to treat her **ingrown toenail** and asked if he could also treat her **infection of the skin beside the nail.**

5. Josh developed a/an **overgrowth of tissue** where his ear was pierced.

6. When Mia developed **a superficial vesiculopustular skin infection,** her mom noticed **superficial elevated lesions containing pus,** as well as **tiny blisters** that were characteristic of the disorder.

7. The school nurse sent a note home that said Laura had **an infestation of lice.**

8. The patient was treated for **an inflammatory disease of the sebaceous glands.**

9. The patient underwent **repeated removal and microscopic examination of tumor layers** until the dermatologist was confident that the **skin cancer of the basal layer of the epidermis** was removed.

10. The patient had a **contagious epithelial growth caused by HPV** on his hand removed with **destruction of tissue through the use of extreme cold.**

11. The burn patient was seen for **a surgical incision into necrotic tissue** and a consultation for a possible **harvest of skin from another human donor for temporary transplant.**

12. Mrs. Mooreland had **a surgical operation to remove wrinkles** and **a surgical repair of the eyelids.**

13. Mr. Kleinfelter was hospitalized for a **sore in the skin over a bony prominence.**

Digestive System

OBJECTIVES

☐ Recognize and use terms related to the anatomy and physiology of the digestive system.

☐ Recognize and use terms related to the pathology of the digestive system.

☐ Recognize and use terms related to the procedures for the digestive system.

ICD-10-CM Example from Tabular
K21 Gastro-esophageal reflux disease
   Excludes1 newborn esophageal reflux **(P78.83)**
   K21.0 Gastro-esophageal reflux disease with esophagitis
   Reflux esophagitis
   K21.9 Gastro-esophageal reflux disease without
       esophagitis
   Esophageal reflux NOS
K22 Other diseases of the esophagus
   Excludes2 esophageal varices **(I85.-)**
   K22.0 Achalasia of cardia
   Achalasia NOS
   Cardiospasm
   Excludes1 congenital cardiospasm **(Q39.5)**

ICD-10-PCS Example from Index
Duodenal ampulla
   see Ampulla of Vater
Duodenectomy
   see Excision, Duodenum **0DB9**
   see Resection, Duodenum **0DT9**
Duodenocholedochotomy
   see Drainage, Gallbladder **0F94**
Duodenocystostomy
   see Bypass, Gallbladder **0F14**
   see Drainage, Gallbladder **0F94**
Duodenoenterostomy
   see Bypass, Gastrointestinal System **0D1**
   see Drainage, Gastrointestinal System **0D9**

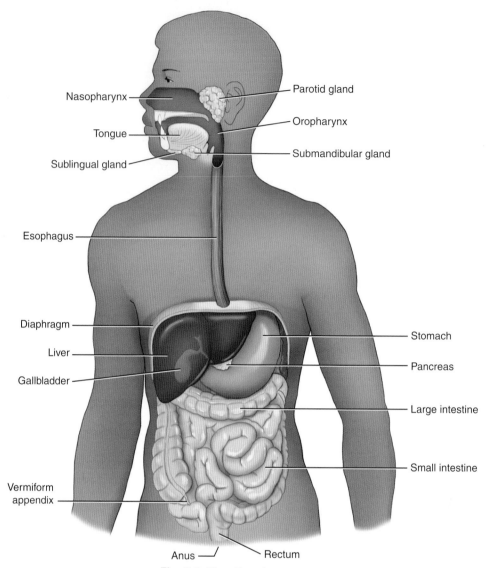

Fig. 5-1 The digestive system.

FUNCTIONS OF THE DIGESTIVE SYSTEM

The **digestive system** (Fig. 5-1) provides the nutrients needed for cells to replicate themselves continually and build new tissue. This is done through several distinct processes: *ingestion,* the intake of food; *digestion,* the mechanical and chemical breakdown of food; *absorption,* the process of extracting nutrients; and *elimination,* the excretion of any waste products. Other names for this system are the **gastrointestinal (GI) tract,** which refers to the two main parts of the system (the stomach and intestines), and the **alimentary canal,** which refers to the function of the tubelike nature of the majority of the digestive system, which starts at the mouth and continues in varying diameters to the anus.

ANATOMY AND PHYSIOLOGY

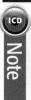

This chapter includes all the anatomy necessary to assign ICD-10 digestive codes, including detail on buccal glands, vermilion borders, and the quadrate lobe. See Appendix H for a complete list of body parts and how they should be coded.

---

gastrointestinal
　gastr/o = stomach
　intestin/o = intestines
　-al = pertaining to

alimentary
　aliment/o = nutrition
　-ary = pertaining to

Overview

The digestive system begins in the **oral cavity,** passes through the thoracic cavity in the **mediastinum,** crosses the **diaphragm** into the **abdominopelvic cavity,** and finally exits at the **anus.** Several glands and organs located in the oral and abdominopelvic cavity are instrumental in carrying out the functions of the digestive system.

Most of the alimentary canal is in four coats, or tunics: the **mucosa,** the **submucosa,** the **muscularis,** and the **serosa** (Fig. 5-2). The inner tunic is the mucosa, which secretes gastric juices, absorbs nutrients, and protects the tissue through the production of mucus, a thick, slimy emission. This membrane is lined with a single layer of epithelial tissue that is attached to a platelike layer of connective tissue, the **lamina propria.** You might want to note that the combining form *lamin/o,* used to mean a "thin plate," appears throughout many body systems. The term *propria* is from Latin and means "one's own," or "special" and is most likely used to designate this particular lamina from the many others in the body. The **submucosa,** the tunic underneath the tunica mucosa, holds blood, lymphatic, and nervous tissues that nourish, protect, and communicate. The next tunic is the muscularis, two layers of circular and longitudinal muscles that contract and relax around the tube in a wavelike movement termed **peristalsis.** If peristalsis is absent or delayed, the movement of food through the tract is impaired, causing disorders like constipation. The outermost tunic has different names in the digestive system, depending on whether it occurs within or outside the peritoneal cavity. If outside, an outer tunic covering that binds a structure together is called the **adventitia** (also **tunica externa).** The tunic within the peritoneal cavity that emits a slippery fluid to counteract friction is termed the **serosa.** The serosa and visceral peritoneum are synonymous. All of these four layers are then attached to the body wall in the peritoneum by a rich vascular membrane, which is an extension of the visceral peritoneum termed the **mesentery.**

submucosa
  sub- = under
  mucos/o = mucus

peristalsis
  peri- = surrounding
  -stalsis = contraction

viscera = **viscer/o**

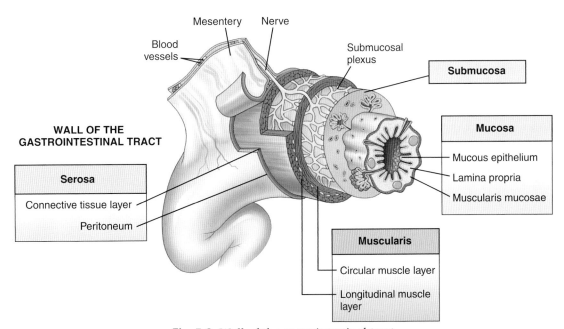

Fig. 5-2 Wall of the gastrointestinal tract.

For a demonstration of peristalsis, click on **Animations.**

Exercise 1: Overview of the Digestive System

Match the anatomy to its function.

_____ 1. muscularis
_____ 2. ingestion
_____ 3. mesentery
_____ 4. peristalsis
_____ 5. serosa
_____ 6. mucosa
_____ 7. lamina propria
_____ 8. absorption
_____ 9. alimentary
_____ 10. digestion
_____ 11. tunic/tunica
_____ 12. submucosa
_____ 13. elimination

A. excretion of waste products
B. process of extracting nutrients
C. breakdown of food
D. vascular extension of visceral peritoneum
E. wavelike movement in digestive tract
F. tunic under tunica mucosa
G. innermost mucus-secreting tunic
H. intake of food
I. small platelike connective tissue in mucosa
J. pertaining to nutrition
K. muscular tunic
L. tunic secreting watery fluid
M. coat, covering

Practice labeling the digestive system by clicking on **Label It.**

Oral Cavity

mouth, oral cavity = or/o, stomat/o, stom/o

Food normally enters the body through the **mouth,** or **oral cavity** (Fig. 5-3). The digestive function of this cavity is to break down the food mechanically by chewing **(mastication)** and lubricate the food to make swallowing **(deglutition)** easier.

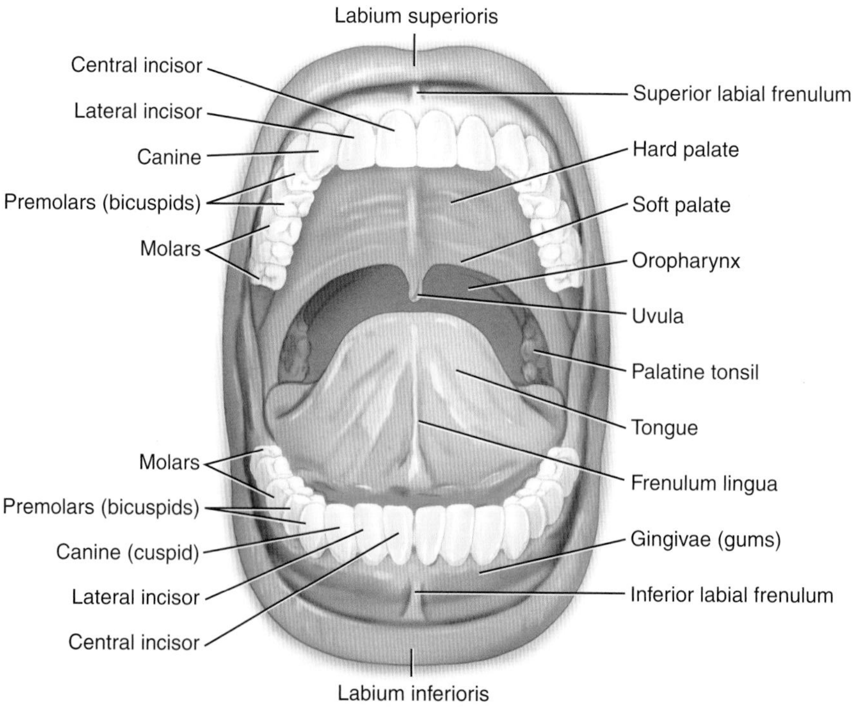

Labium superioris
Central incisor
Lateral incisor
Canine
Premolars (bicuspids)
Molars
Superior labial frenulum
Hard palate
Soft palate
Oropharynx
Uvula
Palatine tonsil
Tongue
Frenulum lingua
Gingivae (gums)
Inferior labial frenulum
Molars
Premolars (bicuspids)
Canine (cuspid)
Lateral incisor
Central incisor
Labium inferioris

Fig. 5-3 The oral cavity.

The oral cavity begins at the **lips,** the two fleshy structures surrounding its opening. The upper lip is termed the **labium superioris** and the lower lip, the **labium inferioris.** The **vermilion borders** of each are the margins between the lip and surrounding skin. The term "vermilion" shares a combining form with the vermiform appendix. Here *verm/o* refers to the dark red color of a worm, while in the appendix, the term is used to describe its shape. The **frenulum** of each lip is the small fold of tissue on the inside of each lip that restrains its movement: the **superior and inferior labial frenula.** (The term *frenulum* is derived from Latin, meaning a "bridle" as one would use to restrain the movement of a horse.) The small vertical depression above the upper lip (and under the nose) is called the **philtrum.**

lips = cheil/o, labi/o

CPT Coding Alert!

CPT specifies a vermilionectomy as a procedure to remove the colored portion of the lips for therapeutic (in the case of actinic cheilitis [inflammation of lips by long-term sun exposure] or cancer) or cosmetic surgery. Also known as a lip shave.

The sides of the face and inside of the mouth are bounded by the cheeks, which are covered by skin on the outside, a mucous membrane on the inside, and muscles, fat, nerves, and glands in between. Several glands secrete mucus in the oral cavity: buccal, molar, palatine, and labial. The **buccal glands** are located throughout the inner cheek wall, while the **molar glands** are on the cheek near the back teeth. The **labial glands** are located inside the lips and surrounding the mouth, and the **palatine glands** surround the soft roof in the back of the mouth.

cheek = bucc/o

The **tongue,** the muscular organ in the oral cavity, is responsible for tasting, chewing, swallowing, and speaking. It is attached in the front to the floor of the mouth by the **frenulum lingua,** a small fold of tissue under the tongue and in the back to the hyoid bone. The tongue is coated in a mucous membrane studded with thousands of tiny projections called **papillae.** In between the papillae are nervelike cells called **taste buds** that have receptors for the five known tastes: sour, sweet, salty, bitter, and savory (umami). The **lingual tonsil** is lymphatic tissue located at the base of the tongue that serves a protective function against pathogens attempting to enter via the mouth. The anterior **hard palate** and posterior **soft palate** form the roof of the mouth. The **uvula** is a tag of flesh that hangs down from the medial surface of the soft palate. It has a role in the production of speech and the initiation of the gag reflex.

tongue = gloss/o, lingu/o

palate = palat/o

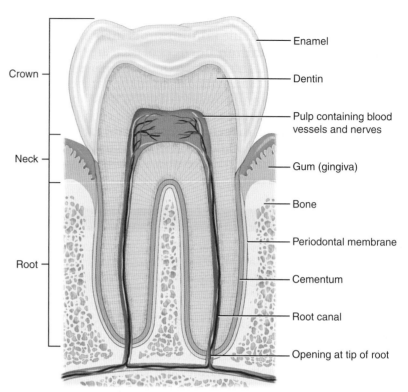

Fig. 5-4 The tooth.

 CPT Coding Alert!

CPT has a code for an operculectomy, an excision of tissue that covers an unerupted or impacted tooth (pericoronal tissues). The combining form opercul/o is from Latin meaning a *lid,* or *covering*.

upper jaw = maxill/o

lower jaw = mandibul/o

teeth = dent/i, odont/o

gums = gingiv/o

alveolus = alveol/o

enamel = amel/o

molar = mol/o

bi- = two

pre- = before

periodontal
  peri- = surrounding
  odont/o = tooth
  -al = pertaining to

salivary gland =
  sialoaden/o

saliva = sial/o, ptyal/o

parotid
  par- = near
  ot/o = ear
  -id = pertaining to

The upper and lower jaws **(maxilla** and **mandible)** hold approximately 32 permanent teeth that are set in the fleshy gums **(gingivae)** of the alveolar ridges of each bone. Each tooth sits in a small space in the bone called an **alveolus**. The thin, hard outer covering of the tooth is the **enamel,** while the **dentin** is the calcified second layer of the tooth (Fig. 5-4). The pulp is the center of the tooth with a blood and nerve supply. **Cementum** is a bonelike substance that covers the part of the tooth that is below the gums. The **crown** of the tooth is the visible enamel, the **root** is the area below the gums, and the **neck** is the area where both of these meet. The teeth are named by their function, location, or appearance. The central and lateral **incisors** are the front teeth that initially tear food to be chewed on the back teeth, the **molars** (derived from Latin for "grinding"). In between the incisors and the molars, the teeth are named for the number of points (cusps), either as **cuspids** or **bicuspids** (also called **premolars** because they are in front of the molars). Another name for the cuspids is the **canines,** because of the perceived similarity to the dentition of dogs. The upper cuspids were also called **eyeteeth,** because in the past, it was thought that the eyes and these teeth shared the same nerve supply. Molars have between 3-5 cusps, but their name is taken from their function, not the number of pointed projections. Periodontal ligaments anchor the teeth in their sockets to the alveolar bone of the upper or lower jaw. Note that the reason that periodontal disease causes a loosening of the teeth is that the tooth/bone bond has been compromised or destroyed.

The three pairs of **salivary glands** provide **saliva,** a substance that moistens the oral cavity and aids in chewing and swallowing. Saliva begins the chemical digestive process by initiating the digestion of starches. The glands are named for their locations: **parotid,** near the ear; **submandibular,** under the lower jaw; and **sublingual,** under the tongue.

Throat

The **throat,** or **pharynx,** is the passageway that connects the oral and nasal cavities with the esophagus (Fig. 5-5). It can be divided into three main parts: the **nasopharynx,** the **oropharynx,** and the **hypopharynx.** The nasopharynx is the most superior part of the pharynx, located behind the nasal cavity. The oropharynx is the part of the throat directly adjacent to the oral cavity, and the hypopharynx (also called the **laryngopharynx** because of its proximity to the larynx, which is the voice box) is the part of the throat directly below the oropharynx. The **piriform recess** (sinus or fossa) is the pear-shaped cavity in the hypopharynx near the opening to the voice box. This site is significant because food has a propensity for becoming lodged there.

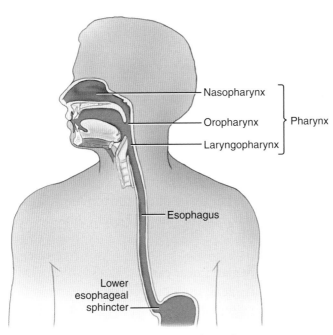

Fig. 5-5 The pharynx and esophagus.

Esophagus

The **esophagus** is a muscular, mucus-lined, approximately 12-inch tube that extends from the throat to the stomach. It carries a masticated lump of food, a **bolus,** from the oral cavity to the stomach by means of peristalsis. The glands in the lining of the esophagus produce mucus, which aids in lubricating and easing the passage of the bolus to the stomach. The muscle that must relax before the food enters the stomach is known by three names: the **lower esophageal sphincter (LES),** the **gastroesophageal sphincter,** or the **cardiac sphincter** (so named because of its proximity to the heart). Sphincters are ringlike muscles that appear throughout the digestive and other body systems. These muscles may be either voluntary or involuntary in their action.

submandibular
  sub- = under
  mandibul/o = lower jaw, mandible
  -ar = pertaining to

sublingual
  sub- = under
  lingu/o = tongue
  -al = pertaining to

pharynx (throat) = **pharyng/o**

nasopharynx
  nas/o = nose
  pharyng/o = pharynx (throat)

oropharynx
  or/o = mouth
  pharyng/o = pharynx (throat)

hypopharynx
  hypo- = below
  pharyng/o = pharynx (throat)

laryngopharynx
  laryng/o = larynx (voice box)
  pharyng/o = pharynx (throat)

esophagus = **esophag/o**

bolus = **bol/o**

Exercise 2: Oral Cavity, Throat, and Esophagus

Match the combining forms with the following definitions.

____ 1. teeth	____ 9. saliva	A. esophag/o	I. gloss/o, lingu/o
____ 2. gums	____ 10. throat	B. bucc/o	J. sial/o, ptyal/o
____ 3. roof of mouth	____ 11. esophagus	C. mandibul/o	K. pharyng/o
____ 4. tongue	____ 12. lower jaw	D. or/o, stom/o, stomat/o	L. dent/i, odont/o
____ 5. mouth	____ 13. molar	E. laryng/o	M. sialoaden/o
____ 6. lips	____ 14. upper jaw	F. palat/o	N. maxill/o
____ 7. cheek	____ 15. voice box	G. labi/o, cheil/o	O. mol/o
____ 8. salivary gland		H. gingiv/o	

 Exercise 3: Oral Cavity, Throat, and Esophagus

Match the term with its correct definition.

____ 1. deglutition

____ 2. frenulum lingua

____ 3. uvula

____ 4. mastication

____ 5. vermilion border

____ 6. cementum

____ 7. hypopharynx

____ 8. gingivae

____ 9. enamel

____ 10. premolars

____ 11. cardiac sphincter

____ 12. maxilla

____ 13. submandibular gland

____ 14. sublingual gland

____ 15. labial frenula

____ 16. cuspid

____ 17. pulp

____ 18. oropharynx

____ 19. parotid gland

____ 20. esophagus

A. chewing

B. lower esophageal sphincter

C. small fold of tissue under the tongue

D. muscular, mucus-lined 12-inch tube between throat and stomach

E. upper jaw

F. salivary gland near ear

G. salivary gland under lower jaw

H. swallowing

I. part of throat adjacent to oral cavity

J. part of throat below oral cavity, also termed laryngopharynx

K. margin between lip and surrounding skin

L. tag of flesh hanging from soft palate

M. gums

N. thin, hard outer covering of the tooth

O. salivary gland under tongue

P. pointed tooth; canine or eyetooth

Q. bonelike substance covering part of tooth below gums

R. center of tooth with blood and nerve supply

S. teeth in front of molars; bicuspids

T. fold of skin on the middle inside of top and bottom lips that restricts their movement

Practice labeling the oral cavity and the pharynx by clicking on **Label It.**

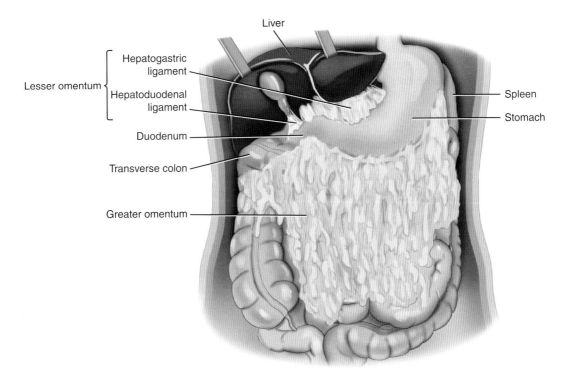

Liver

Lesser omentum { Hepatogastric ligament / Hepatoduodenal ligament

Spleen

Stomach

Duodenum

Transverse colon

Greater omentum

Fig. 5-6 The peritoneal cavity.

Peritoneum

The **peritoneum** is a double-sided membrane that holds many of the organs inside the abdominopelvic cavity. The outer side of the membrane, near the body wall, is termed the **parietal peritoneum,** whereas the inner side, near the organs, is the **visceral peritoneum.** The visceral peritoneum is the serosal layer that coats the abdominopelvic viscera with its serous fluid, facilitating movement between the organs. Ascites, for example, is an abnormal accumulation of this peritoneal fluid in the abdominopelvic cavity.

Not all of the organs in the abdominopelvic cavity lie within the peritoneum. Some—for example, the aorta, kidneys, ureters, duodenum, and pancreas—are outside and behind the peritoneum in the **retroperitoneum.**

The organs that are within the peritoneum (intraperitoneal), however, have additional structures that serve to support and supply them: **mesenteries, (visceral) ligaments,** and **folds.** The mesenteries are extensions of the visceral peritoneum that stretch out to hold many of the abdominal organs and serve as a channel for blood vessels, nerves, and lymphatic vessels traveling to and from the organs in question. Mesenteries are named for the organs that they hold (e.g., mesocolon—mesentery that surrounds the colon, mesoappendix—mesentery that surrounds the appendix). Ligaments and folds attach one structure to another or provide support for organs in the peritoneal cavity.

The **peritoneal cavity** is divided into two main regions: the **greater sac** and the **lesser sac.** These two regions are connected by an opening termed the **epiploic foramen** (also called the **foramen of Winslow).** The greater sac is the main cavity of the peritoneal cavity, while the lesser sac is formed by two separate folds termed **omenta.** The omenta (*sing.* omentum) are folds of peritoneum that extend from the stomach, further compartmentalizing the peritoneal cavity and serving as sites of fat deposition, protecting against trauma and infection, and providing an immune support function (Fig. 5-6). The **greater omentum** extends from the greater curvature of the stomach, covers the intestines, and merges into the parietal peritoneum. The **lesser omentum** (also termed the omental bursa) extends from the lesser curvature of the stomach and connects to the liver.

peritoneum = **peritone/o**

abdominopelvic
  abdomin/o = abdomen
  pelv/i = pelvis

retroperitoneum
  retro- = behind
  peritone/o = peritoneum
  -um = structure

omentum = **epiplo/o,** **oment/o**

Stomach

The **stomach,** an expandable saclike vessel located between the esophagus and the small intestines, has three main functions (Fig. 5-7). It begins the process of digesting proteins by storing the swallowed food and mixing it with gastric juices and hydrochloric acid to further the digestive process chemically. This mixture is called **chyme.** The smooth muscles of the stomach contract to aid in the mechanical digestion of the food. A continuous coating of mucus protects the stomach and the rest of the digestive system from the acidic nature of the gastric juices. Finally, the partially digested mixture is moved to the small intestines.

The stomach is divided into three main sections: the **fundus,** the **body,** and the **pylorus** (also called the **gastric antrum).** The fundus is the area of the stomach that abuts the diaphragm. This section of the stomach has no acid-producing cells, unlike the remainder of the stomach. The body, or corporis, is the central part of the stomach, and the pylorus *(pl.* pylori) is at the distal end of the stomach, where the small intestine begins. The pylorus is divided into the pyloric antrum, the pyloric canal, and the pyloric sphincter. The **pyloric sphincter** regulates the gentle release of food from the stomach into the small intestine. The portion of the stomach that surrounds the esophagogastric connection is the **cardia** (so named because of its proximity to the heart). When the stomach is empty, it has an appearance of being lined with many ridges. These ridges, or wrinkles, are called **rugae** *(sing.* ruga).

stomach = gastr/o

fundus = fund/o

body = corpor/o

pylorus = pylor/o

antrum = antr/o

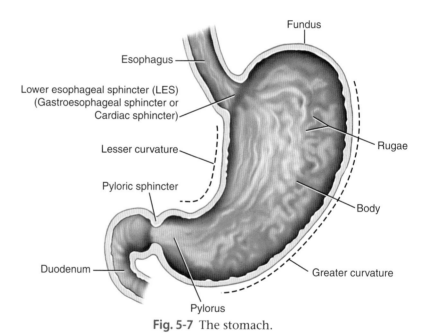

Fig. 5-7 The stomach.

> ⊗ **Be Careful!**   *Don't confuse the term* **ilium,** *meaning* part of the hip bone, *with* **ileum,** *meaning* part of the small intestine.

Small Intestine

Once the chyme has been formed in the stomach, the pyloric sphincter relaxes a bit at a time to release portions of it into the first part of the **small intestine,** called the **duodenum** (Fig. 5-8). The small intestine gets its name not because of its length (it is about 20 feet long), but because of the diameter of its **lumen** (a tubular cavity within the body). The second part of the small intestine is the **jejunum** and the distal part is the **ileum.** The **duodenojejunal flexure** is the border between the first two sections of the small intestines.

Multiple circular folds in the small intestines, called **plicae,** contain thousands of tiny projections called **villi** *(sing.* villus), which contain blood capillaries that absorb the products of carbohydrate and protein digestion. The villi

small intestine = enter/o

duodenum = duoden/o

lumen = lumin/o

jejunum = jejun/o

ileum = ile/o

fold, plica = plic/o

villus = vill/o

also contain lymphatic vessels known as **lacteals** that absorb lipid substances from the chyme.

The suffix *-ase* is used to form the name of an enzyme. It is added to the name of the substance upon which the enzyme acts: for example, **lipase,** which acts on lipids, or **amylase,** which acts on starches. The chemical suffix *-ose* indicates that a substance is a carbohydrate, such as **glucose.**

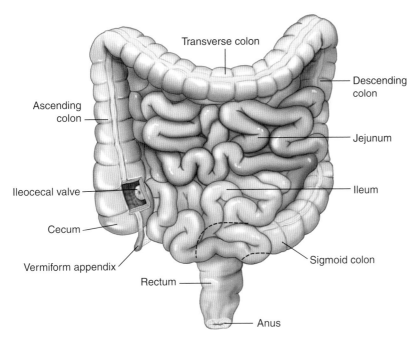

Fig. 5-8 Small and large intestines.

Large Intestine

In contrast to the small intestine, the **large intestine** (see Fig. 5-8) is only about 5 feet long, but it is much wider in diameter. The primary function of the large intestine is the elimination of waste products from the body. Some synthesis of vitamins occurs in the large intestine, but unlike the small intestine, the large intestine has no villi and is not well suited for absorption of nutrients. The **ileocecal valve** is the exit from the small intestine and the entrance to the colon. The first part of the large intestine, the **cecum,** has a wormlike appendage, called the **vermiform appendix** *(pl.* appendices), dangling from it. Although this organ does not seem to have any direct function related to the digestive system, it is thought to have a possible immunological defense mechanism.

No longer called *chyme,* whatever has not been absorbed by the small intestines is now called **feces.** The feces pass from the cecum to the **ascending colon,** bending at the hepatic flexure to cross the abdomen at the **transverse colon,** bending downward at the splenic flexure to become the **descending colon,** and then on to the S-shaped **sigmoid colon.** The **teniae coli** are the muscular bands that contract lengthwise and form the haustra—the bulges in the colon. The **rectosigmoid junction** marks the beginning of the last straight part of the large intestine, the **rectum** and its junction with the **anus** (the anorectal junction), where the feces are held until released from the body completely through the external and internal anal sphincters. The **internal sphincter** is an involuntary muscle, while the **external sphincter** is voluntary. The process of releasing feces from the body is called **defecation** or a **bowel movement** (BM).

---

lipid, fat = lipid/o, lip/o

amylase
    amyl/o = starch
    -ase = enzyme

glucose, sugar = gluc/o, glyc/o

large intestine, colon = col/o, colon/o

ileocecal
    ile/o = ileum
    cec/o = cecum
    -al = pertaining to

cecum = cec/o

appendix = appendic/o, append/o

feces = fec/a

sigmoid colon = sigmoid/o

rectum = rect/o

anus = an/o

rectum and anus = proct/o

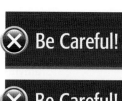 **Be Careful!** The combining form **gastr/o** refers only to the stomach. The combining forms **abdomin/o, lapar/o,** and **celi/o** refer to the abdomen.

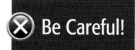 **Be Careful!** Do not confuse **-cele,** the suffix meaning herniation, with **celi/o,** a combining form for abdomen.

Be Careful! Do not confuse **an/o,** the combining form for anus, with **ana-,** the prefix meaning up or apart, and **an-,** the prefix meaning no, not, or without.

Exercise 4: The Peritoneum, Stomach, Small Intestine, and Large Intestine

A. Match the following combining forms and body parts with their terms.

____ 1. lip/o   A. rectum and anus
____ 2. plic/o   B. first part of large intestines
____ 3. col/o   C. structure hanging from cecum
____ 4. jejun/o   D. small intestines
____ 5. ile/o   E. double-sided membrane that holds organs inside the abdominopelvic cavity
____ 6. rect/o   F. stomach
____ 7. an/o   G. second part of small intestines
____ 8. duoden/o   H. fat
____ 9. gastr/o   I. folds
____ 10. cec/o   J. first part of small intestines
____ 11. sigmoid/o   K. section between stomach and first part of small intestines
____ 12. peritone/o   L. last straight part of colon
____ 13. enter/o   M. large intestines
____ 14. pylor/o   N. distal part of small intestines
____ 15. proct/o   O. final sphincter in GI tract
____ 16. appendic/o   P. S-shaped part of large intestine

B. Match the term with the correct definition.

____ 1. mixture of swallowed food, gastric juices, and hydrochloric acid   A. fundus
____ 2. area of the stomach that abuts the diaphragm   B. duodenum
____ 3. exit from the small intestine and entrance to the colon   C. rugae
____ 4. first part of the small intestine   D. ileum
____ 5. regulates release of food from the stomach to small intestines   E. corporis
____ 6. where the rectum and the anus come together   F. ileocecal valve
____ 7. first part of the large intestines   G. pyloric sphincter
____ 8. central part of the stomach   H. jejunum
____ 9. second part of the small intestines   I. cecum
____ 10. stomach wrinkles   J. chyme
____ 11. distal part of the small intestines   K. anorectal junction

 Practice labeling the stomach and intestines by clicking on **Label It**

Accessory Organs (Adnexa)

The **accessory organs** are the **gallbladder** (GB), **liver,** and **pancreas** (Fig. 5-9). These organs secrete fluid into the GI tract but are not a direct part of the tube itself. Sometimes accessory structures are referred to as **adnexa.**

The four **lobes** (right, left, quadrate, caudate) that form the liver virtually fill the right upper quadrant of the abdomen and extend partially into the left upper quadrant directly inferior to the diaphragm.

The liver forms a substance called **bile,** which emulsifies, or mechanically breaks down, fats into smaller particles so that they can be chemically digested. Bile is composed of **bilirubin,** the waste product formed by the normal breakdown of hemoglobin in red blood cells at the end of their life spans, and **cholesterol,** a fatty substance found only in animal tissues (Fig. 5-10). Bile is released from the liver through the right and left hepatic ducts, which join to form the **hepatic duct.** The **cystic duct** carries bile to and from the gallbladder. When the hepatic and cystic ducts merge, they form the **common bile duct,** which empties into the **duodenum.** Collectively, all of these ducts are termed **bile vessels.** Bile is stored in the **gallbladder,** a small sac found on the underside of the right lobe of the liver. When fatty food enters the duodenum, a hormone called **cholecystokinin** is secreted, causing a contraction of the gallbladder to move bile out into the cystic duct, then the common bile duct, and finally into the duodenum. The pancreatic and common bile ducts join and empty into the duodenum. These joined ducts are surrounded by muscular tissue (the sphincter of Oddi) that opens into the ampulla of Vater (hepatopancreatic ampulla). An ampulla is a bottle-shaped dilation in a tube-like structure or cavity.

The **pancreas** is a gland located in the upper left quadrant. It is involved in the digestion of the three types of food molecules: carbohydrates, proteins, and lipids. The pancreatic enzymes are carried through the pancreatic duct, which empties into the common bile duct. Pancreatic involvement in food digestion is an **exocrine** function because the secretion is into a duct. Pancreatic **endocrine** functions (secretion into blood and lymph vessels) are discussed in Chapter 15.

accessory = adnex/o

lobe = lob/o

liver = hepat/o

bile = chol/e, bil/i

cholesterol = cholesterol/o

common bile duct = choledoch/o

bile vessel = cholangi/o

gallbladder = cholecyst/o

movement substance = -kinin

pancreas = pancreat/o

exocrine
 exo- = outside
 -crine = to secrete

endocrine
 endo- = within
 -crine = to secrete

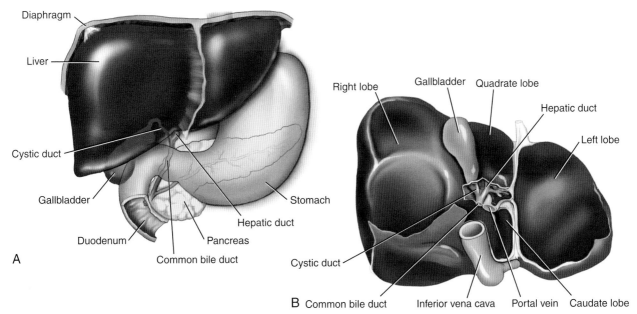

Fig. 5-9 **Accessory organs. A,** Anterior view; **B,** Posterior view.

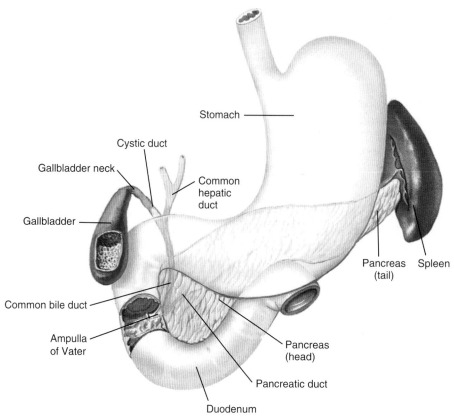

Fig. 5-10 Sources of intestinal secretions.

 Exercise 5: **Accessory Organs**

Matching.

____	1. pancreas	A. lob/o
____	2. gallbladder	B. chol/e, bil/i
____	3. lobe	C. hepat/o
____	4. liver	D. cholecyst/o
____	5. bile	E. cholangi/o
____	6. bile vessels	F. choledoch/o
____	7. common bile duct	G. pancreat/o
____	8. another word for accessory organs	H. adnexa
____	9. substance that breaks down fats	I. gallbladder
____	10. carries bile to and from the gallbladder	J. pancreas
____	11. where bile is stored	K. cystic duct
____	12. hormone that causes gallbladder contraction	L. cholecystokinin
____	13. gland that assists in digestion of carbohydrates, proteins, and lipids	M. bile

Ⓔ

Practice labeling the accessory organs by clicking on **Label It.**

You can review the anatomy of the digestive system by clicking on **Body Spectrum Electronic Anatomy Coloring Book** then **Digestive.**

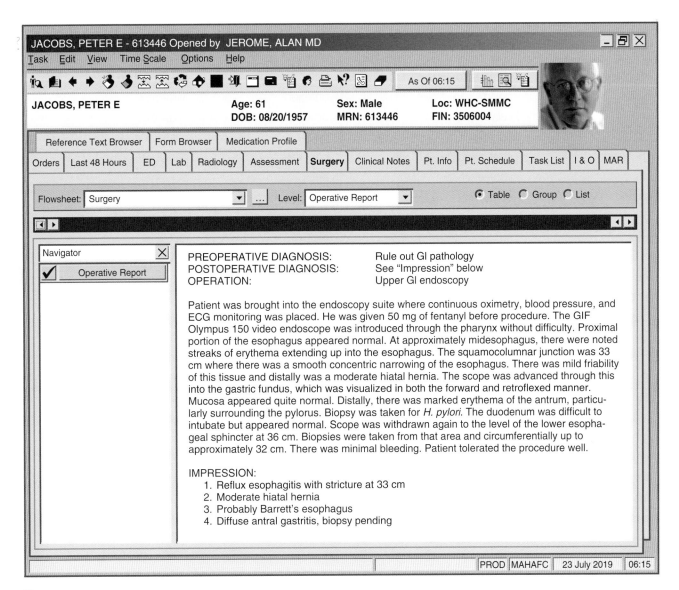

Exercise 6: Operative Report

Using the operative report above, answer the following questions. Use a dictionary as needed for this exercise.

1. What was the route of the endoscope? _____

2. The portion of the esophagus that appeared normal was *(close to/far from)* the mouth. Underline one.

3. The mucosa was normal in which part of the stomach? _____

4. What are synonyms for the "lower esophageal sphincter"?_____

Combining Forms for the Anatomy of the Digestive System

Meaning	Combining Form	Meaning	Combining Form
abdomen	abdomin/o, celi/o, lapar/o	lobe	lob/o
accessory	adnex/o	lower jaw	mandibul/o
anus	an/o	lumen	lumin/o
appendix	appendic/o, append/o	mouth, oral, cavity	or/o, stom/o, stomat/o
bile	chol/e, bil/i	mucus	mucos/o
bile vessel	cholangi/o	nose	nas/o, rhin/o
bolus	bol/o	nutrition	aliment/o
cecum	cec/o	omentum	epiplo/o
cheek	bucc/o	palate	palat/o
cholesterol	cholesterol/o	pancreas	pancreat/o
common bile duct	choledoch/o	peritoneum	peritone/o
corporis, body	corpor/o	pharynx, throat	pharyng/o
duodenum	duoden/o	pylorus	pylor/o
enamel	amel/o	rectum	rect/o
esophagus	esophag/o	rectum and anus	proct/o
fat, lipid	lip/o,lipid/o	rugae	rug/o
feces	fec/a	saliva	sial/o, ptyal/o
fold, plica	plic/o	salivary duct	sialodoch/o
fundus	fund/o	salivary gland	sialoaden/o
gallbladder	cholecyst/o	sigmoid colon	sigmoid/o
glucose, sugar	gluc/o, glyc/o	small intestine	enter/o
gums	gingiv/o	starch	amyl/o
ileum	ile/o	stomach	gastr/o
intestines	intestin/o	teeth	dent/i, odont/o
jejunum	jejun/o	tongue	gloss/o, lingu/o
large intestine, colon	col/o, colon/o	upper jaw	maxill/o
lips	cheil/o, labi/o	uvula	uvul/o
liver	hepat/o	villus	vill/o

Prefixes for the Anatomy of the Digestive System

Prefix	Meaning
endo-	within
exo-	outside
hypo-	below
par-	near
peri-	surrounding
retro-	behind
sub-	under

Suffixes for the Anatomy of the Digestive System

Suffix	Meaning
-al, -ar, -ary, -eal, -id, -ine, -ous, -ic	pertaining to
-ase	enzyme
-crine	to secrete
-kinin	movement substance
-stalsis	contraction

PATHOLOGY

Terms Related to Symptoms and Signs Involving the Digestive System and Abdomen (R1Ø-R19)

Term	Word Origin	Definition
ascites		Excessive intraperitoneal fluid.
diarrhea	*dia-* through, complete *-rrhea* discharge, flow	Abnormal discharge of watery, semisolid stools.
dysphagia	*dys-* difficult, bad *-phagia* condition of swallowing, eating	Difficulty with swallowing that may be due to an obstruction (e.g., a tumor) or a motor disorder (e.g., a spasm).
eructation		Release of air from the stomach through the mouth. Eructation may be caused by rapid eating or by intentionally or unintentionally swallowing air (aerophagia). Also called **burping** or **belching.**
flatulence		Gas expelled through the anus. Also called **flatus.**
gastralgia	*gastr/o* stomach *-algia* pain	Abdominal pain. Also called **gastrodynia.**
halitosis	*halit/o* breath *-osis* abnormal condition	Bad-smelling breath.
hepatomegaly	*hepat/o* liver *-megaly* enlargement	Enlargement of the liver.
jaundice		Yellowing of the skin and sclerae (whites of the eyes) caused by elevated levels of bilirubin. Also called **icterus.**
nausea		Sensation that accompanies the urge to vomit but does not always lead to vomiting. The abbreviation N&V refers to nausea and vomiting. The term is derived from a Greek word meaning *seasickness.*
pyrosis	*pyr/o* fire *-osis* abnormal condition	Painful burning sensation in esophagus, usually caused by reflux of stomach contents, hyperactivity, or peptic ulcer. Also known as **heartburn.**
vomiting		Forcible or involuntary emptying of the stomach through the mouth. The material expelled is called **vomitus** or **emesis.**

Exercise 7: Symptoms and Signs Involving the Digestive System and Abdomen

Match the terms to their definitions.

____ 1. flatulence	A. forcible emptying of stomach through the mouth
____ 2. nausea	B. excessive intraperitoneal fluid
____ 3. jaundice	C. gas expelled through the anus
____ 4. diarrhea	D. sensation accompanying the urge to vomit
____ 5. eructation	E. release of air from the stomach through the mouth
____ 6. vomiting	F. abnormal discharge of watery, semisolid stools
____ 7. pyrosis	G. heartburn; painful burning sensation in the esophagus
____ 8. ascites	H. yellowing of skin and sclerae

Build the terms.

9. pain in the stomach _____

10. condition of difficulty with swallowing _____

11. abnormal condition of the breath _____

Terms Related to Diseases of Oral Cavity and Salivary Glands (KØØ-K14)

Term	Word Origin	Definition
amelogenesis imperfecta	*amel/o* enamel *-genesis* production, origin	An abnormal formation of tooth enamel, resulting in separation from the dentin beneath.
anodontia	*an-* no, not, without *odont/o* teeth *-ia* condition	Either complete or partial lack of teeth. Also referred to as **edentulous.**
aphthous stomatitis	*aphth/o* ulceration *-ous* pertaining to *stomat/o* mouth *-itis* inflammation	Recurring condition characterized by small erosions (ulcers), which appear on the mucous membranes of the mouth. Also called a **canker sore** (Fig. 5-11).
cheilitis	*cheil/o* lip *-itis* inflammation	Inflammation of the lips.
dental caries	*dent/i* teeth *-al* pertaining to	Plaque disease caused by an interaction between food and bacteria in the mouth, leading to tooth decay. Also called **cavities.**

Continued

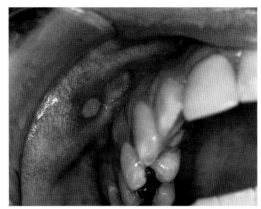

Fig. 5-11 Aphthous stomatitis.

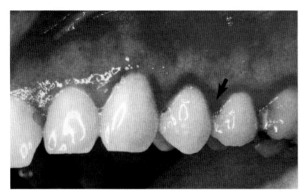

Fig. 5-12 Gingivitis.

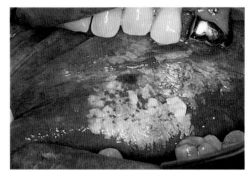

Fig. 5-13 Leukoplakia.

Terms Related to Diseases of Oral Cavity and Salivary Glands (KØØ-K14)—cont'd

Term	Word Origin	Definition
gingivitis	*gingiv/o* gums *-itis* inflammation	Inflammatory disease of the gums characterized by redness, swelling, and bleeding (Fig. 5-12).
glossitis	*gloss/o* tongue *-itis* inflammation	Inflammation of the tongue.
oral mucositis	*or/o* mouth *-al* pertaining to *mucos/o* mucus *-itis* inflammation	Inflammation of the mucous membranes of the mouth. Gastrointestinal mucositis may be an adverse effect of chemotherapy and can occur throughout the GI tract.
oral leukoplakia	*or/o* mouth *-al* pertaining to *leuk/o* white *-plakia* condition of patches	Condition of white patches that may appear on the lips and buccal mucosa (Fig. 5-13). It usually is associated with tobacco use and may be precancerous.
periodontal disease	*peri-* surrounding *odont/o* tooth *-al* pertaining to	Pathological condition of the tissues surrounding the teeth.

Terms Related to Diseases of Oral Cavity and Salivary Glands (KØØ-K14)—cont'd

Term	Word Origin	Definition
ptyalism	*ptyal/o* saliva *-ism* condition	Condition of excessive salivation.
sialoadenitis	*sialoaden/o* salivary gland *-itis* inflammation	Inflammation of a salivary gland.
sialolithiasis	*sial/o* saliva *lith/o* stone *-iasis* presence of, condition	Condition of stones in a salivary gland or duct.

Exercise 8: Diseases of the Oral Cavity and Salivary Glands

Match the terms to their definitions.

____ 1. ptyalism
____ 2. aphthous stomatitis
____ 3. sialolithiasis
____ 4. periodontal disease
____ 5. amelogenesis imperfecta
____ 6. mucositis
____ 7. dental caries
____ 8. leukoplakia

A. plaque disease leading to tooth decay
B. canker sore
C. inflammation of mucous membrane
D. excessive salivation
E. abnormal formation of enamel
F. stones in a salivary gland
G. disease of tissue surrounding teeth
H. white patches on lips and buccal mucosa

Translate the terms.

9. gingivitis _____

10. glossitis _____

11. anodontia _____

12. sialoadenitis _____

13. cheilitis _____

Terms Related to Diseases of Esophagus, Stomach, and Duodenum (K2Ø -K31)

Term	Word Origin	Definition
achalasia	*a-* without *-chalasia* condition of relaxation	Impairment of esophageal peristalsis along with the lower esophageal sphincter's inability to relax. Also called **cardiospasm, esophageal aperistalsis,** and **megaesophagus.**
dyspepsia	*dys-* abnormal, bad *-pepsia* digestion condition	Feeling of epigastric discomfort that occurs shortly after eating. The discomfort may include feelings of nausea, fullness, heartburn, and/or bloating. Also called **indigestion.**

Continued

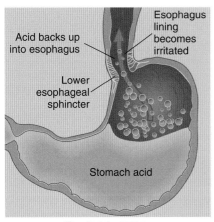

Fig. 5-14 GERD.

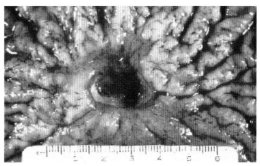

Fig. 5-15 Chronic peptic ulcer.

Terms Related to Diseases of Esophagus, Stomach, and Duodenum (K2Ø-K31)—cont'd

Term	Word Origin	Definition
esophagitis	*esophag/o* esophagus *-itis* inflammation	Inflammation of the esophagus.
gastritis	*gastr/o* stomach *-itis* inflammation	Acute or chronic inflammation of the stomach that may be accompanied by anorexia (lack of appetite), nausea and vomiting, or indigestion.
gastroesophageal reflux disease (GERD)	*gastr/o* stomach *esophag/o* esophagus *-eal* pertaining to *re-* back *-flux* flow	Flowing back, or return, of the contents of the stomach to the esophagus caused by an inability of the lower esophageal sphincter (LES) to contract normally; characterized by pyrosis with or without regurgitation of stomach contents to the mouth (Fig. 5-14). **Barrett's esophagus** is a condition caused by chronic reflux from the stomach. It is associated with an increased risk of cancer.
peptic ulcer disease (PUD)		An erosion of the protective mucosal lining of the stomach or duodenum (Fig. 5-15). Also called a **gastric** or **duodenal ulcer**, depending on the site.

 Exercise 9: Diseases of the Esophagus, Stomach, and Duodenum

Match the terms.

____ 1. dyspepsia   A. erosion of the mucosal lining of the stomach or duodenum
____ 2. GERD   B. indigestion
____ 3. achalasia   C. esophageal aperistalsis
____ 4. PUD   D. return of contents of stomach to esophagus

Translate the terms.

5. gastritis _____

6. achalasia _____

7. dyspepsia _____

8. esophagitis _____

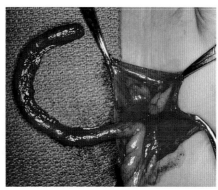

Fig. 5-16 Appendicitis. Note the darker pink color of the appendix, indicating the inflammation.

Terms Related to Diseases of Appendix (K35-K38)

Term	Word Origin	Definition
appendicitis	*appendic/o* appendix *-itis* inflammation	Inflammation of the vermiform appendix (Fig. 5-16). May be acute or chronic, with or without peritonitis.

Terms Related to Hernias (K4Ø-K46)

All hernias are protrusions (bulges) of organs and/or tissues from their normal cavity. Most are named for their location (e.g. **inguinal,**" in the groin," and **umbilical,**" at the navel") and are enclosed in the lining of the cavity from which they are protruding.

Additional terms are used to describe associated complications. **Incarcerated** (also termed **irreducible**) **hernias** are those in which a loop of bowel becomes occluded (blocked) so that solids cannot pass. If a hernia is termed **reducible,** it means that the contents of the protrusion can be returned to their original location manually or spontaneously. **Strangulation,** the constriction of a tubular structure, can lead to an inhibition of circulation, resulting in a lack of blood supply **(ischemia).** If a hernia is strangulated, the lack of blood flow can lead to **gangrene,** necrotic (dead) tissue that is a result of diminished blood flow.

Term	Word Origin	Definition
femoral hernia	*femor/o* femur *-al* pertaining to	Protrusion of a loop of intestine through the femoral canal into the groin. Also called a **crural hernia.**
hiatal hernia	*hiat/o* an opening *-al* pertaining to	Protrusion of a portion of the stomach through the diaphragm. Also known as a **diaphragmatic hernia** and **diaphragmatocele** (Fig. 5-17).

Continued

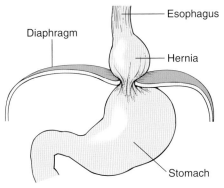

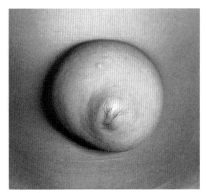

Fig. 5-17 Hiatal hernia.   Fig. 5-18 Umbilical hernia.

Terms Related to Hernias (K40-K46)—cont'd

Term	Word Origin	Definition
inguinal hernia	*inguin/o* groin *-al* pertaining to	Protrusion of a loop of intestine into the inguinal canal. May be indirect (through a normal internal passage) or direct (through a muscle wall).
umbilical hernia	*umbilic/o* umbilicus *-al* pertaining to	Protrusion of the intestine and omentum through a weakness in the abdominal wall at the navel (Fig. 5-18). An **omphalocele**, a herniation of the umbilicus, is a congenital condition.
ventral hernia	*ventr/o* belly *-al* pertaining to	Protrusion of intestines and omentum through the abdominal wall except at the umbilicus. May be epigastric (above the stomach) or incisional (at the site of a previous surgery in the abdominal area).

 Be Careful!   *Note that the suffix **-cele** means a herniation or protrusion.*

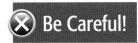 Exercise 10: **Hernias**

Match the hernias to their definitions.

____ 1. hiatal hernia

____ 2. umbilical hernia

____ 3. strangulation

____ 4. gangrene

____ 5. incarcerated hernia

____ 6. inguinal hernia

____ 7. femoral hernia

____ 8. reducible hernia

A. protrusion that can be manually or spontaneously corrected

B. protrusion of part of the intestines and omentum through the abdominal wall at the navel

C. irreducible hernia

D. protrusion of intestine in the inguinal canal

E. protrusion of intestine through the femoral canal

F. constriction of a tubular structure

G. diaphragmatocele

H. necrotic tissue

Terms Related to Noninfective Enteritis and Colitis (K5Ø-K52)

Term	Word Origin	Definition
colitis	*col/o* colon *-itis* inflammation	Inflammation of the large intestine.
Crohn's disease		Inflammation of the ileum or the colon that is of idiopathic origin. Also called **regional** or **granulomatous enteritis.**
ulcerative colitis	*col/o* colon *-itis* inflammation	Chronic inflammation of the colon and rectum manifesting with bouts of profuse, watery diarrhea. Both Crohn's disease and ulcerative colitis are types of **inflammatory bowel disease (IBD).**

Terms Related to Other Diseases of the Intestines (K55-K63)

Term	Word Origin	Definition
anal fissure	*an/o* anus *-al* pertaining to	Cracklike lesion of the skin around the anus.
anorectal abscess	*an/o* anus *rect/o* rectum *-al* pertaining to	Circumscribed area of inflammation in the anus or rectum, containing pus.
anorectal fistula	*an/o* anus *rect/o* rectum *-al* pertaining to	Abnormal channel between the rectum and the anus. Fistulas may occur between organs or between an organ and the surface of the body.
constipation		Infrequent, incomplete, or delayed bowel movements. Obstipation is intractable (difficult to manage) constipation or an intestinal obstruction.
diverticulitis	*diverticul/o* diverticulum *-itis* inflammation	Inflammation occurring secondary to the occurrence of diverticulosis.
diverticulosis	*diverticul/o* diverticulum *-osis* abnormal condition	Development of diverticula, pouches in the lining of the intestines (Fig. 5-19), both large and small. Usually the diverticula are asymptomatic, but sometimes they can become inflamed or infected.
ileus		Obstruction. **Paralytic ileus** is lack of peristaltic movement in the intestinal tract. Also called **adynamic ileus.**
intussusception		Inward telescoping of the intestines (Fig. 5-20, *A*).
irritable bowel syndrome (IBS)		Diarrhea, gas, and/or constipation resulting from stress with no underlying disease.
polyp of colon		Benign growth on the mucous membrane of large intestine.

Continued

Terms Related to Other Diseases of the Intestines (K55-K63)—cont'd

Term	Word Origin	Definition
proctitis	*proct/o* rectum and anus *-itis* inflammation	Inflammation of the rectum and anus. Also called **rectitis.**
proctoptosis	*proct/o* rectum and anus *-ptosis* drooping, prolapse	Prolapse of the rectum outside of the anus.
volvulus		Twisting of the intestine (see Fig. 5-20, *B*).

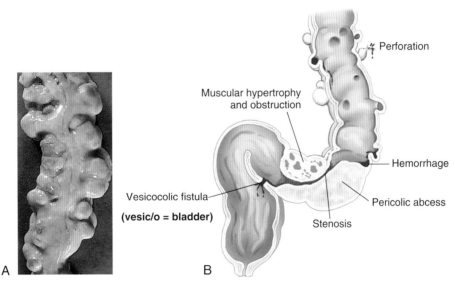

Fig. 5-19 **A,** Diverticulosis. Diverticulosis can lead to diverticulitis and subsequent complications **(B).**

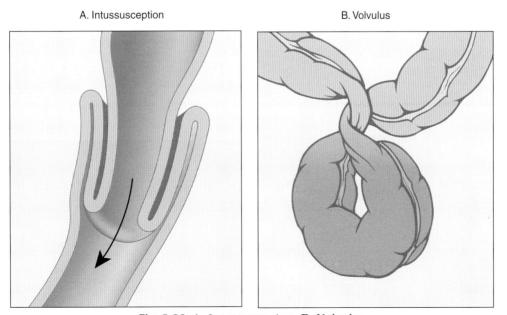

Fig. 5-20 **A,** Intussusception. **B,** Volvulus.

Exercise 11: Noninfective Enteritis and Colitis; Other Diseases of the Intestines

Match the terms to their definitions.

____ 1. ileus	A. growth on mucous membrane of large intestine
____ 2. constipation	B. syndrome of diarrhea, gas, and/or constipation
____ 3. Crohn's disease	C. cracklike lesion around anus
____ 4. volvulus	D. chronic inflammation of the colon and rectum
____ 5. ulcerative colitis	E. circumscribed area (in rectum or anus) of inflammation containing pus
____ 6. intussusception	F. inflammation of the ileum or colon that is of idiopathic origin
____ 7. anal fissure	G. abnormal channel between the rectum and anus
____ 8. IBS	H. infrequent bowel movements
____ 9. anorectal fistula	I. inward telescoping of the intestines
____ 10. anorectal abscess	J. obstruction
____ 11. polyp of colon	K. twisting of the intestines

Build the terms.

12. drooping of the rectum and anus _____

13. inflammation of a diverticulum _____

14. inflammation of the rectum and anus _____

15. abnormal condition of a diverticulum _____

Terms Related to Diseases of Peritoneum and Retroperitoneum (K65-K68) and Diseases of Liver (K7Ø-K77)

Term	Word Origin	Definition
cirrhosis	*cirrh/o* orange-yellow *-osis* abnormal condition	Chronic degenerative disease of the liver, commonly associated with alcohol abuse, chronic liver disease, and biliary tract disorders (Fig. 5-21).
peritonitis	*peritone/o* peritoneum *-itis* inflammation	Inflammation of the peritoneum that most commonly occurs when an inflamed appendix ruptures. An additional code is needed to identify an infectious agent.

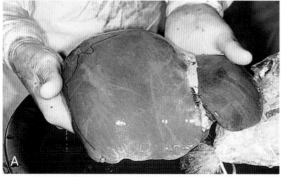 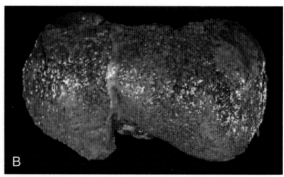

Fig. 5-21 A, Normal liver. **B,** Cirrhosis of the liver is indicated by nodules on the surface.

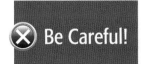 Liver diseases often require additional codes. For example: alcoholic liver diseases need codes to describe alcohol abuse and dependence, while toxic liver disease requires a code to identify the drug or toxic agent.

Viral hepatitis is coded to the Infectious and Parasitic Diseases chapter.

⊗ Be Careful! *Don't confuse **peritone/o,** a combining form for the membrane that lines the abdominal cavity, with **perone/o,** which is a combining form for the fibula, and **perine/o,** a combining form for the space between the anus and external reproductive organs.*

Terms Related to Diseases of Gallbladder, Biliary Tract, and Pancreas (K8Ø-K87)

Term	Word Origin	Definition
cholangitis	*cholangi/o* bile vessel *-itis* inflammation	Inflammation of the bile vessels.
cholecystitis	*cholecyst/o* gallbladder *-itis* inflammation	Inflammation of the gallbladder, either acute or chronic. May be caused by choledocholithiasis or cholelithiasis.
choledocholithiasis	*choledoch/o* common bile duct *lith/o* stones *-iasis* presence of	Presence of stones in the common bile duct (Fig. 5-22).
cholelithiasis	*chol/e* gall, bile *lith/o* stones *-iasis* presence of	Presence of stones (calculi) in the gallbladder, sometimes characterized by right upper quadrant pain **(biliary colic)** with nausea and vomiting (Fig. 5-23).
pancreatitis	*pancreat/o* pancreas *-itis* inflammation	Inflammation of the pancreas, which may be acute or chronic.

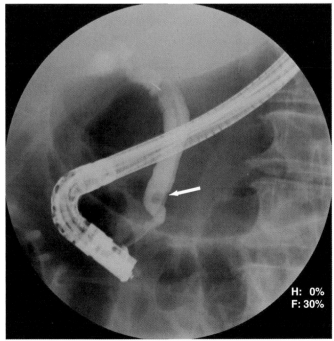

Fig. 5-22 Cholangiogram showing stones in the common bile duct (choledocholithiasis).

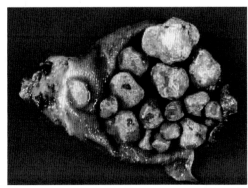

Fig. 5-23 Cholelithiasis (stones in the gallbladder).

Terms Related to Other Diseases of Digestive System (K9Ø-K94)

Term	Word Origin	Definition
celiac disease	*celi/o* abdomen *-ac* pertaining to	Inability of intestines to absorb wheat proteins. Also called **celiac sprue.**
hematemesis	*hemat/o* blood *-emesis* vomiting	Vomiting of blood. If bright red, it is referred to as frank blood. **Coffee-grounds emesis** is dark brown or black.
melena	*melan/o* black, dark	Black, tarry stools caused by the presence of partially digested blood.

Terms Related to Viral Infections Characterized by Skin and Mucous Membranes (BØØ-BØ9) and Viral Hepatitis (B15-B19)

Term	Word Origin	Definition
herpetic stomatitis	*stomat/o* mouth *-itis* inflammation	Inflammation of the mouth caused by the herpes simplex virus (HSV). Also known as a **cold sore** or **fever blister.**
hepatitis	*hepat/o* liver *-itis* inflammation	Inflammatory disease of the liver that is caused by an increasing number of viruses. Currently named by letter, hepatitis A to G, the means of viral transmission is not the same for each form. The most common forms, A to C, are discussed below.
hepatitis A (HAV)	*hepat/o* liver *-itis* inflammation	Virus transmitted through direct contact with fecally contaminated food or water.
hepatitis B (HBV)	*hepat/o* liver *-itis* inflammation	Virus transmitted through contaminated blood or sexual contact.
hepatitis C (HCV)	*hepat/o* liver *-itis* inflammation	Virus transmitted through blood transfusion, percutaneous inoculation, or sharing of infected needles.

Exercise 12: Diseases of Gallbladder, Biliary Tract, Pancreas, Peritoneum, Retroperitoneum, Liver, Digestive System; and Viral Infections

Match the terms to their definitions.

____ 1. cirrhosis
____ 2. hepatitis A
____ 3. hepatitis B
____ 4. hepatitis C
____ 5. cholelithiasis
____ 6. herpetic stomatitis
____ 7. celiac disease
____ 8. melena

A. hepatitis caused by contaminated blood or sexual contact
B. chronic degenerative liver disease, commonly associated with alcohol abuse, chronic liver disease, and biliary tract disorders
C. hepatitis caused by direct contact with fecally contaminated food or water
D. hepatitis caused by blood transfusions or infected needles
E. inflammation of the mouth caused by HSV
F. stones in the gallbladder
G. inability of intestines to absorb wheat proteins
H. black, tarry stools caused by presence of partially digested blood

Build the terms.

9. inflammation of the gallbladder _____

10. inflammation of the liver _____

11. presence of stones in the common bile duct _____

12. inflammation of the bile vessels _____

13. inflammation of the peritonum _____

14. inflammation of the pancreas _____

15. vomiting of blood _____

Terms Related to Benign Neoplasms (D1Ø-D36)

Term	Word Origin	Definition
cystadenoma	*cyst/o* bladder, cyst *aden/o* gland *-oma* tumor	Glandular tumors that are filled with cysts; these are the most common benign tumors in the pancreas.
odontogenic tumor	*odont/o* tooth *-genic* pertaining to produced by	Benign tumors that arise around the teeth and jaw (Fig. 5-24).
polyps, adenomatous or hyperplastic	*aden/o* gland *-omatous* pertaining to tumor *hyper-* excessive *plas/o* formation, growth *-tic* pertaining to	Adenomatous (growths that arise from glandular tissue, have potential to become malignant) or hyperplastic (generally, small growths that have no tendency to become malignant) tumors occurring throughout the digestive tract. Polyps may be sessile (flat) or pedunculated (having a stalk) (Fig. 5-25).

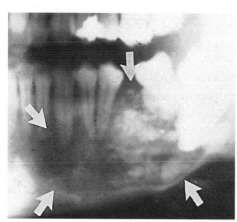

Fig. 5-24 Odontogenic tumor of the teeth and jaw.

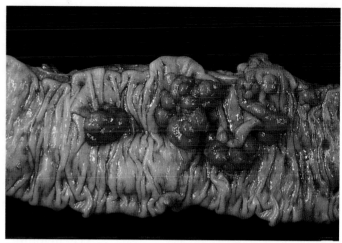

Fig. 5-25 Multiple adenomatous polyps of the large intestine.

Terms Related to Malignant Neoplasms (CØØ-C96)

Term	Word Origin	Definition
adenocarcinoma	*aden/o* gland *-carcinoma* cancerous tumor of epithelial origin	A malignant tumor of epithelial origin that either originates from glandular tissue or has a glandular appearance. Adenocarcinomas occur throughout the gastrointestinal tract, but especially in the esophagus, stomach, pancreas, and colon.
hepatocellular carcinoma/ hepatoma	*hepat/o* liver *cellul/o* cell *-ar* pertaining to	Malignant tumors of epithelial origin that originate in the liver cells. Hepatocellular carcinoma (also called **hepatoma**) is the most common type of primary liver cancer worldwide.
squamous cell carcinoma	*squam/o* scaly *-ous* pertaining to	Cancers that have a scalelike appearance. Squamous cell carcinomas arise from the cells that cover the surfaces of the body. These occur throughout the digestive system.

Please note: Metastatic carcinoma is the most common form of liver cancer, and the liver is the most common site of all metastases. Just remember this is not a primary tumor, but one that has spread from another site.

 ## Exercise 13: Neoplasms

Fill in the blank.

1. What type of benign growth is described as either sessile or pedunculated? _____

2. What is the most common type of liver cancer? _____

3. Which type of cancer occurs throughout the GI tract, but especially in the esophagus, stomach, pancreas, and colon? _____

4. What is the term for a benign tumor that arises from around the teeth and jaw? _____

PROCEDURES

Terms Related to Laboratory Tests

Term	Word Origin	Definition
alanine transaminase (ALT)		Increased measurement of this particular enzyme usually indicates cirrhosis or pancreatitis. ALT was formerly referred to as **SGPT (serum glutamic-pyruvic transaminase)**.
albumin		A blood test that reveals decreased measurement of this protein formed by the liver. May be low when liver disease occurs.
alkaline phosphatase (ALP)		An increase in this liver enzyme may indicate liver or gallbladder disease. A decrease may indicate malnutrition.
aspartate transaminase (AST)		Increased measurement of AST may indicate liver disease or pancreatitis. A decreased amount may mean uncontrolled diabetes mellitus with ketoacidosis. AST was formerly referred to as SGOT (serum glutamic oxaloacetic acid transaminase).
gamma-glutamyl transferase (GGT)		Blood test to detect increased enzymes that can indicate cirrhosis, hepatitis, acute pancreatitis, acute cholecystitis, or nephrosis, and to test for *Helicobacter pylori* antibodies.
gastric analysis	*gastr/o* stomach *-ic* pertaining to *ana-* up, apart *-lysis* breakdown	Examination to determine the amount of blood, bile, bacteria, and hydrochloric acid in the stomach. Decreased hydrochloric acid may indicate stomach cancer.
hepatitis-associated antigen (HAA)		Blood test to detect the hepatitis B virus.
liver function tests (LFTs)		A collection of tests to determine the health of the liver. Includes albumin, total bilirubin, prothrombin time, ALP, ALT, and GGT.
prothrombin time (PT)	*pro-* before *thromb/o* clot *-in* substance	Blood test to measure the time it takes blood to clot. Prothrombin is a protein that is instrumental in the clotting process and is formed in the liver. Liver disease can decrease the production of prothrombin, which can cause an increased clotting time.
rapid urease test		A test to detect the presence of *Helicobacter pylori (H. pylori)*. A gastroscopic biopsy is taken from the gastric antrum. Also termed a **CLO test (Campylobacter-like organism test)**.
stool culture		Fecal exam to test for microorganisms in the feces, such as worms, amoebae, bacteria, and protozoa.
stool guaiac, hemoccult test	*hem/o* blood *-occult* hidden	Fecal specimen exam to detect hidden blood, which may indicate gastrointestinal bleeding. Also referred to as a **fecal occult blood test (FOBT)**.
total bilirubin		Blood test to detect possible jaundice (yellowing of the skin), cirrhosis, or hepatitis.

Exercise 14: Laboratory Tests

Match the laboratory test with its definition.

____ 1. LFTs
____ 2. albumin
____ 3. HAA
____ 4. ALP
____ 5. GGT
____ 6. AST
____ 7. total bilirubin
____ 8. rapid urease test
____ 9. stool culture
____ 10. ALT

A. blood test to detect the hepatitis B virus

B. test to detect the presence of *H. pylori,* also termed *CLO test*

C. formerly called *SGOT;* increased measures may indicate liver disease or pancreatitis

D. fecal exam for microorganisms

E. low levels of this protein may indicate liver disease

F. collection of tests to determine liver health

G. increased levels of this enzyme may indicate liver or gallbladder disease; decreased levels may indicate malnutrition

H. increased enzymes in this blood test may indicate cirrhosis, hepatitis, acute pancreatitis, acute cholecystitis, or nephrosis. May also be used to test for *H. pylori* antibodies.

I. blood test to detect possible jaundice, cirrhosis, or hepatitis

J. formerly called *SGPT;* increased levels may indicate cirrhosis or pancreatitis

Terms Related to Upper GI Procedures

Term	Word Origin	Definition
barium swallow (BS)		Radiographic imaging done after oral ingestion of a barium sulfate suspension; used to detect abnormalities of the esophagus and stomach (Fig. 5-26).
esophagoesophagostomy	*esophag/o* esophagus *esophag/o* esophagus *-stomy* making a new opening	A rejoining of two ends of a cut esophagus, usually as a result of surgery to remove an esophageal defect.
esophagogastroduodenoscopy (EGD)	*esophag/o* esophagus *gastr/o* stomach *duoden/o* duodenum *-scopy* viewing	Viewing the esophagus, stomach, and first part of the duodenum to aid in the diagnosis of reasons for digestive bleeding, vomiting, and weight loss.
frenotomy, frenulotomy	*fren/o, frenul/o* frenulum *- tomy* cutting	Cutting a frenulum of the tongue to treat ankyloglossia.
fundoplication, gastroesophageal	*fund/o* fundus *-plication* folding	Folding the fundus of the stomach around the distal end of the esophagus. Done to treat gastroesophageal reflux.
gastroduodenostomy	*gastr/o* stomach *duoden/o* duodenum *- stomy* making a new opening	A new opening between the stomach and the duodenum (Fig. 5-27). The figure also demonstrates an **anastomosis,** a new connection between two (usually hollow) structures.
gastroplasty	*gastr/o* stomach *-plasty* surgically forming	Surgically forming the stomach for the purpose of repair or reshaping. Usually performed as a type of bariatric (weight reduction) surgery. The stomach may be banded, stapled, or cut to reduce its size.

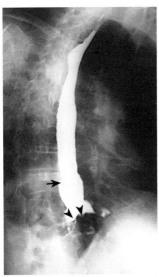

Fig. 5-26 Barium swallow.

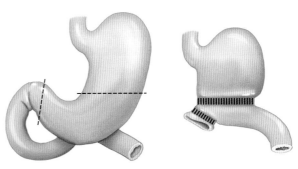

Fig. 5-27 Gastroduodenostomy. Part of the stomach has been cut out and the duodenum has been anastomosed to the remaining stomach.

Terms Related to Upper GI Procedures—cont'd

Term	Word Origin	Definition
gastrostomy	*gastr/o* stomach *-stomy* making a new opening	A new opening in the stomach. A **percutaneous endoscopic gastrostomy (PEG)** is an opening in the stomach for the purpose of placing a tube for enteral feeding.
gingivectomy	*gingiv/o* gums *-ectomy* cutting out	Cutting out part or all of the gums, usually as part of a treatment for periodontal disease.
glossorrhaphy	*gloss/o* tongue *-rrhaphy* suturing	Suturing the tongue, usually to repair a lesion or wound.
hyperalimentation	*hyper-* excessive *aliment/o* nutrition *-ation* process of	The therapeutic use of nutritional supplements that exceed recommended daily requirements.
manometry, esophageal	*man/o* pressure *-metry* measuring	Test that measures the motor function (muscle pressure) of the esophagus. A **manometer** is the instrument used to measure pressure.
odontectomy	*odont/o* tooth *-ectomy* cutting out	Extraction of a tooth.
palatoplasty	*palat/o* palate *-plasty* surgically forming	Surgical correction of the roof of the mouth. May be done to correct a cleft palate or as part of a procedure to treat snoring.
pyloromyotomy	*pylor/o* pylorus *my/o* muscle *-tomy* cutting	An incision of the pyloric sphincter to correct an obstruction, such as pyloric stenosis.

Terms Related to Upper GI Procedures—cont'd

Term	Word Origin	Definition
sialoadenectomy	*sialoaden/o* salivary gland *-ectomy* cutting out	Removal of a salivary gland (usually the submandibular) due to inflammation of the gland, stones, or cancer.
sialodochoplasty	*sialodoch/o* salivary duct *-plasty* surgically forming	Surgical correction of a salivary duct, often following the removal of a stone in a salivary gland.
stomatoplasty	*stomat/o* mouth *-plasty* surgically forming	Surgical reconstruction of the mouth to correct malformation due to trauma, disease, or congenital causes.
uvulectomy	*uvul/o* uvula *-ectomy* cutting out	Removal of part or all of the uvula, usually to correct snoring.

 PCS Guideline Alert

B3.6A Bypass procedures are coded by identifying the body part bypassed "from" and the body part bypassed "to." The fourth character body part specifies the body part bypassed from, and the qualifier specifies the body part bypassed to. Example: Gastrojejunostomy, a bypass from stomach to jejunum—stomach is the body part and jejunum is the qualifier.

 PCS Guideline Alert

B3.8 PCS contains specific body parts for anatomical subdivisions of a body part, such as lobes of the lungs or liver and regions of the intestines. Resection of the specific body part is coded whenever all of the body part is cut out or off, rather than coding Excision of a less specific body part.

 Exercise 15: **Upper GI Procedures**

Match the procedures to their definitions.

_____ 1. barium swallow
_____ 2. esophagoesophagostomy
_____ 3. frenotomy
_____ 4. fundoplication
_____ 5. gingivectomy
_____ 6. gastroduodenostomy
_____ 7. odontectomy
_____ 8. glossorrhaphy
_____ 9. pyloromyotomy
_____ 10. sialoadenectomy

A. incision of the pyloric sphincter to correct an obstruction
B. cutting a frenulum of the tongue
C. rejoining of two ends of a cut esophagus
D. radiographic imaging done after oral ingestion of a barium sulfate suspension
E. cutting out part or all of the gums
F. cutting out a salivary gland
G. folding the fundus of the stomach around the distal end of the esophagus
H. extraction of a tooth
I. suturing the tongue
J. making a new opening between the stomach and the duodenum

Translate the terms.

11. palatoplasty _____

12. esophagogastroduodenoscopy _____

13. gastroplasty _____

14. stomatoplasty _____

Terms Related to Lower GI Procedures

Term	Word Origin	Definition
appendectomy	*append/o* appendix *-ectomy* cutting out	Cutting out the vermiform appendix. If termed an **incidental appendectomy,** the removal was secondary to another surgery.
barium enema (BE)		Introduction of a barium sulfate suspension through the rectum for imaging of the lower digestive tract to detect obstructions, tumors, and other abnormalities.
cecopexy	*cec/o* cecum *-pexy* suspension	Fixation of the cecum to prevent or correct volvulus of the cecum.
colonoscopy	*colon/o* colon, large intestine *-scopy* viewing	Viewing the lining of large intestine for screening for cancer, diverticulitis, or other abnormalities.
colostomy	*col/o* colon, large intestine *-stomy* making a new opening	Surgical redirection of the bowel to a **stoma,** an artificial opening, on the abdominal wall (Fig. 5-28).
diverticulectomy	*diverticul/o* pouch, diverticulum *-ectomy* cutting out	Cutting out a diverticulum

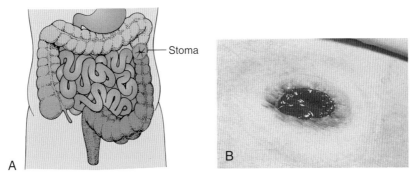

— Stoma

A   B

Fig. 5-28 A, Colostomy. **B,** Stoma.

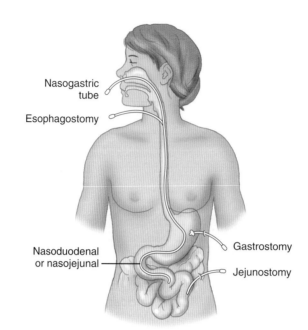

Fig. 5-29 Common placement locations for enteral feeding tubes.

Terms Related to Lower GI Procedures—cont'd

Term	Word Origin	Definition
enteral nutrition	*enter/o* small intestine *-al* pertaining to	Nutrition introduced through a digestive structure (Fig. 5-29).
herniorrhaphy	*herni/o* hernia *-rrhaphy* suturing	Suturing a hernia. Approaches may be through an open incision or laparoscopically and may be simply sutured or include a mesh.
ileoureterostomy	*ile/o* ileum *ureter/o* ureter *-stomy* making a new opening	New opening between (anastomosis) the ileum and the ureters in order to conduct urine into the third section of the small intestines when the bladder and urethra are not functional.
jejunostomy	*jejun/o* jejunum *-stomy* making a new opening	New opening of the jejunum to the surface of the abdomen for the placement of a feeding tube.
omentectomy, omentumectomy	*oment/o* omentum *-ectomy* cutting out	Cutting out part or all of the omentum. Done as part of treatment for ovarian cancer to remove cancer cells that have spread there.
peritoneocentesis	*peritone/o* peritoneum *-centesis* surgical puncture	Surgical puncture of the peritoneum to remove fluid. Often used to treat ascites.
polypectomy, GI	*polyp/o* polyp *-ectomy* cutting out	Cutting out sessile or pedunculated polyps from the gastrointestinal system.

Continued

Terms Related to Lower GI Procedures—cont'd

Term	Word Origin	Definition
proctoclysis	*proct/o* rectum and anus *-clysis* washing	Cleansing the rectum and anus. An enema.
proctoscopy	*proct/o* rectum and anus *-scopy* viewing	Process of viewing the rectum and anus. Used to view hemorrhoids or rectal polyps.
sigmoidoscopy	*sigmoid/o* sigmoid colon *-scopy* viewing	Process of viewing the sigmoid colon.
total parenteral nutrition (TPN)	*par-* near, beside *enter/o* small intestine *-al* pertaining to	Nutrition introduced through a structure outside of the alimentary canal, usually by IV because the GI tract is nonfunctional. Enteral nutrition provides sustenance through a feeding tube to the stomach or intestines.

 Exercise 16: Lower GI Procedures

Match the procedures with their definitions.

_____ 1. cecopexy
_____ 2. barium enema
_____ 3. colonoscopy
_____ 4. ileoureterostomy
_____ 5. enteral nutrition
_____ 6. TPN
_____ 7. jejunostomy

A. introduction of a barium sulfate suspension through the rectum for imaging of the lower digestive tract
B. nutrition introduced through a digestive structure
C. making a new opening between the ileum and the ureters
D. nutrition introduced through a structure outside the alimentary canal
E. suspending the cecum
F. making a new opening of the jejunum to the surface of the abdomen
G. viewing the large intestine.

Translate the terms.

8. appendectomy _____

9. colonoscopy _____

10. colostomy _____

11. peritoneocentesis _____

12. proctoclysis _____

13. herniorrhaphy _____

Terms Related to Procedures of the Adnexa

Term	Word Origin	Definition
cholangiography	*cholangi/o* bile vessel *-graphy* recording	Process of recording the bile vessels. Radiographic procedure that captures images of the common bile vessel through injection of a contrast medium into the bile duct, after which a series of images is taken.
cholecystectomy	*cholecyst/o* gallbladder *-ectomy* cutting out	Cutting out the gallbladder. If done laparoscopically, the gallbladder is removed through the use of small incisions in the abdomen (Fig. 5-30).
choledochectomy	*choledoch/o* common bile duct *-ectomy* cutting out	Cutting out part or all of the common bile duct as part of a procedure to treat cancer in the proximal duodenum
choledocholithotomy	*choledoch/o* common bile duct *-lithotomy* cutting out a stone	Cutting out a stone from the common bile duct. May be done via an open or a laparoscopic approach.

Continued

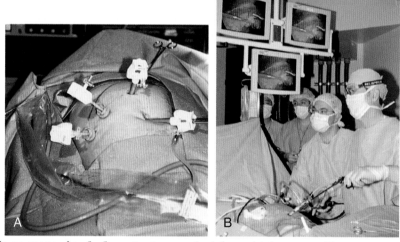

Fig. 5-30 Four-port laparoscopic cholecystectomy. A, A lensed telescope with camera and long instruments are introduced into small incisions. **B,** The camera image is projected to central monitors.

To watch how a cholecystectomy is performed, click on **Animations.**

Terms Related to Procedures of the Adnexa—cont'd

Term	Word Origin	Definition
endoscopic retrograde cholangiopancreatography (ERCP)	*endo-* within *-scopic* pertaining to viewing *cholangi/o* bile vessel *pancreat/o* pancreas *-graphy* recording	Recording the bile vessels and pancreas (Fig. 5-31). An x-ray of the pancreas and bile ducts that is enhanced through the use of radio-opaque dyes; used to diagnose stones, strictures (narrowings), and neoplasms.
hepatectomy	*hepat/o* liver *-ectomy* cutting out	Cutting out part or all of the liver. A total hepatectomy is performed for the purpose of a liver transplant. A partial hepatectomy is done for treatment of neoplasms (Fig. 5-32).

CPT Coding Alert!

CPT specifies a code for endoscopic retrograde cholangiopancreatography (ERCP) with a pressure measurement of the sphincter of Oddi.

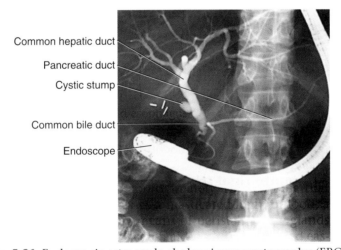

Common hepatic duct
Pancreatic duct
Cystic stump
Common bile duct
Endoscope

Fig. 5-31 Endoscopic retrograde cholangiopancreatography (ERCP).

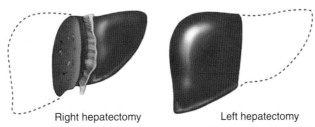

Right hepatectomy   Left hepatectomy

Fig. 5-32 Commonly performed major hepatic resections are indicated by shaded areas.

Exercise 17: Adnexa Procedures

Build the terms.

1. recording of a bile vessel _____

2. cutting out the common bile duct _____

3. cutting out the liver _____

4. cutting out a stone from the common bile duct _____

5. cutting out the gallbladder _____

PHARMACOLOGY

anorexiants: Appetite suppressants designed to aid in weight control, often in an attempt to treat **morbid obesity** (an amount of body fat that threatens normal health). Examples of anorexiants are phendimetrazine (Bontril PDM) and phentermine (Adipex-P).

antacids: A buffer (neutralizer) of hydrochloric acid in the stomach to temporarily relieve symptoms of GERD, pyrosis, and ulcers. Examples include calcium carbonate (Tums, Rolaids), and aluminum hydroxide with magnesium hydroxide (Maalox).

antidiarrheals: Provide relief from diarrhea by reducing intestinal motility, inflammation, or loss of fluids and nutrients. Examples include loperamide (Imodium), bismuth subsalicylate (Pepto-Bismol), and diphenoxylate with atropine (Lomotil).

antiemetics: Prevent or alleviate nausea and vomiting. Examples include scopolamine (Transderm Scop), ondansetron (Zofran), and promethazine (Promethegan).

gastrointestinal stimulants: Promote motility of smooth muscles in gastrointestinal tract. An example is metoclopramide (Reglan).

histamine-2 receptor antagonists (H2RAs) or **H2-blockers:** Block the histamine-2 receptors in the stomach to reduce hydrochloric stomach acid production for moderate-lasting acid suppression. Reduce hydrochloric acid production in the stomach for moderate-lasting acid suppression. Examples include famotidine (Pepcid) and ranitidine (Zantac).

irritable bowel syndrome (IBS) agents: Provide relief from constipation or diarrhea symptom effects of irritable bowel syndrome. This class includes multiple modes of action affecting the GI system. Examples include eluxadoline (Viberzi), linaclotide (Linzess), and alosetron (Lotronex).

laxatives: Promote evacuation of the bowel by increasing the bulk of the feces, softening the stool, or lubricating the intestinal wall. Examples include psyllium (Metamucil) and docusate (Colace). Stimulant laxatives cause more direct bowel evacuation by stimulating peristalsis. Examples include sennosides (Ex-Lax) and bisacodyl (Dulcolax).

proton pump inhibitors: Block gastric proton pump to reduce production of stomach acid for long-lasting acid suppression for treatment of disorders like GERD. Examples include esomeprazole (Nexium) and lansoprazole (Prevacid).

antiemetic
anti- = against
-emetic = pertaining to vomiting

Exercise 18: **Pharmacology**

Match each disorder with the type of drug that is used to treat it.

____ 1. nausea and vomiting   ____ 4. excessive weight gain   A. laxative

____ 2. chronic GERD   ____ 5. constipation   B. antidiarrheal

____ 3. short-term dyspepsia   ____ 6. intestinal cramping and   C. proton pump inhibitor
                                         loose, watery stools   D. antacid
                                                                 E. antiemetic
                                                                 F. anorexiant

RECOGNIZING SUFFIXES FOR PCS

Now that you've finished reading about the procedures for the digestive system, take a look at this review of the *suffixes* used in their terminology. Each of these suffixes is associated with one or more root operations in the medical surgical section or one of the other categories in PCS.

Suffixes and Root Operations for the Digestive System

Suffix	Root Operation
-centesis	Drainage
-ectomy	Excision, resection
-lithotomy	Extirpation
-pexy	Repair, reposition
-plasty	Repair, supplement, replacement
-plication	Restriction
-rrhaphy	Repair, supplement
-scopy	Inspection
-stomy	Bypass, drainage
-tomy	Drainage, release, division

Abbreviations

Abbreviation	Meaning	Abbreviation	Meaning
BE	barium enema	HBV	hepatitis B virus
BM	bowel movement	HCV	hepatitis C virus
BS	barium swallow	HSV	herpes simplex virus
CLO	Campylobacter-like organism test	IBD	inflammatory bowel disease
EGD	esophagogastroduodenoscopy	IBS	irritable bowel syndrome
ERCP	endoscopic retrograde cholangiopancreatography	LES	lower esophageal sphincter
		N&V	nausea and vomiting
FOBT	fecal occult blood test	PEG	percutaneous endoscopic gastrostomy
GB	gallbladder		
GERD	gastroesophageal reflux disease	PUD	peptic ulcer disease
GI	gastrointestinal	TPN	total parenteral nutrition
HAV	hepatitis A virus		

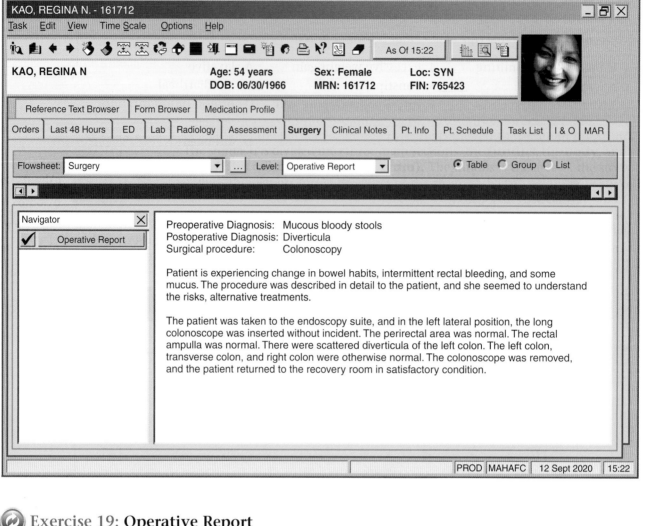

KAO, REGINA N. - 161712

Task   Edit   View   Time Scale   Options   Help

KAO, REGINA N   Age: 54 years   Sex: Female   Loc: SYN
                     DOB: 06/30/1966   MRN: 161712   FIN: 765423

Reference Text Browser | Form Browser | Medication Profile

Orders | Last 48 Hours | ED | Lab | Radiology | Assessment | **Surgery** | Clinical Notes | Pt. Info | Pt. Schedule | Task List | I & O | MAR

Flowsheet: Surgery   Level: Operative Report   ● Table ○ Group ○ List

Navigator   ✓ Operative Report

Preoperative Diagnosis: Mucous bloody stools
Postoperative Diagnosis: Diverticula
Surgical procedure: Colonoscopy

Patient is experiencing change in bowel habits, intermittent rectal bleeding, and some mucus. The procedure was described in detail to the patient, and she seemed to understand the risks, alternative treatments.

The patient was taken to the endoscopy suite, and in the left lateral position, the long colonoscope was inserted without incident. The perirectal area was normal. The rectal ampulla was normal. There were scattered diverticula of the left colon. The left colon, transverse colon, and right colon were otherwise normal. The colonoscope was removed, and the patient returned to the recovery room in satisfactory condition.

PROD | MAHAFC | 12 Sept 2020 | 15:22

Exercise 19: Operative Report

Using the operative report above, answer the following questions.

1. What diagnostic procedure was performed? _____

2. What instrument was used? _____

3. What diagnosis was determined from the procedure? _____

4. What is the "perirectal" area? _____

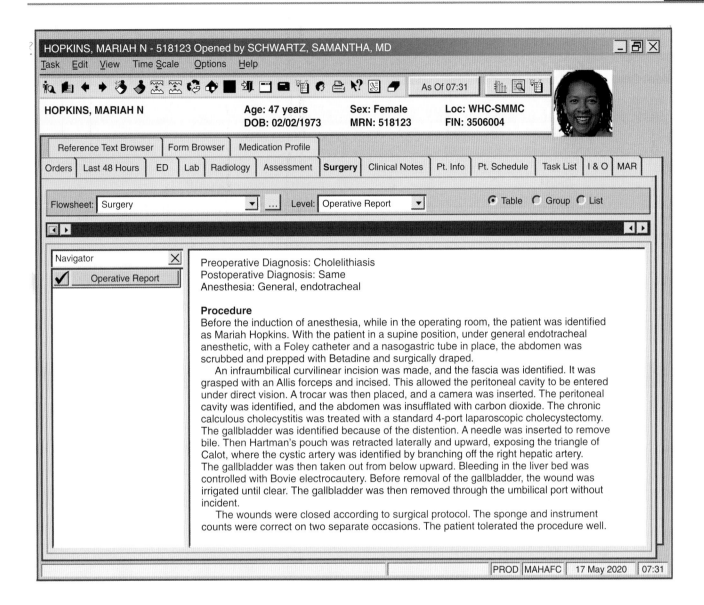

Preoperative Diagnosis: Cholelithiasis
Postoperative Diagnosis: Same
Anesthesia: General, endotracheal

Procedure
Before the induction of anesthesia, while in the operating room, the patient was identified as Mariah Hopkins. With the patient in a supine position, under general endotracheal anesthetic, with a Foley catheter and a nasogastric tube in place, the abdomen was scrubbed and prepped with Betadine and surgically draped.

An infraumbilical curvilinear incision was made, and the fascia was identified. It was grasped with an Allis forceps and incised. This allowed the peritoneal cavity to be entered under direct vision. A trocar was then placed, and a camera was inserted. The peritoneal cavity was identified, and the abdomen was insufflated with carbon dioxide. The chronic calculus cholecystitis was treated with a standard 4-port laparoscopic cholecystectomy. The gallbladder was identified because of the distention. A needle was inserted to remove bile. Then Hartman's pouch was retracted laterally and upward, exposing the triangle of Calot, where the cystic artery was identified by branching off the right hepatic artery. The gallbladder was then taken out from below upward. Bleeding in the liver bed was controlled with Bovie electrocautery. Before removal of the gallbladder, the wound was irrigated until clear. The gallbladder was then removed through the umbilical port without incident.

The wounds were closed according to surgical protocol. The sponge and instrument counts were correct on two separate occasions. The patient tolerated the procedure well.

 Exercise 20: **Operative Report**

Using the operative report above, answer the following questions.

1. How do you know that Ms. Hopkins has gallstones? _____

2. Which term tells you that her gallbladder was inflamed? _____

3. Her gallbladder was removed through an endoscopic procedure called a/an _____

4. To say that the patient was in a supine position means that she was lying on her _____

Go to the Evolve website to interactively build terms, label images, memorize word parts and practice using digestive terms in context.

Match the word parts to their definitions.

WORD PART DEFINITIONS

Suffix		Definition
-chalasia	1. _____	discharge, flow
-emesis	2. _____	viewing
-iasis	3. _____	making a new opening
-pepsia	4. _____	condition of relaxation
-phagia	5. _____	suturing
-rrhaphy	6. _____	vomiting
-rrhea	7. _____	presence of
-scopy	8. _____	condition of swallowing, eating
-stalsis	9. _____	contraction
-stomy	10. _____	digestion condition

Combining Form		Definition
an/o	11. _____	tongue
bil/i	12. _____	gums
bucc/o	13. _____	fat, lipid
cheil/o	14. _____	bile
cholangi/o	15. _____	esophagus
choledoch/o	16. _____	saliva
cholecyst/o	17. _____	bile vessel
col/o	18. _____	common bile duct
enter/o	19. _____	mouth
epiplo/o	20. _____	omentum
esophag/o	21. _____	stomach
gastr/o	22. _____	rectum and anus
gingiv/o	23. _____	lips
gloss/o	24. _____	liver
hepat/o	25. _____	cheek
lip/o	26. _____	tooth
lumin/o	27. _____	anus
odont/o	28. _____	gallbladder
pharyng/o	29. _____	throat
proct/o	30. _____	lumen
sial/o	31. _____	large intestine
stomat/o	32. _____	small intestines

WORDSHOP

Prefixes	Combining Forms	Suffixes
an-	an/o	-al
dys-	cholecyst/o	-clysis
per-	choledoch/o	-eal
peri-	col/o	-ectomy
	duoden/o	-ia
	esophag/o	-iasis
	gastr/o	-itis
	gloss/o	-megaly
	hepat/o	-phagia
	lith/o	-plasty
	odont/o	-rrhaphy
	proct/o	-scopy
	sialoaden/o	-stomy
	sialodoch/o	

Build digestive terms by combining the word parts above. Some word parts may be used more than once. Some may not be used at all. The number in parentheses indicates the number of word parts needed.

Definition	Term
1. pertaining to the stomach and esophagus (3)	
2. surgically forming the stomach (2)	
3. pertaining to surrounding the teeth (3)	
4. inflammation of the stomach (2)	
5. making a new opening in the colon (2)	
6. washing the rectum and anus (2)	
7. viewing the esophagus, stomach, and duodenum (4)	
8. cutting out the gallbladder (2)	
9. making a new opening in the stomach (2)	
10. condition of painful, difficult swallowing (2)	
11. enlargement of the liver (2)	
12. surgically forming the salivary duct (2)	
13. suturing the tongue (2)	
14. condition of stones in the common bile duct (3)	
15. condition of without teeth (3)	

Sort the terms below into their correct categories.

TERM SORTING

Anatomy and Physiology	Pathology	Procedures

achalasia	defecation	ileum
anodontia	deglutition	ileus
anorectal fistula	duodenum	mastication
aphthous stomatitis	dyspepsia	omentum
appendectomy	enteral nutrition	peristalsis
appendicitis	ERCP	peritoneocentesis
ascites	esophagus	philtrum
BE	femoral hernia	plicae
cecopexy	frenulum	ptyalism
cheilitis	gastroplasty	retroperitoneum
chyme	glossorrhaphy	rugae
cholangiography	halitosis	sialoadenectomy
cholelithiasis	herniorrhaphy	stomatoplasty
cirrhosis	hyperalimentation	total bilirubin

Replace the highlighted words with the correct terms.

TRANSLATIONS

1. After having a **viewing of the large intestine**, the patient needed a **cutting out of a polyp.**

2. The patient was tested for **an inflammation of the liver** due to **yellowing of the skin and sclerae.**

3. The patient's **protrusion of a loop of the intestine into the inguinal canal** was corrected with a **suturing of the hernia.**

4. A **fecal exam to detect hidden blood** was used to determine if the patient had bleeding in his gastrointestinal tract.

5. The patient was diagnosed with **the presence of stone in the gallbladder** and underwent a **cutting out of the gallbladder.**

6. Ross underwent a **surgical redirection of the bowel to a stoma** when his **inflammation of the ileum or the colon that is of idiopathic origin** became too severe.

7. The patient had **gas expelled through the anus** and an **abnormal discharge of watery, semisolid stools.**

8. Delay in treating the patient's **inflammation of the appendix** led to a nearly fatal case of **inflammation of the peritoneum.**

9. The dentist told Ava she had **inflammatory disease of the gums,** which could eventually lead to **pathologic condition of the tissue surrounding the teeth.**

10. The last patient of the day had complaints of **indigestion, abdominal pain,** and **heartburn.**

11. The patient underwent **surgical puncture of the peritoneum to remove fluid** to treat his **excessive intraperitoneal fluid.**

12. The surgeon created a/an **new connection between two structures** when he performed a **new opening between the stomach and duodenum.**

ICD-10-CM Example from Tabular

N30 Cystitis

Use additional code to identify infectious agent
(B95-B97)

Excludes1 prostatocystitis (N41.3)

N30.0 Acute cystitis

Excludes1 irradiation cystitis (N30.4-)

trigonitis (N30.3-)

N30.00 Acute cystitis without hematuria

N30.01 Acute cystitis with hematuria

N30.1 Interstitial cystitis (chronic)

N30.10 Interstitial cystitis (chronic) without hematuria

N30.11 Interstitial cystitis (chronic) with hematuria

N30.2 Other chronic cystitis

N30.20 Other chronic cystitis without hematuria

N30.21 Other chronic cystitis with hematuria

N30.3 Trigonitis

Urethrotrigonitis

N30.30 Trigonitis without hematuria

N30.31 Trigonitis with hematuria

N30.4 Irradiation cystitis

N30.40 Irradiation cystitis without hematuria

N30.41 Irradiation cystitis with hematuria

N30.8 Other cystitis

Abscess of bladder

N30.80 Other cystitis without hematuria

N30.81 Other cystitis with hematuria

N30.9 Cystitis, unspecified

N30.90 Cystitis, unspecified without hematuria

N30.91 Cystitis, unspecified with hematuria

ICD-10-PCS Example from Index

Pyelography
- *– see* Plain Radiography, Urinary System **BT0**
- *– see* Fluoroscopy, Urinary System **BT1**

Pyeloileostomy, urinary diversion
- *– see* Bypass, Urinary System **0T1**

Pyeloplasty
- *– see* Repair, Urinary System **0TQ**
- *– see* Replacement, Urinary System **0TR**
- *– see* Supplement, Urinary System **0TU**

Pyelorrhaphy
- *– see* Repair, Urinary System **0TQ**

Pyeloscopy
- **0TJ58ZZ**

Pyelostomy
- *– see* Bypass, Urinary System **0T1**
- *– see* Drainage, Urinary System **0T9**

Pyelotomy
- *– see* Drainage, Urinary System **0T9**

CHAPTER OUTLINE

Urinary System

FUNCTIONS OF THE URINARY SYSTEM

ANATOMY AND PHYSIOLOGY

PATHOLOGY

PROCEDURES

PHARMACOLOGY

RECOGNIZING SUFFIXES FOR PCS

ABBREVIATIONS FOR THE URINARY SYSTEM

Male Reproductive System

FUNCTIONS OF THE MALE REPRODUCTIVE SYSTEM

ANATOMY AND PHYSIOLOGY

PATHOLOGY

PROCEDURES

PHARMACOLOGY

RECOGNIZING SUFFIXES FOR PCS

ABBREVIATIONS FOR THE MALE REPRODUCTIVE SYSTEM

Female Reproductive System

FUNCTIONS OF THE FEMALE REPRODUCTIVE SYSTEM

ANATOMY AND PHYSIOLOGY

PATHOLOGY

PROCEDURES

PHARMACOLOGY

RECOGNIZING SUFFIXES FOR PCS

ABBREVIATIONS FOR THE FEMALE REPRODUCTIVE SYSTEM

OBJECTIVES

☐ Recognize and use terms related to the anatomy and physiology of the genitourinary system.

☐ Recognize and use terms related to the pathology of the genitourinary system.

☐ Recognize and use terms related to the procedures for the genitourinary system.

URINARY SYSTEM

FUNCTIONS OF THE URINARY SYSTEM

The major function of the urinary system is to continually maintain a healthy balance of the amount and content of **extracellular fluids** within the body. Biologists use the term *homeostasis* to describe this important process. The process of metabolism changes food and liquid (with its requisite fats, carbohydrates, and proteins) into building blocks, energy sources, and waste products. To operate efficiently, the body needs to constantly monitor and rebalance the amounts of these substances in the bloodstream. The breakdown of proteins and amino acids in the liver leaves chemical wastes, such as urea, creatinine, and uric acid. These wastes are toxic, nitrogenous substances that must be excreted in the urine. The act of releasing urine is called **urination, voiding,** or **micturition.**

ANATOMY AND PHYSIOLOGY

The urinary system is composed of two kidneys, two ureters, a urinary bladder, and a urethra (Figs. 6-1 and 6-2). The work of the urinary system is done by a specialized tissue in the **kidneys** called *parenchymal tissue.* The kidneys function to filter the blood and eliminate waste through the passage of urine. The **ureters** are thin, muscular tubes that move urine in peristaltic waves from the kidneys to the bladder. The urinary **bladder** is the sac that stores the urine until it is excreted. The bladder is lined with an epithelial mucous membrane of transitional cells. Underneath, a layer termed the *lamina propria* is composed of connective tissue that holds the blood vessels and nerves. The detrusor muscle is the

extracellular
  extra- = outside
  cellul/o = cell
  -ar = pertaining to

urination
  urin/o = urine, urinary system
  -ation = process of

⊗ Be Careful!

-uria is a *suffix that means* urinary condition; **urea** is a *chemical waste product.*

kidney = **nephr/o, ren/o**

parenchymal
  par- = near, beside
  en- = in
  chym/o = juices
  -al = pertaining to

ureter = **ureter/o**

bladder = **cyst/o, vesic/o**

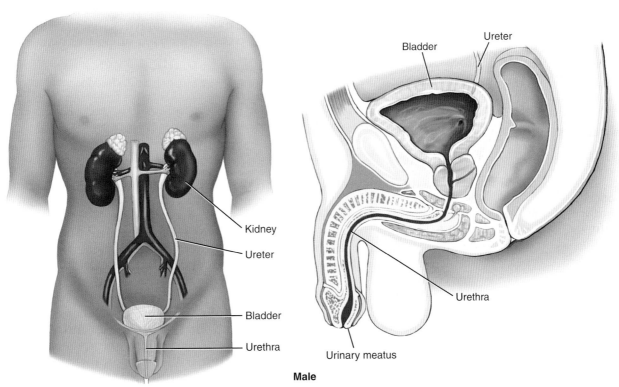

Male

Fig. 6-1 Male urinary system.

urethra = urethr/o

meatus = meat/o

trigone = trigon/o

stromal tissue = strom/o

retroperitoneal
  retro- = behind
  peritone/o =
    peritoneum
  -al = pertaining to

cortex = cortic/o

medulla = medull/o

renal pelvis = pyel/o

renal calyx = calic/o,
  cali/o, calyc/o

hilum = hil/o

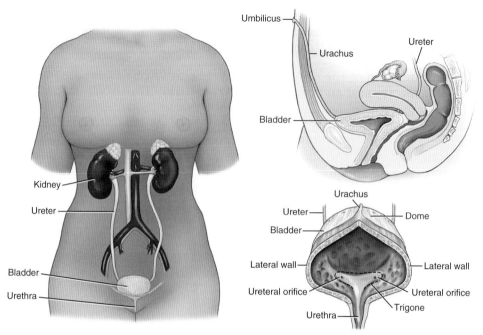

Fig. 6-2 Female urinary system.

final coat; it normally contracts to expel urine. The **urethra** is the tube that conducts the urine out of the bladder. Two sphincters (ringlike muscles) surrounding the urethra are instrumental in the release of urine. The internal sphincter is involuntary, while the external one is voluntary. The opening of the urethra is called the **urinary meatus.** The triangular area in the bladder between the ureters' entrance and the urethral outlet is called the **trigone.** When this area is stretched by the filling of the bladder with urine, a signal is sent to the brain for the urge to urinate. Other trigones (three point structures) occur throughout the body, but the one in the bladder is the most commonly referred to. The ureters, bladder, and urethra are all **stromal tissue,** which is a supportive tissue.

ICD Note This chapter includes all the anatomy necessary to assign ICD-10 urinary system codes, including detail on the renal calyx, the trigone, and the ureteropelvic junction. See Appendix H for a complete list of body parts and how they should be coded.

The Kidney

Because the kidneys are primarily responsible for the functioning of the urinary system, it is helpful to look at them in greater detail. Each of the two kidneys is located high in the posterior abdominal area, tucked under the ribs in the back and behind the lining of the abdominal area **(retroperitoneal).** The normal human kidney is about the size of a fist. The tough outer covering of the kidney is the **renal capsule.** If a kidney were sliced open, the outer portion, the **cortex** *(pl.* cortices), and the inner portion, called the **medulla** *(pl.* medullae), would be visible (Fig. 6-3). The **renal pelvis** and **calyces** *(sing.* calyx) are an extension of the ureter inside the kidney. The **renal pyramids** are triangular sections that extend from the renal medulla toward the renal pelvis. The downward point of the pyramid is referred to as the **papilla.** The term *renal* means "pertaining to the kidneys." The **ureteropelvic junction (UPJ)** is the area where the ureter joins the renal pelvis. It is a common site of obstruction of the outward flow of urine from the kidney.

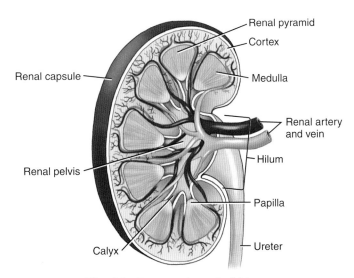

Fig. 6-3 Cross section of a kidney.

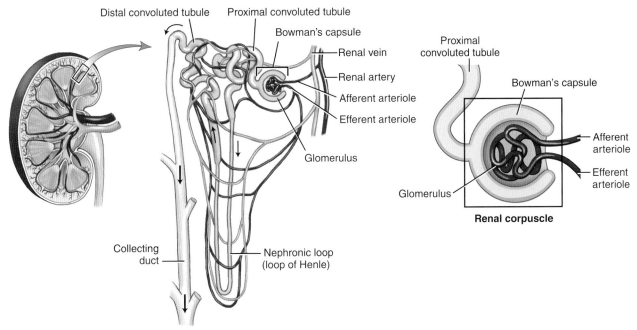

Fig. 6-4 The nephron.

The **renal hilum** *(pl.* hila) is the location on the kidney where the ureter and renal vein leave the kidney and the renal artery enters. The cortex contains tissue with millions of microscopic units called **nephrons** (Fig. 6-4). Here in the tiny neph- rons, blood passes through a continuous system of urinary filtration, reabsorp- tion, and secretion that measures, monitors, and adjusts the levels of substances in the extracellular fluid.

The Nephron

The nephrons filter all the blood in the body approximately every 5 minutes. The **renal afferent arteries** transport unfiltered blood to the kidneys. Once in the kidneys, the blood travels through small arteries called **arterioles** and finally into tiny balls of renal capillaries, called **glomeruli** *(sing.* glomerulus). These glomeruli cluster at the entrance to each nephron. It is here that the process of filtering the blood to form urine begins.

artery = arteri/o

glomerulus = glomerul/o

The nephron consists of four parts: (1) the **renal corpuscle,** which is composed of the glomerulus and its surrounding Bowman's capsule; (2) a **proximal convoluted tubule;** (3) the **nephronic loop,** also known as the loop of Henle; and (4) the **distal convoluted tubule.** As blood flows through the capillaries, water, electrolytes, glucose, and nitrogenous wastes are passed through the glomerular membrane and collected. The most common electrolytes are sodium (Na), chloride (Cl), and potassium (K). Blood cells and proteins are too large to pass through a healthy glomerular membrane. Selective filtration and reabsorption continue along the renal tubules, with the end result of **urine** concentration and subsequent dilution occurring in the renal medulla. From there, the urine flows to the calyces and exits the kidney, flowing through the ureter into the bladder, where it is stored until it can be expelled from the body through the urethra.

urine = ur/o, urin/o

To see how urine is formed, click on **Animations.**

 Exercise 1: The Urinary System

Match the combining form with its term.

_____ 1. opening of the urethra
_____ 2. tubes connecting kidneys and bladder
_____ 3. tube conducting urine out of the bladder
_____ 4. same as ren/o
_____ 5. sac that stores urine
_____ 6. area between ureters coming in and urethra going out in the sac that stores urine
_____ 7. urine, urinary system
_____ 8. renal pelvis
_____ 9. outer portion of the kidney
_____ 10. inner portion of the kidney
_____ 11. artery
_____ 12. renal calyx
_____ 13. location where ureter and renal vein leave kidney and renal artery enters

A. nephr/o
B. urin/o
C. meat/o
D. urethr/o
E. vesic/o
F. ureter/o
G. trigon/o
H. medull/o
I. calyc/o
J. cortic/o
K. hil/o
L. pyel/o
M. arteri/o

Translate the terms.

14. transurethral _____

15. paranephric _____

16. retroperitoneal _____

17. suprarenal _____

18. perivesical _____

To practice labeling the urinary system, click on **Label It.**

Combining Forms for the Anatomy of the Urinary System

Meaning	Combining Form	Meaning	Combining Form
artery	arteri/o	medulla	medull/o
bladder	cyst/o, vesic/o	parenchyma	parenchym/o
calyx	calic/o, cali/o, calyc/o	peritoneum	peritone/o
cell	cellul/o	renal pelvis	pyel/o
cortex	cortic/o	stroma	strom/o
glomerulus	glomerul/o	trigone	trigon/o
hilum	hil/o	ureter	ureter/o
kidney	nephr/o, ren/o	urethra	urethr/o
meatus	meat/o	urine, urinary system	urin/o, ur/o

Prefixes for the Anatomy of the Urinary System

Prefix	Meaning
extra-	outside
en-	in
par-	beside, near
retro-	backward

Suffixes for the Anatomy of the Urinary System

Suffix	Meaning
-al, -ar, -ic	pertaining to
-ation, -ion	process of

You can review the anatomy of the urinary system by clicking on **Body Spectrum Electronic Anatomy Coloring Book,** then **Urinary.**

PATHOLOGY

Terms Related to Symptoms and Signs Involving the Genitourinary System (R30-R39)

Term	Word Origin	Definition
anuria	*an-* without *-uria* urinary condition	Condition of no urine.
dysuria	*dys-* painful, abnormal *-uria* urinary condition	Condition of painful urination.
enuresis	*en-* in *ur/o* urine *-esis* state of	Also commonly known as "bed-wetting," enuresis can be nocturnal (at night) or diurnal (during the day).

Continued

Terms Related to Symptoms and Signs Involving the Genitourinary System (R30-R39)—cont'd

Term	Word Origin	Definition
extrarenal uremia	*extra-* outside *ren/o* kidney *-al* pertaining to *ur/o* urine *-emia* blood condition	Excessive urea in blood (uremia) due to kidney failure caused by disease outside the kidney (e.g., congestive heart failure).
extravasation of urine	*extra-* outside *vas/o* vessel *-ation* process of	Condition of urine leaking outside the bladder and into surrounding tissues. May be due to trauma or a stone formed within and blocking the urinary tract.
hematuria	*hemat/o* blood *-uria* urinary condition	Blood in the urine.
incontinence, urinary		Inability to hold urine.
nocturia	*noct/i* night *-uria* urinary condition	Condition of excessive urination at night.
oliguria	*olig/o* scanty, few *-uria* urinary condition	Condition of scanty urination.
polyuria	*poly-* excessive, frequent *-uria* urinary condition	Condition of excessive urination.
retention, urinary		Inability to release urine.
vesical tenesmus	*vesic/o* bladder *-al* pertaining to	Bladder spasms.

Terms Related to Glomerular Diseases (N00-N08)

Term	Word Origins	Definition
acute nephritic syndrome	*nephr/o* kidney *-itic* pertaining to	Hypertension, hematuria, and proteinuria (protein in the urine) resulting from damage to the glomeruli.
nephrotic syndrome	*nephr/o* kidney *-tic* pertaining to	Abnormal group of signs in the kidney, characterized by proteinuria, hypoalbuminemia (abnormally low levels of albumin in the blood), and edema; may occur in glomerular disease and as a complication of many systemic diseases (e.g., diabetes mellitus). Also called **nephrosis**.

Terms Related to Renal Tubulo-interstitial Diseases (N10-N16)

Term	Word Origin	Definition
hydronephrosis	*hydr/o* water *nephr/o* kidney *-osis* abnormal condition	Dilation of the renal pelvis and calices of one or both kidneys resulting from obstruction of the flow of urine.
pyelonephritis	*pyel/o* renal pelvis *nephr/o* kidney *-itis* inflammation	Bacterial or viral infection of the kidneys and renal pelvis.

Terms Related to Renal Tubulo-interstitial Diseases (N10-N16)—cont'd

Term	Word Origin	Definition
pyonephrosis	*py/o* pus *nephr/o* kidney *-osis* abnormal condition	Pyogenic (pus-producing) infection of the kidney.
vesicoureteral reflux	*vesic/o* urinary bladder *ureter/o* ureter *-al* pertaining to *re-* back *-flux* flow	Abnormal backflow of urine from the bladder to the ureter, usually associated with a urinary tract disorder and caused by congenital urethral malformation.

Terms Related to Acute Kidney Failure and Chronic Kidney Failure (N17-N19)

Term	Word Origin	Definition
renal failure	*ren/o* kidney *-al* pertaining to	Inability of the kidneys to excrete wastes, concentrate urine, and conserve electrolytes. May be acute or chronic.
acute renal failure (ARF)		Sudden inability of the kidneys to excrete wastes, resulting from hemorrhage, trauma, burns, toxic injury to the kidney, pyelonephritis or glomerulonephritis, or lower urinary tract obstruction. Characterized by oliguria and rapid azotemia.
chronic kidney disease (CKD) (formerly chronic renal failure)		CKD is measured in stages of increasing severity, from 1 (mild damage with a normal glomerular filtration rate) to 5 (complete kidney failure requiring either dialysis or a renal transplant). Stage 5 is also called end-stage renal disease (ESRD) and is the most extreme form of CKD.

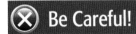 **Be Careful!**

Don't confuse *pyelonephritis*, an inflammation of the kidneys and renal pelvis, with *pyonephrosis*, a pus-producing inflammation of the kidneys.

 CM Guideline Alert

14A CHRONIC KIDNEY DISEASE

1) Stages of Chronic Kidney Disease (CKD)
The ICD-10-CM classifies CKD based on severity. The severity of CKD is designated by stages 1-5. Stage 2, code N18.2, equates to mild CKD; stage 3, code N18.3, equates to moderate CKD; and stage 4, code N18.4, equates to severe CKD. Code N18.6, end-stage-renal disease (ESRD), is assigned when the provider has documented ESRD. If both a stage of CKD and ESRD are documented, assign code N18.6 only.

2) CHRONIC KIDNEY DISEASE AND KIDNEY TRANSPLANT STATUS
Patients who have undergone kidney transplant may still have some form of CKD because the kidney transplant may not fully restore kidney function. Therefore, the presence of CKD alone does not constitute a transplant complication. Assign the appropriate N18 code for the patient's stage of CKD and code Z94.0, Kidney transplant status. If a transplant complication such as failure or rejection or other transplant complication is documented, see section I.C.19.g for information on coding complications of a kidney transplant. If the documentation is unclear as to whether the patient has a complication of the transplant, query the provider.

3) CHRONIC KIDNEY DISEASE WITH OTHER CONDITIONS
Patients with CKD may also suffer from other serious conditions, most commonly diabetes mellitus and hypertension. The sequencing of the CKD code in relationship to codes for other contributing conditions is based on the conventions in the Tabular List. *See I.C.9. Hypertensive chronic kidney disease. See I.C.19. Chronic kidney disease and kidney transplant complications.*

Exercise 2: Signs and Symptoms; Glomerular Diseases, Tubulointerstitial Diseases; Acute Kidney Failure; and Chronic Kidney Failure

_____ 1. vesical tenesmus

_____ 2. extravasation of urine

_____ 3. extrarenal uremia

_____ 4. hematuria

_____ 5. enuresis

_____ 6. urinary incontinence

_____ 7. urinary retention

_____ 8. anuria

_____ 9. oliguria

_____ 10. nocturia

_____ 11. acute nephritic syndrome

_____ 12. nephrotic syndrome

_____ 13. pyonephrosis

_____ 14. vesicoureteral reflux

_____ 15. ARF

_____ 16. ESRD

A. inability to hold urine

B. blood in the urine

C. condition of scanty urination

D. abnormal group of signs in the kidney, characterized by proteinuria, hypoalbuminemia, and edema

E. abnormal backflow of urine from the bladder to the ureter

F. inability to release urine

G. excessive urea in blood due to kidney failure caused by some disease outside the kidney

H. sudden inability of the kidneys to excrete wastes

I. hypertension, hematuria, and proteinuria resulting from damage to the glomeruli

J. pus-producing infection of the kidney

K. spasms of the bladder

L. condition of excessive urination at night

M. bed-wetting

N. condition of no urine

O. condition of urine leaking out of the bladder and into surrounding tissues

P. stage 5 CKD

Build the terms.

17. painful urinary condition _____.

18. excessive (frequent) urinary condition _____.

19. abnormal condition of water in the kidney _____.

Terms Related to Urolithiasis (N20-N23)

Term	Word Origin	Definition
urolithiasis	_ur/o_ urine, urinary system _lith/o_ stone _-iasis_ condition, presence of	Stones (calculi) anywhere in the urinary tract, but usually in the renal pelvis or urinary bladder. Depending on where the stone is located, the term is **nephrolithiasis** (kidney), **ureterolithiasis** (ureter), **cystolithiasis** (urinary bladder), or **urethrolithiasis** (urethra). Usually formed in patients with an excess of the mineral calcium. Also called **urinary calculi** (Fig. 6-5).

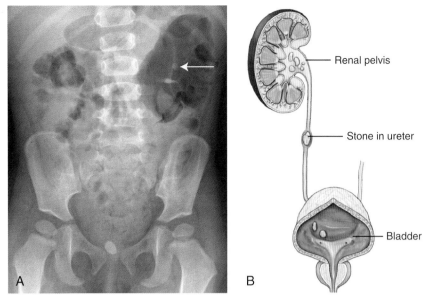

Fig. 6-5 **A,** X-ray showing nephrolithiasis and cystolithiasis. **B,** Locations of ureteral calculi.

Terms Related to Other Disorders of the Kidney and Ureter (N25-N29)

Term	Word Origin	Definition
nephrogenic diabetes insipidus	*nephr/o* kidney *-genic* pertaining to producing	A form of diabetes insipidus caused by a defect in the renal tubules causing them to be unresponsive to antidiuretic hormone (ADH). This not the same as diabetes insipidus, which is a lack of secretion of ADH.
nephropathy	*nephr/o* kidney *-pathy* disease process	Disease of the kidneys; a general term that does not specify a disorder.
nephroptosis	*nephr/o* kidney *-ptosis* drooping, sagging	Prolapse or sagging of the kidney that occurs when the patient stands from a sitting position. Also called **renal ptosis**.

Terms Related to Other Diseases of the Urinary System (N30-N39)

Term	Word Origin	Definition
cystitis	*cyst/o* bladder *-itis* inflammation	Inflammation of the urinary bladder.
interstitial cystitis (IC)	*inter-* between *stiti/o* space *–al* pertaining to *cyst/o* bladder *-itis* inflammation	A painful inflammation of the wall of the bladder. Symptoms include urinary frequency and urgency.
trigonitis	*trigon/o* trigone *-itis* inflammation	Inflammation of the bladder between the inlet of the ureters and outlet of the urethra.
urethral stricture	*urethr/o* urethra *-al* pertaining to	Narrowing of the urethra. Also called **urethral stenosis**.

Continued

Terms Related to Other Diseases of the Urinary System (N30-N39)-cont'd

Term	Word Origin	Definition
urethritis	*urethr/o* urethra *-itis* inflammation	Inflammation of the urethra.
urinary tract infection (UTI)	*urin/o* urine, urinary system	Infection anywhere in the urinary system, caused most commonly by bacteria, but also by parasites, yeast, and protozoa (sing. protozoon). Most frequently occurring disorder in the urinary system.

Terms Related to Benign Neoplasms (D30 and D41)

Term	Word Origin	Definition
renal adenoma	*ren/o* kidney *-al* pertaining to *aden/o* gland *-oma* tumor, mass	Small, slow-growing, glandular, noncancerous tumors of the kidney, usually found at autopsy.
renal oncocytoma	*onc/o* tumor *cyt/o* cell *-oma* tumor, mass	The most common benign solid renal tumor. These tumors are without signs or symptoms and are often discovered incidentally (by accident) on diagnostic imaging for another disorder.
transitional cell papilloma	*papill/o* nipple *-oma* tumor, mass	Also referred to as bladder papilloma. Although this type of tumor is benign when found, recurrences are occasionally malignant.

Terms Related to Malignant Neoplasms (C64-C68)

Term	Word Origin	Definition
nephroblastoma	*nephr/o* kidney *blast/o* embryonic *-oma* tumor	Also called **Wilms' tumor**, these tumors develop from kidney cells that did not develop fully before a child's birth. These cancerous tumors of the kidney occur mainly in children (Fig. 6-6, *A*).
renal cell carcinoma	*ren/o* kidney *-al* pertaining to *carcinoma* cancerous tumor of epithelial origin	Also referred to as **hypernephroma** or **adenocarcinoma** of the kidney, this is one of the most common cancers. Although the cause is unknown, risk factors include smoking and obesity.
transitional cell carcinoma (TCC) of the bladder	*carcinoma* cancerous tumor of epithelial origin	These malignant tumors account for approximately 90% of all bladder cancers and arise from the cells lining the bladder (Fig. 6-6, *B*).

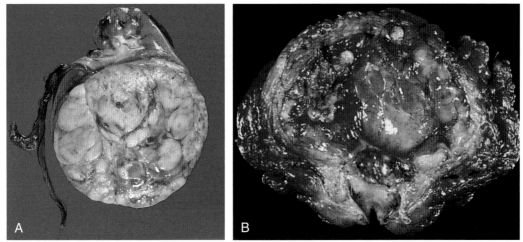

Fig. 6-6 **A,** Wilms' tumor (nephroblastoma) of the kidney. **B,** Transitional cell carcinoma of the bladder.

 ### Exercise 3: Urolithiasis; Other Disorders of Kidney and Ureter; Other Diseases of the Urinary System; and Neoplasms

Matching.

_____ 1. nephrolithiasis
_____ 2. nephrogenic diabetes insipidus
_____ 3. nephropathy
_____ 4. interstitial cystitis
_____ 5. trigonitis
_____ 6. urethritis
_____ 7. urethral stricture
_____ 8. UTI
_____ 9. renal adenoma
_____ 10. renal oncocytoma
_____ 11. transitional cell papilloma
_____ 12. renal cell carcinoma
_____ 13. TCC

A. bladder inflammation located between the inlet of the ureters and outlet of the urethra
B. diabetes insipidus caused by a defect in the renal tubules
C. urethral stenosis
D. most common benign, solid renal tumor
E. kidney disease
F. bladder papilloma
G. infection anywhere in the urinary system
H. kidney stones
I. inflammation of the urethra
J. hypernephroma
K. small, slow-growing, noncancerous tumor of the kidney
L. painful inflammation of the bladder wall
M. tumor that arises from the cells lining the bladder

Translate the terms.

14. nephroptosis_____

15. cystitis_____

16. nephroblastoma_____

PROCEDURES

Terms Related to Procedures

Term	Word Origin	Definition
cystectomy	*cyst/o* bladder *-ectomy* cutting out	Cutting out part or all of the urinary bladder.
cystolithotomy	*cyst/o* bladder *-lithotomy* cutting out a stone	Incision to cut a stone out of the urinary bladder.
cystoscopy	*cyst/o* bladder *-scopy* viewing	Visual examination of the urinary bladder using a **cystoscope** (Fig. 6-7).
lithotripsy	*lith/o* stone *-tripsy* crushing	Process of crushing stones either to prevent or clear an obstruction in the urinary system; crushing may be done manually, by high-energy shock waves, or by pulsed dye laser. In each case, the fragments may be expelled naturally or washed out (Fig. 6-8). Use of shock waves is termed **extracorporeal shock wave lithotripsy (ESWL).**
meatotomy	*meat/o* meatus *-tomy* cutting	Incision of the urinary meatus to widen the opening.

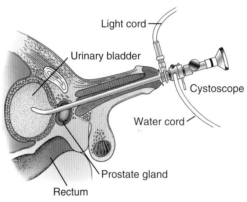

Fig. 6-7 Cystoscopy.

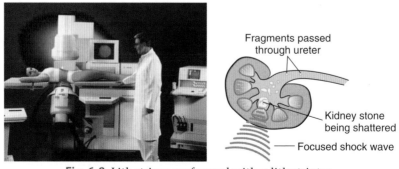

Fig. 6-8 Lithotripsy performed with a lithotripter.

Terms Related to Procedures—cont'd

Term	Word Origin	Definition
nephrectomy	*nephr/o* kidney *-ectomy* cutting out	Resection of the kidney.
nephrolithotomy	*nephr/o* kidney *-lithotomy* cutting out a stone	Incision of the kidney for removal of a kidney stone.
nephropexy	*nephr/o* kidney *-pexy* suspension	Suspension or fixation of the kidney.
nephrostomy	*nephr/o* kidney *-stomy* making a new opening	New opening and/or dilation of opening made in the kidney so that a catheter can be inserted.
nephrotomy	*nephr/o* kidney *-tomy* cutting	Incision of the kidney.
pyeloplasty	*pyel/o* renal pelvis *-plasty* surgically forming	Surgical operation to repair a blockage between the renal pelvis and a ureter.
renal dialysis	*ren/o* kidney *-al* pertaining to *dia-* through, complete *-lysis* breaking down	Process of diffusing blood across a semipermeable membrane to remove substances that a healthy kidney would eliminate, including poisons, drugs, urea, uric acid, and creatinine.
continuous ambulatory peritoneal dialysis (CAPD)	*peritone/o* peritoneum *-al* pertaining to *dia-* through, complete *-lysis* breaking down	Type of renal dialysis in which an indwelling catheter in the abdomen permits fluid to drain into and out of the peritoneal cavity to cleanse the blood (Fig. 6-9).

Continued

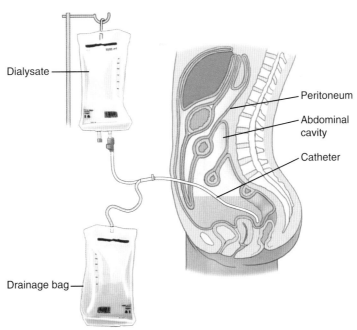

Fig. 6-9 Continuous ambulatory peritoneal dialysis (CAPD).

Terms Related to Procedures—cont'd

Term	Word Origin	Definition
hemodialysis (HD)	*hem/o* blood *dia-* through, complete *-lysis* breaking down	Type of renal dialysis that cleanses the blood by shunting it from the body through a machine for diffusion and ultrafiltration and then returning it to the patient's circulation (Fig. 6-10).
renal transplant	*ren/o* kidney *-al* pertaining to *trans-* across	Surgical transfer of a complete kidney from a donor to a recipient (Fig. 6-11).
urethrolysis	*urethr/o* urethra *-lysis* breaking down	Destruction of adhesions of the urethra.
urinalysis (UA)	*urin/o* urinary system, urine *-lysis* breaking down	The physical, chemical, and/or microscopic examination of urine.
blood urea nitrogen (BUN)		Blood test that measures the amount of nitrogenous waste in the circulatory system; an increased level is an indicator of kidney dysfunction.

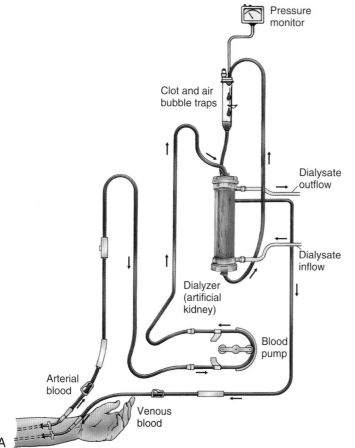
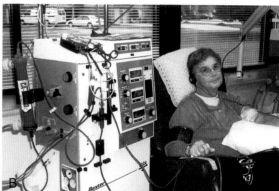

Fig. 6-10 A, Hemodialysis circuit. **B,** Hemodialysis machine.

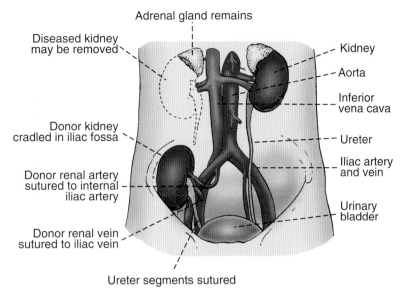

Fig. 6-11 Kidney transplant.

Terms Related to Procedures—cont'd

Term	Word Origin	Definition
creatinine clearance test		Test of kidney function that measures the rate at which nitrogenous waste is removed from the blood by comparing its concentration in the blood and urine over a 24-hour period.
glomerular filtration rate (GFR)		The amount of blood that is filtered by the glomeruli of the kidneys. This rate is decreased when the kidneys are dysfunctional.
vesicotomy	*vesic/o* bladder *-tomy* cutting	Incision of the urinary bladder.

Exercise 4: Procedures

____ 1. cystolithotomy	A. incision of the urinary meatus to widen the opening
____ 2. meatotomy	B. resection of the kidney
____ 3. CAPD	C. incision of the urinary bladder
____ 4. renal transplant	D. type of renal dialysis that occurs in the peritoneal cavity
____ 5. nephrectomy	E. opening made in the kidney so that a catheter can be inserted
____ 6. nephropexy	F. destruction of urethral adhesions
____ 7. nephrostomy	G. fixation of the kidney
____ 8. nephrotomy	H. surgical transfer of a complete kidney from a donor to a recipient
____ 9. vesicotomy	I. incision of the kidney
____ 10. urethrolysis	J. cutting a stone out of the urinary bladder

Build the terms.

11. cutting out the bladder_____.

12. complete breaking down of the blood_____.

13. removing a kidney stone_____.

14. crushing a stone_____.

PHARMACOLOGY

anti- = against

urinary pH modifiers: Increase (alkalinizers) or decrease (acidifiers) the pH of the urine to prevent kidney stones, treat acidosis, or promote excretion of some drugs and toxins. Examples of acidifiers include methionine and ammonium chloride, but are more commonly used in animals. Examples of alkalinizers include sodium bicarbonate (Neut) and potassium citrate (Urocit-K).

anticholinergics: Help control urinary incontinence by delaying the urge to void, increasing the bladder capacity, and relaxing the bladder muscles. Examples include tolterodine (Detrol), darifenacin (Enablex), and oxybutynin (Ditropan).

antidiuretics: Suppress urine formation. Examples include vasopressin (also known as antidiuretic hormone, ADH) and desmopressin (DDAVP).

antiinfectives: Fight infection in the urinary system, such as antibiotics, antiseptics, or antifungals. Nitrofurantoin (Macrobid), sulfamethoxazole-trimethoprim (Septra, Bactrim), and levofloxacin (Levaquin) are common examples of antiinfectives used for conditions of the urinary tract.

antispasmodics: Anticholinergic drugs that relax the bladder for the treatment of incontinence. Examples include flavoxate (Urispas) and dicyclomine (Bentyl).

diuretics: Increase the formation of urine by promoting excretion of water and sodium. These drugs are often used to treat high blood pressure, congestive heart failure, and peripheral edema. Examples include hydrochlorothiazide (Hydro-Diuril, also found in many combinations), furosemide (Lasix), and triamterene (Dyrenium, also found in many combinations).

Exercise 5: **Pharmacology**

Match the pharmacology terms with their definitions.

___ 1. diuretic
___ 2. antiinfective
___ 3. alkalinizer
___ 4. anticholinergic
___ 5. acidifier
___ 6. antidiuretic

A. increases the pH of urine
B. suppresses urine formation
C. decreases the pH of urine
D. increases formation of urine
E. antibiotics, antifungals, antiseptics
F. helps control urinary incontinence

RECOGNIZING SUFFIXES FOR PCS

Now that you've finished reading about the procedures for the urinary system, take a look at this review of the *suffixes* used in their terminology. Each of these suffixes is associated with one or more root operations in the medical surgical section or one of the other categories in PCS.

Suffixes and Root Operations for the Urinary System

Suffix	Root Operation
-ectomy	Excision, resection
-lithotomy	Extirpation
-lysis	Release
-pexy	Repair, reposition
-scopy	Inspection
-stomy	Bypass, drainage
-tomy	Drainage, division
-tripsy	Fragmentation

Abbreviations for the Urinary System

Abbreviation	Definition	Abbreviation	Definition
ADH	antidiuretic hormone	GFR	glomerular filtration rate
ARF	acute renal failure	HD	hemodialysis
BUN	blood urea nitrogen	IC	interstitial cystitis
CAPD	continuous ambulatory peritoneal dialysis	K	potassium
		Na	sodium
Cl	chloride	TCC	transitional cell carcinoma
CKD	chronic kidney disease	UA	urinalysis
ESRD	end-stage renal disease	UPJ	ureteropelvic junction
ESWL	extracorporeal shock wave lithotripsy	UTI	urinary tract infection

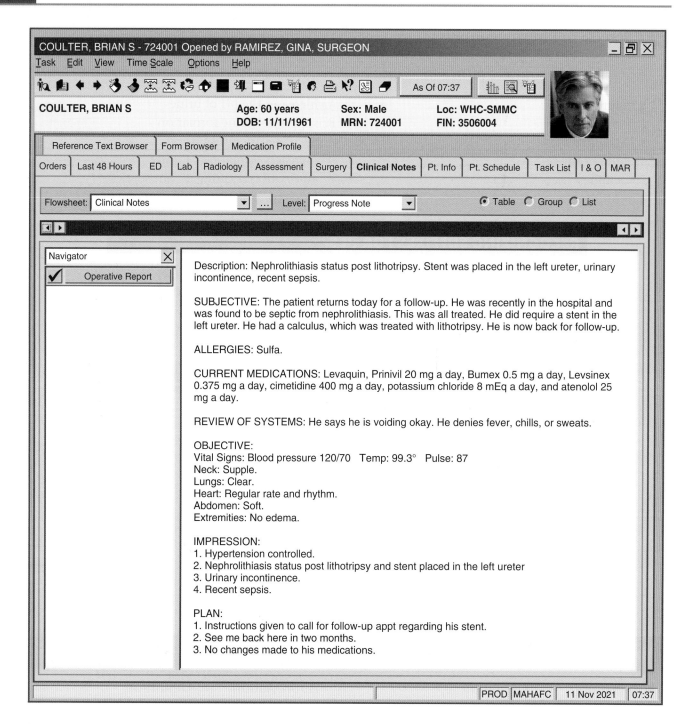

COULTER, BRIAN S - 724001 Opened by RAMIREZ, GINA, SURGEON

Task   Edit   View   Time Scale   Options   Help

As Of 07:37

COULTER, BRIAN S

Age: 60 years   Sex: Male   Loc: WHC-SMMC
DOB: 11/11/1961   MRN: 724001   FIN: 3506004

Reference Text Browser | Form Browser | Medication Profile

Orders | Last 48 Hours | ED | Lab | Radiology | Assessment | Surgery | **Clinical Notes** | Pt. Info | Pt. Schedule | Task List | I & O | MAR

Flowsheet: Clinical Notes   ...   Level: Progress Note   ○ Table   ○ Group   ○ List

Navigator
✓   Operative Report

Description: Nephrolithiasis status post lithotripsy. Stent was placed in the left ureter, urinary incontinence, recent sepsis.

SUBJECTIVE: The patient returns today for a follow-up. He was recently in the hospital and was found to be septic from nephrolithiasis. This was all treated. He did require a stent in the left ureter. He had a calculus, which was treated with lithotripsy. He is now back for follow-up.

ALLERGIES: Sulfa.

CURRENT MEDICATIONS: Levaquin, Prinivil 20 mg a day, Bumex 0.5 mg a day, Levsinex 0.375 mg a day, cimetidine 400 mg a day, potassium chloride 8 mEq a day, and atenolol 25 mg a day.

REVIEW OF SYSTEMS: He says he is voiding okay. He denies fever, chills, or sweats.

OBJECTIVE:
Vital Signs: Blood pressure 120/70   Temp: 99.3°   Pulse: 87
Neck: Supple.
Lungs: Clear.
Heart: Regular rate and rhythm.
Abdomen: Soft.
Extremities: No edema.

IMPRESSION:
1. Hypertension controlled.
2. Nephrolithiasis status post lithotripsy and stent placed in the left ureter
3. Urinary incontinence.
4. Recent sepsis.

PLAN:
1. Instructions given to call for follow-up appt regarding his stent.
2. See me back here in two months.
3. No changes made to his medications.

PROD | MAHAFC | 11 Nov 2021 | 07:37

 Exercise 6: Progress Note

Using the progress note above, answer the following questions.

1. How do you know that the patient is being seen after his treatment for stones in the kidney?

_____.

2. Which term(s) tell you that the patient had an inability to hold his urine? _____.

3. The stone was lodged in the tube between the kidney and the urinary bladder called a _____.

4. Which term tells you that the stones were crushed?_____.

5. What indicates the patient had no difficulty with urination?_____.

6. What is the term that indicates the patient has no swelling? _____.

MALE REPRODUCTIVE SYSTEM

FUNCTIONS OF THE MALE REPRODUCTIVE SYSTEM

The function of the male reproductive system is to reproduce. In the process of providing half of the genetic material (in the form of spermatozoa) necessary to form a new person—and then successfully storing, transporting, and delivering this material to fertilize the female counterpart, the ovum—the species survives.

ANATOMY AND PHYSIOLOGY

Both male and female anatomy can be divided into two parts: parenchymal, or primary, tissue, which produces sex cells for reproduction; and stromal, or secondary, tissue, which includes all of the glands, nerves, ducts, and other tissues that serve a supportive function in producing, maintaining, and transmitting these sex cells. Together these types of reproductive tissue, in either sex, are called **genitalia.** The parenchymal organs that produce the sex cells in both sexes are called **gonads.** The sex cells themselves are called **gametes.**

This chapter includes all the anatomy necessary to assign ICD-10 male reproductive system codes, including detail on the corpus spongiosum, the glans penis, and the epididymis. See Appendix H for a complete list of body parts and how they should be coded.

In the male, the gonads are the **testes** *(sing.* testis) or **testicles,** paired organs that produce the gametes called **spermatozoa** *(sing.* spermatozoon). The testes are suspended in a sac called the **scrotum** *(pl.* scrota) outside the body's trunk (Fig. 6-12).

At **puberty,** the stage of life in which males and females become functionally capable of sexual reproduction, the interstitial cells in the testicles begin to produce **testosterone,** a sex hormone responsible for the growth and development of male sex characteristics. The spermatozoa are formed in a series of tightly coiled, tiny tubes in each testis called the **seminiferous tubules.** The formation of sperm is called **spermatogenesis.** The serous membrane that surrounds the front and sides of the testicle is called the **tunica vaginalis testis.** From the seminiferous tubules, the formed spermatozoa travel to the **epididymis** *(pl.* epididymides), where they are stored.

When the seminal fluid is about to be ejected from the urethra **(ejaculation),** the spermatozoa travel through the left and right **vas deferens,** also called the **ductus deferens,** from the epididymides, around the bladder. The **spermatic cord** is an enclosed sheath that includes the vas deferens, along with arteries, veins, and nerves.

parenchymal
   par- = near
   en- = in
   chym/o = juice
   -al = pertaining to

stromal tissue = strom/o

gonad = gonad/o

testis, testicle = test/o,
   testicul/o, orchi/o,
   orchid/o, orch/o

spermatozoon =
   sperm/o, spermat/o

scrotum = scrot/o

testosterone
   test/o = testis
   ster/o = steroid
   -one = substance that
      forms

seminiferous
   semin/i = semen
   -ferous = pertaining to
      carrying

spermatogenesis
   spermat/o =
      spermatozoon
   -genesis = production

epididymis = epididym/o

**vas deferens, ductus
   deferens** = vas/o

To see how spermatogenesis occurs, click on **Animations.**

Be Careful!

Don't confuse **vesic/o,** *which means* the urinary bladder, *and* **vesicul/o,** *which means* the seminal vesicle.

 Be Careful!

Don't confuse **phall/o,** *which means* penis, *and* **phalang/o,** *which is a* bone in the finger or toe.

 Be Careful!

Don't confuse **urethr/o,** *which means* urethra, *and* **ureter/o,** *which means* the ureter.

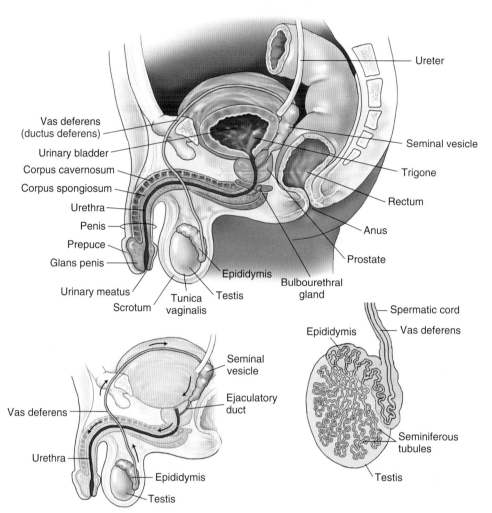

Fig. 6-12 Male reproductive system with inset of sperm production (spermatogenesis).

Note Many of the male reproductive organs are paired, so they need to be coded for left, right, or bilateral disorders.

To survive and thrive, the sperm are nourished by fluid from a series of glands. The **seminal vesicles, Cowper's** (or **bulbourethral) glands,** and the **prostate gland** provide fluid either to nourish or to aid in motility and lubrication. The sperm and the fluid together make up a substance called **semen.** The **ejaculatory duct** begins where the seminal vesicles join the vas deferens, and this "tube" joins the urethra. Once the sperm reach the **urethra,** they travel out through the shaft, or body, of the **penis,** which is composed of three columns of highly vascular erectile tissue. There are two columns of **corpora cavernosa** and one of **corpus spongiosum** that fill with blood through the dorsal veins during sexual arousal. Two leglike extensions of the corpus cavernosa, the **crura,** attach the penis to the pubic bone on either side. During ejaculation, the sperm exit through the enlarged tip of the penis, the **glans penis.** At birth, the glans penis is surrounded by a fold of skin called the **prepuce,** or foreskin. The removal of this skin is termed **circumcision.**

When ejaculation occurs during sexual intercourse **(coitus** or **copulation),** the sperm then are propelled toward the female sex cell, or ovum. If a specific sperm penetrates and unites with the ovum, **conception** takes place, and formation of an embryo begins.

seminal vesicle = vesicul/o

prostate = prostat/o

semen = semin/i

urethra = urethr/o

penis = pen/i, phall/o

glans penis = balan/o

prepuce, foreskin = preputi/o, posth/o

Exercise 7: Anatomy of the Male Reproductive System

Match the word parts with their meanings.

____ 1. penis
____ 2. prostate
____ 3. seminal vesicle
____ 4. scrotum
____ 5. prepuce
____ 6. semen

____ 7. urethra
____ 8. glans penis
____ 9. ductus deferens
____ 10. spermatozoon
____ 11. epididymis
____ 12. testis

A. vesicul/o
B. preputi/o, posth/o
C. orchid/o
D. phall/o
E. epididym/o
F. spermat/o

G. scrot/o
H. vas/o
I. semin/i
J. urethr/o
K. prostat/o
L. balan/o

 To practice labeling the male reproductive system, click on **Label It.**

Combining Forms for the Anatomy of the Male Reproductive System

Meaning	Combining Form	Meaning	Combining Form
epididymis	epididym/o	seminal vesicle	vesicul/o
glans penis	balan/o	spermatozoon	sperm/o, spermat/o
gonad	gonad/o	steroid	ster/o
juices	chym/o	stroma	strom/o
penis	pen/i, phall/o	testis, testicle	test/o, testicul/o, orchid/o, orch/o
prepuce, foreskin	preputi/o, posth/o		
prostate	prostat/o	urethra	urethr/o
scrotum	scrot/o	vas deferens, ductus deferens	vas/o
semen	semin/i		

Prefixes for the Anatomy of the Male Reproductive System

Prefix	Meaning
en-	in
par-	near, beside

Suffixes for the Anatomy of the Male Reproductive System

Suffix	Meaning
-al, -ous, -ar, -ile, -atic, -ic	pertaining to
-ferous	pertaining to carrying
-genesis	production
-one	substance that forms

 You can review the anatomy of the male reproductive system by clicking on **Body Spectrum Electronic Anatomy Coloring Book,** then **Reproductive,** then **Male Reproductive.**

PATHOLOGY

Terms Related to Diseases of Male Genital Organs (N40-N53)

Term	Word Origin	Definition
azoospermia	*a-* no, not, without *zo/o* animal *sperm/o* sperm *-ia* condition	Condition of no living sperm in the semen. This may be a desired condition, as when it follows a vasectomy.
balanitis	*balan/o* glans penis *-itis* inflammation	Inflammation of the glans penis.
balanoposthitis	*balan/o* glans penis *posth/o* foreskin *-itis* inflammation	Inflammation of the glans penis and the foreskin.
benign prostatic hyperplasia (BPH)	*prostat/o* prostate *-ic* pertaining to *hyper-* excessive *-plasia* formation	Abnormal enlargement of the prostate gland surrounding the urethra, leading to difficulty with urination (Fig. 6-13). Also known as **benign prostatic hypertrophy and enlarged prostate. PSA** (prostate-specific antigen) is a blood test used to diagnose BPH. Very high levels may indicate prostate cancer.
epididymitis	*epididym/o* epididymis *-itis* inflammation	Inflammation of the epididymis, usually as a result of an ascending infection through the genitourinary tract.
erectile dysfunction (ED)		Inability to achieve or sustain a penile erection for sexual intercourse. Also known as **impotence.**
hydrocele	*hydr/o* water, fluid *-cele* herniation, protrusion	Accumulation of fluid in the tunica vaginalis testis (Fig. 6-14). If the the sac is still open it is called **communicating;** if the sac has already closed it is called **noncommunicating.**
induration penis plastica	*indur/o* to make hard *-ation* process of	A hardening of the corpus cavernosa of the penis that can cause painful erections. Idiopathic in nature. Also called **Peyronie's disease**.

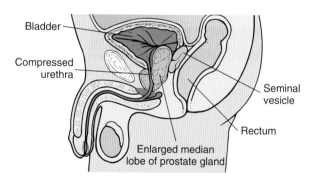

Fig. 6-13 Benign prostatic hyperplasia (BPH).

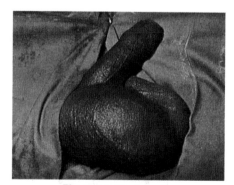

Fig. 6-14 Hydrocele.

Terms Related to Diseases of Male Genital Organs (N40-N51)—cont'd

Term	Word Origin	Definition
oligospermia	*olig/o* scanty, few *sperm/o* sperm *-ia* condition	Condition of temporary or permanent deficiency of sperm in the seminal fluid; related to azoospermia.
orchitis	*orch/o* testis *-itis* inflammation	Inflammation of the testicles; may or may not be associated with the mumps virus. Also known as **testitis**.
phimosis		Condition of tightening of the prepuce around the glans penis so that the foreskin cannot be retracted. May also be congenital.
priapism		An abnormally prolonged erection.
prostatitis	*prostat/o* prostate *-itis* inflammation	Inflammation of the prostate gland.
spermatocele of epididymis	*spermat/o* sperm *-cele* herniation, protrusion	A swelling of the epididymis that contains sperm. Also called a **spermatic cyst**, it is usually painless.
testicular torsion	*testicul/o* testicle *-ar* pertaining to	Twisting of a testicle on its spermatic cord, usually caused by trauma. May lead to ischemia of the testicle. Also called **torsion of testis** (Fig. 6-15).
vesiculitis	*vesicul/o* seminal vesicle *-itis* inflammation	Inflammation of a seminal vesicle, usually associated with prostatitis.

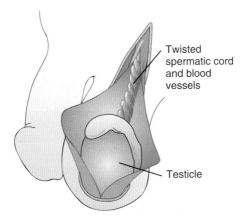

Twisted spermatic cord and blood vessels

Testicle

Fig. 6-15 Testicular torsion.

Exercise 8: Male Reproductive Disorders

Match the terms to their definitions.

____ 1. spermatocele of epididymis	A. inflammation of the testicles
____ 2. balanoposthitis	B. inflammation of a seminal vesicle
____ 3. induration penis plastica	C. inability to achieve or sustain a penile erection for sexual intercourse
____ 4. BPH	
____ 5. hydrocele	D. swelling of the epididymis that contains sperm
____ 6. testicular torsion	E. twisting of the testicle on its spermatic cord, usually caused by trauma
____ 7. epididymitis	
____ 8. orchitis	F. inflammation of the glans penis and the foreskin
____ 9. azoospermia	G. condition of tightening of the prepuce around the glans penis so that the foreskin cannot be retracted
____ 10. phimosis	
____ 11. priapism	H. hardening of the corpus cavernosa of the penis
____ 12. vesiculitis	I. inflammation of the epididymis
____ 13. ED	J. abnormal enlargement of the prostate gland
	K. condition of no living sperm in the semen
	L. accumulation of fluid in the tunica vaginalis testis
	M. an abnormally prolonged erection

Build the terms.

14. inflammation of the glans penis_____.

15. condition of no living sperm (in the semen)_____.

16. inflammation of the prostate_____.

17. herniation of water_____.

18. inflammation of the glans penis and foreskin_____.

Terms Related to Sexually Transmitted Diseases (STDs)

The pathogens that cause STDs are various, but what they have in common is that all are most efficiently transmitted by sexual contact. The other term for STDs is **venereal disease**, abbreviated VD. Note that some of these are coded in the Certain Infectious and Parasite Diseases chapter.

Term	Word Origin	Definition
gonorrhea	*gon/o* seed *-rrhea* flow, discharge	Disease caused by the gram-negative diplococcus *Neisseria gonorrhoeae* bacterium (Gc), which manifests itself as inflammation of the urethra, prostate, rectum, or pharynx (Fig. 6-16). The cervix and fallopian tubes may also be involved in females, although they may be asymptomatic, meaning "without symptoms." Diagnosed with a Gram stain test, a method of staining microorganisms as either gram-negative or gram-positive.

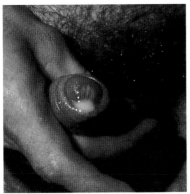

Fig. 6-16 Gonorrhea in a male patient.

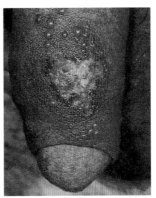

Fig. 6-17 Genital herpes.

Terms Related to Sexually Transmitted Diseases (STDs)—cont'd

Term	Word Origin	Definition
herpes genitalis (herpes simplex virus, HSV-2)		Form of the herpesvirus transmitted through sexual contact, causing recurring painful vesicular eruptions (Fig. 6-17).
human papillomavirus (HPV)		Virus that causes common warts of the hands and feet and lesions of the mucous membranes of the oral, anal, and genital cavities. A genital wart is referred to as a **condyloma** (*pl.* condylomata).
nongonococcal urethritis (NGU)	*urethr/o* urethra *-itis* inflammation	Inflammation of the urethra caused by *Chlamydia trachomatis, Mycoplasma genitalium,* or *Ureaplasma urealyticum.*
syphilis		Multistage STD caused by the spirochete *Treponema pallidum.* A highly infectious **chancre**, a painless red ulcer, appears in the first stage, usually on the genitals. Diagnosed with a VDRL (Venereal Disease Research Laboratory) test and/or an FTA-ABS (fluorescent treponemal antibody absorption) test.

 Exercise 9: Sexually Transmitted Diseases

Fill in the blanks with one of the following terms.

condylomata   **chancres**   **syphilis**
asymptomatic   **herpes simplex virus-2**   **gonorrhea**
human papillomavirus **nongonococcal urethritis**

1. HPV causes genital warts that are referred to as_____.

2. Which STD has multiple stages?_____.

3. Inflammation of the urethra not caused by the gonorrhea bacterium is called_____.

4. An STD caused by gram-negative bacteria is called_____.

5. Syphilitic lesions that are painless ulcers are called_____.

6. When a patient has no symptoms, he is considered to be _____.

7. Genital warts are caused by the _____.

8. A viral infection that results in painful, recurring vesicular eruptions is called _____.

Terms Related to Benign Neoplasms (D29)

Term	Word Origin	Definition
Leydig and Sertoli cell tumors		These testicular tumors arise from the stromal tissue of the testes, which produces hormones. They are usually benign.

Terms Related to Malignant Neoplasms (C60-C63)

Term	Word Origin	Definition
adenocarcinoma of the prostate	*aden/o* gland *-carcinoma* cancer of epithelial origin	Prostate cancer is diagnosed in one of every six men. With early detection, however, this cancer is treatable (Fig. 6-18).
nonseminoma	*non-* not *semin/i* semen *-oma* tumor, mass	Nonseminoma is a type of germ cell tumor (GCT). It accounts for the majority of testicular cancer cases and occurs in younger men, usually between the ages of 15 and 35.
seminoma	*semin/i* semen *-oma* tumor, mass	This malignancy is one type of GCT that develops from the cells that form sperm (Fig. 6-19).
teratoma, malignant	*terat/o* deformity *-oma* tumor, mass	This tumor is a type of nonseminoma that is usually benign in children. Because these tumors are created from germ cells, they have half of the necessary genetic information to form an individual. A synonym is the term **dermoid cyst**.

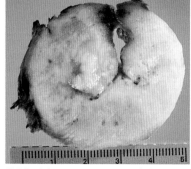

Fig. 6-18 Adenocarcinoma of the prostate.

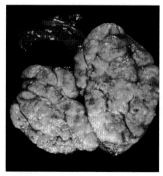

Fig. 6-19 Seminoma of the testicle.

Exercise 10: Neoplasms

Match the neoplasms with their definitions.

_____ 1. nonseminoma

_____ 2. teratoma

_____ 3. seminoma

_____ 4. adenocarcinoma of the prostate

_____ 5. Leydig and Sertoli cell tumors

A. benign tumors that arise from testicular stromal tissue

B. prostate cancer

C. majority of germ cell tumors

D. germ cell tumor developing from cells that form sperm

E. synonym is dermoid cyst

Build the terms.

6. tumor of semen_____.

7. glandular cancerous tumor of epithelial origin_____.

Terms Related to Procedures

Term	Word Origin	Definition
balanoplasty	*balan/o* glans penis *-plasty* surgically forming	Surgically correcting a defect of the glans penis.
circumcision	*circum-* around *-cision* cutting	Surgical procedure in which the prepuce of the penis (or that of the clitoris of the female) is excised.
epididymotomy	*epididym/o* epididymis *tomy* cutting	Incision of the epididymis to drain a cyst.
epididymovesiculography	*epididym/o* epididymis *vesicul/o* seminal vesicle *-graphy* recording	Imaging of the epididymis and seminal vesicle using a contrast medium (Fig. 6-20).
orchidectomy	*orchid/o* testis *-ectomy* cutting out	Cutting out part or all of one or both testicles, usually for removal of a tumor or cyst. Also called **orchectomy** and **orchiectomy**.
orchiopexy	*orchi/o* testis *-pexy* suspension	Surgical procedure to mobilize an undescended testicle, attaching it to the scrotum. Usually performed to correct a congenital condition.
phalloplasty	*phall/o* penis *-plasty* surgically forming	Surgically correcting a defect of the penis. Usually performed to correct a congenital condition.
prostatectomy	*prostat/o* prostate *-ectomy* cutting out	Removal of the prostate gland. In a radical prostatectomy, the seminal vesicles and area of vas ampullae of the vas deferens are also removed.
transurethral resection of the prostate (TUR, TURP)	*trans-* through *urethr/o* urethra *-al* pertaining to	Cutting out the prostate in sections through a urethral approach (Fig. 6-21). This procedure is the most common type of prostatectomy. The approach may be through the urethra (transurethral), above the pubic bone (suprapubic), or through the perineum (perineal).
transurethral incision of the prostate (TUIP)	*trans-* through *urethr/o* urethra *-al* pertaining to	Form of prostate surgery involving tiny incisions of the prostate. The prostate is not removed (Fig. 6-22). TUIP is considered a minimally invasive surgical treatment.

Continued

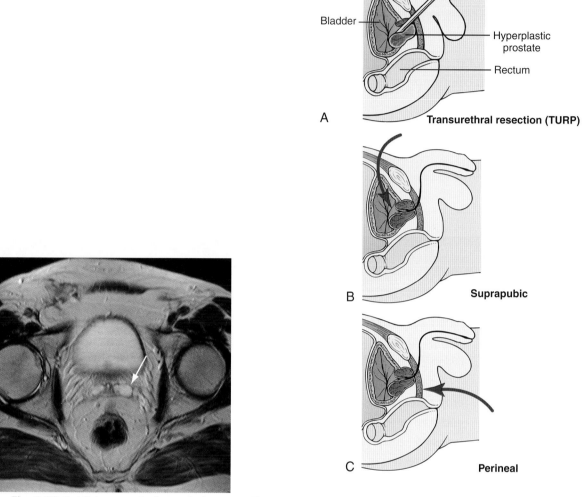

A **Transurethral resection (TURP)**

B **Suprapubic**

C **Perineal**

Fig. 6-21 **Prostatectomy.** The approach may be, **A,** through the urethra (transurethral), **B,** above the pubic bone (suprapubic), or, **C,** through the perineum (perineal).

Fig. 6-20 Epididymovesiculography.

Terms Related to Procedures—cont'd

Term	Word Origin	Definition
transurethral microwave thermotherapy (TUMT)	*therm/o* heat *–therapy* treatment	Minimally invasive procedure to destroy excess prostatic tissue with heat.
vasovasostomy	*vas/o* vas deferens *vas/o* vas deferens *-stomy* making a new opening	Anastomosis of the ends of the vas deferens as a means of reconnecting them to reverse the sterilization procedure.
vasectomy	*vas/o* vas deferens *-ectomy* cutting out	Incision, ligation, and cauterization of both of the vas deferens for the purpose of male sterilization (Fig. 6-23).

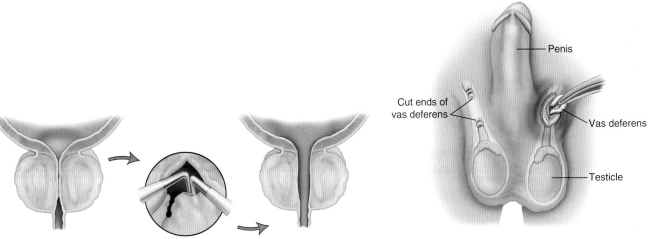

Fig. 6-22 Transurethral incision of the prostate (TUIP).

Fig. 6-23 Vasectomy.

Terms Related to Procedures—cont'd

Term	Word Origin	Definition
vasography	*vas/o* vessel *-graphy* recording	Imaging of the vas deferens to visualize possible blockages.
vasoligation	*vas/o* vessel *-ligation* tying	A tying of the vas deferens as a sterilization procedure.
vesiculectomy	*vesicul/o* seminal vesicle *-ectomy* cutting out	Cutting out the seminal vesicle.

⊗ Be Careful!   *If the suffix* **-cision** *is used with the prefix* **ex-,** *it will be an excision, not a resection.*

Exercise 11: Procedures

Match the terms to their definitions.

_____ 1. circumcision
_____ 2. epididymotomy
_____ 3. orchiectomy
_____ 4. phalloplasty
_____ 5. prostatectomy
_____ 6. TURP
_____ 7. vasovasostomy
_____ 8. vesiculectomy
_____ 9. TUIP
_____ 10. vasectomy
_____ 11. vasography

A. cutting out part or all of a testicle
B. incision of the epididymis to drain a cyst
C. cutting out the prostate in sections through a urethral approach
D. removal of the prostate gland
E. form of prostate surgery involving tiny incisions of the prostate
F. surgical procedure in which the prepuce of the penis is excised
G. anastomosis of the ends of the vas deferens to reverse a sterilization
H. incision, ligation, and cauterization of the vas deferens for the purpose of male sterilization
I. imaging of the vas deferens
J. cutting out the seminal vesicle
K. surgically correcting a defect of the penis

Build the terms.

12. forming the glans penis_____.
13. suspending a testis_____.
14. recording the epididymis and seminal vesicle_____.
15. tying a vessel_____.

andr/o = male

anti- = against

PHARMACOLOGY

alpha blockers: Improve urinary flow by blocking alpha-1 adrenergic receptors to relax smooth muscle in prostate. Examples include tamsulosin (Flomax) and terazosin (Hytrin).

androgens: Stimulate male characteristics and/or organ development to treat impotence or hormonal imbalances. Examples include fluoxymesterone (Androxy) and testosterone (Androgel).

androgen antagonists: Block receptors or inhibit synthesis of androgen hormones. Finasteride (Proscar) and dutasteride (Avodart) block the conversion of testosterone to the more potent hormone 5-alpha-dihydrotestosterone (DHT) to suppress growth of and even shrink the enlarged prostate. Saw palmetto *(Serenoa repens)* is an alternative medicine that may be effective in treating symptoms of BPH.

antibiotics: Treat bacterial infection. Penicillin G, tetracycline (Sumycin), and doxycycline (Vibramycin) all can be used to treat syphilis.

antiimpotence agents: Used to alleviate erectile dysfunction. Sildenafil (Viagra) and tadalafil (Cialis) are examples of oral agents. Alprostadil (Caverject) is injected directly into the corpus cavernosum of the penis.

antivirals: Treat viral infections. Acyclovir (Zovirax) is used to treat genital herpes virus.

 Exercise 12: **Pharmacology**

Match the pharmacology terms with their definitions.

___ 1. class of drug used to treat bacterial infection

___ 2. class of drug used to treat viral infections

___ 3. class of drug used to treat erectile dysfunction

___ 4. an example of a drug used to treat BPH

___ 5. class of drug used to improve urine flow in patients with BPH

A. antivirals

B. antiimpotence agents

C. alpha blockers

D. antibiotics

E. finasteride

RECOGNIZING SUFFIXES FOR PCS

Now that you've finished reading about the procedures for the male reproductive system, take a look at this review of the *suffixes* used in their terminology. Each of these suffixes is associated with one or more root operations in the medical surgical section or one of the other categories in PCS.

Suffixes and Root Operations for the Male Reproductive System

Suffix	Root Operation
-cision	Resection
-ectomy	Excision, resection
-ligation	Occlusion
-pexy	Repair, reposition
-plasty	Repair, supplement
-stomy	Repair
-therapy	Destruction
-tomy	Drainage

Abbreviations for the Male Reproductive System

Abbreviation	Definition	Abbreviation	Definition
BPH	benign prostatic hyperplasia/hypertrophy	TUIP	transurethral incision of the prostate
ED	erectile dysfunction	TUMT	transurethral microwave thermotherapy
FTA-ABS	fluorescent treponemal antibody absorption	TUR	transurethral resection (of the prostate)
Gc	gonococcus	TURP	transurethral resection of the prostate
GCT	germ cell tumor		
HPV	human papillomavirus	VD	venereal disease
HSV-2	herpes simplex virus-2, herpes genitalis	VDRL	Venereal Disease Research Laboratory
NGU	nongonococcal urethritis		
PSA	prostate-specific antigen		
STD	sexually transmitted disease		

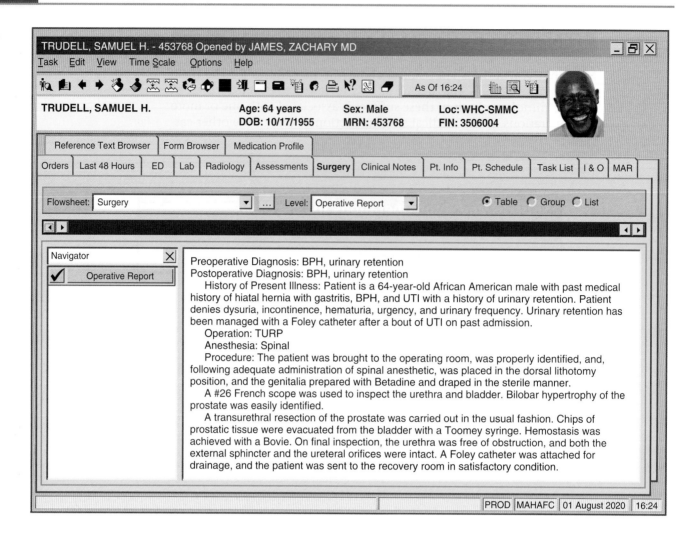

 Exercise 13: **Operative Report**

Using the operative report above, answer the following questions.

1. The patient's past medical history included BPH. Describe this condition.

_____

2. Explain what the patient does *not* complain of:

A. dysuria _____   C. urinary frequency _____

B. incontinence _____   D. hematuria _____

3. How many lobes of the prostate were enlarged?_____

4. What does the abbreviation for the patient's surgery, TURP, mean?_____

5. If this patient had had periprostatic lesions, where would they have been?

_____

FEMALE REPRODUCTIVE SYSTEM

FUNCTIONS OF THE FEMALE REPRODUCTIVE SYSTEM

The role of the female reproductive system is to keep one's genetic material in the world's gene pool. Through sexual reproduction, the 23 pairs of chromosomes of the female must join with 23 pairs of chromosomes from a male to create new life. To do this, the system must produce the hormones necessary to provide a hospitable environment for the **ovum** (OH vum) *(pl. ova)*, the female gamete, to connect with the spermatozoon, the male gamete, for fertilization to occur. Once an egg is fertilized, it is nurtured throughout its growth process until the delivery of the neonate (newborn).

ANATOMY AND PHYSIOLOGY

Internal Anatomy

Because the primary function of the female reproductive system is to create new life through the successful fertilization of an ovum, discussion of this system begins with this very important germ cell.

This chapter includes all the anatomy necessary to assign ICD-10 female reproductive system codes, including detail on the myometrium, the mammary ducts, and the rectouterine pouch. See Appendix H for a complete list of body parts and how they should be coded.

Ova and Ovaries

From **menarche,** the first menstrual period, to **menopause** (the climacteric), the cessation of menstruation, mature ova are produced by the female gonads, the **ovaries** (Fig. 6-24). The ovaries are small, almond-shaped, paired organs located on either side of the uterus in the female pelvic cavity. They are attached to the uterus by the ovarian ligaments and lie close to the opening of the **fallopian tubes,** the ducts that convey the ova from the ovaries to the uterus. Approximately every 28 days, in response to hormonal stimulation, the ovaries alternate releasing one ovum (Fig. 6-25). This egg matures in one of the **follicles,** which are tiny secretory sacs within an ovary. Graafian follicles are the result of a monthly maturation of these structures that occurs between puberty and menopause. The pituitary gland, an endocrine gland located in the cranial cavity, secretes two hormones that influence the activity of the ovaries. **Follicle-stimulating hormone (FSH)** causes the ovarian follicles to begin to mature and secrete estrogen. Because of the increase of estrogen in the bloodstream, **luteinizing hormone (LH)** is released by the anterior lobe of the pituitary gland. LH then stimulates the follicle to mature and release its ovum **(ovulation)** and aids in the development of the **corpus luteum.** The corpus luteum, a tiny yellow endocrine structure, is then responsible for secreting **estrogen** and **progesterone,** hormones responsible for female secondary sex characteristics and the cyclical maintenance of the uterus for pregnancy.

If two eggs are released and fertilized, the resulting twins will be termed *fraternal,* because they will be no more or less alike in appearance than brothers (or sisters) occurring in sequential pregnancies. If, however, one of the fertilized eggs divides and forms two infants, these are *identical* twins, who share the same appearance and genetic material.

Fallopian Tubes

Once the mature ovum has been released, it is drawn into the **fimbriae** *(sing. fimbria),* the feathery ends of the fallopian tube (see Fig. 6-24). These tubes, about the width of a pencil, and about as long (10 to 12 cm), transport the ovum

---

female = gynec/o

ovum, egg = o/o, ov/o, ov/i

 Be Careful!

*The term **germ** comes from the Latin word for sprout or fetus, here referring to its reproductive nature; however, it can also mean a type of microorganism that can cause disease.*

menarche
  men/o = menstruation
  -arche = beginning

menopause
  men/o = menstruation
  -pause = stop, cease

menstruation = **men/o, menstru/o**

ovary = **oophor/o, ovari/o**

uterus = **hyster/o, metri/o, metr/o, uter/o**

fallopian tube = **salping/o, -salpinx**

follicle = **follicul/o**

ovulation
  ovul/o = egg
  -ation = process of

 Be Careful!

*Do not confuse **ureter/o,** which means the ureter, with **uter/o ,** which means uterus.*

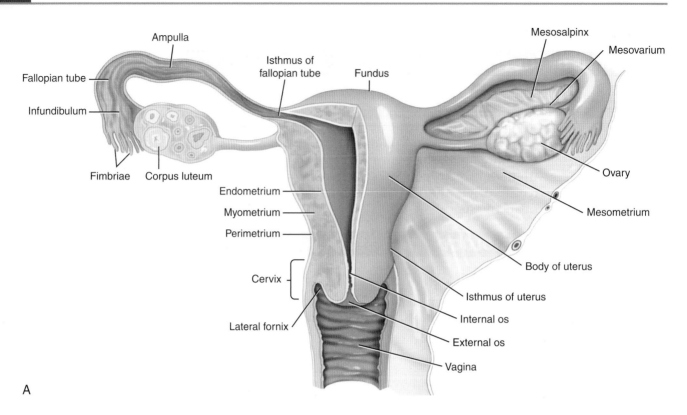

A

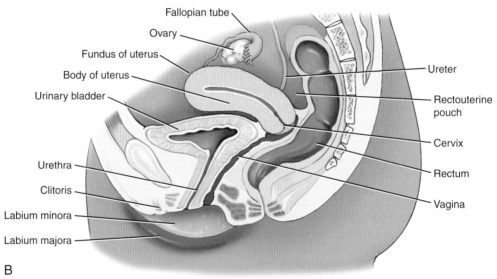

B

Fig. 6-24 Female reproductive organs. **A,** Frontal view. **B,** Sagittal view.

fimbria = fimbri/o

perimetrium = perimetri/o

myometrium = myometri/o

endometrium = endometri/o

to the uterus. Along the length of the tube are structures with names that indicate their shape or location: the **infundibulum** is the funnel-shaped area adjacent to each fimbria; the **ampulla** follows, named for its bottle shape, and the **fallopian isthmus** is the narrowed area close to the uterus. The fallopian tubes (also called *oviducts* or *uterine tubes)* and the ovaries make up what is called the **uterine adnexa,** or accessory organs of the uterus.

Uterus

Once the ovum has traversed the fallopian tube, it is secreted into the **uterus,** or **womb,** a pear-shaped organ that is designed to nurture a developing embryo/fetus (see Fig. 6-24). The uterus is composed of three layers: the outer layer, called the **perimetrium,** or serosa; the **myometrium,** or muscle layer; and the **endometrium,** the lining of the uterus. Disorders that involve the layers of the uterus

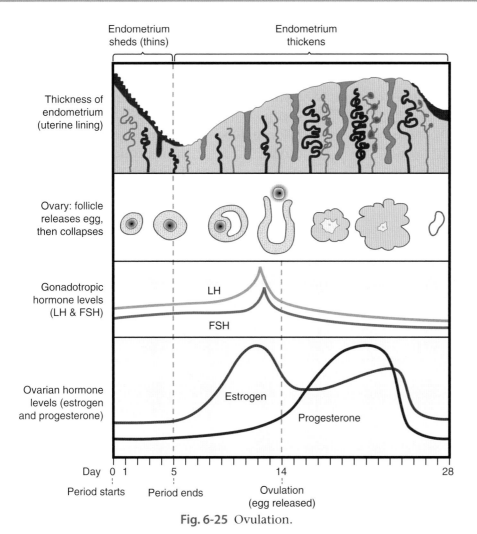

Fig. 6-25 Ovulation.

are termed **intramural.** As a whole, the uterus can be divided into several areas. The **corpus** (which means *body* in Latin) is the large central area; the **fundus** is the raised area at the top of the uterus between the outlets for the fallopian tubes; and the **cervix (cx)** is the narrowed lower area, often referred to as the "neck" of the uterus. Note that there are two openings of the cervix: the **internal os** and the **external os.** The area in between is termed the **cervical canal.**

Rectouterine Pouch

An area associated with the female reproductive system that does not play a direct role in its function, the **rectouterine pouch,** is also called **Douglas' cul-de-sac,** a space in the pelvic cavity between the uterus and the rectum.

Vagina

If the ovum does not become fertilized by a spermatozoon, the corpus luteum stops producing estrogen and progesterone, and the lining of the uterus is shed through the muscular, tubelike vagina by the process of **menstruation (menses).** The vagina extends from the uterine cervix to the vulva (the external genitalia). *Vagin/o* is from Latin and literally means a "sheath." This is important to note because male anatomy includes the **tunica vaginalis**—a membrane that partially covers the testicles.

Mesentery

The fallopian tubes, ovaries, and uterus are held in place by folds of **mesentery** termed the **mesosalpinx,** the **mesovarium,** and the **mesometrium.**

---

intramural
   intra- = within
   mur/o = wall
   -al = pertaining to

fundus = fund/o

cervix = cervic/o, trachel/o

rectouterine pouch = culd/o

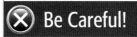 Be Careful!

*Don't confuse **culd/o,** which means the rectouterine pouch, with **colp/o,** which means vagina.*

vagina = colp/o, vagin/o

Exercise 14: Combining Forms for Internal Female Genitalia

Match the following. Answers may be used more than once.

____ 1. culd/o
____ 2. oophor/o
____ 3. metr/o
____ 4. hyster/o
____ 5. colp/o
____ 6. ov/o
____ 7. salping/o

____ 8. trachel/o
____ 9. ovari/o
____ 10. uter/o
____ 11. vagin/o
____ 12. men/o
____ 13. fimbri/o

A. uterus
B. vagina
C. fallopian tube
D. cervix

E. rectouterine pouch
F. ovary
G. female germ cell
H. menstruation, menses
I. fimbria

Translate the terms.

14. supracervical_____.

15. intrauterine_____.

16. premenstrual_____

17. transvaginal_____

vulva = vulv/o, episi/o

hymen = hymen/o

labia = labi/o

clitoris = clitorid/o

perineum = perine/o

Bartholin's gland
   =bartholin/o

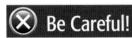 **Be Careful!**

*The combining form **cervic/o** has two meanings: the neck and the cervix (the neck of the uterus).*

External Genitalia

The external female genitalia collectively are called the **vulva** (Fig. 6-26). The vulva consists of the vaginal opening, or **orifice;** the membrane covering the opening, or **hymen;** the two folds of skin surrounding the opening, or **labia majora** (the larger folds) and **labia minora** (the smaller folds); the **clitoris,** which is sensitive, erectile tissue; and the **perineum,** the area between the opening of the vagina and the anus. The **vestibular glands,** located in or near the opening of the vagina, are divided into two types. The greater vestibular glands (also called **Bartholin's glands)** are the paired glands in the vulva that secrete a mucous lubricant for the vagina. The lesser vestibular glands (also called **Skene's** or **paraurethral glands)** are located in the vagina near the outlet of the urethra and have a function similar to the male prostate, providing fluid during ejaculation. The **mons pubis** is a mound of fatty tissue covering the pubic area.

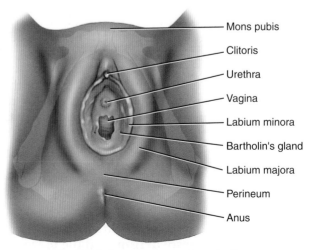

Fig. 6-26 Female external genitalia.

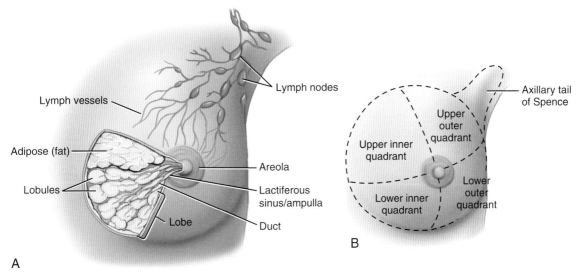

Fig. 6-27 The breast.

CPT Coding Alert!

CPT uses the term "Skene's glands" for the lesser vestibular glands (also called periurethral or paraurethral glands). These glands are the subject of surgeries to treat cystic formations and infections that affect them.

The Breast

The **breasts,** or mammary glands, are composed of fatty (adipose) tissue, fibrous connective tissue, milk-producing glands and ducts, lymphatic tissue, and blood vessels (Fig. 6-27). Pectoral muscles lie beneath the breast tissue and the suspensory (Cooper's) ligaments attach the breast to the chest wall.

The **nipple** of the breast is the **mammary papilla** *(pl.* papillae), and the darker-colored skin surrounding the nipple is the areola *(pl.* areolae). Internally, the breast is composed of 15 to 20 sections that radiate around the nipple. Each of the sections is made up of several segments called **lobules,** each of which ends in a bulblike cavity termed an **alveolus.** Thin passageways called **ducts** carry milk from the lobules to the nipple. Small dilations of the duct close to the nipple that serve to hold milk prior to being expressed are termed **lactiferous sinuses** or **ampullae.**

ICD-10 coding for breast cancers asks for specificity as to where the tumor is located. Locations with separate codes are each of the quadrants, the axillary tail, the nipple, areola, the skin, and the central portion of the breast (the area under the areola). Note that the axillary tail of Spence (also called the tail of Spence, axillary process, and axillary tail) is the part of the breast that extends into the axilla (armpit).

Lymph vessels surround and drain the breast into axillary and mediastinal lymph nodes. **Prolactin,** released by the anterior pituitary, is the main hormone associated with the formation and production of milk **(lactogenesis),** whereas the hormone **oxytocin** is produced by the posterior lobe of the pituitary and is responsible for the release of the milk produced.

breast = mast/o, mamm/o

nipple = papill/o, thel/e

milk = lact/o, galact/o

Exercise 15: External Female Genitalia and the Breast

Match the following combining forms with their meanings. There may be more than one answer.

___ 1. vulva
___ 2. nipple
___ 3. hymen
___ 4. milk
___ 5. labia

___ 6. breast
___ 7. perineum
___ 8. Bartholin's glands
___ 9. clitoris

A. galact/o
B. episi/o
C. bartholin/o
D. papill/o
E. mamm/o
F. thel/e
G. hymen/o

H. perine/o
I. lact/o
J. vulv/o
K. mast/o
L. labi/o
M. clitorid/o

Translate the terms.

10. interlabial_____.

11. intramammary_____.

Combining Forms for the Anatomy and Physiology of the Female Reproductive System

Meaning	Combining Form	Meaning	Combining Form
Bartholin's gland	bartholin/o	mesentery	mesenter/o
breast	mamm/o, mast/o	milk	lact/o, galact/o
cervix	cervic/o, trachel/o	myometrium	myometri/o
clitoris	clitorid/o	nipple	papill/o, thel/e
endometrium	endometri/o	ovary	oophor/o, ovari/o
fallopian tube	salping/o, fallopi/o	ovum, egg	ov/o, ov/i, ovul/o, o/o
female	gynec/o	perimetrium	perimetri/o
fimbria	fimbri/o	perineum	perine/o
follicle	follicul/o	rectouterine pouch	culd/o
fundus	fund/o	uterus	hyster/o, metri/o, metr/o, uter/o
hymen	hymen/o		
labia	labi/o	vagina	colp/o, vagin/o
menstruation, menses	men/o, menstru/o	vulva	vulv/o, episi/o

Suffixes for the Anatomy and Physiology of the Female Reproductive System

Suffix	Meaning
-arche	beginning
-ation	process of
-pause	stop, cease
-salpinx	fallopian tube

You can review the anatomy of the female reproductive system by clicking on **Body Spectrum Electronic Anatomy Coloring Book**, then **Reproductive**, then **Female Reproductive**.

PATHOLOGY

Terms Related to Disorders of Breast (N60-N65)

Term	Word Origin	Definition
benign mammary dysplasia	*mamm/o* breast *-ary* pertaining to *dys-* abnormal *-plasia* formation	Any noncancerous, abnormal formation of breast tissue.
galactorrhea	*galact/o* milk *-rrhea* flow, discharge	An abnormal discharge of milk from the breasts.
gynecomastia	*gynec/o* female *mast/o* breast *-ia* condition	Enlargement of either unilateral or bilateral breast tissue in the male. The *gynec/o* is a reference to the appearance of the breast, not to a female. Note that this diagnosis is under the heading "hypertrophy of the breast" and shares the code number with excessive breast development in women, listed separately as "hypertrophy of breast, NOS."
mastodynia	*mast/o* breast *-dynia* pain	Breast pain. May be cyclical (associated with menstruation) or noncyclical. Also called **mastalgia**.
mastoptosis	*mast/o* breast *-ptosis* drooping, sagging	Downward displacement of the breasts. Also referred to as ptosis of breast. The code is not subject to laterality specification.

Terms Related to Inflammatory Diseases of Female Pelvic Organs (N70-N77)

Term	Word Origin	Definition
bartholinitis	*bartholin/o* Bartholin's gland *-itis* inflammation	Inflammation of a Bartholin's gland.
cervicitis	*cervic/o* cervix *-itis* inflammation	Inflammation of the cervix.
female pelvic inflammatory disease (PID)		A general term that usually refers to a bacterial infection of the uterus, fallopian tubes, and/or ovaries.
oophoritis	*oophor/o* ovary *-itis* inflammation	Inflammation of an ovary.
salpingitis	*salping/o* fallopian tubes *-itis* inflammation	Inflammation of the fallopian tubes.
vulvitis	*vulv/o* vulva *-itis* inflammation	Inflammation of the external female genitalia.

Exercise 16: Disorders of Breast and Inflammatory Disease of Female Pelvic Organs

Translate the terms.

1. galactorrhea_____.

2. gynecomastia_____.

3. mastodynia_____.

4. mastoptosis_____.

5. bartholinitis_____.

6. cervicitis_____.

7. oophoritis_____.

8. salpingitis_____.

9. vulvitis _____.

Terms Related to Noninflammatory Disorders of Female Genital Tract (N80-N98)		
Term	**Word Origin**	**Definition**
amenorrhea	*a-* without *men/o* menses *-rrhea* discharge, flow	Lack of menstrual flow. This is a normal, expected condition before puberty, after menopause, and during pregnancy.
cervical intraepithelial neoplasia (CIN) I and II	*cervic/o* cervix *-al* pertaining to *intra-* within *epitheli/o* epithelium *-al* pertaining to *neo-* new *-plasia* condition of development, formation	Precancerous changes in the tissue lining the cervix. Measured in grades to indicate the degree of change away from normal formation.
cystocele	*cyst/o* urinary bladder *-cele* herniation	Herniation of the urinary bladder into the vagina (Fig. 6-28).
dysfunctional uterine bleeding (DUB)		Abnormal uterine bleeding not caused by a tumor, inflammation, or pregnancy.
dysmenorrhea	*dys-* painful *men/o* menses *-rrhea* discharge, flow	Painful menstrual flow, cramps.

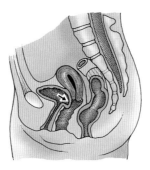

Fig. 6-28 Cystocele.

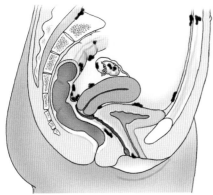

Fig. 6-29 Black spots indicate common sites of endometriosis.

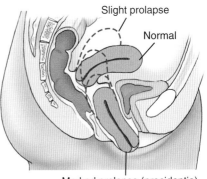

Fig. 6-30 Prolapse of uterus.

Terms Related to Noninflammatory Disorders of Female Genital Tract (N80-N98)—cont'd

Term	Word Origin	Definition
dyspareunia	*dys-* painful, abnormal *-pareunia* intercourse	Painful intercourse.
endometrial hyperplasia	*endometri/o* endometrium *-al* pertaining to *hyper-* excessive *-plasia* condition of development, formation	An excessive development of cells in the lining of the uterus; this condition is benign but can become malignant.
endometriosis	*endometri/o* endometrium *-osis* abnormal condition	Condition in which the tissue that makes up the lining of the uterus, the endometrium, is found ectopically (outside the uterus). Causes are unknown (Fig. 6-29).
hematosalpinx	*hemat/o* blood *-salpinx* fallopian tubes	Condition of blood in the fallopian tubes.
hysteroptosis	*hyster/o* uterus *-ptosis* drooping, sagging	Falling or sliding of the uterus from its normal location in the body. Also called **uterine prolapse** (Fig. 6-30).

Continued

Terms Related to Noninflammatory Disorders of Female Genital Tract (N80-N98)—cont'd

Term	Word Origin	Definition
menometrorrhagia	*men/o* menses *metr/o* uterus *-rrhagia* bursting forth	Both excessive menstrual flow and uterine bleeding other than that caused by menstruation.
menorrhagia	*men/o* menses *-rrhagia* bursting forth	Abnormally heavy or prolonged menstrual period; may be an indication of fibroids.
metrorrhagia	*metr/o* uterus *-rrhagia* bursting forth	Uterine bleeding other than that caused by menstruation. May be caused by uterine lesions.
mittelschmerz		Pain during ovulation; midcycle pain.
oligomenorrhea	*olig/o* scanty, few *men/o* menses *-rrhea* discharge, flow	Abnormally light or infrequent menstrual flow; menorrhea refers to the normal discharge of blood and tissue from the uterus.
ovarian cyst	*ovari/o* ovary *-an* pertaining to	Benign, fluid-filled sac. Can be either a follicular cyst, which occurs when a follicle does not rupture at ovulation, or a cyst of the corpus luteum, caused when it does not continue its transformation (Fig. 6-31).
polymenorrhea	*poly-* many *men/o* menses *-rrhea* discharge, flow	Abnormally frequent menstrual flow. Frequency is less than 21 days per cycle.
postmenopausal bleeding (PMB)		Dysfunctional uterine bleeding (DUB) after menopause. May be due to fibroids or cancer.

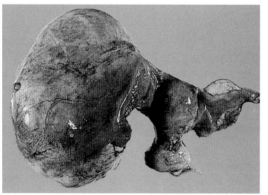
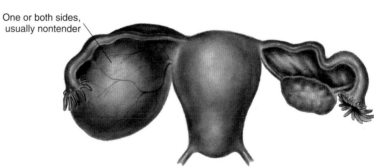

One or both sides, usually nontender

Fig. 6-31 Ovarian cyst.

Terms Related to Noninflammatory Disorders of Female Genital Tract (N80-N98)—cont'd

Term	Word Origin	Definition
premenstrual tension syndrome (PMS)	*pre-* before *menstru/o* menses *-al* pertaining to *syn-* together *-drome* run	Poorly understood group of symptoms that occur in some women on a cyclic basis: Breast pain, irritability, fluid retention, headache, and lack of coordination are some of the symptoms.
rectocele	*rect/o* rectum *-cele* herniation, protrusion	A protrusion of the rectum into the vagina.
retroflexion of uterus	*retro-* backward *flex/o* bend *-ion* process	Condition in which the fundus of the uterus is bent backward, forming an angle with the cervix. Retroversion is when the entire uterus is bent backward.
vulvodynia	*vulv/o* vulva *-dynia* pain	Idiopathic syndrome of nonspecific complaints of pain of the vulva.

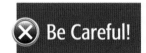 **Be Careful!** Do not confuse PMS, premenstrual tension syndrome, with PMDD, premenstrual dysphoric disorder, which is a major depressive disorder.

 Exercise 17: Noninflammatory Disorders of Female Genital Tract

Fill in the blank with the correct term from the list below.

amenorrhea   **menometrorrhagia**   **metrorrhagia**   **polymenorrhea**
dysmenorrhea   **menorrhagia**   **oligomenorrhea**

1. An abnormally frequent menstrual flow is_____.

2. Excessive menstrual flow and uterine bleeding not caused by menstruation is_____.

3. _____ is the lack of menstrual flow.

4. Uterine bleeding not caused by menstruation is_____.

5. _____ is abnormally heavy or prolonged menstrual bleeding.

6. Abnormally light or infrequent menstrual flow is_____.

7. Another term for cramps is_____.

Write out the following abbreviations.

8. DUB_____.

9. PMS_____.

10. PMB_____.

11. CIN_____.

Build the following terms.

12. herniation of the urinary bladder_____.

13. painful intercourse_____.

14. pertaining to excessive formation of the endometrium (2 words) _____.

15. abnormal condition of the endometrium_____.

16. blood in the fallopian tubes_____.

17. drooping uterus_____.

18. herniation of the rectum_____.

19. pain of the vulva_____.

Terms Related to Benign Neoplasms (D06, D24, D25)

Term	Word Origin	Definition
cervical intraepithelial neoplasia (CIN) III	*cervic/o* cervix *-al* pertaining to *neo-* new *-plasia* formation, development	Also termed **cervical dysplasia**, this abnormal cell growth may or may not develop into cancer. Grade III is the most severe.
fibroadenoma of the breast	*fibr/o* fiber *aden/o* gland *-oma* tumor, mass	Noncancerous breast tumors composed of fibrous and glandular tissue (Fig. 6-32).
leiomyoma of the uterus	*leiomy/o* smooth muscle *-oma* tumor, mass	Also termed **fibroids**, these smooth muscle tumors of the uterus are usually nonpainful growths, which may be removed surgically (Fig. 6-33).

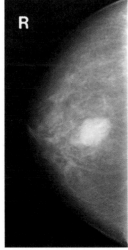

Fig. 6-32 Fibroadenoma in the right (R) breast.

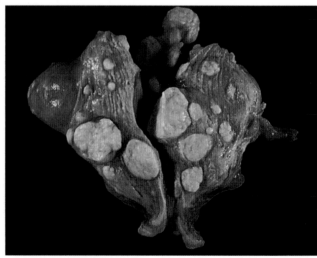

Fig. 6-33 Leiomyoma of the uterus.

Terms Related to Malignant Neoplasms (C50 and C51-C58)

Term	Word Origin	Definition
endometrial adenocarcinoma	*endometri/o* endometrium *-al* pertaining to *aden/o* gland *-carcinoma* cancer of epithelial origin	By far the most common cancer of the uterus, this type develops from the cells that line the uterus.
epithelial ovarian cancer (EOC)	*epitheli/o* epithelium *-al* pertaining to *ovari/o* ovary *-an* pertaining to	An inherited mutation of the *BRCA1* or *BRCA2* gene is linked to the risk of this malignancy and breast cancer.
infiltrating ductal carcinoma (IDC)	*duct/o* carry *-al* pertaining to *carcinoma* cancer of epithelial origin	The most common type of breast cancer, infiltrating ductal carcinoma arises from the cells that line the milk ducts (Fig. 6-34).
leiomyosarcoma	*leiomy/o* smooth muscle *-sarcoma* cancerous tumor of connective tissue	A rare type of cancer of the smooth muscle of the uterus.
lobular carcinoma	*lobul/o* small lobe *-ar* pertaining to *carcinoma* cancer of epithelial origin	About 15% of breast cancers are lobular carcinomas. These tumors begin in the glandular tissue of the breast at the ends of the milk ducts (Fig. 6-35).
mature teratoma of the ovary	*terat/o* deformity *-oma* tumor, mass	Also termed **dermoid cysts**, these usually noncancerous ovarian growths arise from germ cells.
Paget's disease of the breast		A rare form of cancer, this malignancy of the nipple can occur in men and women.
squamous cell carcinoma of the cervix	*squam/o* scaly *-ous* pertaining to *-carcinoma* cancer of epithelial origin	The most common type of cervical cancer. Thought to be caused by the human papillomavirus (HPV), it is also one of the most curable cancers if detected in its early stage.

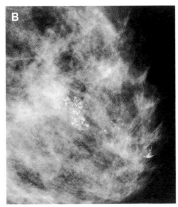

Fig. 6-34 Infiltrating ductal carcinoma (IDC).

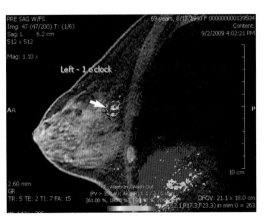

Fig. 6-35 MRI breast image using contrast and demonstrating lobular carcinoma in the left breast *(arrow)*.

Exercise 18: Neoplasms

Match the neoplasms with their definitions.

____ 1. CIN III	A. fibroid
____ 2. fibroadenoma of breast	B. dermoid cyst
____ 3. mature teratoma of ovary	C. benign breast tumors of fibrous and glandular tissue
____ 4. leiomyoma of uterus	D. the most severe form of cervical dysplasia
____ 5. endometrial adenocarcinoma	E. most common cancer of the uterus
____ 6. lobular carcinoma	F. rare smooth muscle tumor of uterus
____ 7. Paget's disease of the breast	G. breast cancer arising from ends of milk ducts
____ 8. infiltrating ductal carcinoma	H. most common type of cervical cancer
____ 9. EOC	I. inherited mutation linked to this form of ovarian cancer
____ 10. squamous cell carcinoma of the cervix	J. most common type of breast cancer arising from cells that line milk ducts
____ 11. leiomyosarcoma of the uterus	K. malignancy of nipple

PROCEDURES

Terms Related to Procedures

Term	Word Origin	Definition
cervicectomy	*cervic/o* cervix *-ectomy* cutting out	Resection (removal) of the uterine cervix.
clitoridectomy	*clitorid/o* clitoris *-ectomy* cutting out	Removal of the clitoris. Referred to as "female circumcision" in some cultures.
colpopexy	*colp/o* vagina *-pexy* suspension	Fixation of the vagina to an adjacent structure to hold it in place.
colpoplasty	*colp/o* vagina *-plasty* surgically forming	Surgical repair of the vagina.
colposcopy	*colp/o* vagina *-scopy* viewing	Endoscopic procedure used for viewing the cervix and vagina. The instrument used is called a **colposcope** (Fig. 6-36).
culdoscopy	*culd/o* cul-de-sac *-scopy* viewing	Endoscopic procedure used for biopsy of Douglas' cul-de-sac. The instrument used is called a culdoscope.
dilation and curettage (D&C)		Procedure involving widening (dilation) of the cervix until a curette, a sharp scraping tool, can be inserted to remove the lining of the uterus (curettage). Used to treat and diagnose conditions such as heavy menstrual bleeding or to empty the uterus of the products of conception.
fimbrioplasty	*fimbri/o* fimbria *-plasty* surgically forming	Surgical repair of the fimbria, usually to facilitate pregnancy.

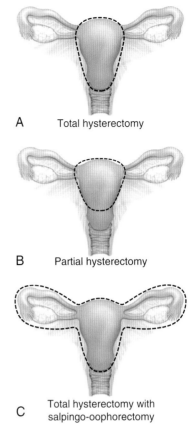

A   Total hysterectomy

B   Partial hysterectomy

C   Total hysterectomy with salpingo-oophorectomy

Fig. 6-37 A, Total hysterectomy. **B,** Partial hysterectomy. **C,** TAH-BSO.

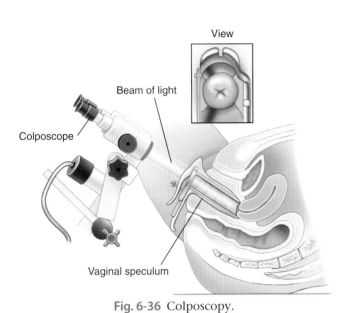

Fig. 6-36 Colposcopy.

To see a demonstration of dilation and curettage, click on **Animations.**

Terms Related to Procedures—cont'd

Term	Word Origin	Definition
hymenotomy	*hymen/o* hymen *-tomy* cutting	Incision of the hymen to enlarge the vaginal opening.
hysterectomy	*hyster/o* uterus *-ectomy* cutting out	Resection (removal) of the uterus; may be partial, pan- (all), or include other organs as well (e.g., **total *a*bdominal hysterectomy with a *b*ilateral *s*alpingo-*o*ophorectomy [TAH-BSO]**). The surgical approach is usually stated: whether it is laparoscopic, vaginal, or abdominal (Fig. 6-37).
hysteropexy	*hyster/o* uterus *-pexy* suspension	Suspension and fixation of a prolapsed uterus.
hysterosalpingography (HSG)	*hyster/o* uterus *salping/o* fallopian tube *-graphy* recording	X-ray procedure in which contrast medium is used to image the uterus and fallopian tubes (Fig. 6-38).

Continued

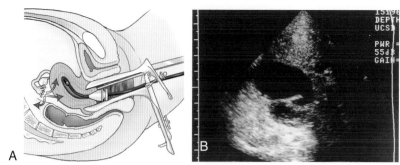

Fig. 6-38 A, Hysterosalpingography. **B,** Resulting hysterosalpingogram demonstrating coronal image of a very dilated fallopian tube. When swollen with fluid, the tube bends and curls.

Terms Related to Procedures—cont'd

Term	Word Origin	Definition
hysterotracheloplasty	*hyster/o* uterus *trachel/o* cervix *-plasty* surgically forming	Plastic surgery of the uterine cervix, usually for repair of a laceration. (The combining form trachel/o for cervix is seldom used, but easy to confuse with trache/o for throat when trying to translate this term.)
loop electrocautery excision procedure (LEEP)	*electr/o* electricity *cauter/i* burning *-y* process of	A procedure done to remove abnormal cells in cervical dysplasia.
mammography	*mamm/o* breast *-graphy* recording	Imaging technique (radiography) for the early detection of breast cancer. The record produced is called a **mammogram** (see Fig. 6-32).
mammoplasty	*mamm/o* breast *-plasty* surgically forming	Surgical or cosmetic repair of the breast. Options may include augmentation, to increase the size of the breasts, or reduction, to reduce the size of the breasts.
mastectomy	*mast/o* breast *-ectomy* cutting out	Removal of the breast; may be unilateral or bilateral.
mastopexy	*mast/o* breast *-pexy* suspension	Reconstructive procedure to lift and fixate the breasts.
oophorectomy	*oophor/o* ovary *-ectomy* cutting out	Removal of an ovary; may be unilateral or bilateral.
Pap smear		Exfoliative cytology procedure useful for the detection of vaginal and cervical cancer (Fig. 6-39).
salpingectomy	*salping/o* fallopian tube *-ectomy* -cutting out	Removal of a fallopian tube, usually because of infection or an ectopic pregnancy.
salpingolysis	*salping/o* fallopian tubes *-lysis* breaking down	Removal of the adhesions in the fallopian tubes to reestablish patency, with the goal of fertility.

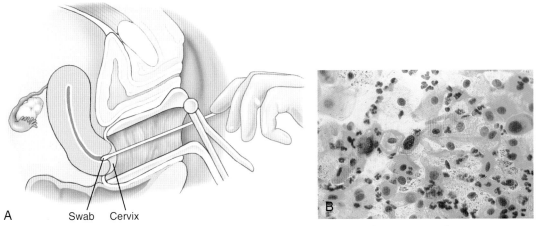

A   Swab   Cervix

Fig. 6-39 **A,** Obtaining a Pap smear. **B,** Malignant cells have enlarged hyperchromatic nuclei in contrast to the small nuclei of normal cells.

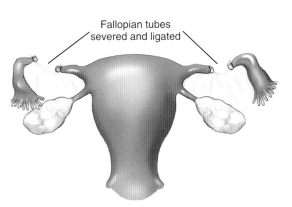

Fallopian tubes severed and ligated

Fig. 6-40 Tubal ligation.

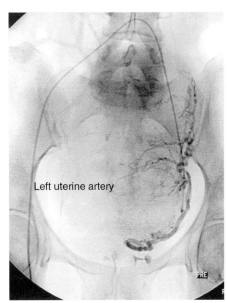

Left uterine artery

Fig. 6-41 Uterine artery embolization (UAE).

Terms Related to Procedures—cont'd

Term	Word Origin	Definition
tubal ligation	**tub/o** tube **-al** pertaining to **ligation** tying	Sterilization procedure in which the fallopian tubes are cut, ligated (tied), and cauterized to prevent released ova from being fertilized by spermatozoa (Fig. 6-40). This is considered an occlusion/blockage in ICD-10.
uterine artery embolization (UAE)		Injection of particles to block a uterine artery supplying blood to a fibroid with resultant death of fibroid tissue. Also termed **uterine fibroid embolization** (Fig. 6-41).
vaginotomy	**vagin/o** vagina **-tomy** cutting	An incision of the vagina. May be incidental (unintentional) during a cesarean section. Also called a **colpotomy**.

CPT Coding Alert!

CPT uses the terminology "tubotubal anastomosis" as the rejoining of a previously occluded fallopian tube (usually performed to restore fertility.

Exercise 19: Disorders of Breast and Inflammatory Disease of Female Pelvic Organs

Match the terms to their definitions.

____	1. vaginotomy	A. resection of an ovary
____	2. cervicectomy	B. removal of the uterine cervix
____	3. clitoridectomy	C. incision of the vagina
____	4. LEEP	D. reconstructive procedure to lift and fixate the breasts
____	5. hymenotomy	E. removal of the breast
____	6. hysterectomy	F. suspension and fixation of a prolapsed uterus
____	7. hysteropexy	G. surgical repair of the vagina
____	8. tubal ligation	H. incision of the hymen to enlarge the vaginal opening
____	9. colpoplasty	I. radiography of the breast
____	10. colposcopy	J. cutting, tying and cauterization of fallopian tubes for the purpose of sterilization
____	11. D&C	K. injection of particles to block a uterine artery to destroy a fibroid
____	12. mammography	L. removal of the clitoris
____	13. UAE	M. endoscopic procedure used to biopsy Douglas' cul-de-sac
____	14. culdoscopy	N. endoscopic procedure used for a biopsy of the cervix or vagina
____	15. oophorectomy	O. procedure done to remove abnormal cells in cervical dysplasia
____	16. mastectomy	P. removal of the uterus
____	17. mastopexy	Q. widening of the cervix and removal of the lining of the uterus

Translate the terms.

18. hysterotracheloplasty_____.

19. colpopexy_____.

20. hysterosalpingography_____.

21. salpingolysis_____.

22. mammoplasty_____.

PHARMACOLOGY

aromatase inhibitors: Block the conversion of androgen into estrogen. Used to treat breast cancer. Examples include anastrazole (Arimidex) and letrozole (Femara).

hormone replacement therapy (HRT) and estrogen replacement therapy (ERT): The healthcare replacement of estrogen alone (ERT) or with progesterone (HRT) perimenopausally in several forms (tablet, transdermal patch, injection, or vaginal suppository) to relieve symptoms of menopause and protect against osteoporosis.

phytoestrogens: An alternative source of estrogen replacement that occurs through the ingestion of certain plants like soybeans. Phytoestrogens act similarly to human estrogens in the body.

prolactin inhibitors: Lower levels of prolactin to prevent breast milk production or treat other conditions related to high levels of prolactin. One example is bromocriptine (Parlodel).

RECOGNIZING SUFFIXES FOR PCS

Now that you've finished reading about the procedures for the genitourinary system, take a look at this review of the *suffixes* used in their terminology. Each of these suffixes is associated with one or more root operations in the medical surgical section or one of the other categories in PCS.

Suffixes and Root Operations for the Female Reproductive System

Suffix	Root Operation
-ectomy	Excision, resection
-ligation	Occlusion
-lysis	Release
-pexy	Repair, reposition
-plasty	Repair, supplement, alteration, replacement
-scopy	Inspection
-tomy	Drainage, division

Abbreviations for the Female Reproductive System

Abbreviation	Definition	Abbreviation	Definition
CIN	cervical intraepithelial neoplasia	LEEP	loop electrocautery excision procedure
CX	cervix	LH	luteinizing hormone
D & C	dilation and curettage	PID	pelvic inflammatory disease
DUB	dysfunctional uterine bleeding	PMB	postmenopausal bleeding
EOC	epithelial ovarian cancer	PMS	premenstrual syndrome
FSH	follicle-stimulating hormone	TAH-BSO	total abdominal hysterectomy with a bilateral salpingo-oophorectomy
HPV	human papillomavirus		
HSG	hysterosalpingography		
IDC	infiltrating ductal carcinoma	UAE	uterine artery embolization

GARCIA, HORTENCIA T.

Age: 27 years   Sex: Female   Loc: WHC-SMMC
DOB: 04/04/1992   MRN: 538437   FIN: 3506004

Reference Text Browser   Form Browser   Medication Profile

Orders   Last 48 Hours   ED   Lab   Radiology   Assessments   **Surgery**   Clinical Notes   Pt. Info   Pt. Schedule   Task List   I & O   MAR

Flowsheet: Surgery   Level: Operative Report   ⊙ Table   ○ Group   ○ List

Navigator

✓   Operative Report

DESCRIPTION: Total abdominal hysterectomy and bilateral salpingo-oophorectomy

PREOPERATIVE DIAGNOSES:
Chronic pelvic pain, dysmenorrhea, dyspareunia, endometriosis, enlarged uterus, menorrhagia

POSTOPERATIVE DIAGNOSES:
Chronic pelvic pain, dysmenorrhea, dyspareunia, endometriosis, enlarged uterus, menorrhagia

PROCEDURE: Total abdominal hysterectomy and bilateral salpingo-oophorectomy.

ESTIMATED BLOOD LOSS: Less than 100 mL.

ANESTHESIA: General.

This 27-year-old white female presented to undergo TAH-BSO secondary to chronic pelvic pain and a diagnosis of endometriosis.

At the time of the procedure, once entering into the abdominal cavity, there was no gross evidence of abnormalities of the uterus, ovaries or fallopian tube. All endometriosis had been identified laparoscopically from a previous surgery. At the time of the surgery, all the tissue was quite thick and difficult to cut as well around the bladder flap and the uterus itself.

DESCRIPTION OF PROCEDURE: The patient was taken to the operating room and placed in supine position, at which time general form of anesthesia was administered by the anesthesia department. The patient was then prepped and draped in the usual fashion for a low transverse incision. Approximately two fingerbreadths above the pubic symphysis, a first knife was used to make a low transverse incision. This was extended down to the level of the fascia. The fascia was nicked in the center and extended in a transverse fashion. The edges of the fascia were grasped with Kocher. Both blunt and sharp dissection both caudally and cephalic was then completed consistent with Pfannenstiel technique. The abdominal rectus muscle was divided in the midline and extended in a vertical fashion. Peritoneum was entered at the high point and extended in a vertical fashion as well. An O'Connor-O'Sullivan retractor was put in place on either side. A bladder blade was put in place as well. Uterus was grasped with a double-tooth tenaculum and large and small colon were packed away cephalically and held in place with free wet lap packs and a superior blade. The bladder flap was released with Metzenbaum scissors and then dissected away caudally. EndoGIA were placed down both sides of the uterus in two bites on each side with the staples reinforced with a medium Endoclip. Two Heaney were placed on either side of the uterus at the level of cardinal ligaments. These were sharply incised and both pedicles were tied off with 1 Vicryl suture.
The uterus was transected at the level of Merz forceps and the uterus and cervix were removed intact. From there, the corners of the vaginal cuff were reinforced with figure-of-eight stitches. Betadine soaked sponge was placed in the vaginal vault and a continuous locking stitch of 0 Vicryl was used to re-approximate the edges with a second layer used to reinforce the first. Bladder flap was created with the use of 3-0 Vicryl and Gelfoam was placed underneath. The EndoGIA was used to transect both the fallopian tube and ovaries at the infundibulopelvic ligament and each one was reinforced with medium clips. The entire area was then re-peritonized and copious amounts of saline were used to irrigate the pelvic cavity. Once this was completed, Gelfoam was placed into the cul-de-sac and the O'Connor-O'Sullivan retractor was removed as well as all the wet lap pack. Edges of the peritoneum were grasped in 3 quadrants with hemostat and a continuous locking stitch of 2-0 Vicryl was used to re-approximate the peritoneum as well as abdominal rectus muscle. The edges of the fascia were grasped at both corners and a continuous locking stitch of 1 Vicryl was used to re-approximate the fascia with overlapping in the center. The subcutaneous tissue was irrigated. Cautery was used to create adequate hemostasis and 3-0 Vicryl was used to re-approximate the tissue and the skin edges were re-approximated with sterile staples. Sterile dressing was applied and Betadine soaked sponge was removed from the vaginal vault and the vaginal vault was wiped clean of any remaining blood. The patient was taken to recovery room in stable condition. Instrument count, needle count, and sponge counts were all correct.

Exercise 20: **Operative Report**

Using the operative report on the previous page, answer the following questions.

1. What is a TAH?_____

2. What term (and abbreviation) tells you that the patient had her left and right fallopian tubes and

   ovaries removed?_____

3. Which term refers to painful intercourse?_____

4. How do you know that she had an abnormal condition of the lining of her uterus?

   _____

5. Which term indicates painful menstrual periods?_____

6. Which term means an excessive amount of bleeding during menstrual periods? _____

7. Which term tells you that the patient was lying on her back for the surgery? _____

8. How do you know that the initial incision was made crosswise above the pubic symphysis?

   _____

Go to the Evolve website to interactively build terms, label images, memorize word parts, and practice using terms that relate to the genitourinary system in context.

Match the word parts for the urinary system to their definitions.

WORD PART DEFINITIONS: URINARY

Suffix
-esis
-iasis
-lithotomy
-lysis
-osis
-pexy
-ptosis
-scopy
-tripsy
-uria

Definition
1. _____ cutting out a stone
2. _____ condition, presence of
3. _____ breaking down
4. _____ crushing
5. _____ abnormal condition
6. _____ viewing
7. _____ suspension
8. _____ drooping, prolapse
9. _____ urinary condition
10. _____ state of

Combining Form
calic/o
cortic/o
cyst/o
glomerul/o
hil/o
hydr/o
lith/o
meat/o
nephr/o
noct/i
olig/o
py/o
pyel/o
ren/o
trigon/o
ur/o
ureter/o
urethr/o
vesic/o

Definition
11. _____ water
12. _____ bladder
13. _____ ureter
14. _____ pus
15. _____ night
16. _____ trigone
17. _____ urethra
18. _____ urine, urinary system
19. _____ stone
20. _____ meatus
21. _____ kidney
22. _____ scanty, few
23. _____ glomerulus
24. _____ kidney
25. _____ calyx
26. _____ renal pelvis
27. _____ hilum
28. _____ bladder
29. _____ cortex

WORDSHOP: URINARY

Prefixes	Combining Forms	Suffixes
a-	cyst/o	-al
an-	glomerul/o	-emia
dia-	hemat/o	-iasis
dys-	hem/o	-itis
per-	lith/o	-lithotomy
peri-	nephr/o	-lysis
poly-	py/o	-oma
pre-	pyel/o	-pathy
	trigon/o	-scope
	ur/o	-scopy
	ureter/o	-stomy
	urethr/o	-tomy
	vesic/o	-tripsy
		-uria

Build urinary terms by combining the word parts above. Some word parts may be used more than once. Some may not be used at all. The number in parentheses indicates the number of word parts needed.

Definition	Term
1. pertaining to surrounding the bladder (3)	
2. cutting out a kidney stone (2)	
3. instrument to view the bladder (2)	
4. inflammation of the trigone (2)	
5. painful, abnormal urinary condition (2)	
6. urinary condition of blood (2)	
7. disease process of the kidney (2)	
8. condition of stone in the ureter (3)	
9. condition of no urination (2)	
10. process of crushing stones (2)	
11. condition of urea in the blood (2)	
12. complete breakdown of the blood (3)	
13. condition of excessive urination (2)	
14. breaking down the urethra (2)	
15. making a new opening in the kidney (2)	

Sort the terms into the correct categories.

TERM SORTING: URINARY

Anatomy and Physiology	Pathology	Procedures

ARF	hydronephrosis	pyonephrosis
BUN	incontinence	renal adenoma
calyx	lithotripsy	renal corpuscle
CAPD	loop of Henle	renal dialysis
CKD	meatotomy	renal pelvis
cortex	medulla	trigone
cystectomy	micturition	urethra
cystitis	nephroblastoma	urethral stricture
cystoscopy	nephrolithotomy	urethrolysis
enuresis	nephron	urinalysis
GFR	nephropexy	urinary meatus
glomeruli	nephroptosis	urine
hematuria	nephrostomy	urolithiasis
hemodialysis	nocturia	UTI
hilum	parenchymal tissue	vesicotomy

Replace the highlighted words with the correct urinary terms.

TRANSLATIONS: URINARY

1. Emily was suffering from **the inability to release urine** and **bladder spasms**.

2. Dr. Garcia ordered a **blood test that measures the amount of nitrogenous waste** and **a test of kidney function that measures the rate at which nitrogenous waste is removed from the blood**.

3. Moumoud was admitted for **blood in the urine** and **stones anywhere in the urinary tract**.

4. Mr. Samuels was treated for his **stones in the kidney** with **process of crushing stones to prevent or clear an obstruction in the urinary system**.

5. Once **an infection anywhere in the urinary system** was ruled out, Rebecca was evaluated for ongoing **bed-wetting**.

6. **An instrument for visual examination of the inside of the bladder** was used to diagnose Alberta's **painful inflammation of the bladder wall**.

7. Mr. Alton's acute renal failure was diagnosed after examination findings that included **condition of scanty urination** and **excessive urea in the blood**.

8. The patient's **prolapsed or sagging of the kidney** was surgically corrected with a **suspension or fixation of the kidney**.

9. The patient was diagnosed with **dilation of the renal pelvis and calices of one or both kidneys**.

10. The patient showed symptoms of **pus-producing infection of the kidney**.

11. Dr. Simons told Marqueta that she had **abnormal backflow of urine from the bladder to the ureter**.

12. After several years of **process of diffusing blood across a semipermeable membrane to remove substances that a healthy kidney would eliminate**, Johnna underwent **a surgical transfer of a complete kidney from a donor**.

Match the word parts for the male and female reproductive systems to their definitions.

WORD PART DEFINITIONS: REPRODUCTIVE

Prefix/Suffix	Definition
a-	1. _____ through
-cele	2. _____ excessive
-genesis	3. _____ fallopian tube
hyper-	4. _____ substance that forms
-ligation	5. _____ flow, discharge
-one	6. _____ bursting forth
-plasia	7. _____ drooping, sagging
-ptosis	8. _____ herniation, protrusion
-rrhagia	9. _____ no, not, without
-rrhea	10. _____ tying
-salpinx	11. _____ production
trans-	12. _____ formation

Combining Form	Definition
balan/o	13. _____ semen
colp/o	14. _____ glans penis
culd/o	15. _____ testis
episi/o	16. _____ foreskin
galact/o	17. _____ seminal vesicle
hyster/o	18. _____ penis
leiomy/o	19. _____ vas deferens
mamm/o	20. _____ scanty, few
men/o	21. _____ cervix
o/o	22. _____ milk
olig/o	23. _____ breast
oophor/o	24. _____ smooth muscle
orchid/o	25. _____ ovum, egg
phall/o	26. _____ menstruation
preputi/o	27. _____ vagina
salping/o	28. _____ uterus
semin/i	29. _____ rectouterine pouch
trachel/o	30. _____ fallopian tube
vas/o	31. _____ ovary
vesicul/o	32. _____ vulva

WORDSHOP: REPRODUCTIVE

Prefixes	Combining Forms	Suffixes
a-	balan/o	-ectomy
an-	colp/o	-graphy
dys-	endometri/o	-ia
e-	epididym/o	-ism
poly-	galact/o	-itis
	hyster/o	-ligation
	mast/o	-osis
	men/o	-pexy
	olig/o	-plasty
	orchid/o	-ptosis
	salping/o	-rrhea
	sperm/o	-stomy
	trachel/o	-tomy
	vas/o	
	vesicul/o	
	zo/o	

Build male and female reproductive terms by combining the word parts above. Some word parts may be used more than once. Some may not be used at all. The number in parentheses indicates the number of word parts needed.

Definition	Term
1. condition of scanty sperm (3)	
2. inflammation of a seminal vesicle (2)	
3. recording the uterus and fallopian tube (3)	
4. surgically forming the glans penis (2)	
5. painful menstrual flow (3)	
6. flow, discharge of milk (2)	
7. drooping, sagging of the breast (2)	
8. tying a vessel (2)	
9. abnormal condition of the endometrium (2)	
10. condition of no animals (life) in the sperm (4)	
11. suspension of the vagina (2)	
12. discharge of many menses (3)	
13. cutting out the epididymis (2)	
14. surgically forming the uterus and cervix (3)	

Sort the terms into the correct categories.

TERM SORTING: REPRODUCTIVE

Anatomy and Physiology	Pathology	Procedures

amenorrhea	hysteropexy	PID
areola	hysteroptosis	prepuce
BPH	leiomyosarcoma	prostatectomy
colposcopy	mammoplasty	puberty
corpora cavernosa	menarche	rectouterine pouch
corpus luteum	menopause	salpingolysis
D & C	menorrhagia	seminoma
endometriosis	menstruation	spermatogenesis
epididymis	mittelschmerz	tubal ligation
epididymitis	mons pubis	TUIP
epididymotomy	oligospermia	tunica vaginalis
epididymo-vesiculography	oophorectomy	vasoligation
gametes	orchiopexy	vasovasostomy
hematosalpinx	ovulation	vulvodynia
HPV	phalloplasty	

Replace the highlighted words with the correct male or female reproductive terms.

TRANSLATIONS: REPRODUCTIVE

1. A sperm analysis revealed **a condition of temporary or permanent deficiency of sperm in the seminal fluid** that caused the couple's infertility.

2. Ms. Costello made an appointment with her gynecologist to discuss her **painful menstrual flow** and **painful intercourse**.

3. Mr. Steinman's **abnormal enlargement of the prostate gland** was treated with a **form of prostate surgery involving tiny incisions of the prostate**.

4. Mrs. Graf had a **cutting out of the breast** to treat her **breast cancer that arises from the cells that line the milk ducts**.

5. The physician suggested **surgical procedure in which the prepuce of the penis is excised** to treat the patient's **condition of tightening of the prepuce around the glans penis**.

6. The doctor ordered an **x-ray procedure in which contrast medium is used to image the uterus and fallopian tubes** to image the patient's **inflammation of the fallopian tubes**.

7. When Ken remarried, he decided to have his **incision, ligation, and cauterization of both of the vas deferens** reversed and was scheduled for a **anastomosis of the ends of the vas deferens as a means of reconnecting them**.

8. Janice had a **resection of the uterus** to treat her **rare cancer of the smooth muscle of the uterus**.

9. Hunter underwent a/an **pertaining to one side removal of a testicle** to treat a **germ cell tumor** in his right testicle.

10. Patient G had **downward displacement of the breasts** with resultant **breast pain**.

11. Robert underwent **imaging of the epididymis and seminal vesicles** to diagnose his **swelling of the epididymis that contains sperm**.

Obstetric, Perinatal and Congenital Conditions

ICD-10-CM Example From Tabular

O30.03 Twin pregnancy, monochorionic/diamniotic

  O30.031 Twin pregnancy, monochorionic/diamniotic; first trimester

  O30.032 Twin pregnancy, monochorionic/diamniotic; second trimester

  O30.033 Twin pregnancy, monochorionic/diamniotic; third trimester

  O30.039 Twin pregnancy, monochorionic/diamniotic; unspecified trimester

O30.04 Twin pregnancy, dichorionic/diamniotic

  O30.041 Twin pregnancy, dichorionic/diamniotic; first trimester

  O30.042 Twin pregnancy, dichorionic/diamniotic; second trimester

  O30.043 Twin pregnancy, dichorionic/diamniotic; third trimester

  O30.049 Twin pregnancy, dichorionic/diamniotic; unspecified trimester

ICD-10-PCS Example From Index

Delivery

  Cesarean—see Extraction, products of conception **10D0**

  Forceps—see Extraction, products of conception **10D0**

  Manually assisted **10E0XZZ**

  Products of conception **10E0XZZ**

  Vacuum assisted —see Extraction, Products of Conception **10D0**

CHAPTER OUTLINE

Childbirth and the Puerperium

ANATOMY AND PHYSIOLOGY OF PREGNANCY

PATHOLOGY

PROCEDURES

PHARMACOLOGY

Perinatal Conditions

Congenital Malformations

RECOGNIZING SUFFIXES FOR PCS

ABBREVIATIONS

OBJECTIVES

☐ Recognize and use terms related to the anatomy and physiology of pregnancy, the perinatal period, and congenital malformations.

☐ Recognize and use terms related to the pathology of pregnancy, perinatal conditions, and congenital malformations of the newborn.

☐ Recognize and use terms related to the procedures for pregnancy and congenital conditions.

CHILDBIRTH AND THE PUERPERIUM

ANATOMY AND PHYSIOLOGY OF PREGNANCY

Pregnancy begins with the fertilization of an ovum by a spermatozoon as the ovum travels toward the uterus through the fallopian tube. This beginning of new life (conception) is usually the result of sexual intercourse (also termed *copulation* or *coitus*). Terms that are used to describe pregnancy are **gravid** or **gravida,** as in a gravid (pregnant) uterus; **gestation,** as in the time period of fetal development; and the suffixes *-gravida* and *-cyesis.* A woman who has never been pregnant is a **nulligravida,** whereas one who is pregnant for the first time is a **unigravida** (or **primigravida).** A woman who has been pregnant two or more times is described as a **multigravida.** The term **obstetrics** comes from the word root *obstetr/o* meaning "midwife," the traditional authority on all matters regarding childbirth. The term **puerperium** is from a Latin term referring to the time immediately following childbirth.

pregnancy = gravid/o, -gravida, -cyesis

nulligravida
   nulli- = none
   -gravida = pregnancy

primigravida
   primi- = first
   -gravida = pregnancy

multigravida
   multi- = many
   -gravida = pregnancy

puerperium
   puerperi/o = childbirth
   -um = structure, thing, membrane

 CM Guideline Alert

15a. GENERAL RULES FOR OBSTETRIC CASES
1) CODES FROM CHAPTER 15 AND SEQUENCING PRIORITY
Obstetric cases require codes from Chapter 15, codes in the range O00-O9A Pregnancy, Childbirth, and the Puerperium. Chapter 15 codes have sequencing priority over codes from other chapters. Additional codes from other chapters may be used in conjunction with Chapter 15 codes to further specify conditions. Should the provider document that the pregnancy is incidental to the encounter, then code Z33.1, Pregnant state, incidental, should be used in place of any Chapter 15 codes. It is the provider's responsibility to state that the condition being treated is not affecting the pregnancy.

2) CHAPTER 15 CODES USED ONLY ON THE MATERNAL RECORD
Chapter 15 codes are to be used only on the maternal record, never on the record of the newborn.

Time periods are important when using the terminology of pregnancy. A normal pregnancy is approximately 38 to 40 weeks, or 9 months. This time period is divided into **trimesters,** three 3-month segments. Specifically, the first trimester is less than 14 weeks 0 days; the second trimester is 14 weeks 0 days to less than 28 weeks 0 days; and the third trimester is 28 weeks 0 days until delivery (Fig. 7-1). Many ICD-10-CM codes require the addition of information as to the specific

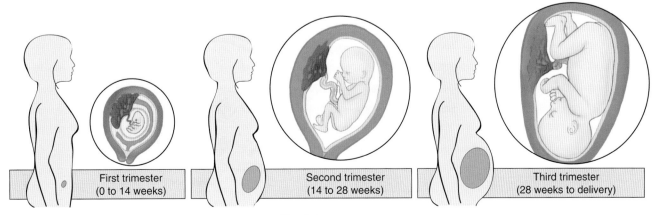

First trimester (0 to 14 weeks)   Second trimester (14 to 28 weeks)   Third trimester (28 weeks to delivery)

Fig. 7-1 Trimesters.

trimester of the patient's pregnancy. The **estimated date of delivery (EDD)** of the infant can be calculated using a formula, Naegeli's rule, that uses the first day of a woman's **last menstrual period (LMP),** subtracts 3 months, and adds 7 days to come up with a "due" date. Note that this is based on 38 weeks (266 days). Forty weeks (280 days) is the standard time period for a pregnancy.

 CM Guideline Alert

3) FINAL CHARACTER FOR TRIMESTER

The majority of codes in Chapter 15 have a final character indicating the trimester of pregnancy. The timeframes for the trimesters are indicated at the beginning of the chapter. If trimester is not a component of a code, it is because the condition always occurs in a specific trimester or the concept of trimester of pregnancy is not applicable. Certain codes have characters for only certain trimesters because the condition does not occur in all trimesters, but it may occur in more than just one.

Assignment of the final character for trimester should be based on the provider's documentation of the trimester (or number of weeks) for the current admission/ encounter. This applies to the assignment of trimester for pre-existing conditions as well as those that develop during or are due to the pregnancy. The provider's documentation of the number of weeks of pregnancy may be used to assign the appropriate code identifying the trimester.

Whenever delivery occurs during the current admission and there is an "in childbirth" option for the obstetric complication being coded, the "in childbirth" code should be assigned.

The one-celled fertilized egg, or **zygote,** carrying the genome (complete set of chromosomal information) divides as it moves through the fallopian tube toward the uterus (Fig. 7-2). In the first few days after fertilization, when the zygote has become a solid ball of cells from repeated divisions, it is called a **morula.** It is termed a *morula,* which is Latin for *mulberry,* because of its similar appearance. As it continues to develop, it moves from the fallopian tube into the uterus and becomes implanted in the uterine wall. At this point, it is identified as a **blastocyst.** Upon implantation, human chorionic gonadotropin (hCG), the pregnancy hormone, is secreted by the blastocyst. The hCG stimulates the corpus luteum in the ovary to continue to produce progesterone and estrogen. The continued secretion of progesterone maintains the endometrial lining to nourish the growing zygote, while the estrogen contributes to

blastocyst

blast/o = embryonic, immature

-cyst = sac

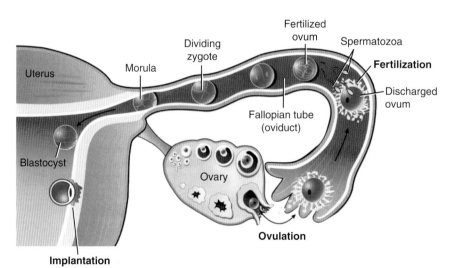

Fig. 7-2 Fertilization and implantation.

increasing the size of the lining of the uterus and the number of blood vessels that it has.

The blastocyst has a hollow outer shell, called the **trophoblast,** and an inner segment called the **inner cell mass.** The trophoblast becomes the membranes that surround and nourish the fetus, whereas the inner mass becomes the embryo and later the fetus. Notice the connection between the meaning of the combining form *troph/o* and its function in the developing embryo.

Twins are the result of a modification of this process. In the case of identical **(monozygotic)** twins, one zygote divides to develop into two genetically identical copies of chromosomes (identical genomes). When two ova are released and fertilized by two different sperm, fraternal **(dizygotic)** twins develop with two different sets of chromosomes (two genomes), making them not identical, but only as similar as siblings. Although a normal zygote has one set of membranes (an outer chorionic and inner amniotic) to support it through the pregnancy, twins may have a different configuration of sacs depending on when their fertilized eggs divide. If the egg divides 3 to 4 days after it is fertilized, the monozygotic twins will develop in two sets of sacs **(dichorionic/diamniotic).** If the division happens 3 to 8 days after fertilization, the twins will share the same outer sac **(monochorionic),** but each will be in its own inner sac **(diamniotic).** If the split occurs from 8 to 13 days after fertilization, they share the same outer and inner sac (monochorionic/monoamniotic). Finally, if the split happens after 13 days, the twins share the same outer and inner sac (monochorionic/monoamniotic), but the division is incomplete and results in **conjoined twins** (Fig. 7-3).

Time is also a component in naming the stages of the developing fetus. For the first 2 weeks, the developing fertilized egg is called a zygote. From weeks 3 to 8, it is termed an **embryo.** For the remainder of the pregnancy, it is labeled a **fetus.** Connecting the time periods of pregnancy with the time periods of the developing fetus, one can see that the progression from zygote to fetus occurs in the first trimester. At the end of the first trimester, the fetus weighs about 1 ounce and is 3 inches long, and the fetal membranes that support the pregnancy are developing. During the second trimester, fetal movement may be felt ("quickening"), the reproductive organs can be seen, and the fetus begins to urinate. At this time, the fetus weighs approximately 11 ounces and is 6 inches long. The third trimester is a time period of rapid weight gain, when the fetus has the best chance to survive premature delivery. At the end of this trimester, the fetus weighs about $7^{1}/_{2}$ pounds and is 18 inches long. At this time, the pregnancy is considered to be at **term.** ICD-10 classifies late pregnancies as **post-term pregnancy** (from 40 to 42 completed weeks) and **prolonged pregnancy** (over 42 weeks).

trophoblast
 troph/o = development, nourishment
 -blast = embryonic, immature

monochorionic
 mono- = one
 chorion/o = chorion, outer fetal sac
 -ic = pertaining to

diamniotic
 di- = two
 amni/o = amnion, inner fetal sac
 -tic = pertaining to

fetus = **fet/o**

Diamniotic/Dichorionic
Cleavage 1-3 days

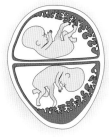

Monochorionic/Diamniotic
Cleavage 4-8 days

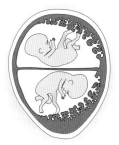

Monochorionic/Monoamniotic
Cleavage 8-13 days

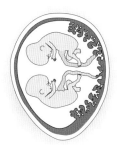

Conjoined twins
Cleavage 13-15 days

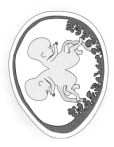

Fig. 7-3 Twins.

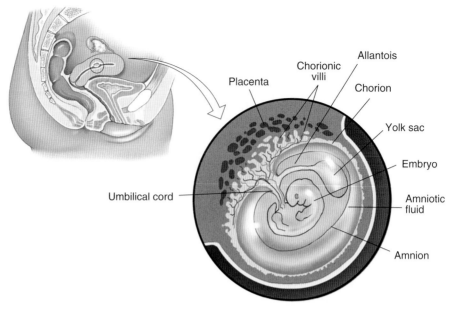

Fig. 7-4 The uterus of the pregnant woman.

chorion = chori/o, chorion/o

placenta = placent/o

amnion = amni/o, amnion/o

umbilicus = umbilic/o, omphal/o

parturition, delivery = part/o, -para, -partum, -tocia

ante- = before

intra- = within

nullipara
nulli- = none
-para = delivery

primipara
primi- = first
-para = delivery

multipara
multi = many
-para = delivery

At the same time that the embryo is developing, extraembryonic membranes are forming to sustain the pregnancy. Two of these, the amnion and the chorion, form the inner and outer sacs that contain the embryo (Fig. 7-4). The outer sac, the **chorion,** forms part of the **placenta,** a highly vascular structure that acts as a physical communication between the mother and the embryo. The **chorionic villi** are small projections that extend from the outer sac to provide a maximum amount of contact with the maternal blood supply. The inner sac, the **amnion** and its amniotic fluid, cushion the embryo, protect it against temperature changes, and allow it to move. On the outer side, the amniotic sac is connected to the yolk sac, the **allantois,** and to the placenta by way of the umbilical cord. The yolk sac, attached to the developing embryo, provides a source of nutrition for the early stage of development. The allantois is an embryonic structure that assists in waste removal and gas exchange. It later develops into the placenta and umbilical cord, which share similar functions. The **umbilical cord** is the tissue that connects the embryo to the placenta (and hence to the mother). When the baby is delivered, the umbilical cord is cut, and the baby is then dependent on his/her own body for all physiological processes. The remaining "scar" is the **umbilicus,** or **navel.**

Documentation regarding the diagnosis of pregnancy may mention the **signs of pregnancy.** These are divided into three types: **presumptive** (subjective symptoms indicative of pregnancy, but may appear in other diagnoses as well), **probable** (objective signs that are recognized by an examiner that may or may not indicate a pregnancy), and **positive** (objective signs recognized by an examiner that are present only in pregnancy).

The terms that describe delivery and childbirth are different from those of pregnancy. **Parturition** is the term for the act of giving birth. Related terms are **antepartum** (before childbirth), **intrapartum** (during childbirth), and **postpartum** (after childbirth). A mother's **parity** is the number of times that she has delivered a child. The terms *nullipara, unipara/primipara,* and *multipara* are similar to those used for pregnancy. They respectively mean: no deliveries, one delivery, and two or more deliveries. ICD-10 categorizes a young primipara as a woman whose EDD is before her 16th birthday. An **elderly primipara** is one whose EDD is after her 35th birthday. ICD-10 also specifies that a code be used to describe **grand multiparity,** a woman who has delivered five or more children. The 6-week time period immediately after delivery is termed the **puerperium,** derived from the Latin for *child* and *bearing*. It is the period when the mother's reproductive system returns to its pregravid state.

 Be Careful! *Stage 1* has three separate phases of labor; *stage 2* is the delivery of the infant; and *stage 3* is the delivery of the placenta.

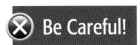 **CM Guideline Alert**

15.0. THE PERIPARTUM AND POSTPARTUM PERIODS
1) PERIPARTUM AND POSTPARTUM PERIODS
The postpartum period begins immediately after delivery and continues for six weeks following delivery. The peripartum period is defined as the last month of pregnancy to five months postpartum.

2) PERIPARTUM AND POSTPARTUM COMPLICATIONS
A postpartum complication is any complication occurring within the six-week period.

3) PREGNANCY-RELATED COMPLICATIONS AFTER 6-WEEK PERIOD
Chapter 15 codes may also be used to describe pregnancy-related complications after the peripartum or postpartum period if the provider documents that a condition is pregnancy related.

Stages of labor: Like the trimesters, labor is also divided into three stages: first, second, and third (Fig. 7-5. The **first stage** is the longest and, again, includes three parts: an early (or latent) phase, an active phase, and a transitional phase. The early phase, the longest, is marked by dilation of the cervix to approximately 4 centimeters and a changeover from irregular to regular contractions. The active phase has the now regular contractions becoming stronger and closer together. The final phase of the first stage, the transition phase, is the

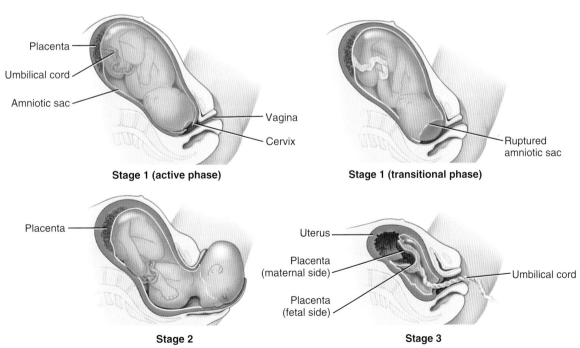

Fig. 7-5 Stages of labor.

time when the cervix dilates to 10 centimeters and the baby moves down into the birth canal. The **second stage** is the time when the actual birth takes place and the umbilical cord is cut and clamped. The **third stage** is the delivery of the placenta.

To practice labeling the uterus of a pregnant woman, click on **Label It** .

To see the process of fetal development, click on **Animations** .

Combining Forms for the Anatomy and Physiology of Pregnancy

Meaning	Combining Form
amnion, inner fetal sac	amni/o, amnion/o
chorion, outer fetal sac	chorion/o, chori/o
development, nourishment	troph/o
embryonic, immature	blast/o
parturition, delivery	part/o
placenta	placent/o
pregnancy	gravid/o
umbilicus	umbilic/o, omphal/o

Prefixes for the Anatomy and Physiology of Pregnancy

Prefix	Meaning
ante-	before
di-	two
intra-	within
mono-	one
multi-	many
neo-	new
nulli-	none
primi-	first

Suffixes for the Anatomy and Physiology of Pregnancy

Suffix	Meaning
-blast	embryonic, immature
-cyst	sac
-gravida, -cyesis	pregnancy
-para, -tocia	delivery

Exercise 1: **Anatomy of Pregnancy**

Match the word parts to their meanings.

____	1.	nulli-	A. two
____	2.	intra-	B. inner fetal membrane
____	3.	uni-, mono-	C. nourishment, development
____	4.	chori/o, chorion/o	D. immature
____	5.	di-	E. none
____	6.	-gravida, -cyesis	F. three
____	7.	blast/o, -blast	G. pregnancy
____	8.	ante-, pre-	H. one
____	9.	multi-	I. before
____	10.	troph/o	J. many, more than one
____	11.	amni/o, amnion/o	K. outer fetal membrane
____	12.	tri-	L. within
____	13.	-para, -tocia	M. delivery

Fill in the blank.

14. A woman who has been pregnant two or more times is termed a/an_____.

15. Once the fertilized egg has implanted in the uterine wall it is called a/an_____.

16. Fraternal twins are called_____ twins, whereas identical twins are called _____twins.

17. A developing fertilized egg is called a/an_____in its first 2 weeks, a/an_____in weeks 3

    to 8, and a/an_____for the remainder of the pregnancy.

18. The inner sac that contains the embryo is called the_____, whereas the outer sac is called

    the_____.

19. The tissue that connects the embryo to the placenta is called the_____.

20. _____is the term for the act of giving birth.

21. A nullipara has delivered how many babies?_____

PATHOLOGY

Terms Related to Pregnancy with Abortive Outcome (O00-O09)

Term	Word Origin	Definition
ectopic pregnancy	*ec-* out *top/o* place *-ic* pertaining to	Implantation of the embryo in any location but the uterus (Fig. 7-6). Most ectopic pregnancies occur in the fallopian tubes and are referred to as **tubal pregnancies.** Ectopic pregnancies cannot come to term successfully.
hydatidiform mole	*hydatid/i* water drop *-form* shape	Rare, cystlike growth of a nonviable embryo (Fig. 7-7).
miscarriage/abortion		Termination of a pregnancy before the fetus is viable. If spontaneous, it may be termed a **miscarriage** or a **spontaneous abortion.** If induced, it can be referred to as a **therapeutic abortion.** A **missed abortion** is fetal death <20 weeks with retention of the dead fetus An **incomplete abortion** includes the retained products of conception after a spontaneous abortion.

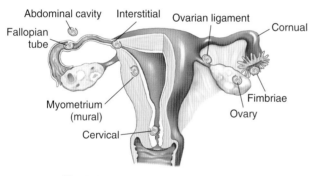
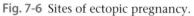

Fig. 7-6 Sites of ectopic pregnancy.

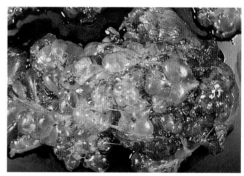

Fig. 7-7 Hydatidiform mole.

Terms Related to Edema, Proteinuria, and Hypertensive Disorders in Pregnancy, Childbirth, and the Puerperium (O10-O16)

Term	Word Origin	Definition
eclampsia in pregnancy		Extremely serious form of hypertension secondary to pregnancy. Patients are at risk from coma, convulsions, and death.
gestational edema	*edema* swelling	An abnormal accumulation of fluid in the body limited to the pregnancy time period.
HELLP syndrome	*hem/o* blood *-lysis* breaking down	Preeclampsia with **h**emolysis (destruction of blood cells), **e**levated **l**iver enzymes, and **l**ow **p**latelet count.
preeclampsia	*pre-* before	Abnormal condition of pregnancy with unknown cause, marked by hypertension, edema, and proteinuria. Also called **toxemia of pregnancy.**

Terms Related to Other Maternal Disorders Predominantly Related to Pregnancy (O20-O29)

Term	Word Origin	Definition
gestational diabetes mellitus		Abnormally high blood glucose levels during pregnancy in women with normal blood glucose levels.
gestational phlebitis	*phleb/o* vein *-itis* inflammation	Inflammation of veins during pregnancy.
hyperemesis gravidarum	*hyper-* excessive *-emesis* vomiting *gravidarum* pregnancy	Excessive vomiting that begins before the 20th week of pregnancy.
pruritic urticarial papules and plaques (PUPP)	*prurit/o* itching *-ic* pertaining to	A common rash of late pregnancy with itchy wheals, papules (bumps), and plaques (patches) that develop on the abdomen, breasts, arms, and legs (Fig. 7-8).

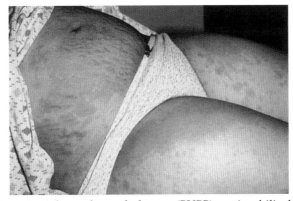

Fig. 7-8 Pruritic urticarial papules and plaques (PUPP): periumbilical striae involved.

CM Guideline Alert!

15.i. GESTATIONAL (PREGNANCY INDUCED) DIABETES

Gestational (pregnancy induced) diabetes can occur during the second and third trimester of pregnancy in women who were not diabetic prior to pregnancy. Gestational diabetes can cause complications in the pregnancy similar to those of pre-existing diabetes mellitus. It also puts the woman at greater risk of developing diabetes after the pregnancy. Codes for gestational diabetes are in subcategory O24.4, Gestational diabetes mellitus. No other code from category O24, Diabetes mellitus in pregnancy, childbirth, and the puerperium, should be used with a code from O24.4.

Terms Related to the Fetus and Amniotic Cavity and Possible Delivery Problems (O30-O48)

Term	Word Origin	Definition
abruptio placentae		Premature separation of the placenta from the uterine wall; may result in a severe hemorrhage that can threaten both infant and maternal lives. Also called **ablatio placentae** (Fig. 7-9).
cephalopelvic disproportion	*cephal/o* head *pelv/i* pelvis *-ic* pertaining to	Condition in which the infant's head is larger than the pelvic outlet it must pass through, thereby inhibiting normal labor and birth. It is one of the indications for a cesarean section.
cervical incompetence	*cervic/o* cervix, neck *-al* pertaining to	Lack of cervical closure during pregnancy. May lead to early termination of pregnancy.
chorioamnionitis	*chori/o* chorion *amnion/o* amnion *-itis* inflammation	Inflammation of the outer and inner membranes (chorion and amnion) surrounding the fetus. This bacterial infection occurs late in pregnancy or during labor.
malpresentation of fetus	*mal-* bad, abnormal	Any fetal position but cephalic for birth. A breech presentation is an example (Fig. 7-10).

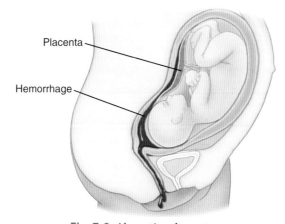

Fig. 7-9 Abruptio placentae.

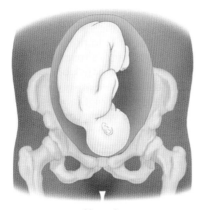
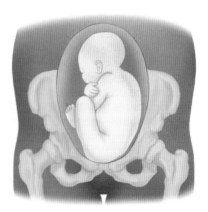

Normal   Breech

Fig. 7-10 Normal and breech presentations.

Terms Related to the Fetus and Amniotic Cavity and Possible Delivery Problems (O30-O48)—cont'd

Term	Word Origin	Definition
oligohydramnios	*olig/o* scanty *hydr/o* water, fluid *-amnios* amnion	Condition of low or missing amniotic fluid.
placenta accreta	*ac-* toward *cret/o* to grow *-a* noun ending	An abnormal attachment of the placenta to the uterine wall.
placenta increta	*in-* in *cret/o* to grow *-a* noun ending	An abnormal attachment of the placenta within the uterine wall.
placenta percreta	*per-* through *cret/o* to grow *-a* noun ending	An abnormal attachment of the placenta through the uterine wall.
placenta previa	*previa* in front of	Placenta that is malpositioned in the uterus, so that it covers the opening of the cervix.
placentitis	*placent/o* placenta *-itis* inflammation	Inflammation of the placenta.
polyhydramnios	*poly-* excessive, many *hydr/o* water, fluid *-amnios* amnion	Condition of excessive amniotic fluid. The most common cause of the disorder is gestational diabetes.
twin-to-twin transfusion syndrome (TTTS)		Complication of blood supply with one twin receiving a deficient amount (the donor) and other receiving too much (the recipient).

Terms Related to Complications of Labor and Delivery (O60 -O77)

Term	Word Origin	Definition
dystocia	*dys-* abnormal, difficult *-tocia* delivery	Abnormal or difficult childbirth. Meconium staining (fetal defecation in utero) indicates fetal distress that may accompany dystocia.
nuchal cord	*nuch/o* neck *-al* pertaining to	Abnormal but common occurrence of the umbilical cord wrapped around the neck of the neonate.

Terms Related to Complication Predominantly Related to the Puerperium(O85-O92)

Term	Word Origin	Definition
agalactia	*a-* without *galact/o* milk *-ia* condition	Condition of mother's inability to produce milk.
galactorrhea	*galact/o* milk *-rrhea* flow, discharge	Abnormal discharge of milk. May occur in men as well as women.
hypogalactia	*hypo-* deficient, below *galact/o* milk *-ia* condition	Abnormally low production of milk.
puerperal sepsis	*puerper/o* puerperium *-al* pertaining to *sepsis* infection	Infection of female reproductive system after delivery.

Terms Related to Malignant Neoplasms (C58)

Term	Word Origin	Definition
choriocarcinoma	*chori/o* chorion *-carcinoma* cancer of epithelial origin	A malignant tumor arising from the chorionic membrane surrounding the fetus.

 CM Guideline Alert

15k. PUERPERAL SEPSIS
Code **O85,** Puerperal sepsis, should be assigned with a secondary code to identify the causal organism (e.g., for a bacterial infection, assign a code from category **B95-B96,** Bacterial infections in conditions classified elsewhere). A code from category **A40,** Streptococcal sepsis, or **A41,** Other sepsis, should not be used for puerperal sepsis. If applicable, use additional codes to identify severe sepsis **(R65.2-)** and any associated acute organ dysfunction.

Exercise 2: Pathology Related to Pregnancy

Match the terms to their definitions.

_____ 1.   placenta accreta
_____ 2.   oligohydramnios
_____ 3.   hydatidiform mole
_____ 4.   eclampsia
_____ 5.   PUPP
_____ 6.   puerperal sepsis
_____ 7.   hyperemesis gravidarum
_____ 8.   placenta percreta
_____ 9.   chorioamnionitis
_____10.   agalactia
_____11.   nuchal cord
_____12.   cephalopelvic
             disproportion
_____13.   abruptio placentae
_____14.   placenta increta

A. excessive vomiting that begins before the 20th week of pregnancy
B. umbilical cord around the neonate's neck
C. condition of low or missing amniotic fluid
D. common rash of late pregnancy
E. inflammation of the outer and inner membranes surrounding the fetus
F. premature separation of the placenta from the uterine wall
G. abnormal attachment of the placenta to the uterine wall
H. abnormal attachment of the placenta within the uterine wall
I. infection of the female reproductive system after delivery
J. condition in which the infant's head is larger than the mother's pelvic outlet
K. serious form of hypertension secondary to pregnancy
L. abnormal attachment of the placenta through the uterine wall
M. condition of mother's inability to produce milk
N. cystlike growth of a nonviable embryo

Translate the terms.

15. choriocarcinoma_____

16. hypogalactia_____

17. polyhydramnios_____

18. placentitis_____

PROCEDURES

Terms Related to Prenatal Diagnosis

Term	Word Origin	Definition
alpha fetoprotein (AFP) test		Maternal serum (blood) alpha fetoprotein test performed between 14 and 19 weeks of gestation; may indicate a variety of conditions, such as neural tube defects (spina bifida is the most common finding) and multiple gestation.
amniocentesis	*amni/o* amnion *-centesis* surgical puncture	Removal and analysis of a sample of the amniotic fluid with the use of a guided needle through the abdomen of the mother into the amniotic sac to diagnose fetal abnormalities (Fig. 7-11).
chorionic villus sampling (CVS)	*chorion/o* chorion *-ic* pertaining to	Removal of a small piece of the chorionic villi that develop on the surface of the chorion, either transvaginally or through a small incision in the abdomen, to test for chromosomal abnormalities (Fig. 7-12).
contraction stress test (CST)		Test to predict fetal outcome and risk of intrauterine asphyxia by measuring fetal heart rate throughout a minimum of three contractions within a 10-minute period.
cordocentesis	*cord/o* cord *-centesis* surgical puncture	A percutaneous surgical puncture of the fetal umbilical cord to obtain blood for testing.
nonstress test (NST)		The fetus is monitored for a normal, expected acceleration of the fetal heart rate. A reactive nonstress test should be followed by a CST and possible ultrasound studies.

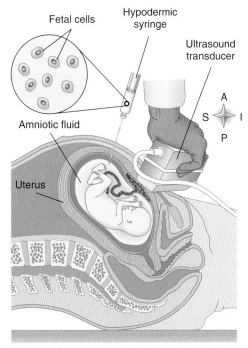

Fig. 7-11 Amniocentesis.

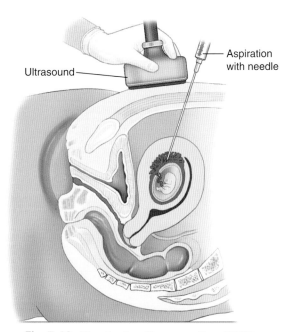

Fig. 7-12 Chorionic villus sampling (CVS).

Terms Related to Prenatal Diagnosis—cont'd

Term	Word Origin	Definition
pelvimetry	*pelv/i* pelvis *-metry* measuring	Measurement of the birth canal. Types of pelvimetry include clinical and x-ray, although x-ray pelvimetry is not commonly done.
pregnancy		Test available in two forms: a standard over-the-counter pregnancy test, which examines urine for the presence of hCG; and a serum (blood) pregnancy test performed in a physician's office or laboratory to get a quantitative hCG. A "triple screen" is a blood test for hCG, AFP, and uE3 (unconjugated estriol).

CPT Coding Alert!

CPT includes a specific code for intrauterine cordocentesis (also called percutaneous umbilical blood sampling or PUBS), an antepartum procedure that tests the cord blood of the fetus while still in utero for abnormalities.

Terms Related to Pregnancy and Delivery Procedures

Term	Word Origin	Definition
cerclage		Suturing the cervix closed to prevent a spontaneous abortion in a woman with an incompetent cervix. The suture is removed when the pregnancy is at full term to allow the delivery to proceed normally (Fig. 7-14).
cesarean section (C-section, CS)		Delivery of an infant through a surgical abdominal incision (Fig. 7-15).
episiotomy	*episi/o* vulva *-tomy* cutting	Incision to widen the vaginal orifice to prevent tearing of the tissue of the vulva during delivery (Fig. 7-16).
external cephalic version (ECV)	*cephal/o* head *-ic* pertaining to *version* turning	Process of turning the fetus so that the head is at the cervical outlet for a vaginal delivery (Fig. 7-13).
vaginal birth after C-section (VBAC)	*vagin/o* vagina *-al* pertaining to	Delivery of subsequent babies vaginally after a C-section. In the past, women were told "once a C-section, always a C-section." Currently, this is being changed by recent developments in technique.
vaginal delivery	*vagin/o* vagina *-al* pertaining to	(Usually) cephalic presentation (head first) through the vagina. Feet or buttock presentation is a breech delivery. Assistance may include instruments, such as forceps or vacuum extraction (Fig. 7-17).

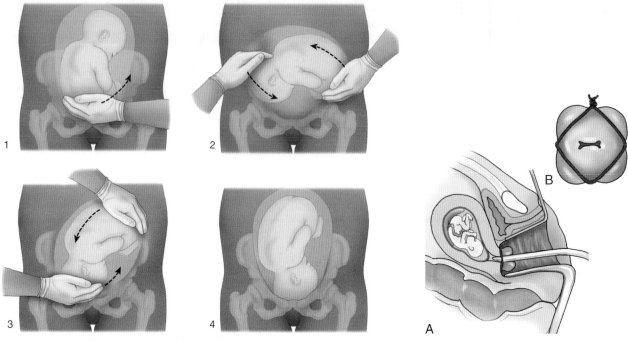

Fig. 7-13 External cephalic version (ECV).

Fig. 7-14 Cerclage.

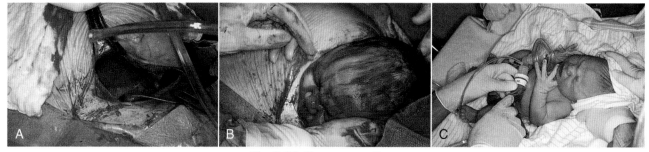

Fig. 7-15 Cesarean section.

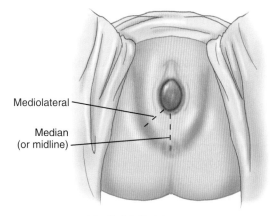

Mediolateral

Median
(or midline)

Fig. 7-16 Episiotomy.

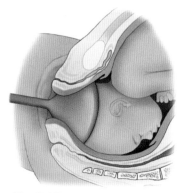

Fig. 7-17 Vacuum extraction.

To see a cesarean section being performed, click on **Animations**.

CPT Coding Alert!

"External cephalic version, with or without tocolysis" is the description of a CPT code to turn the fetus from a breech presentation to a cephalic one, with or without the use of labor-slowing medications.

PCS Guideline Alert

CI Procedures performed on the products of conception are coded to the Obstetrics section. Procedures performed on the pregnant female other than the products of conception are coded to the appropriate root operation in the Medical and Surgical section.

PCS Guideline Alert

C2 Procedures performed following a delivery or abortion for curettage of the endometrium or evacuation of retained products of conception are all coded in the Obstetrics section, to the root operation Extraction and the body part Products of Conception, Retained. Diagnostic or therapeutic dilation and curettage performed during times other than the postpartum or postabortion period are all coded in the Medical and Surgical section, to the root operation Extraction and the body part Endometrium.

Exercise 3: Procedures Related to Prenatal Diagnosis and Pregnancy and Delivery Procedures

Match the terms to their definitions.

_____ 1. cerclage

_____ 2. chorionic villus sampling

_____ 3. external cephalic version

_____ 4. breech delivery

_____ 5. C-section

A. removal of piece of chorionic villi to test for chromosomal abnormalities

B. delivery of an infant through a surgical abdominal incision

C. process of turning the fetus

D. suturing the cervix closed to prevent spontaneous abortion

E. feet or buttock presentation of fetus at birth

Translate the terms.

6. amniocentesis _____

7. episiotomy _____

8. pelvimetry _____

PHARMACOLOGY

Contraceptive Management

abortifacient: Medication that terminates pregnancy. Mifepristone (Mifeprex) and dinoprostone (Prostin E2) may be used as abortifacients.

abstinence: Total avoidance of sexual intercourse as a contraceptive option.

barrier methods: See *diaphragm* and *cervical cap*.

birth control patch: Timed-release contraceptive worn on the skin that delivers hormones transdermally.

cervical cap: Small rubber cup that fits over the cervix to prevent sperm from entering.

contraceptive sponge: Intravaginal barrier with a spermicidal additive.

diaphragm: Soft rubber hemisphere that fits over the cervix, which can be lined with a spermicidal lubricant prior to insertion.

emergency contraception pill (ECP): Medication that can prevent pregnancy after unprotected vaginal intercourse; does not affect existing pregnancies or cause abortions. Plan B (levonorgestrel) is a popular brand-name ECP that is now available without a prescription. Commonly called the "morning-after pill."

female condom: Soft, flexible sheath that fits within the vagina and prevents sperm from entering the vagina.

hormone implant: Timed-release medication placed under the skin of the upper arm, providing long-term protection. The Norplant system is an example.

hormone injection: Contraceptive hormones such as Depo-Provera that may be given every few months to provide reliable pregnancy prevention.

intrauterine device (IUD): Small, flexible device inserted into the uterus that prevents implantation of a zygote.

male condom: Soft, flexible sheath that covers the penis and prevents sperm from entering the vagina. It may also be coated with a spermicide.

oral contraceptive pill (OCP) or birth control pill (BCP): Pill containing estrogen and/or progesterone that is taken daily to fool the body into thinking it is pregnant so that ovulation is suppressed.

procreative and contraceptive management: Term for a variety of medications and techniques that describe the options available for women's reproductive health.

rhythm method: A natural family planning method that involves charting the menstrual cycle to determine fertile and infertile periods.

spermicides: Foam or gel applied as directed prior to intercourse to kill sperm.

vaginal ring: Flexible ring containing contraceptive hormones inserted into the vagina to prevent pregnancy.

---

cervix = cervic/o

intrauterine
intra- = within
uter/o = uterus

spermicide
sperm/o = sperm
-cide = to kill

Exercise 4: Contraceptive Options

Fill in the blanks with the terms provided.

abstinence	**OCP**	**condoms**
rhythm method	**spermicides**	**ECP**
abortifacient	**IUDs**	**barrier methods**

1. A contraceptive oral medication that works by suppressing ovulation is _____

2. Diaphragms and cervical caps are examples of what type of contraceptive method? _____ _____.

3. Soft, flexible sheaths that prevent sperm from entering the vagina are called _____.

4. Small, flexible devices that fit within the uterus to prevent implantation are called _____ _____.

5. A medication intended to terminate a pregnancy is a/an _____.

6. A natural family planning method that has participants chart the woman's menstrual cycle to determine fertile and infertile periods is _____.

7. The only 100% effective contraceptive method is _____.

8. Foams and gels that kill sperm are called _____.

9. An emergency contraceptive measure that prevents pregnancy but does not affect an existing pregnancy is called a/an _____

Fertility Drugs

All of the following fertility drugs support or trigger ovulation and may be referred to as *ovulation stimulants:*

bromocriptine (Parlodel): Oral medication typically used with in vitro fertilization to reduce prolactin levels (which suppresses ovulation).

clomiphene (Clomid, Serophene): Oral medication that stimulates the pituitary gland to produce the hormones that trigger ovulation.

gonadotropin-releasing hormone (GRH) agonist (Lupron): Agent injected or inhaled nasally to prevent premature release of eggs.

human chorionic gonadotropin (hCG) (Pregnyl): Hormone given intramuscularly to trigger ovulation, typically administered with another hormone that will stimulate the release of developed eggs.

human menopausal gonadotropins (hMG or menotropins) (Menopur): Dual gonadotropins that both stimulate the production of egg follicles and cause the eggs to be released once they are developed. These are given by intramuscular or subcutaneous injection.

lutropin alfa (Luveris): A gonadotropin that stimulates the production of egg follicles.

ovulation stimulants: Support or trigger ovulation. Examples include clomiphene (Clomid), human chorionic gonadotropin (Pregnyl) and follicle-stimulating hormone (Bravelle).

urofollitropin (Bravelle): Hormone given subcutaneously that mimics follicle-stimulating hormone (FSH) to directly stimulate the ovaries to produce egg follicles.

Drugs to Manage Delivery

oxytocic: Medication given to induce labor by mimicking the body's natural release of the oxytocin hormone or to manage postpartum uterine hemorrhage. Oxytocin (Pitocin) is the most commonly used agent to induce labor. Another available oxytocic agent is methylergonovine (Methergine).

tocolytic: Medication given to slow down or stop preterm labor by inhibiting uterine contractions. Various drugs such as magnesium sulfate, terbutaline (Brethine), nifedipine (Procardia), or indomethacin (Indocin) may be used for this purpose.

Exercise 5: Fertility and Delivery Drugs

Underline the correct answer in parentheses.

1. Bromocriptine, clomiphene, and hMG all are used to *(increase, decrease)* fertility.

2. Oxytocin is used to *(inhibit, induce)* labor.

3. Medications given to slow down or stop labor are called *(tocolytics, oxytocics).*

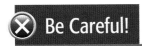 **Be Careful!** *Do not confuse* **oxytocin,** *a labor-inducing drug, with* **oxytocia,** *which means rapid birth.*

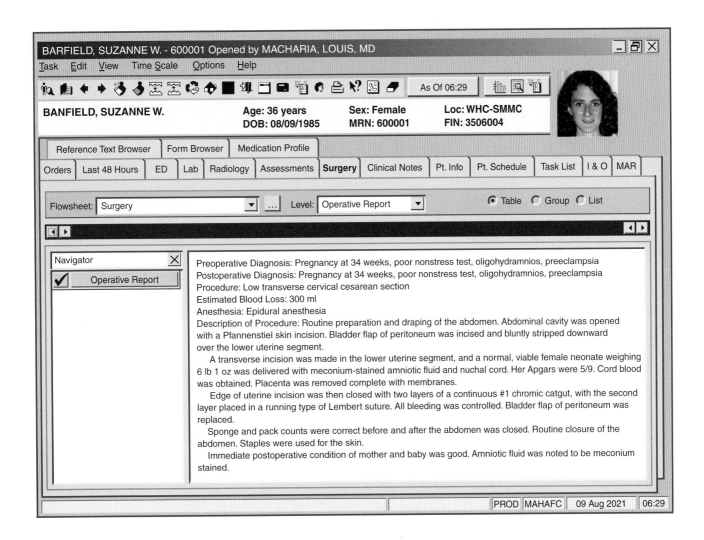

BARFIELD, SUZANNE W. - 600001 Opened by MACHARIA, LOUIS, MD

Task   Edit   View   Time Scale   Options   Help

As Of 06:29

BANFIELD, SUZANNE W.

Age: 36 years   Sex: Female   Loc: WHC-SMMC
DOB: 08/09/1985   MRN: 600001   FIN: 3506004

Reference Text Browser | Form Browser | Medication Profile

Orders | Last 48 Hours | ED | Lab | Radiology | Assessments | **Surgery** | Clinical Notes | Pt. Info | Pt. Schedule | Task List | I & O | MAR

Flowsheet: Surgery   Level: Operative Report   ⦿ Table   ○ Group   ○ List

Navigator   ✕

✓ Operative Report

Preoperative Diagnosis: Pregnancy at 34 weeks, poor nonstress test, oligohydramnios, preeclampsia
Postoperative Diagnosis: Pregnancy at 34 weeks, poor nonstress test, oligohydramnios, preeclampsia
Procedure: Low transverse cervical cesarean section
Estimated Blood Loss: 300 ml
Anesthesia: Epidural anesthesia
Description of Procedure: Routine preparation and draping of the abdomen. Abdominal cavity was opened
with a Pfannenstiel skin incision. Bladder flap of peritoneum was incised and bluntly stripped downward
over the lower uterine segment.
      A transverse incision was made in the lower uterine segment, and a normal, viable female neonate weighing
6 lb 1 oz was delivered with meconium-stained amniotic fluid and nuchal cord. Her Apgars were 5/9. Cord blood
was obtained. Placenta was removed complete with membranes.
      Edge of uterine incision was then closed with two layers of a continuous #1 chromic catgut, with the second
layer placed in a running type of Lembert suture. All bleeding was controlled. Bladder flap of peritoneum was
replaced.
      Sponge and pack counts were correct before and after the abdomen was closed. Routine closure of the
abdomen. Staples were used for the skin.
      Immediate postoperative condition of mother and baby was good. Amniotic fluid was noted to be meconium
stained.

PROD | MAHAFC | 09 Aug 2021 | 06:29

Exercise 6: Operative Report

Using the operative report above, answer the following questions.

1. An infant born at 34 weeks of gestation is born in what trimester?_____

   _____

2. What does the term *oligohydramnios* mean?_____

3. What is a nuchal cord?_____

4. In what direction was the incision made?_____

5. What does the term *preeclampsia* mean?_____

   _____

PERINATAL CONDITIONS

While the "O" codes are designated for the mother, the "P" and "Q" codes are for the baby's chart. Remember: when coding, *you must be sure to separate the codes for the maternal and neonatal charts.* Terminology can help, so be sure to memorize the word parts that indicate one or the other.

 ## CM Guideline Alert

For coding and reporting purposes the perinatal period is defined as before birth through the 28th day following birth. The following guidelines are provided for reporting purposes:

16.a.1 USE OF CHAPTER 16 CODES
Codes in this chapter are <u>never</u> for use on the maternal record. Codes from Chapter 15, the obstetric chapter, are never permitted on the newborn record. Chapter 16 codes may be used throughout the life of the patient if the condition is still present.

 ## CM Guideline Alert

16.a.2 PRINCIPAL DIAGNOSIS FOR BIRTH RECORD
When coding the birth episode in a newborn record, assign a code from category Z38, Liveborn infants according to place of birth and type of delivery, as the principal diagnosis. A code from category Z38 is assigned only once, to a newborn at the time of birth. If a newborn is transferred to another institution, a code from category Z38 should not be used at the receiving hospital. A code from category Z38 is used only on the newborn record, not on the mother's record.

The combining form *nat/o,* meaning "birth" or "born," is often used to describe the time period around the birth of the child. It can be used to describe the newborn infant **(neonate)** or descriptors about the time before, around, or after birth (prenatal/antenatal, perinatal, postnatal).

Terms that are specific to neonates are related to weights (measured in grams) and weeks (referred to as **immaturity).** Birth weight is measured in categories of extremely low birth weight (<500 to 999 grams) and low birth weight (1000 to 2499 grams). Immaturity is categorized as "extreme" (<24 to 27 weeks) and "other" (28 to <37 weeks). At the other end of the spectrum are high weight and long gestation. High-birth-weight neonates are classified as "exceptionally large" newborns (>4500 grams) and "other heavy for gestational age" (4000 to 4499 grams). The term **macrosomia** may be used for neonates over 4000 grams. Long gestation is categorized as late newborn, not heavy for gestational age; post-term is 40 to 42 weeks, and prolonged gestation is >42 weeks.

neonate
  neo- = new
  nat/o = birth

pre- = before

peri- = around, surrounding

post- = after

macrosomia
  macro- = large
  som/o = body
  -ia = condition, state of

CM Guideline Alert

16d. PREMATURITY AND FETAL GROWTH RETARDATION

Providers utilize different criteria in determining prematurity. A code for prematurity should not be assigned unless it is documented. Assignment of codes in categories **P05,** Disorders of newborn related to slow fetal growth and fetal malnutrition, and **P07,** Disorders of newborn related to short gestation and low birth weight, not elsewhere classified, should be based on the recorded birth weight and estimated gestational age. Codes from category **P05** should not be assigned with codes from category **P07.**

When both birth weight and gestational age are available, two codes from category **P07** should be assigned, with the code for birth weight sequenced before the code for gestational age.

16e. LOW BIRTH WEIGHT AND IMMATURITY STATUS

Codes from category **P07,** disorders of newborn related to short gestation and low birth weight, not elsewhere classified, are for use for a child or adult who was premature or had a low birth weight as a newborn, which is affecting the patient's current health status.

 When both birth weight and gestational age of the newborn are available, both should be coded, with birth weight sequenced before gestational age.

Newborn weights are termed "light for gestational age" (LGA) and "small for gestational age" (SGA). Light for gestational age means that the baby has a weight in the lowest 10th percentile, but a length above the 10th percentile. Small for gestational age means that the baby is below the 10th percentile in both weight and length.

Although newborn weights are one indicator of the state of the health of a newborn, the **Apgar score** rates the physical health of the infant with a set of criteria assessed at 1 minute and 5 minutes after birth. The five criteria are conveniently summarized as **A**ppearance, **P**ulse, **G**rimace, **A**ctivity, **R**espiration.

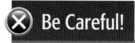 **Be Careful!**   **LGA** *is an abbreviation that has in the past meant "large for gestational age" but which now means "light for gestational age."*

Codes denoting the size and length of gestation (with synonyms in the definition column) are categorized as follows:

Disorders of Newborn Related to Length of Gestation and Fetal Growth (PØ5-PØ8)

Term	Word Origin	Definition
disorders of newborn related to long gestation and high birth weight		Includes exceptionally large newborn baby, late newborn, not heavy for gestational age, post-term newborn, prolonged gestation of newborn
disorders of newborn related to short gestation and low birth weight, not elsewhere classified		Includes low birth weight, extreme immaturity, preterm
disorders of newborn related to slow fetal growth and fetal malnutrition		Newborn light for gestational age Newborn light for dates Newborn small for gestational age Newborn small and light for dates Newborn small for dates

Respiratory and Cardiovascular Disorders Specific to the Perinatal Period (P19-P29) and Infections Specific to the Perinatal Period (P35-P39)

Term	Word Origin	Definition
hyaline membrane syndrome		A respiratory distress syndrome in newborn infants, usually premature infants with insufficient pulmonary surfactants.
neonatal aspiration		Condition in which neonate inhales meconium, amniotic fluid, blood, milk, or regurgitated food.
neonatal hypertension	*hyper-* excessive, above *-tension* process of stretching, pressure	High blood pressure (hypertension) in the newborn.
omphalitis of newborn	*omphal/o* umbilicus *-itis* inflammation	Inflammation of the umbilicus.
ophthalmia neonatorum	*ophthalm/o* eye *-ia* condition	Acute conjunctival inflammation in the newborn, usually caused by *Neisseria gonorrhoeae*. The baby's eyes are contaminated during passage through the birth canal.
transient tachypnea of the newborn (TTN)	*tachy-* fast, rapid *-pnea* breathing	Abnormal increase in respiratory rate in the newborn. It is self-limiting and attributed to the delayed fetal lung fluid clearance. Occurs most often in cesarean section delivery.

Hemorrhagic and Hematological Disorders of Newborn (P50-P61) and Digestive System Disorders of Newborn (P76-P78) and Conditions Involving the Integument and Temperature Regulation of Newborn (P80-P83)

Term	Word Origin	Definition
erythroblastosis fetalis	*erythr/o* red (blood cell) *blast/o* immature *-osis* abnormal condition	Condition in which the mother is Rh negative and her fetus is Rh positive, causing the mother to form antibodies to the Rh-positive factor. Subsequent Rh-positive pregnancies will be in jeopardy because the mother's anti-Rh antibodies will cross the placenta and destroy fetal blood cells (Fig. 7-18). Also called **hemolytic disease of the newborn (HDN).**
hydrops fetalis, NOS		A serious neonatal condition in which there is an inability to manage the accumulation of fluid in two or more areas of the body.
hypothermia of newborn	*hypo-* deficient, below, under, decreased *therm/o* temperature *-ia* condition, state of	A condition of an abnormally low body temperature, usually below 35.5°C (95.9°F)
kernicterus		Neonatal brain damage as the result of extreme jaundice. "Kern" is from a word root for "nucleus," a section of the brain damaged by the icterus (jaundice).
meconium plug syndrome		A delayed passage of meconium (first feces of the newborn), usually due to immaturity of the colon or diabetes in the neonate.

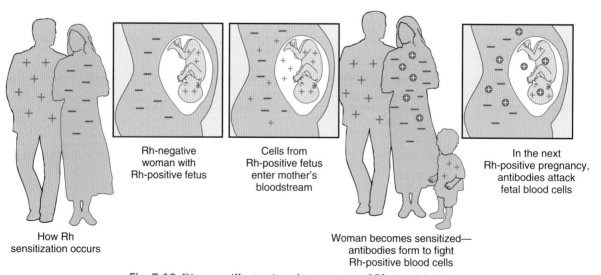

How Rh sensitization occurs

Rh-negative woman with Rh-positive fetus

Cells from Rh-positive fetus enter mother's bloodstream

Woman becomes sensitized— antibodies form to fight Rh-positive blood cells

In the next Rh-positive pregnancy, antibodies attack fetal blood cells

Fig. 7-18 Diagram illustrating the concept of Rh sensitization.

Other Disorders Originating in the Perinatal Period (P90-P96)

Term	Word Origin	Definition
congenital hypotonia	*hypo-* deficient, below, under, decreased *ton/o* tension, tone *-ia* condition, state of	A lack of normal muscle tone in the neonate. Also known as "floppy baby syndrome."
meconium staining		Evidence of release of meconium in the amniotic fluid before birth. Usually a sign of stress to the fetus. This is NOT the same as meconium aspiration.
neonatal craniotabes	*crani/o* skull *-tabes* wasting	A condition of a softening of the skull bones. May be a normal condition unless associated with rickets or osteogenesis imperfecta.

Combining Forms for the Perinatal Period

Meaning	Combining Form
blast/o	immature, embryonic
crani/o	skull, cranium
erythr/o	red
nat/o	birth
omphal/o	umbilicus
som/o	body
spir/o	to breathe, breathing
stom/o	mouth
therm/o	temperature
ton/o	tension, tone

Prefixes for the Perinatal Period

Meaning	Combining Form
a-	no, not, without, lack of
hyper-	excessive, above
hypo-	deficient, below, under, decreased
macro-	large
neo-	new
peri-	around, surrounding
post-	after
pre-	before
tachy-	rapid, fast

Suffixes for the Perinatal Period	
Meaning	**Combining Form**
-ation	process of
-ia	condition, state of
-itis	inflammation
-osis	abnormal condition
-pnea	breathing, to breathe
-tabes	wasting

! CM Guideline Alert

16g. STILLBIRTH
Code P95, Stillbirth, is only for use in institutions that maintain separate records for stillbirths. No other code should be used with P95. Code P95 should not be used on the mother's record.

 ## Exercise 7: Perinatal Conditions

Match the term to the definition.

____ 1. neonate	A. pertaining to after birth
____ 2. prenatal	B. newborn
____ 3. perinatal	C. pertaining to around birth
____ 4. postnatal	D. pertaining to before birth

Build the terms.

5. inflammation of the umbilicus _____

6. abnormal condition of immature red (blood cells) _____ fetalis.

7. condition of large body _____

Exercise 8: Perinatal Conditions

Fill in the blanks using the terms from the list below.

hyaline membrane syndrome   **neonatal hypertension**   **ophthalmia neonatorum**
neonatal craniotabes   **meconium staining**   **kernicterus**
hydrops fetalis   **hypothermia of newborn**   **congenital hypotonia**

1. neonatal brain damage as the result of extreme jaundice _____

2. high blood pressure in the neonate _____

3. respiratory distress syndrome in newborn infants because of insufficient pulmonary surfactants

   _____

4. acute conjunctival inflammation usually caused by *Neisseria gonorrhoeae* _____

5. condition of softening of the skull bones _____

6. inability of neonate to manage accumulation of fluid in two or more areas of the body _____

7. evidence of release of meconium in amniotic fluid before birth _____

8. lack of normal muscle tone in neonate _____

9. condition of abnormally low body temperature _____

CONGENITAL CONDITIONS

As can be gathered from the ICD-10-CM guidelines, congenital conditions are coded not only for conditions that are present at birth, but also for congenital conditions that may be diagnosed or treated throughout the lifetime of the patient. Some of the conditions (hydrocephalus, for example) may be present at birth or may be acquired later in life. Depending on when (or how) it was acquired, the code may appear in different chapters.

 ICD-0-CM Guideline Alert

Assign an appropriate code(s) from categories Q00-Q99, Congenital malformations, deformations, and chromosomal abnormalities when a malformation/deformation or chromosomal abnormality is documented. A malformation/deformation or chromosomal abnormality may be the principal/first-listed diagnosis on a record or a secondary diagnosis.

When a malformation/deformation or chromosomal abnormality does not have a unique code assignment, assign additional code(s) for any manifestations that may be present.

When the code assignment specifically identifies the malformation/deformation or chromosomal abnormality, manifestations that are an inherent component of the anomaly should not be coded separately. Additional codes should be assigned for manifestations that are not an inherent component.

Codes from Chapter 17 may be used throughout the life of the patient. If a congenital malformation or deformity has been corrected, a personal history code should be used to identify the history of the malformation or deformity. Although present at birth, malformation/deformation or chromosomal abnormality may not be identified until later in life. Whenever the condition is diagnosed by the physician, it is appropriate to assign a code from codes Q00-Q99. For the birth admission, the appropriate code from category Z38, Liveborn infants, according to place of birth and type of delivery, should be sequenced as the principal diagnosis, followed by any congenital anomaly codes, Q00-Q99.

Terms Related to Congenital Malformations, Deformations, and Chromosomal Abnormalities (Q00-Q99)

Musculoskeletal System		
Term	**Word Origin**	**Definition**
achondroplasia	*a-* no, not, without *chondr/o* cartilage *-plasia* condition of formation	Disorder of the development of cartilage at the epiphyses of the long bones and skull, resulting in dwarfism.
polydactyly	*poly-* many, much *dactyl/o* fingers, toes *-y* process of	Condition of more than five fingers or toes on each hand or foot (Fig. 7-19).
spina bifida occulta	*spin/o* spine *bi-* two *-fida* to split *occulta* hidden	Congenital malformation of the bony spinal canal without involvement of the spinal cord.
syndactyly	*syn-* joined, together *dactyl/o* fingers, toes *-y* process of	Condition of the joining of the fingers or toes, giving them a webbed appearance (Fig. 7-20).
talipes		Deformity resulting in an abnormal twisting of the foot. Also called **clubfoot** (Fig. 7-21). May also be acquired.
torticollis		Prolonged congenital or acquired condition that manifests itself as a contraction of the muscles of the neck. Also called **wryneck**.

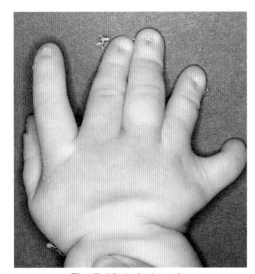

Fig. 7-19 Polydactyly.

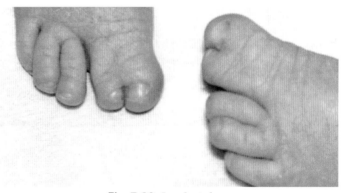

Fig. 7-20 Syndactyly.

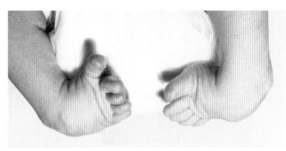

Fig. 7-21 Talipes.

Digestive System		
Term	**Word Origin**	**Definition**
ankyloglossia	*ankyl/o* stiffening *gloss/o* tongue *-ia* condition	An inability to move the tongue freely as a result of a congenital shortened frenulum. Also referred to as being "tongue-tied."
cleft palate		Failure of the palate to close during embryonic development, creating an opening in the roof of the mouth. Cleft palate often is accompanied by a cleft lip (Fig. 7-22). Corrected with **palatoplasty**, the surgical repair of the palate.
esophageal atresia	*esophag/o* esophagus *-eal* pertaining to *a-* no, not, without *-tresia* condition of an opening	Esophagus that ends in a blind pouch and therefore lacks an opening into the stomach (Fig. 7-23). May be corrected with an esophagogastrostomy.
gastroschisis	*gastr/o* stomach *-schisis* split	A congenital opening in the anterior abdominal wall.
Hirschsprung's disease		Congenital absence of normal nervous function in part of the colon, which results in an absence of peristaltic movement, accumulation of feces, and an enlarged colon. Also called **congenital megacolon**.
macrostomia	*macro-* large *stom/o* a mouth, an opening *-ia* condition, state of	A congenital condition of an abnormally large (wide) mouth that results in either unilateral or bilateral facial cleft(s).
omphalocele	*omphal/o* umbilicus *-cele* herniation, protrusion	A congenital herniation at the umbilicus. Also called **exomphalos**.
pyloric stenosis	*pylor/o* pylorus *-ic* pertaining to *stenosis* narrowing	Condition in which the muscle between the stomach and the small intestine narrows or fails to open adequately to allow partially digested food into the duodenum. Corrected by a **pyloromyotomy**, an incision of the pyloric sphincter.

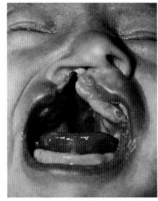

Fig. 7-22 Cleft palate and cleft lip.

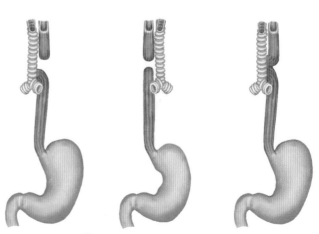

Fig. 7-23 Esophageal atresia.

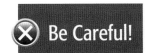 **Be Careful!** *Do not confuse **macrostomia** (a congenital malformation of an abnormally wide mouth) with **macrosomia** (an abnormally large birth weight).*

Male Reproductive System		
Term	Word Origin	Definition
anorchism	*an-* no, not, without *orch/o* testis *-ism* condition	Condition of being born without a testicle. May also be an acquired condition due to trauma or disease. Also termed **monorchism**.
chordee, congenital	*chord/o* cord	Congenital defect resulting in a downward (ventral) curvature of the penis due to a fibrous band (cord) of tissue along the corpus spongiosum. Often associated with hypospadias (Fig. 7-24).
cryptorchidism	*crypt-* hidden *orchid/o* testis *-ism* condition	Condition in which the testicles fail to descend into the scrotum before birth. Also called **cryptorchidism** (Fig. 7-25). Corrected by **orchiopexy**, surgical procedure to mobilize an undescended testicle, attaching it to the scrotum.
epispadias	*epi-* above *-spadias* a rent or tear	Urethral opening on the dorsum (top) of the penis rather than on the tip. Also called **hyperspadias**. Corrected by **balanoplasty**, the surgical repair of the glans penis.
hypospadias	*hypo-* below *-spadias* a rent or tear	Urethral opening on the ventral surface (underside) of the penis instead of on the tip (Fig. 7-26). May be acquired as a result of a disease process. Corrected by **balanoplasty**, the surgical repair of the glans penis.

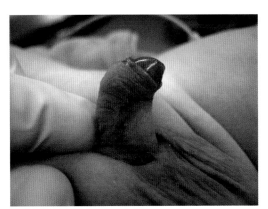

Fig. 7-24 Chordee.

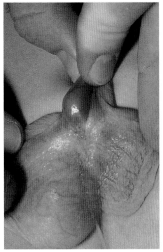

Fig. 7-25 Cryptorchidism in left testicle of a neonate.

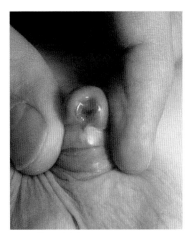

Fig. 7-26 Hypospadias.

Circulatory System		
Term	**Word Origin**	**Definition**
coarctation of the aorta		Congenital cardiac anomaly characterized by a localized narrowing of the aorta. Coarctation is another term for a narrowing (Fig. 7-27).
dextrocardia	*dextr/o* right *-cardia* heart condition	Congenital condition in which the heart is located in the right (instead of left) side of the thoracic cavity.
levocardia	*levo-* left *-cardia* heart condition	Condition whereby the heart is in the normal left side of the thoracic cavity, but the remaining organs are transposed to the side opposite to their normal position.
patent ductus arteriosus (PDA)		Abnormal opening between the pulmonary artery and the aorta caused by failure of the fetal ductus arteriosus to close after birth, most often in premature infants. *Patent* means "open." *Occluded* means "closed." Because the ductus arteriosus is also referred to as *Botallo's duct,* a synonym is **patent ductus Botallo.**
septal defect	*sept/o* septum, wall *-al* pertaining to	Any abnormality of the walls between the heart chambers. **Atrial septal defect (ASD)** is an abnormal opening in the wall between the upper chambers of the heart. **Ventricular septal defect (VSD)** is that same abnormal opening in the wall between the lower two chambers of the heart. These defects can be either congenital or acquired (Fig. 7-28).
tetralogy of Fallot	*tetra-* four *-logy* study of	Congenital cardiac anomaly that consists of four defects: pulmonic stenosis; ventricular septal defect; malposition of the aorta, so that it arises from the septal defect or the right ventricle; and right ventricular hypertrophy.

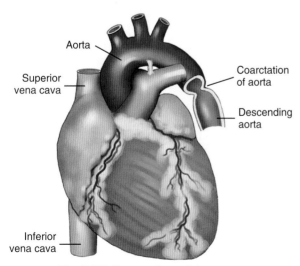

Fig. 7-27 Coarctation of the aorta.

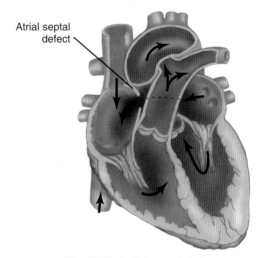

Fig. 7-28 Atrial septal defect.

Respiratory System		
Term	Word Origin	Definition
tracheoesophageal fistula	*trache/o* trachea, windpipe *esophag/o* esophagus *-eal* pertaining to	A congenital abnormal opening between the trachea and the esophagus. Can be acquired.
tracheomalacia	*trache/o* trachea, windpipe *-malacia* softening	Congenital softening of the tissues of the trachea. Can also result from chronic ventilator use.
tracheostenosis	*trache/o* trachea, windpipe *-stenosis* narrowing	Congenital narrowing of the windpipe. Can be acquired.

Nervous System		
Term	Word Origin	Definition
anencephaly	*an-* no, not, without *encephal/o* brain *-y* condition, process of	A congenital lack of formation of major portions of the brain. Along with microcephaly, anencephaly can also be caused by the Zika virus.
craniorachischisis	*crani/o* skull, cranium *rach/i* vertebra *-schisis* split	A failure of the skull and vertebral column to fuse during fetal development.
hydrocephalus	*hydr/o* water *-cephalus* head	Condition of abnormal accumulation of fluid in the ventricles of the brain; may or may not result in intellectual disabilities. Although usually diagnosed in babies, may also occur in adults as a result of stroke, trauma, or infection (Fig. 7-29). Treatment includes **ventriculocisternostomy, ventriculoperitoneostomy** and/or **endoscopic ventriculostomy** (see Ch 11 for more information).
microcephaly	*micro-* small *cephal/o* head *-y* condition, process of	Abnormal smallness of the brain. Can be caused by the Zika virus.
spina bifida	*spin/o* spine *bi-* two *-fida* split	Condition in which the spinal column has an abnormal opening that allows protrusion of the meninges and/or the spinal cord. This saclike protrusion is termed a **meningocele** or **meningomyelocele** (Fig. 7-30).

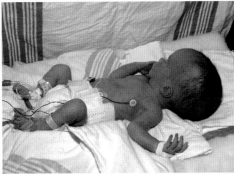

Fig. 7-29 Hydrocephalus.

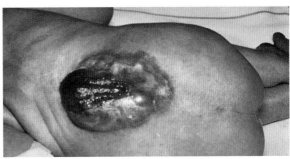

Fig. 7-30 Meningomyelocele.

The Ear		
Term	**Word Origin**	**Definition**
macrotia	*macro-* large *ot/o* ear *-ia* condition	A condition of abnormally large auricles. Can be corrected by performing **otoplasty.**
microtia	*micro-* small, tiny *ot/o* ear *-ia* condition	A condition of abnormally small auricles.

Exercise 9: **Congenital Disorders of the Musculoskeletal, Digestive, and Male Reproductive Systems**

Match the congenital disorder with its description.

___ 1. torticollis
___ 2. talipes
___ 3. spina bifida occulta
___ 4. cleft palate
___ 5. Hirschsprung's disease
___ 6. esophageal atresia
___ 7. pyloric stenosis
___ 8. chordee

A. clubfoot
B. congenital defect resulting in a ventral curvature of the penis
C. malformation of the bony spinal canal without involvement of the spinal cord
D. narrowing of the muscle between the stomach and small intestine
E. congenital megacolon; lack of peristaltic movement in the colon
F. wryneck
G. esophagus ending in a blind pouch
H. congenital opening in the roof of the mouth

Build the terms.

9. process of joined fingers/toes _____

10. condition of formation without cartilage _____

11. process of many fingers/toes _____

Translate the terms.

12. gastroschisis _____

13. omphalocele _____

14. ankyloglossia _____

Build the terms.

15. condition of hidden testis _____

16. condition of no testis _____

17. condition of a rent or tear above _____

18. condition of a rent or tear below _____

Exercise 10: Congenital Conditions of the Circulatory, Respiratory, and Nervous Systems and the Ear

Match the congenital disorders with their definitions.

___ 1. patent ductus arteriosus

___ 2. septal defect

___ 3. coarctation of the aorta

___ 4. tetralogy of Fallot

___ 5. tracheoesophageal fistula

___ 6. spina bifida

A. cardiac anomaly consisting of four defects

B. abnormal opening between the pulmonary artery and the aorta

C. hole in the wall between the upper or lower chambers of the heart

D. narrowing of the largest artery of the body

E. an abnormal opening between the trachea and esophagus

F. An abnormal opening of the spinal column that allows protrusion of the meninges and/or spinal cord

Translate the terms.

7. levocardia _____

8. dextrocardia _____

9. tracheomalacia _____

10. craniorachischisis _____

11. anencephaly _____

Build the terms.

12. narrowing of the windpipe _____

13. water in the head _____

14. condition of large ear _____

15. condition of small ear _____

 CPT Coding Alert!

Corrections of congenital anomalies are not always listed as a "congenital repair." For example, repair of hypospadias is listed with several code options for repair of penis. Fetal Doppler electrocardiograms, however, do have a listing in the index for cardiac anomalies.

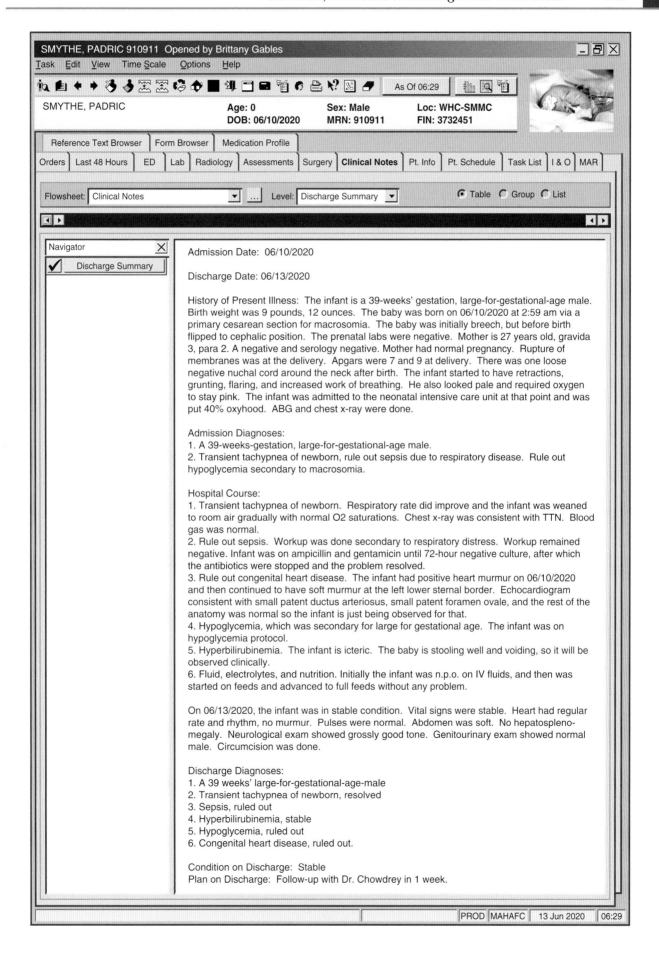

SMYTHE, PADRIC 910911 Opened by Brittany Gables

Task   Edit   View   Time Scale   Options   Help

SMYTHE, PADRIC

Age: 0
DOB: 06/10/2020

Sex: Male
MRN: 910911

Loc: WHC-SMMC
FIN: 3732451

Reference Text Browser | Form Browser | Medication Profile

Orders | Last 48 Hours | ED | Lab | Radiology | Assessments | Surgery | **Clinical Notes** | Pt. Info | Pt. Schedule | Task List | I & O | MAR

Flowsheet: Clinical Notes   Level: Discharge Summary   ○ Table ○ Group ○ List

Navigator
✓ Discharge Summary

Admission Date: 06/10/2020

Discharge Date: 06/13/2020

History of Present Illness: The infant is a 39-weeks' gestation, large-for-gestational-age male.
Birth weight was 9 pounds, 12 ounces. The baby was born on 06/10/2020 at 2:59 am via a
primary cesarean section for macrosomia. The baby was initially breech, but before birth
flipped to cephalic position. The prenatal labs were negative. Mother is 27 years old, gravida
3, para 2. A negative and serology negative. Mother had normal pregnancy. Rupture of
membranes was at the delivery. Apgars were 7 and 9 at delivery. There was one loose
negative nuchal cord around the neck after birth. The infant started to have retractions,
grunting, flaring, and increased work of breathing. He also looked pale and required oxygen
to stay pink. The infant was admitted to the neonatal intensive care unit at that point and was
put 40% oxyhood. ABG and chest x-ray were done.

Admission Diagnoses:
1. A 39-weeks-gestation, large-for-gestational-age male.
2. Transient tachypnea of newborn, rule out sepsis due to respiratory disease. Rule out
hypoglycemia secondary to macrosomia.

Hospital Course:
1. Transient tachypnea of newborn. Respiratory rate did improve and the infant was weaned
to room air gradually with normal O2 saturations. Chest x-ray was consistent with TTN. Blood
gas was normal.
2. Rule out sepsis. Workup was done secondary to respiratory distress. Workup remained
negative. Infant was on ampicillin and gentamicin until 72-hour negative culture, after which
the antibiotics were stopped and the problem resolved.
3. Rule out congenital heart disease. The infant had positive heart murmur on 06/10/2020
and then continued to have soft murmur at the left lower sternal border. Echocardiogram
consistent with small patent ductus arteriosus, small patent foramen ovale, and the rest of the
anatomy was normal so the infant is just being observed for that.
4. Hypoglycemia, which was secondary for large for gestational age. The infant was on
hypoglycemia protocol.
5. Hyperbilirubinemia. The infant is icteric. The baby is stooling well and voiding, so it will be
observed clinically.
6. Fluid, electrolytes, and nutrition. Initially the infant was n.p.o. on IV fluids, and then was
started on feeds and advanced to full feeds without any problem.

On 06/13/2020, the infant was in stable condition. Vital signs were stable. Heart had regular
rate and rhythm, no murmur. Pulses were normal. Abdomen was soft. No hepatosplenomegaly. Neurological exam showed grossly good tone. Genitourinary exam showed normal
male. Circumcision was done.

Discharge Diagnoses:
1. A 39 weeks' large-for-gestational-age-male
2. Transient tachypnea of newborn, resolved
3. Sepsis, ruled out
4. Hyperbilirubinemia, stable
5. Hypoglycemia, ruled out
6. Congenital heart disease, ruled out.

Condition on Discharge: Stable
Plan on Discharge: Follow-up with Dr. Chowdrey in 1 week.

PROD | MAHAFC | 13 Jun 2020 | 06:29

Exercise 11: **Discharge Record**

1. What does LGA mean? _____

2. The respiratory diagnosis means that the infant had a temporary condition

   of_____rapid breathing.

3. Which two congenital heart defects were named? _____

4. The term icteric means that the infant exhibited what? _____

5. Macrosomia is a synonym for which term? _____

6. What does TTN stand for? _____

RECOGNIZING SUFFIXES FOR PCS

Take a quick look at a summary of the suffixes used in the procedures covered for this chapter. Two of them are root operations in the medical/surgical section *(-centesis* and *-tomy),* whereas one is from the remaining categories in the PCS *(-metry).* Learning to associate suffixes with their possible root operations and categories will help you locate your codes much more quickly.

Suffixes and Root Operations for Obstetric, Perinatal and Congenital Conditions

Suffix	Root Operation(s) and Categories
-centesis	Drainage (products of conception)
-metry	Measurement
-pexy	Repair, reposition
-plasty	Repair, replacement, supplement
-stomy	Bypass
-tomy	Division
-version, version	Reposition

Abbreviations

Abbreviation	Definition	Abbreviation	Definition
AFP	alpha fetoprotein test	NST	nonstress test
ASD	atrial septic defect	PUPP	pruritic urticarial papules and plaques
CS	cesarean section		
CST	contraction stress test	Rh	Rhesus factor
CVS	chorionic villus sampling	SGA	small for gestational age
EDD	estimated date of delivery	TTN	transient tachypnea of the newborn
ECV	external cephalic version		
hCG	human chorionic gonadotropin	TTTS	twin-to-twin transfusion syndrome
HELLP	hemolytic elevated liver enzymes low platelet (count)	uE3	unconjugated estriol
		VBAC	vaginal birth after C-section
LGA	light for gestational age	VSD	ventricular septic defect
LMP	last menstrual period		

Go to the Evolve website to interactively study word parts, build terms, label images, and use medical terms in context.

Match the word parts to their definitions.

WORD PART DEFINITIONS: PREGNANCY AND THE PERINATAL PERIOD

Prefix/Suffix		Definition
-amnios	1. _____	first
ante-	2. _____	new
-gravida	3. _____	delivery
-metry	4. _____	measuring
multi-	5. _____	many
neo-	6. _____	none
nulli-	7. _____	around, surrounding
-para	8. _____	flow, discharge
peri-	9. _____	delivery
post-	10. _____	before
primi-	11. _____	amnion
-rrhea	12. _____	after
-tocia	13. _____	pregnancy

Combining Form		Definition
amni/o	14. _____	embryonic, immature
blast/o	15. _____	pregnancy
cephal/o	16. _____	milk
chori/o	17. _____	to grow
cret/o	18. _____	birth
episi/o	19. _____	head
galact/o	20. _____	itching
gravid/o	21. _____	inner fetal sac
hydatid/i	22. _____	vulva
hydr/o	23. _____	development, nourishment
nat/o	24. _____	water drop
olig/o	25. _____	scanty
omphal/o	26. _____	delivery
part/o	27. _____	outer fetal sac
pelv/i	28. _____	pelvis
placent/o	29. _____	umbilicus
prurit/o	30. _____	placenta
troph/o	31. _____	water, fluid

WORDSHOP: PREGNANCY AND THE PERINATAL PERIOD

Prefixes	Combining Forms	Suffixes
a-	amni/o	-al
di-	amnion/o	-amnios
dys-	blast/o	-blast
ec-	cephal/o	-clast
mono-	chori/o	-cyst
multi-	chorion/o	-gravida
nulli-	episi/o	-ia
poly-	galact/o	-ic
post-	hydr/o	-itis
primi-	nat/o	-para
	olig/o	-tic
	pelv/i	-tocia
	top/o	-tomy
	troph/o	

Build pregnancy and perinatal terms by combining the word parts above. Some word parts may be used more than once. Some may not be used at all. The number in parentheses indicates the number of word parts needed.

Definition	Term
1. embryonic development (2)	
2. pertaining to two amnions (3)	
3. pertaining to out of place (3)	
4. no pregnancy (2)	
5. pertaining to after birth (3)	
6. first delivery (2)	
7. pertaining to head and pelvis (3)	
8. inflammation of the chorion and amnion (3)	
9. scanty amnion water (3)	
10. excessive amnion water, fluid (3)	
11. abnormal, difficult childbirth (2)	
12. condition of without milk (3)	
13. cutting the vulva (2)	
14. embryonic sac (2)	
15. pertaining to one chorion (3)	

Sort the terms below into the correct categories.

TERM SORTING: PREGNANCY AND THE PERINATAL PERIOD

Anatomy and Physiology	Pathology	Procedures

abruptio placentae	dystocia	oligohydramnios
AFP	EDD	parturition
allantois	embryo	pelvimetry
amniocentesis	episiotomy	placenta accreta
amnion	erythroblastosis fetalis	placenta
blastocyst	gestation	placentitis
cephalic version	gravida	preeclampsia
cerclage	hCG	puerperium
chorioamnionitis	HELLP syndrome	PUPP
choriocarcinoma	hydatidiform mole	TTTS
chorion	hyperemesis gravidarum	VBAC
C-section	hypogalactia	zygote
CST	LMP	
CVS	morula	

Replace the highlighted words with the correct terms.

TRANSLATIONS: PREGNANCY AND THE PERINATAL PERIOD

1. The patient underwent **measurement of the birth canal** to diagnose **a condition in which the infant's head is larger than the pelvic outlet**.

   _____

2. Anna Walker's obstetrician scheduled her for **a removal and analysis of a sample of amniotic fluid**.

   _____

3. The **newborn** was born with **an umbilical cord around his neck**.

   _____

4. Olivia suffered from **excessive vomiting in pregnancy** in the first trimester and **inflammation of veins during pregnancy** in the third trimester.

   _____

5. After discerning that the baby was in a **buttocks-first position**, Dr. Trivinsky performed a **process of turning the fetus so the head is at the cervical outlet**.

   _____

6. After her third **implantation of the embryo in any location but the uterus**, the patient requested a tubal ligation.

   _____

7. The 42-year-old **woman who was pregnant for the first time** had to undergo **suturing of the cervix closed due to an incompetent cervix**.

   _____

8. Because the patient was experiencing **premature separation of the placenta from the uterine wall**, she had to undergo a **delivery of an infant through a surgical abdominal incision**.

   _____

9. Mrs. Wallen's obstetrician told her that her twins were suffering from **complication of blood supply with one twin receiving a deficient amount of blood and the other receiving too much**.

   _____

10. To prevent tearing during delivery, Wendy underwent an **incision to widen the vaginal orifice**.

    _____

11. After her baby was born, Ms. Yarborough experienced **abnormally low production of milk**.

    _____

12. After **a difficult childbirth**, Maria contracted **infection of female reproductive system after delivery**.

WORD PART DEFINITIONS: CONGENITAL CONDITIONS

Prefix/Suffix	Definition
a-, an-	1. _____ small
-cardia	2. _____ many, much
-cele	3. _____ herniation
crypt-	4. _____ four
epi-	5. _____ together
hypo-	6. _____ heart condition
levo-	7. _____ softening
macro-	8. _____ hidden
-malacia	9. _____ no, not, without
micro-	10. _____ split
poly-	11. _____ abnormal condition of narrowing
-schisis	12. _____ rent or tear
-spadias	13. _____ above
-stenosis	14. _____ large
syn-	15. _____ left
tetra-	16. _____ deficient, under

Combining Form	Definition
ankyl/o	17. _____ skull
cephal/o	18. _____ stiffening
chondr/o	19. _____ right
crani/o	20. _____ windpipe
dactyl/o	21. _____ ear
dextr/o	22. _____ stomach
encephal/o	23. _____ cartilage
gastr/o	24. _____ head
omphal/o	25. _____ umbilicus
orch/o	26. _____ brain
ot/o	27. _____ testis
trache/o	28. _____ finger or toe

WORDSHOP: CONGENITAL CONDITIONS

Prefixes	Combining Forms	Suffixes
a-	amni/o	-al
an-	amnion/o	-amnios
crypt-	ankyl/o	-blast
di-	blast/o	-cardia
dys-	cephal/o	-cele
ec-	chondr/o	-clast
epi-	dactyl/o	-ia
levo-	encephal/o	-ism
macro-	gastr/o	-malacia
poly-	gloss/o	-plasia
	omphal/o	-schisis
	orch/o	-spadias
	ot/o	-stenosis
	trache/o	-us
		-y

Build congenital condition terms by combining the word parts above. Some word parts may be used more than once. Some may not be used at all. The number in parentheses indicates the number of word parts needed.

Definition	Term
1. condition of left heart (2)	
2. softening of the windpipe (2)	
3. condition of large ear (3)	
4. split of the stomach (2)	
5. herniation of the umbilicus (2)	
6. condition of without brain (3)	
7. condition of many fingers or toes (3)	
8. condition of lack of development of cartilage (3)	
9. condition of stiffening tongue (3)	
10. condition of water in head (3)	
11. condition of narrowed windpipe (2)	
12. condition of no testis (3)	
13. condition of hidden testis (3)	
14. condition of rent below (2)	
15. condition of right heart (2)	

Sort the terms below into the correct categories.

TERM SORTING: CONGENITAL CONDITIONS

Digestive	Circulatory	Musculoskeletal	Male Repro

achondroplasia

ankyloglossia

anarchism

chordee

coarctation of the aorta

cryptorchidism

dextrocardia

epispadias

esophageal atresia

gastroschisis

Hirschsprung's disease

hypospadias

levocardia

omphalocele

PDA

polydactyly

pyloric stenosis

septal defect

spina bifida occulta

syndactyly

talipes

tetralogy of Fallot

torticollis

Replace the highlighted words with the correct terms.

TRANSLATIONS: CONGENITAL CONDITIONS

1. The baby was born with **condition of more than five fingers on her hand** and **condition of the joining of the toes**.

2. Enrique was diagnosed with **congenital malformation of the spinal canal without spinal cord involvement**.

3. The infant was born with **failure of the palate to close during embryonic development**, which was corrected with **surgical repair of the palate**.

4. Hunter underwent a/an **suspension of a testicle** to correct his **condition in which a testicle fails to descend into the scrotum before birth**.

5. Monique LaPlante was born with **abnormal opening between the pulmonary artery and the aorta**.

6. The child's **congenital cardiac anomaly that consists of four defects** was discovered using echocardiography.

7. The baby's **condition in which there is an abnormal opening in the spinal column** resulted in a **saclike protrusion of the meninges**.

8. Bhani was born with **abnormally large auricles**, which was corrected with **surgical repair of the ears**.

9. Henri was born with **a condition in which the muscle between the stomach and the small intestine narrows or fails to open adequately**. It was corrected by **incision of the pyloric sphincter**.

10. Baby Phillip was born with **a urethral opening on the ventral surface of the penis**, which was corrected by **the surgical repair of the glans penis**.

11. Sonia's mother was devastated to hear her baby was born with **condition of abnormal accumulation of fluid in the ventricles of the brain**. The baby was treated by **making a new opening in a ventricle and peritoneum**.

Blood, Blood-Forming Organs, and the Immune Mechanism

ICD-10-CM Examples from Tabular

D72.82 Elevated white blood cell count

Excludes1 eosinophilia (D72.1)

D72.820 Lymphocytosis (symptomatic)

Elevated lymphocytes

D72.821 Monocytosis (symptomatic)

Excludes1 infectious mononucleosis (B27.-)

D72.822 Plasmacytosis

D72.823 Leukemoid reaction

Basophilic leukemoid reaction

Leukemoid reaction NOS

Lymphocytic leukemoid reaction

Monocytic leukemoid reaction

Myelocytic leukemoid reaction

Neutrophilic leukemoid reaction

D72.824 Basophilia

D72.825 Bandemia

Bandemia without diagnosis of specific infection

Excludes1 confirmed infection—code to infection

leukemia (C91.-, C92.-, C93.-, C94.-, C95.-)

D72.828 Other elevated white blood cell count

D72.829 Elevated white blood cell count, unspecified

Elevated leukocytes, unspecified

Leukocytosis, unspecified

D72.89 Other specified disorders of white blood cells

Abnormality of white blood cells NEC

ICD-10-PCS Example from Index

Pheresis

Erythrocytes **6A55**

Leukocytes **6A55**

Plasma **6A55**

Platelets **6A55**

Stem cells

Cord blood **6A55**

Hematopoietic **6A55**

CHAPTER OUTLINE

FUNCTIONS OF THE BLOOD AND IMMUNE SYSTEMS

ANATOMY AND PHYSIOLOGY

HEMATIC SYSTEM

IMMUNE SYSTEM

PATHOLOGY

PROCEDURES

PHARMACOLOGY

RECOGNIZING SUFFIXES FOR PCS

ABBREVIATIONS

OBJECTIVES

☐ Recognize and use terms related to the anatomy and physiology of the blood and immune systems.

☐ Recognize and use terms related to the pathology of the blood and immune systems.

☐ Recognize and use terms related to the procedures for the blood and immune systems.

FUNCTIONS OF THE BLOOD AND IMMUNE SYSTEMS

Homeostasis, or a "steady state," is a continual balancing act of the body systems to provide an internal environment that is compatible with life. The two liquid tissues of the body, the **blood** and **lymph,** have separate but interrelated functions in maintaining this balance. They combine with a third system, the **immune** system, to protect the body against **pathogens** that could threaten the organism's viability.

The **blood** is responsible for the following:

- Transportation of gases (oxygen [O_2] and carbon dioxide [CO_2]), chemical substances (hormones, nutrients, salts), and cells that defend the body.
- Regulation of the body's fluid and electrolyte balance, acid-base balance, and body temperature.
- Protection of the body from infection.
- Protection of the body from loss of blood by the action of clotting.

The **lymph system** is responsible for the following:

- Cleansing the cellular environment.
- Returning proteins and tissue fluids to the blood (drainage).
- Providing a pathway for the absorption of fats and fat-soluble vitamins into the bloodstream.
- Defending the body against disease.
- The lymphatic system is discussed in Chapter 9 as part of the circulatory system. Explaining its role in protecting the body against disease, however, requires a discussion of how it interacts with the hematic and immune systems.

The **immune system** is responsible for the following:

- Defending the body against disease via the immune response.

Fig. 8-1 is a Venn diagram of the interrelationship among the three systems, with the shared goals of homeostasis and protection at the intersection of the three circles.

ANATOMY AND PHYSIOLOGY

The **hematic** and **lymphatic** systems flow through separate yet interconnected and interdependent channels. Both are systems composed of vessels and the liquids that flow through them. The **immune** system, a very complex set of levels of protection for the body, includes blood and lymph cells.

Fig. 8-2 shows the relationship of the lymphatic vessels to the circulatory system. Note the close relationship between the distribution of the lymphatic vessels and the venous blood vessels. Tissue fluid is drained by the lymphatic capillaries and is transported by a series of larger lymphatic vessels toward the heart.

The organs in the lymphatic system are the spleen, the thymus gland, the tonsils, the appendix, and Peyer's patches. The spleen is located in the upper left quadrant and serves to filter, store, and produce blood cells; remove red blood cells (RBCs); and activate B lymphocytes. The thymus gland is located in the mediastinum and is instrumental in the development of T lymphocytes (T cells). The tonsils are lymphatic tissue (lingual, pharyngeal, and palatine) that helps protect the entrance to the respiratory and digestive systems. The vermiform appendix and Peyer's patches are lymphoid tissue in the intestines, both with protective functions in the digestive system.

The clearest path to understanding the interconnected roles of these three systems is to look at the hematic system first.

---

homeostasis
    home/o = same
    -stasis = controlling, stopping

blood = **hem/o, hemat/o**

lymph = **lymph/o, lymphat/o**

pathogen
    path/o = disease
    -gen = producing

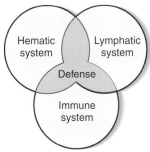

Fig. 8-1 Diagram of interrelationships among the hematic, lymphatic, and immune systems.

safety, protection = **immun/o**

spleen = **splen/o**

thymus gland = **thym/o**

tonsil = **tonsill/o**

appendix = **append/o, appendic/o**

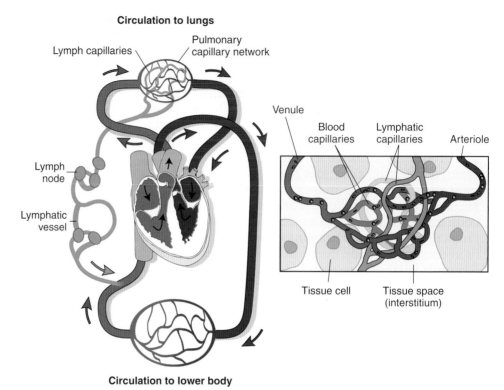

Fig. 8-2 Relationship of the lymphatic vessels to the circulatory system.

This chapter includes all the anatomy necessary to assign ICD-10 blood-forming organs and immune mechanism codes, including detail on agglutinogens, hemosiderin, and polymorphonucleocytes. See Appendix H for a complete list of body parts and how they should be coded.

HEMATIC SYSTEM

The hematic system is composed of blood and the vessels that carry the blood throughout the body. The formation of blood, **hematopoiesis,** begins in the bone marrow with a single type of cell, a multipotential (pluripotent) hematopoietic stem cell (HSC), or **hemocytoblast.** This cell divides into cells that mature in lymphatic tissue (band T lymphocytes) and cells that mature in the bone marrow. Refer to Fig. 8-3 to follow the development from the stem cell to specialized mature blood cells.

Whole blood is composed of a solid portion that consists of formed elements, or cells, and a liquid portion called **plasma.** Blood cells make up 45% of the total blood volume, and plasma makes up the other 55% (Fig. 8-4).

$$(\text{whole}) \text{ blood} = \text{cells } (45\%) + \text{plasma} (55\%)$$

hematopoiesis
   hemat/o = blood
   -poiesis = formation

hemocytoblast
   hem/o = blood
   cyt/o = cell
   -blast = embryonic,
      immature

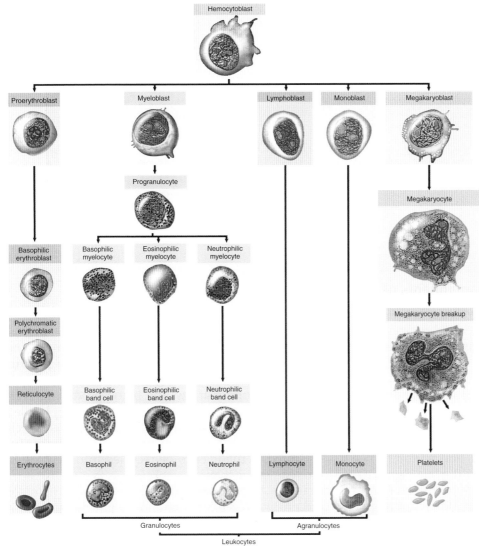

Fig. 8-3 Formation of blood cells. The hematopoietic stem cell serves as the original stem cell from which all formed elements of the blood are derived. Note that all five precursor cells are derived from a stem cell called a *hemocytoblast*.

The solid portion of blood is composed of three different types of cells:
1. **Erythrocytes,** also called red blood cells **(RBCs).**
2. **Leukocytes,** also called white blood cells **(WBCs).**
3. **Thrombocytes,** also called clotting cells, cell fragments, or **platelets (plats).**
    In a milliliter of blood, there are 4.2 million to 5.8 million RBCs, 250,000 to 400,000 platelets, and 5000 to 9000 WBCs. These cells together account for approximately 8% of body volume. Converted to more familiar liquid measure, there are about 10.5 pints (5 liters) of blood in a 150-lb (68-kg) person.

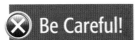 **Be Careful!**   **Hgb, HB, Hb,** *and* **HG** *are all abbreviations for hemoglobin.* **Hg** *is the abbreviation for mercury.*

Click on **Animations** to watch a demonstration of the different types of blood cells.

erythrocyte
    erythr/o = red
    -cyte = cell

leukocyte
    leuk/o = white
    -cyte = cell

thrombocyte
    thromb/o = clotting, clot
    -cyte = cell

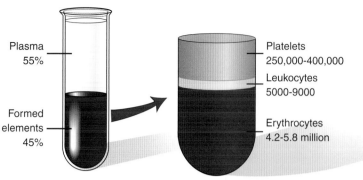

Fig. 8-4 Composition of blood.

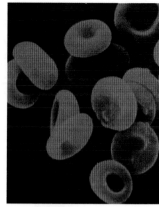

Fig. 8-5 Erythrocytes, or red blood cells.

Components of Blood

Erythrocytes (Red Blood Cells)

The erythrocytes (which are normally present in the millions) have the important function of transporting O_2 and CO_2 throughout the body (Fig. 8-5). The vehicle for this transportation is a protein-iron pigment called **hemoglobin.** When combined with oxygen, it is termed **oxyhemoglobin.**

The formation of RBCs in the red bone marrow, the blood-producing cavities found in many bones, is stimulated by a hormone from the kidneys called **erythropoietin.** RBCs have a life span of approximately 120 days, after which they decompose into **hemosiderin,** an iron pigment resulting from **hemolysis,** and bilirubin. The iron is stored in the liver to be recycled into new RBCs, and the bile pigments are excreted via the liver.

Abnormal RBCs can be named by their **morphology,** the study of shape or form. RBCs normally have a biconcave, disclike shape and are anuclear (without a nucleus). (Although the center is depressed, there is not an actual hole.) Those that are shaped differently often have difficulty in carrying out their function. "Abnormal" can also be used to describe the level of maturity of the cell. As seen in Fig. 8-3, reticulocytes are immature red blood cells. Although the appearance of these is normal in a count of red blood cells, a greater than normal proportion can be an indication of increased bone marrow activity, possibly signaling anemia.

For example, sickle cell anemia is a hereditary condition characterized by erythrocytes (RBCs) that are abnormally shaped. They resemble a crescent or sickle. An abnormal hemoglobin found inside these erythrocytes causes sickle cell anemia in a number of Africans and African Americans.

CPT Coding Alert!

CPT has a variety of codes for counting reticulocytes. A manual count is differentiated from automated counting.

Leukocytes (White Blood Cells)

Although there are fewer leukocytes (thousands, not millions), there are different types with different functions. In general, WBCs protect the body from invasion by pathogens. The different types of cells provide this defense in a number of different ways. There are two main types of WBCs: granulocytes and agranulocytes.

---

hemoglobin
  hem/o = blood
  -globin = protein
    substance

oxyhemoglobin
  oxy- = oxygen
  hem/o = blood
  -globin = protein
    substance

bone marrow = myel/o

erythropoietin
  erythr/o = red
  -poietin = forming
    substance

hemosiderin
  hem/o = blood
  -siderin = iron
    substance

hemolysis
  hem/o = blood
  -lysis = breaking down

morphology
  morph/o = shape, form
  -logy = study of

granulocyte
  granul/o = little grain
  -cyte = cell

polymorphonucleocyte
  poly- = many
  morph/o = shape, form
  nucle/o = nucleus
  -cyte = cell

Granulocytes (Polymorphonucleocytes)

Named for their appearance, **granulocytes,** also called **polymorphonucleocytes** (PMNs, or polys) are white blood cells that have small grains within the cytoplasm and multilobed nuclei. These names are used interchangeably.

There are three types of granulocytes, each with its own function. Each of them is named for the type of dye that it attracts.

1. **Eosinophils** (eosins) are cells that absorb an acidic dye, which causes them to appear reddish. An increase in eosinophils is a response to a need for their function in defending the body against allergens and parasites.

2. **Neutrophils** (neuts), the most numerous WBCs, are cells that do not absorb either an acidic or a basic dye and consequently are a purplish color. They are also called **phagocytes** because they specialize in **phagocytosis** and generally combat bacteria in pyogenic infections. This means that these cells are drawn to the site of a pathogenic "invasion," where they consume the enemy and remove the debris resulting from the battle. Because the nucleus in immature neutrophils has a long "bandlike" shape, these cells are often referred to as **band cells**. They are also called *stabs;* the name is from the German word for *rods* because of their rodlike appearance. As the cells continue to mature, the bands divide, and the adult cells are renamed *segs* because now the nuclei are divided into clumps (*seg*mented).

3. **Basophils** (basos) are cells that absorb a basic (or alkaline) dye and stain a bluish color. Especially effective in combating parasites, they release histamine (a substance that initiates an inflammatory response) and heparin (an **anticoagulant**), both of which are instrumental in healing damaged tissue.

Agranulocytes (Mononuclear Leukocytes)

Agranulocytes are white blood cells named for their lack of granules. The alternative name **mononuclear leukocytes** is so given because the cells have one nucleus. The two names are used interchangeably. Although these cells originate in the bone marrow, they mature after entering the lymphatic system. There are two types of these WBCs:

1. **Monocytes:** These cells, named for their single large nucleus, transform into **macrophages,** which eat pathogens (phagocytosis) and are effective against severe infections.

2. **Lymphocytes** (lymphs): These cells are key in what is called the *immune response,* which involves the "recognition" of dangerous, foreign (viral) substances and the manufacture of their neutralizers. The foreign substances are called **antigens**, and the neutralizers are called **antibodies.**

Granulocytes are also known as **polymorphonucleocytes,** *abbreviated* **PMNs** *or* **polys.** *However, one type of granulocyte, the neutrophil, is also commonly referred to as a* **polymorph (PMN, poly)** *because it has the greatest degree of nuclear polymorphism, in addition to being the most common type of leukocyte.*

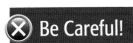 *Don't confuse* **cyt/o,** *meaning* cell, *with* **cyst/o,** *meaning a bladder or a sac.*

---

eosinophil
  eosin/o = rosy-colored
  -phil = attraction

neutrophil
  neutr/o = neutral
  -phil = attraction

phagocyte
  phag/o = eat, swallow
  -cyte = cell

band cell = **band/o**

basophil
  bas/o = base
  -phil = attraction

agranulocyte
  a- = no, not, without
  granul/o = little grain
  -cyte = cell

monocyte
  mono- = one
  -cyte = cell

lymphocyte
  lymph/o = lymph
  -cyte = cell

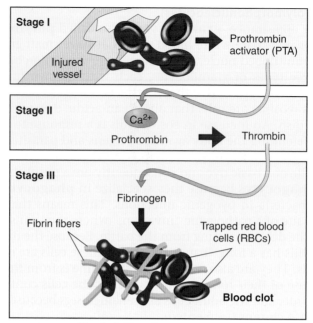

Fig. 8-6 The clotting process.

---

thrombocyte
  thromb/o = clot, clotting
  -cyte = cell

prothrombin
  pro- = before
  -thrombin = clotting
    substance

fibrinogen
  fibrin/o = fibrous
    substance
  -gen = producing

hemostasis
  hem/o = blood
  -stasis = stopping,
    controlling

plasma = **plasm/o**

serum = **ser/o**

Thrombocytes (Platelets)

Platelets (also known as *thrombocytes* or *plats*) have a round or oval shape and are so named because they look like small plates. Platelets aid in **coagulation**, the process of changing a liquid to a solid. When blood cells escape their normal vessels, they **agglutinate**, or clump together, by the following process: First, they release **factor X** (formerly called *thrombokinase*), which, in the presence of calcium, reacts with the blood protein **prothrombin** to form **thrombin.** Thrombin then converts another blood protein, **fibrinogen,** to **fibrin,** which eventually forms a meshlike fibrin clot (blood clot), achieving **hemostasis** (control of blood flow; that is, stopping the bleeding). See Fig. 8-6 for a visual explanation of the clotting process.

⊗ Be Careful! *Don't confuse* **hemostasis,** *meaning* control of blood flow, *with* **homeostasis,** *meaning a* steady state.

Plasma

Plasma, the liquid portion of blood, is composed of the following:
1. Water, or H_2O (90%)
2. Inorganic substances (calcium, potassium, sodium)
3. Organic substances (glucose, amino acids, fats, cholesterol, hormones)
4. Waste products (urea, uric acid, ammonia, creatinine)
5. Plasma proteins (serum albumin, serum globulin, and two clotting proteins: fibrinogen and prothrombin)

Serum *(pl.* sera) is plasma minus the clotting proteins. Serology is the branch of laboratory medicine that studies blood serum for evidence of infection by evaluating antigen-antibody reactions in vitro. In vitro means outside the body, as in a test tube.

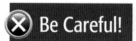

Serum = Plasma − (Prothrombin + Fibriongen)

Exercise 1: **The Hematic System**

A. Match the following combining forms with their meanings.

____ 1. blood   ____ 8. lymph   A. thromb/o   H. immun/o
____ 2. red   ____ 9. shape, form   B. phag/o   I. hem/o, hemat/o
____ 3. same   ____ 10. white   C. leuk/o   J. erythr/o
____ 4. clotting, clot   ____ 11. safety, protection   D. morph/o   K. path/o
____ 5. fibrous substance ____ 12. rosy-colored   E. home/o   L. granul/o
____ 6. disease   ____ 13. eat, swallow   F. lymph/o, lymphat/o M. fibrin/o
____ 7. little grain   ____ 14. bone marrow   G. eosin/o   N. myel/o

B. Match the following suffixes with their meanings.

____ 1. -stasis   ____ 6. -phil   A. cell   F. clotting substance
____ 2. -cyte   ____ 7. -globin   B. attraction   G. protein substance
____ 3. -poiesis   ____ 8. -gen   C. iron substance   H. breaking down
____ 4. -lysis   ____ 9. -siderin   D. producing   I. forming substance
____ 5. -poietin   ____ 10. -thrombin   E. formation   J. controlling, stopping

Translate the terms.

11. polynuclear _____

12. agranulocytic _____

13. lymphatic _____

14. anuclear _____

15. polymorphic _____

Blood Type	Antigen (RBC membrane)	Antibody (plasma)	Can receive blood from	Can donate blood to
A (40%)	A antigen	Anti-B antibodies	A, O	A, AB
B (10%)	B antigen	Anti-A antibodies	B, O	B, AB
AB (4%)	A antigen B antigen	No antibodies	A, B, AB, O	AB
O (46%)	No antigen	Both anti-A and anti-B antibodies	O	O, A, B, AB

Fig. 8-7 ABO blood groups.

Blood Groups

Human blood is divided into four major types: A, B, AB, and O. See Fig. 8-7 for a table of blood types, agglutinogens, and agglutinins. The differences are due to antigens present on the surface of the red blood cells. **Antigens** are substances that produce an immune reaction by their nature of being perceived as foreign to the body. In response, the body produces substances called **antibodies** that nullify or neutralize the antigens. In blood, these antigens are called **agglutinogens** because their presence can cause the blood to clump. The antibody is termed an **agglutinin.** For example, type A blood has A antigen, type B has B antigen, type AB has both A and B antigens, and type O has neither A nor B antigens. If an individual with type A blood is transfused with type B blood, the A antigens will form anti-B antibodies because they perceive B blood as being foreign. Following the logic of each of these antigen-antibody reactions, an individual with type AB blood would be a universal recipient, and an individual with type O blood would be a universal donor. The presence or absence of yet another antigen, the Rh factor, doubles the number of groups from four to eight, however. Individuals with this antigen add a + (positive) to their type (A+, B+, AB+, O+) and those without it add a – (negative) to their type (A–, B–, AB–, O–). Hence, each of the groups is divided into those with and without the Rh antigen. Universal donors are O types without the antigen, or O–. Universal recipients are AB types with the antigen, or AB+.

The **Rh factor,** is important in pregnancy because a mismatch between the fetus and the mother can cause erythroblastosis fetalis, or hemolytic disease of the newborn (HDN) (see Fig. 7-18). In this disorder, a mother with a negative Rh factor will develop antibodies to an Rh+ fetus during the first pregnancy. If another pregnancy occurs with an Rh+ fetus, the antibodies will destroy the fetal blood cells.

antigen
  anti- = against
  -gen = producing

agglutinogen
  agglutin/o = clumping
  -gen = producing

agglutinin
  agglutin/o = clumping
  -in = substance

haemolytic
  hem/o = blood
  -lytic = pertaining to breaking down

Exercise 2: Blood Groups

1. The four blood types are _____

2. Not all blood types are interchangeable because of _____

3. A person with type A blood can donate blood to people with which blood type? _____

4. Type O blood type is the *universal* _____, whereas type AB is the *universal* _____

5. HDN is an example of an antigen-antibody reaction of what blood factor? _____

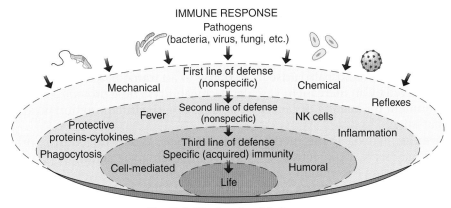

Fig. 8-8 The levels of defense.

IMMUNE SYSTEM

The immune system is composed of organs, tissues, cells, and chemical messengers that interact to protect the body from external invaders and its own internally altered cells. The chemical messengers are **cytokines,** which are secreted by cells of the immune system that direct immune cellular interactions. Lymphocytes (leukocytes that are categorized as either **B cells** or **T cells)** secrete lymphokines. Monocytes and macrophages secrete monokines. **Interleukins** are a type of cytokine that sends messages among leukocytes to direct protective action.

The best way to understand this system is through the body's various levels of defense. The goal of pathogens is to breach these levels to enter the body, reproduce, and, subsequently, exploit healthy tissue, causing harm. The immune system's task is to stop them.

Fig. 8-8 illustrates the levels of defense. The two outside circles represent **nonspecific immunity** and its two levels of defense. The inner circle represents the various mechanisms of **specific immunity,** which can be **natural (genetic)** or **acquired** in four different ways. Most pathogens can be contained by the first two lines of nonspecific defense. However, some pathogens deserve a "special" means of protection, which is discussed in the section titled "Specific Immunity."

Nonspecific Immunity

Nonspecific immunity refers to the various ways that the body protects itself from many types of pathogens, without having to "recognize" them.

1. The *first line of defense* in nonspecific immunity (the outermost layer) consists of the following methods of protection:
   - **Mechanical:** Examples include the skin, which acts as a barrier, and the sticky mucus on mucous membranes, which serves to trap pathogens.
   - **Physical:** Examples include coughing, sneezing, vomiting, and diarrhea. Although not pleasant, these serve to expel pathogens that have gotten past the initial barriers**.**
   - **Chemical:** Examples include tears, saliva, and perspiration. These have a slightly acidic nature that deters pathogens from entering the body while also washing them away. In addition, stomach acids and enzymes kill germs.
2. The *second line of defense* in nonspecific immunity comes into play if the pathogens make it past the first line. Defensive measures include certain processes, proteins, and specialized cells. Defensive processes include the following:
   - **Phagocytosis:** Phagocytosis is the process of cells "eating" and destroying microorganisms. Pathogens that make it past the first line of defense

cytokine
  cyt/o = cell
  -kine = movement

lymphokine
  lymph/o = lymph
  -kine = movement

monokine
  mono- = one
  -kine = movement

interleukin
  inter- = between
  -leukin = white
     substance

phagocytosis
  phag/o = eat, swallow
  cyt/o = cell
  -osis = abnormal
     Condition

and enter into the bloodstream may be consumed by neutrophils and monocytes.

- **Inflammation:** Acquiring its name from its properties, inflammation is a protective response to irritation or injury. The characteristics (heat, swelling, redness, and pain) arise in response to an immediate vasoconstriction, followed by an increase in vascular permeability. These provide a good environment for healing. If caused by a pathogen, the inflammation is called an *infection.*

pyrexia
pyr/o = fever, fire
-exia = condition

- **Pyrexia:** Pyrexia is the medical term for fever. When infection is present, fever may serve a protective function by increasing the action of phagocytes and decreasing the viability of certain pathogens.

The **protective proteins** are part of the second line of defense. These include **interferons,** which get their name from their ability to "interfere" with viral replication and limit a virus's ability to damage the body. The **complement proteins,** a second protein type, exist as inactive forms in blood circulation that become activated in the presence of bacteria, enabling them to lyse (destroy) the organisms.

Finally the last of the "team" in the second line of defense are the **natural killer (NK) cells.** This special kind of lymphocyte acts nonspecifically to kill cells that have been infected by certain viruses and cancer cells.

Specific Immunity

Specific immunity may be either **genetic**—an inherited ability to resist certain diseases because of one's species, race, sex, or individual genetics—or **acquired.** Specific immunity depends on the body's ability to identify a pathogen and prepare a specific response (antibody) to only that invader (antigen). Antibodies are also referred to as **immunoglobulins (Ig).** The acquired form can be further divided into natural and artificial forms, which in turn can each be either active or passive. After the specific immune process is described, each of the four types is discussed.

Specific immunity depends on the agranulocytes (lymphocytes and monocytes) for its function. The monocytes metamorphose into macrophages, which dispose of foreign substances. The lymphocytes differentiate into either T lymphocytes (they mature in the thymus) or B lymphocytes (they mature in the bone marrow or fetal liver). Although both types of lymphocytes take part in specific immunity, they do so in different ways.

humoral
humor/o = liquid
-al = pertaining to

The T cells neutralize their enemies through a process of **cell-mediated immunity.** This means that they attack antigens directly. They are effective against fungi, cancer cells, protozoa, and, unfortunately, organ transplants. B cells use a process of **humoral immunity** (also called **antibody-mediated immunity).** This means that they secrete antibodies to "poison" their enemies, either during the attack (plasma B cells) or in subsequent attacks (memory B cells).

Types of Acquired Immunity
Acquired immunity is categorized as *active* or *passive* and then is further subcategorized as *natural* or *artificial.* All describe ways that the body has acquired antibodies to specific diseases.

Active acquired immunity can take either of the following two forms:
1. Natural: Development of memory cells to protect the individual from a second exposure.
2. Artificial: Vaccination (immunization) that uses a greatly weakened form of the antigen, thus enabling the body to develop antibodies in response to this intentional exposure. Examples are the DTP and MMR vaccines.

Passive acquired immunity can take either of the following two forms:
1. Natural: Passage of antibodies through the placenta or breast milk.
2. Artificial: Use of immunoglobulins harvested from a donor who developed resistance against specific antigens.

Exercise 3: Immune System

1. How do nonspecific and specific immunity differ?

_____

2. Name examples of first-line defenses.

_____

3. Name examples of second-line defenses.

_____

Choose from the following types of acquired immunity to fill in the blanks.

active natural   active artificial   passive natural   passive artificial

4. If a child has an immunization against measles, he/she has what type of immunity? _____

5. If an individual receives maternal antibodies, then this is a type of _____ immunity.

6. If an individual receives a mixture of antibodies from a donor, he/she has received _____ immunity.

7. Acquiring a disease and producing memory cells for that disease is a type of _____ immunity.

Match the following word parts with their meanings.

____ 8. fever, fire	____ 13. liquid	A. humor/o	F. phag/o
____ 9. eat, swallow	____ 14. not	B. pyr/o	G. non-
____ 10. substance	____ 15. movement	C. leuk/o	H. -kine
____ 11. between	____ 16. one	D. -in	I. mono-
____ 12. white	____ 17. cell	E. inter-	J. cyt/o

Combining Forms for the Anatomy and Physiology of Blood and the Immune System

Meaning	Combining Form	Meaning	Combining Form
appendix	append/o, appendic/o	lymph	lymph/o, lymphat/o
base	bas/o	nucleus	nucle/o
blood	hem/o, hemat/o	oxygen	ox/i, ox/o
bone marrow	myel/o	plasma	plasm/a, plasm/o
cell	cyt/o	red	erythr/o
clotting, clot	thromb/o	rosy-colored	eosin/o
clumping	agglutin/o	safety, protection	immun/o
disease	path/o	same	home/o
eat, swallow	phag/o	serum	ser/o
fever, fire	pyr/o	shape	morph/o
fiber	fibr/o	spleen	splen/o
fibrous substance	fibrin/o	thymus	thym/o
liquid	humor/o	tonsil	tonsill/o
little grain	granul/o	white	leuk/o

Prefixes for the Anatomy and Physiology of the Blood and Immune Systems

Prefix	Meaning	Prefix	Meaning
a-	without	oxy-	oxygen
anti-	against	poly-	many
inter-	between	pro-	before
mono-	one		

Suffixes for the Anatomy and Physiology of the Blood and Immune Systems

Suffix	Meaning	Suffix	Meaning
-cyte	cell	-osis	abnormal condition
-exia	condition	-phil	attraction
-gen	producing	-poiesis	formation
-globin	protein substance	-poietin	forming substance
-in	substance	-siderin	iron substance
-kine	movement	-stasis	controlling, stopping
-leukin	white substance	-thrombin	clotting substance
-lysis	breaking down		

PATHOLOGY

Terms Related to Nutritional Anemias (D5Ø-D53)

Term	Word Origin	Definition
B_{12} deficiency anemia		Insufficient blood levels of cobalamin, also called **vitamin B_{12},** which is essential for red blood cell maturation. Condition may be caused by inadequate dietary intake, as in some extreme vegetarian diets, or it may result from absence of intrinsic factor, a substance in the GI system essential to vitamin B_{12} absorption.
folate deficiency anemia		Anemia as a result of a lack of folate from dietary, drug-induced, congenital, or other causes.
pernicious anemia	*an-* no, not, without *-emia* blood condition	Progressive anemia that results from a lack of intrinsic factor essential for the absorption of vitamin B_{12}.
sideropenia	*sider/o* iron *-penia* condition of deficiency	Condition of having reduced numbers of RBCs because of chronic blood loss, inadequate iron intake, or unspecified causes. A type of iron-deficiency anemia.

Terms Related to Hemolytic Anemias (D55-D59)

Term	Word Origin	Definition
autoimmune acquired hemolytic anemia	*auto-* self *immune* safety, protection *hem/o* blood *-lytic* pertaining to destruction *an-* no, not *-emia* blood condition	Anemia caused by the body's destruction of its own RBCs by serum antibodies.
glucose-6-phosphate-dehydrogenase(G6PD)		An inherited enzyme deficiency that causes hemolytic anemia.
hemoglobinopathy	*hem/o* blood *globin/o* protein *-pathy* disease process	A general term for genetic defects of hemoglobin.
hemolytic anemia	*hem/o* blood *-lytic* pertaining to destruction	A group of anemias caused by destruction of red blood cells.
hereditary spherocytosis	*spher/o* sphere, globe *-cytosis* condition of abnormal increase in cells	Condition in which red blood cells have a round shape (instead of biconcave disc-shape) because of a fragile membrane.
nonautoimmune acquired hemolytic anemia	*non-* not *hem/o* blood *-lytic* pertaining to destruction *an-* no, not *-emia* blood condition	Anemia that may be drug induced or may be caused by an infectious disease, in which the RBCs are destroyed.
sickle cell disorders		**Sickle cell trait** is a condition in which an individual has one gene that is for normal hemoglobin and one for sickle hemoglobin. Those who have the trait do not exhibit symptoms of sickle cell disease. **Sickle cell anemia** is an inherited anemia characterized by crescent-shaped RBCs. This abnormality in morphology causes RBCs to block small-diameter capillaries, thereby decreasing the oxygen supply to the cells (Fig. 8-9). A **sickle cell crisis** is an acute, painful exacerbation of sickle cell anemia.
thalassemia	*thalass/o* sea *-emia* blood condition	Group of inherited disorders of people of Mediterranean, African, and Southeast Asian descent, in which the anemia is the result of a decrease in the synthesis of hemoglobin, resulting in decreased production and increased destruction of RBCs.

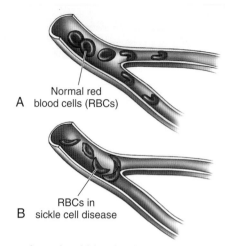

A Normal red blood cells (RBCs)

B RBCs in sickle cell disease

Fig. 8-9 A, Normal, donut-shaped red blood cells bend to fit through capillaries. **B,** Sickled red blood cells cannot bend and therefore block the flow of blood through the vessel.

Terms Related to Aplastic and Other Anemias and Other Bone Marrow Failure Syndromes (D60-D64)

Term	Word Origin	Definition
acute posthemorrhagic anemia	*post-* after *hem/o* blood *-rrhagic* pertaining to bursting forth *an-* no, not *-emia* blood condition	RBC deficiency caused by blood loss.
aplastic anemia	*a-* no, not, without *plast/o* formation *-ic* pertaining to *an-* no, not, without *-emia* blood condition	Suppression of bone marrow function leading to a reduction in RBC production. Although causes of this often fatal type of anemia may be hepatitis, radiation, or cytotoxic agents, most causes are idiopathic. Also called **hypoplastic anemia** (Fig. 8-10).
erythroblastopenia	*erythr/o* red *blast/o* embryonic, immature *-penia* condition of deficiency	Deficiency of immature red blood cells. Significant in that they indicate a future lack of mature blood cells
myelophthisis	*myel/o* bone marrow *-phthisis* wasting	Wasting of bone marrow, usually with replacement by cancer cells. The term **phthisis** by itself usually refers to a condition of tuberculosis of the lungs.
pancytopenia	*pan-* all *cyt/o* cell *-penia* condition of deficiency	Deficiency of all blood cells caused by dysfunctional stem cells (Fig. 8-11).

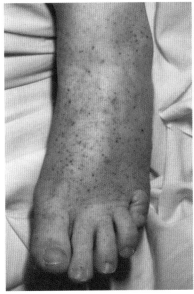

Fig. 8-10 Petechiae on left foot as a result of aplastic anemia.

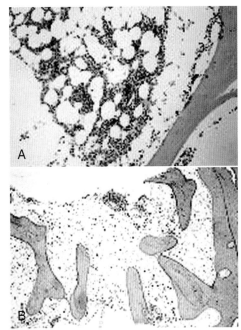

Fig. 8-11 **A,** Normal cellularity. **B,** Hypocellularity in pancytopenia.

 Exercise 4: Nutritional, Hemolytic, Aplastic, and Other Anemias and Bone Marrow Failure Syndromes

Match the terms to their definitions.

_____ 1. B$_{12}$ deficiency
_____ 2. aplastic anemia
_____ 3. pernicious anemia
_____ 4. thalassemia
_____ 5. G6PD
_____ 6. hemolytic anemia
_____ 7. hereditary spherocytosis
_____ 8. acute posthemorrhagic anemia
_____ 9. sickle cell trait
_____ 10. sickle cell anemia
_____ 11. sickle cell crisis

A. hemolytic anemia caused by inherited enzyme deficiency
B. condition in which red blood cells have a round shape
C. reduction of RBC production caused by suppression of bone marrow function
D. progressive anemia caused by lack of intrinsic factor
E. a condition in which a person has one gene for normal hemoglobin and one gene for sickle cell disease
F. anemia caused by a decrease in the synthesis of hemoglobin
G. an acute, painful exacerbation of sickle cell anemia
H. group of anemias caused by destruction of red blood cells
I. an inherited anemia characterized by crescent-shaped RBCs
J. RBC deficiency caused by blood loss
K. insufficient blood levels of cobalamin

Build the terms.

12. condition of iron deficiency _____

13. disease process of blood protein _____

14. condition of red embryonic, immature deficiency _____

15. wasting of bone marrow _____

16. condition of all cell deficiency _____

Terms Related to Coagulation Defects, Purpura, and Other Hemorrhagic Conditions (D65-D69)

Term	Word Origin	Definition
disseminated intravascular coagulopathy (DIC)	*intra-* within *vascul/o* vessel *-ar* pertaining to *coagul/o* clotting *-pathy* disease process	A disorder of clotting mechanisms that results in bleeding at scattered sites in the body. Causes may be severe trauma or infection, and treatment can include blood transfusions along with oxygen therapy.
hemophilia	*hem/o* blood *-philia* condition of attraction	Group of inherited bleeding disorders characterized by a deficiency of one of the factors (factor VIII) necessary for the coagulation of blood (Fig. 8-12).
purpura	*purpur/o* purple *-a* noun ending	Bleeding disorder characterized by hemorrhage into the tissues (Fig. 8-13).
thrombocytopenia	*thromb/o* clot, clotting *cyt/o* cell *-penia* condition of deficiency	Deficiency of platelets that causes an inability of the blood to clot. The most common cause of bleeding disorders.
thrombophilia	*thromb/o* clot *-philia* condition of attraction	An increase in the body's tendency to form clots.

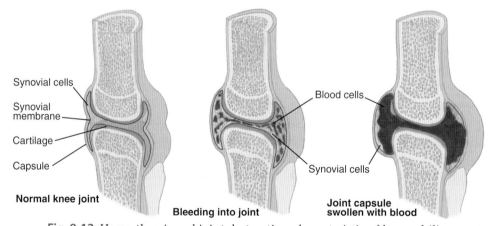

Fig. 8-12 Hemarthrosis and joint destruction characteristic of hemophilia.

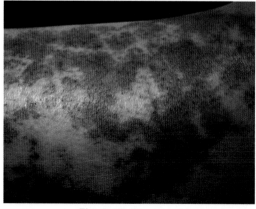

Fig. 8-13 Purpura.

Terms Related to Other Disorders of Blood and Blood-Forming Organs (D7Ø-D77)

Term	Word Origin	Meaning
asplenia	*a-* without *splen/o* spleen *-ia* condition	Absence of the spleen, either congenital or acquired due to surgical removal.
bandemia	*band/o* bands *-emia* blood condition	An increase in the number of immature neutrophils (band cells) in the blood. Increases of band cells may indicate infection.
basophilia	*bas/o* base *-philia* condition of attraction	Excessive basophils in the blood.
eosinophilia	*eosin/o* rosy-colored *-philia* condition of attraction	An increase in the number of eosinophils in the blood.
erythrocytosis	*erythr/o* red *-cytosis* condition of abnormal increase of cells	An excessive number of red blood cells in the blood.
hypersplenism	*hyper-* excessive *splen/o* spleen *-ism* condition	Increased function of the spleen, resulting in hemolysis (Fig. 8-14). Usually secondary to splenomegaly, treatment often involves removal of the spleen.
leukocytosis	*leuk/o* white *-cytosis* condition of abnormal increase in cells	Abnormal increase in WBCs. Abnormal increases in each type of granulocyte are termed **eosinophilia, basophilia,** and **neutrophilia,** where the suffix -philia denotes a slight increase. Abnormal increases in the number of each type of agranulocyte are termed **lymphocytosis** and **monocytosis.**
leukopenia	*leuk/o* white *-penia* condition of deficiency	Abnormal decrease in WBCs. Specific deficiencies are termed **neutropenia, eosinopenia, monocytopenia,** and **lymphocytopenia.** Also called **leukocytopenia.**
lymphocytopenia	*lymph/o* lymph *cyt/o* cell *-penia* condition of deficiency	Deficiency of lymphocytes caused by infectious mononucleosis, malignancy, nutritional deficiency, or a hematological disorder.
methemoglobinemia	*met(a)-* change *hem/o* blood *globin/o* protein *-emia* blood condition	Abnormal condition in which red blood cells are unable to carry hemoglobin. May be hereditary or acquired.
monocytosis	*mono-* one *-cytosis* abnormal increase of cells	Excessive monocytes in the blood.

Continued

Terms Related to Other Disorders of Blood and Blood-Forming Organs (D70-D77)—cont'd

Term	Word Origin	Meaning
myelofibrosis	*myel/o* bone marrow *fibr/o* fiber *-osis* abnormal condition	Abnormal condition of fibrous tissue development in the bone marrow due to a chromosomal abnormality (Fig. 8-15).
neutropenia	*neutr/o* neutral *-penia* condition of deficiency	Abnormal decrease in neutrophils due to disease process. Formerly called **agranulocytosis**.
plasmacytosis	*plasm/a* plasma *-cytosis* abnormal increase of cells	Excessive plasma cells in the blood.
splenitis	*splen/o* spleen *-itis* inflammation	Inflammation of the spleen.

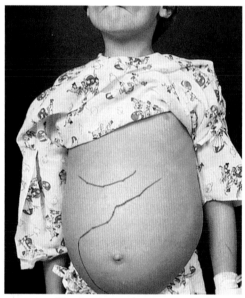

Fig. 8-14 Hypersplenism.

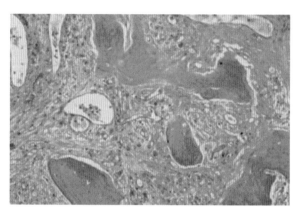

Fig. 8-15 Myelofibrosis.

Terms Related to Systemic Infections of the Blood

Term	Word Origin	Definition
sepsis, severe		Severe sepsis is sepsis complicated by acute organ dysfunction.
septicemia	*septic/o* infection *-emia* blood condition	Systemic infection with pathological microbes in the blood as the result of an infection that is spread from elsewhere in the body. The term **sepsis** means infection.
septic shock	*sept/o* infection *-ic* pertaining to	Inadequate systemic blood flow to the body caused by an overwhelming infection and resultant low blood pressure. Organs fail and death may occur. Septic shock may or may not be present with severe sepsis.
systemic inflammatory response syndrome (SIRS)		SIRS is an inflammatory state affecting the whole body. SIRS can be caused by trauma, ischemia, or infection.

CM Guideline Alert

1.D.1.B SEVERE SEPSIS
The coding of severe sepsis requires a minimum of 2 codes: first a code for the underlying systemic infection, followed by a code from subcategory R65.2, Severe sepsis. If the causal organism is not documented, assign code A41.9, Sepsis, unspecified organism, for the infection Additional code(s) for the associate acute organ dysfunction are also required.

   Due to the complex nature of severe sepsis, some cases may require querying the provider prior to assignment of the codes.

 CM Guideline Alert

1.D.2.A SEPTIC SHOCK
Septic shock generally refers to the circulatory failure associated with severe sepsis, and therefore, it represents a type of acute organ dysfunction.

   For all cases of septic shock, the code for the systemic infection should be sequenced first, followed by code R65.21, Severe sepsis with septic shock, or code T81.12, Postprocedural septic shock. Any additional codes for the other acute organ dysfunctions should also be assigned. As noted in the sequencing instructions in the Tabular List, the code for septic shock cannot be assigned as a principal diagnosis.

 Exercise 5: **Coagulation Defects, Hemorrhagic Conditions, Disorders of Blood and Blood-Forming Organs, and Systemic Infections of the Blood**

Match the terms to their definitions.

____ 1. hemophilia

____ 2. purpura

____ 3. DIC

____ 4. lymphocytopenia

____ 5. bandemia

____ 6. hypersplenism

____ 7. methemoglobinemia

____ 8. erythrocytosis

____ 9. myelofibrosis

____ 10. leukocytosis

____ 11. leukopenia

____ 12. neutropenia

____ 13. SIRS

____ 14. septic shock

____ 15. severe sepsis

A. bleeding disorder characterized by a deficiency of blood coagulation factor

B. abnormal decrease in neutrophils

C. inadequate systemic blood flow caused by an infection

D. bleeding disorder characterized by hemorrhage into the tissues

E. clotting mechanism disorder that results in bleeding at different places in the body

F. abnormal decrease in WBCs

G. excessive number of red blood cells

H. deficiency of lymphocytes

I. abnormal condition in which red blood cells are unable to carry hemoglobin

J. abnormal condition of fibrous tissue development in bone marrow

K. increased function of the spleen

L. an inflammatory response affecting the whole body. Caused by an infection, trauma, or ischemia

M. abnormal increase in WBCs

N. increase in the number of immature neutrophils

O. a systemic infection associated with organ dysfunction

Translate the terms.

16. thrombocytopenia _____

17. eosinophilia _____

18. plasmacytosis _____

19. asplenia _____

20. septicemia _____

Terms Related to Certain Disorders Involving the Immune Mechanism (D8Ø-D89)

Term	Word Origin	Definition
autoimmune lymphoproliferative syndrome (ALPS)	*auto-* self *immun/o* safety, protection *syn-* together *-drome* run	Inherited disorder of the immune system with unusually high numbers of lymphocytes that accumulate in the lymph nodes, liver, and spleen.
graft-versus-host disease (GVHD)		Disorder occurring when donated tissue cells attack the cells of the recipient.
hypogammaglobulinemia	*hypo-* deficiency *gamma* *globulin/o* protein *-emia* blood condition	A lack of antibodies (immunoglobulin G) in the blood. Also called **agammaglobulinemia**. An inherited immunodeficiency disorder.
sarcoidosis	*sarc/o* flesh *-oid* like *-osis* abnormal condition	An inflammatory disorder in which small fleshlike tumors develop throughout the body.

Terms Related to Other Immune Disorders

Term	Word Origin	Definition
acquired immunodeficiency syndrome (AIDS)	*immun/o* safety, protection	Syndrome caused by the human immunodeficiency virus (HIV) and transmitted through body fluids. Fig. 8-16 demonstrates the life cycle of HIV.
autoimmune disease	*auto-* self *immun/o* safety, protection	Condition in which a person's T cells attack his/her own cells, causing extensive tissue damage and organ dysfunction. Examples of resultant autoimmune diseases include myasthenia gravis, rheumatoid arthritis, systemic lupus erythematosus, and multiple sclerosis.
infectious mononucleosis	*mono-* one *nucle/o* nucleus *-osis* abnormal condition	Named for its characteristic proliferation of monocytes, this common disorder is caused by the Epstein-Barr virus (EBV). Spread through the saliva, the symptoms include sore throat, fever, and fatigue. Commonly known as **mono** or **the kissing disease**.

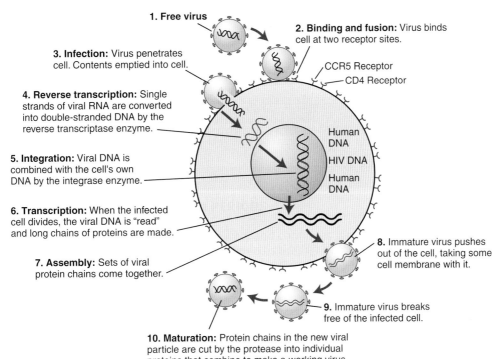

1. Free virus

2. Binding and fusion: Virus binds cell at two receptor sites.

3. Infection: Virus penetrates cell. Contents emptied into cell.

CCR5 Receptor
CD4 Receptor

4. Reverse transcription: Single strands of viral RNA are converted into double-stranded DNA by the reverse transcriptase enzyme.

Human DNA
HIV DNA
Human DNA

5. Integration: Viral DNA is combined with the cell's own DNA by the integrase enzyme.

6. Transcription: When the infected cell divides, the viral DNA is "read" and long chains of proteins are made.

8. Immature virus pushes out of the cell, taking some cell membrane with it.

7. Assembly: Sets of viral protein chains come together.

9. Immature virus breaks free of the infected cell.

10. Maturation: Protein chains in the new viral particle are cut by the protease into individual proteins that combine to make a working virus.

Fig. 8-16 HIV life cycle.

 Exercise 6: **Disorders Involving the Immune Mechanism**

Match the terms to their definitions.

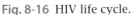

____ 1. AIDS	A. lack of antibodies in the blood
____ 2. hypogammaglobulinemia	B. disorder that occurs when donated tissue cells attack recipient cells
____ 3. sarcoidosis	
____ 4. GVHD	C. Inherited disorder in which high number of lymphocytes accumulate in lymph nodes, liver, and spleen
____ 5. ALPS	
____ 6. autoimmune disease	D. condition in which a person's T cells attack his or her own body
	E. syndrome caused by HIV
	F. inflammatory disorder in which small fleshlike tumors develop throughout the body

Terms Related to Benign Neoplasms

Term	Word Origin	Definition
myelodysplastic syndrome	*myel/o* bone marrow *dys-* abnormal *-plastic* pertaining to forming	Group of disorders that result from a defect in the bone marrow. Also referred to as **preleukemia.**
polycythemia vera	*poly-* many, much *cyt/o* cell *-(h)emia* blood condition *vera* true	Condition in which the bone marrow produces an excessive number of blood cells. A rare form of a slow-growing cancer of the blood. Coded as a neoplasm of uncertain behavior. If documented as benign, secondary, or familial, it is coded as an unspecified disease of blood and blood-forming organs.
thymoma	*thym/o* thymus gland *-oma* tumor, mass	Noncancerous tumor of epithelial origin that is often associated with myasthenia gravis.

Terms Related to Malignant Neoplasms

Term	Word Origin	Definition
acute lymphocytic leukemia (ALL)	*lymph/o* lymph *cyt/o* cell *-ic* pertaining to *leuk/o* white *-emia* blood condition	Also termed **acute lymphoblastic leukemia,** this cancer is characterized by the uncontrolled proliferation of immature lymphocytes. It is the most common type of leukemia for individuals under the age of 19 (Fig. 8-17).
acute myelogenous leukemia (AML)	*myel/o* bone marrow *-genous* pertaining to originating from *leuk/o* white *-emia* blood condition	This rapidly progressive form of leukemia develops from immature bone marrow stem cells.
chronic lymphocytic leukemia (CLL)	*lymph/o* lymph *cyt/o* cell *-ic* pertaining to *leuk/o* white *-emia* blood condition	A slowly progressing form of leukemia in which immature lymphocytes proliferate. Occurs most frequently in middle age (or older) adults, rarely in children.
chronic myelogenous leukemia (CML)	*myel/o* bone marrow *-genous* pertaining to originating from *leuk/o* white *-emia* blood condition	A slowly progressing form of leukemia in which immature bone marrow cells proliferate. Like CLL, it occurs most frequently in middle age (or older) adults, rarely in children.
Hodgkin lymphoma	*lymph/o* lymph *-oma* tumor, mass	Also termed **Hodgkin disease,** this cancer is diagnosed by the detection of a type of cell specific only to this disorder: Reed-Sternberg cells.
myeloma, multiple	*myel/o* bone marrow *-oma* tumor, mass	Also termed **plasma cell dyscrasia** or **myelomatosis,** this rare malignancy of the plasma cells is formed from B lymphocytes. It is called "multiple" myeloma because the tumors are found in many bones. If it occurs in only one bone, the tumor is referred to as a **plasmacytoma** (Fig. 8-18).

Terms Related to Malignant Neoplasms—cont'd

Term	Word Origin	Definition
non-Hodgkin lymphoma	*lymph/o* lymph *-oma* tumor, mass	A collection of all other lymphatic cancers but Hodgkin lymphomas. This type is the most common of the two lymphomas and is the sixth most common type of cancer in the United States.
thymoma, malignant	*thym/o* thymus gland *-oma* tumor, mass	Also termed **thymic carcinoma,** this rare malignancy of the thymus gland is particularly invasive and, unlike its benign form, is not associated with autoimmune disorders.

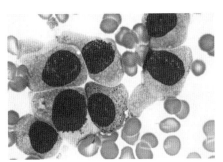

Fig. 8-17 Micrograph of leukemia.

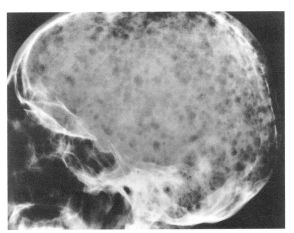

Fig. 8-18 Multiple myeloma. Diffuse, punched-out osteolytic lesions are scattered throughout the skull.

Exercise 7: Neoplasms

Match the neoplasms with their definitions.

_____ 1. non-Hodgkin lymphoma
_____ 2. ALL
_____ 3. thymoma
_____ 4. CLL
_____ 5. CML
_____ 6. multiple myeloma
_____ 7. AML
_____ 8. malignant thymoma
_____ 9. Hodgkin lymphoma
_____ 10. polycythemia vera

A. rapidly progressive form of leukemia due to immature bone marrow stem cells

B. benign tumor of thymus gland

C. cancer of lymphatic system detected by presence of Reed-Sternberg cells

D. slowly progressing form of leukemia with proliferation of immature lymphocytes

E. thymic carcinoma

F. slowly progressing form of leukemia in which immature bone marrow cells proliferate

G. a collection of all lymphatic cancers except Hodgkin lymphoma

H. plasma cell dyscrasia; tumors are found in many bones

I. form of leukemia characterized by uncontrolled proliferation of immature lymphocytes

J. condition in which bone marrow produces too many blood cells

PROCEDURES

Terms Related to Laboratory Tests

Term	Word Origin	Definition
AIDS tests—ELISA, Western blot		Tests to detect the presence of HIV types 1 and 2 (Fig. 8-19).
basic metabolic panel (BMP)		Group of blood tests to measure calcium; glucose; electrolytes such as sodium (Na), potassium (K), and chloride (Cl); creatinine; and blood urea nitrogen (BUN).
blood cultures		Blood samples are submitted to propagate microorganisms that may be present. Cultures may be indicated for bacteremia or septicemia, or to discover other pathogens (fungi, viruses, or parasites) (Fig. 8-20).

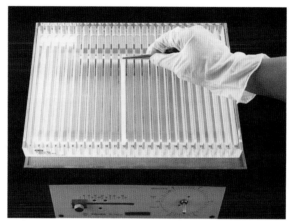

Fig. 8-19 Western blot test. A technician is placing a Western blot strip in a test tray. If present, antigens will bind to this sheet and later be detected.

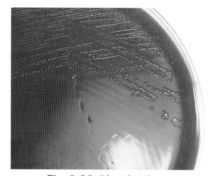

Fig. 8-20 Blood culture.

Terms Related to Laboratory Tests—cont'd

Term	Word Origin	Definition
complete blood cell count (CBC)		Twelve tests, including RBC (red blood cell count), WBC (white blood cell count), Hb (hemoglobin), Hct/PCV (hematocrit/packed-cell volume), and diff (WBC differential).
comprehensive metabolic panel (CMP)		Set of 14 blood tests that adds protein and liver function tests to the BMP. Glucose is also measured with a different method than in the basic panel.
Coombs antiglobulin test	*anti-* against *-globulin* protein substance	Blood test to diagnose hemolytic disease of the newborn (HDN), acquired hemolytic anemia, or a transfusion reaction.
diff count		Measure of the numbers of the different types of WBCs.
erythrocyte sedimentation rate (ESR)	*erythr/o* red *-cyte* cell	Measurement of time for mature RBCs to settle out of a blood sample after an anticoagulant is added. An increased ESR indicates inflammation.
hematocrit (Hct), packed-cell volume (PCV)	*hemat/o* blood *-crit* separate	Measure of the percentage of RBCs in the blood.
hemoglobin (Hgb, Hb)	*hem/o* blood *-globin* protein substance	Measurement of the iron-containing pigment of RBCs that carries oxygen to tissues.
mean corpuscular hemoglobin (MCH)	*hem/o* blood *-globin* protein substance	Test to measure the average weight of hemoglobin per RBC. Useful in diagnosing anemia.
mean corpuscular hemoglobin concentration (MCHC)		Test to measure the concentration of hemoglobin in RBCs. This test is useful for measuring a patient's response to treatment for anemia.
partial thromboplastin time (PTT)	*thromb/o* clot, clotting *-plastin* forming substance	Test of blood plasma to detect coagulation defects of the intrinsic system; used to detect hemophilia.
prothrombin time (PT)	*pro-* before *-thrombin* clotting substance	Test that measures the amount of time taken for clot formation. It is used to determine the cause of unexplained bleeding, to assess levels of anticoagulation in patients taking warfarin or with vitamin K deficiency, and to assess the ability of the liver to synthesize blood-clotting proteins.
Schilling test		Nuclear medicine test used to diagnose pernicious anemia and other metabolic disorders.
serology testing	*ser/o* serum	Test to examine blood for presence and level of antibodies as a result of exposure to a disease.
white blood cell count (WBC)		Measurement of the number of leukocytes in the blood. An increase may indicate the presence of an infection; a decrease may be caused by radiation or chemotherapy.

Exercise 8: **Laboratory Tests**

Matching. Some answers may be used more than once.

____ 1. Coombs antiglobulin

____ 2. Schilling test

____ 3. PTT

____ 4. PCV

____ 5. ESR

____ 6. blood culture

____ 7. WBC

____ 8. Western blot

____ 9. Hct

____ 10. ELISA

____ 11. MCH

____ 12. MCHC

____ 13. PT

A. % RBCs

B. if increased, inflammation indicated

C. anemia

D. HIV

E. response to anemia treatment

F. determines cause of bleeding

G. hemophilia

H. pernicious anemia

I. HDN, transfusion reaction

J. microorganisms

K. number of leukocytes in the blood

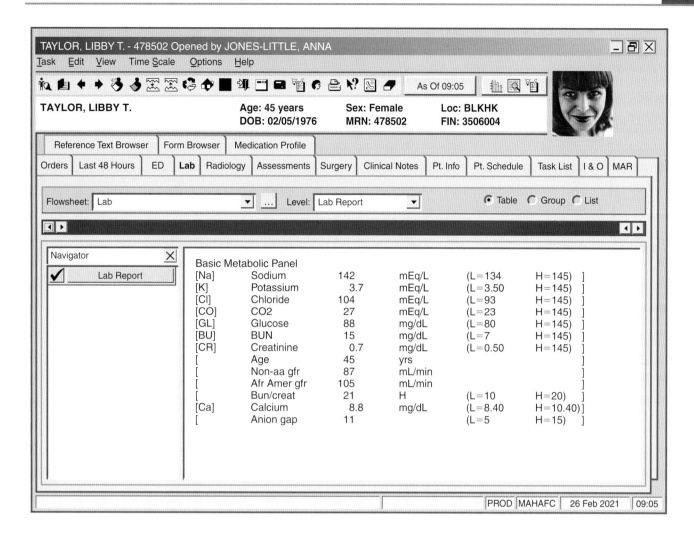

Exercise 9: Lab Report

Using the lab report above, answer the following questions.

1. What is the patient's potassium level? _____

2. What is the sodium level? _____

3. What is the patient's blood urea nitrogen? _____

Terms Related to Blood and Bone Marrow Procedures

Term	Word Origin	Definition
apheresis	*-apheresis* removal	Temporary removal of blood from a donor, in which one or more components are removed and the rest of the blood is reinfused into the donor. Examples include **leukapheresis,** removal of WBCs; **plasmapheresis,** removal of plasma; and **plateletpheresis,** removal of thrombocytes. Also called **pheresis**.

Continued

Terms Related to Blood and Bone Marrow Procedures—cont'd

Term	Word Origin	Definition
autologous bone marrow transplant	*auto-* self *log/o* study *-ous* pertaining to	Harvesting of patient's own healthy bone marrow before treatment for reintroduction later.
autologous transfusion	*auto-* self *log/o* study *-ous* pertaining to *trans-* across *-fusion* pouring	Process in which the donor's own blood is removed and stored in anticipation of a future need.
autotransfusion	*auto-* self *trans-* across *-fusion* pouring	Process in which the donor is transfused with his/her own blood, after anticoagulation and filtration, from an active bleeding site in cases of major surgery or trauma.
blood transfusion	*trans-* across *-fusion* pouring	Intravenous transfer of blood from a donor to a recipient, giving either whole blood or its components (Fig. 8-21).
bone marrow transplant (BMT)		The transplantation of bone marrow to stimulate production of normal blood cells.
hemostasis	*hem/o* blood *-stasis* stopping, controlling	The control of bleeding by mechanical or chemical means.
homologous bone marrow transplant	*homo-* same (species) *log/o* study *-ous* pertaining to	Transplantation of healthy bone marrow from a donor to a recipient to stimulate formation of new blood cells.

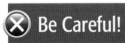 **Be Careful!** *Do not confuse* **-apheresis,** *meaning* removal of blood, *with* **-poiesis,** *which means* formation.

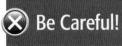 **Be Careful!** *Do not confuse* **hemostasis,** *meaning* the control of bleeding, *with* **homeostasis,** *which means* the body's process of balance.

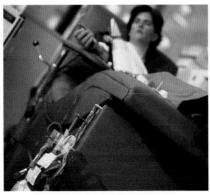

Fig. 8-21 Blood transfusion.

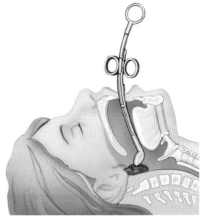

Fig. 8-22 Adenoidectomy.

Terms Related to Lymphatic and Immune System Interventions

Term	Word Origin	Definition
adenoidectomy	*adenoid/o* adenoid *-ectomy* cutting out	Removal of the adenoids (pharyngeal tonsils) (Fig. 8-22).
biopsy (bx) of lymphatic structures	*bi/o* life *-opsy* viewing *lymphat/o* lymph *-ic* pertaining to	Removal of the lymph nodes or lymphoid tissue as a means of diagnosis and treatment.
lymphadenectomy	*lymphaden/o* lymph gland *-ectomy* cutting out	Removal of a lymph node.
splenectomy	*splen/o* spleen *-ectomy* cutting out	Removal of the spleen.

Exercise 10: Procedures

Match the interventions with their definitions.

_____ 1. autologous transfusion
_____ 2. homologous bone marrow transplant
_____ 3. apheresis
_____ 4. autologous bone marrow transplant
_____ 5. biopsy of lymphatic structures
_____ 6. autotransfusion

A. harvesting of patient's own bone marrow to be reintroduced later
B. donor is transfused with his own blood from an active bleeding site
C. temporary removal of blood from a donor with removal of one or more components and subsequent reinfusion
D. transplantation of healthy bone marrow from donor
E. donor is reinfused with her own stored blood
F. removal of lymph nodes for examination

Build the terms.

7. cutting out the spleen _____

8. cutting out the pharyngeal tonsils _____

9. stopping blood _____

10. cutting out a lymph node _____

PHARMACOLOGY

Blood Drugs

anti- = against

anticoagulants: Prevent or delay the coagulation of blood and the formation of thrombi. Examples include heparin, warfarin (Coumadin), enoxaparin (Lovenox), and apixaban (Eliquis).

antifibrinolytics: Stop bleeding by blocking plasmin formation. Examples include aminocaproic acid (Amicar) and tranexamic acid (Cyklokapron).

antiplatelets: Inhibit the function of platelets or destroy them. Examples include aspirin, clopidogrel (Plavix), dipyridamole (Persantine), and ticagrelor (Brilinta).

blood-flow modifiers: Promote blood flow by keeping platelets from clumping or decreasing blood viscosity. Examples include the prescription medications cilostazol (Pletal) and pentoxifylline (Trental) and the herbal product ginkgo biloba.

colony-stimulating factors (CSFs): Stimulate the production of white blood cells in the bone marrow. The two kinds are granulocyte CSF (G-CSF) and granulocyte-macrophage CSF (GM-CSF). Available synthetic agents of each type are filgrastim (Neupogen) and sargramostim (Leukine), respectively.

erythropoietic
erythr/o = red
-poietic = pertaining to formation

erythropoietic agents: Increase production of red blood cells (RBCs) by stimulating erythro- poiesis. Two available agents are epoetin alfa (Epogen, Procrit) and darbepo- etin alfa (Aranesp).

hematinics: Increase the number of erythrocytes and/or hemoglobin concentration in the erythrocytes, usually to treat iron-deficiency anemia. Examples are iron supplements, folate, and B-complex vitamins.

hematopoietic
hemat/o = blood
-poietic = pertaining to formation

hematopoietic agents: Stimulate blood cell production. Subdivisions of this class include colony-stimulating factors, erythropoietic agents, and thrombopoietic factors.

hemostatic
hem/o = blood
-static = pertaining to stopping or controlling

thrombopoietic factors: Stimulate the production of thrombocytes or platelets. Oprelvekin (Neumega) is an available agent. Platelet-stimulating agents include romiplostim (Nplate) and eltrombopag (Promacta).

Immune Drugs

antineoplastics: Treat cancer by preventing growth or promoting destruction of tumor cells. Numerous drugs, including methotrexate (Trexall), ibrutinib (Imbruvica), and rituximab (Rituxan), fall into this category.

antiretrovirals: Minimize the replication of HIV and its progression into AIDS. Examples include zidovudine or AZT (Retrovir), tenofovir (Viread), and efavirenz (Sustiva).

corticosteroids: Steroids that suppress the immune system and reduce inflammation. Examples include triamcinolone (Triesence), hydrocortisone (Cortizone), and prednisone (Rayos).

cytotoxic agents: Damage or destroy cells to treat cancer; often act as immunosuppressants or antineoplastics.

immunomodulators: Reduce the impact of immune system disorders. Dimethyl fumarate Tecfidera and peginterferon beta-1a (Plegridy) are examples of these drugs used to treat multiple sclerosis.

immunosuppressants: Minimize the immune response. Examples include azathioprine (Imuran), cyclosporine (Sandimmune), secukinumab (Cosentyx), and tacrolimus (Prograf).

protease inhibitors: Antiretrovirals used to treat HIV infection. By blocking the production of an essential enzyme called protease, these drugs keep the virus from replicating. Examples are indinavir (Crixivan), nelfinavir (Viracept), and saquinavir (Invirase).

vaccines: Modified disease-causing microbial components administered to induce immunity or reduce the pathological effects of a disease. Examples are the measles, mumps, rubella, tetanus vaccine (MMR); diphtheria, and pertussis vaccine (DTaP); and the chicken pox (Varicella) vaccine. A **vaccination** is an injection, inhalation, or oral solution derived from dead or weakened (attenuated) virus. You may have heard the terms *vaccination* and *immunization* used interchangeably. A vaccine is the *substance* that produces immunity from a given disease. It can be introduced into the body orally, intranasally, or by injection using a needle (usually intramuscular). A *vaccination* is the introduction itself, and *immunization* is the entire process of providing protection against the organism introduced.

CPT Coding Alert!

CPT requires specificity as to the exact vaccine with the route of administration and often the age of the patient.

Click on **Animations** to see how vaccinations protect the body from pathogens.

Exercise 11: Pharmacology

Match each drug group with its action.

____	1. erythropoietic agents	A. damage or destroy cells to treat cancer
____	2. antiplatelets	B. delay clotting of blood
____	3. hematopoietic agents	C. inhibit clotting, destroy thrombocytes
____	4. hematinics	D. help induce immunity
____	5. anticoagulants	E. increase blood cell production
____	6. cytotoxic agents	F. stop the flow of blood
____	7. immunosuppressants	G. decrease tumor cells
____	8. antineoplastics	H. lessen the immune response
____	9. hemostatics	I. increase RBC or Hgb concentration
____	10. vaccines	J. increase production of RBCs

RECOGNIZING SUFFIXES FOR PCS

Now that you've finished reading about the procedures for the blood, blood-forming organs, and immune mechanisms, take a look at this review of the *suffixes* used in their terminology. Each of these suffixes is associated with one or more root operations in the medical surgical section or one of the other categories in PCS.

Suffixes and Root Operations for the Blood, Blood-Forming Organs, and Immune Mechanisms

Suffix	Root Operation
-apheresis	Perfusion
-ectomy	Excision, resection

Black Hawk Hospital
1400 Washington Ave.
Waterloo, IA 50707

MEDICAL LETTER

Sally C. Quinn, MD
Student Health Center
Black Hawk Hospital
1400 Washington Avenue
Waterloo, IA 50707

Allen B. Corwin, MD
River City Physician Practice
7777 S. Shore Dr.
Mason City, IA 50428

Re: Manny Ochoa

Dear Dr. Quinn,

Please find the enclosed summary of treatment for Manny Ochoa, date of birth 8/3/1993, a college student whom I treated in my office last month. He requested that I forward this to you as his primary care physician in his hometown; I understand he will be returning home this summer.

This 27-year-old college student had a 2-week history of a sore throat, stiffness and tenderness of his neck, and extreme fatigue. On examination, he was mildly pyrexic with posterior cervical lymphadenopathy, palatal petechiae, and pharyngeal inflammation without an exudate. Abdominal examination showed marked splenomegaly. There was no evidence of a skin rash or jaundice.

The clinical diagnosis of infectious mononucleosis was confirmed on investigation with more than 50% of the lymphocytes showing atypical lymphocytosis. His serum contained IgM antibodies to the Epstein-Barr viral antigen. Liver function test results were normal.

He was treated symptomatically and was advised to avoid strenuous activity until his splenomegaly has completely resolved because of the danger of splenic rupture. He was also advised to abstain from alcohol for at least 6 months because many patients show clinical or biochemical evidence of liver involvement.

Sincerely,

Allen B. Corwin, MD

 Exercise 12: **Medical Letter**

Using the medical letter above, answer the following questions.

1. How do you know that the patient had a slight fever? _____

2. On examination, what phrase might explain why his throat was sore? _____

3. Translate "cervical lymphadenopathy." _____

4. How do you know that the patient's spleen was enlarged? _____

5. What term tells you that test results showed an increase in the number of lymphocytes? _____

Abbreviations

Abbreviation	Meaning
A, B, AB, O	blood types
AIDS	acquired immunodeficiency syndrome
ALL	acute lymphocytic leukemia
ALPS	autoimmune lymphoproliferative syndrome
AML	acute myelogenous leukemia
basos	basophils
BMP	basic metabolic panel
BMT	bone marrow transplant
BUN	blood urea nitrogen
bx	biopsy
CBC	complete blood cell count
Cl	chloride
CLL	chronic lymphocytic leukemia
CML	chronic myelogenous leukemia
CMP	comprehensive metabolic panel
CO_2	carbon dioxide
DIC	disseminated intravascular coagulopathy
diff	differential WBC count
EBV	Epstein-Barr virus
eosins	eosinophils
ESR	erythrocyte sedimentation rate
G6PD	glucose-6-phosphate-dehydrogenase
GVHD	graft-versus-host disease

Abbreviation	Meaning
Hb, Hgb	hemoglobin
Hct	hematocrit, packed-cell volume
HDN	hemolytic disease of the newborn
HIV	human immunodeficiency virus
HSC	hematopoietic stem cell
Ig	immunoglobulin
K	potassium
lymphs	lymphocytes
MCH	mean corpuscular hemoglobin
MCHC	mean corpuscular hemoglobin concentration
Na	sodium
neuts	neutrophils
NK	natural killer cells
PCV	packed-cell volume, hematocrit
plats	platelets, thrombocytes
PMNs, polys	polymorphonucleocytes
PT	prothrombin time
PTT	partial thromboplastin time
RBC	red blood cell (count)
segs	segmented neutrophils
SIRS	systemic inflammatory response syndrome
stabs	band cells
WBC	white blood cell (count)

Go to the Evolve website to interactively build terms, label images, memorize word parts and practice using blood and immune terms in context.

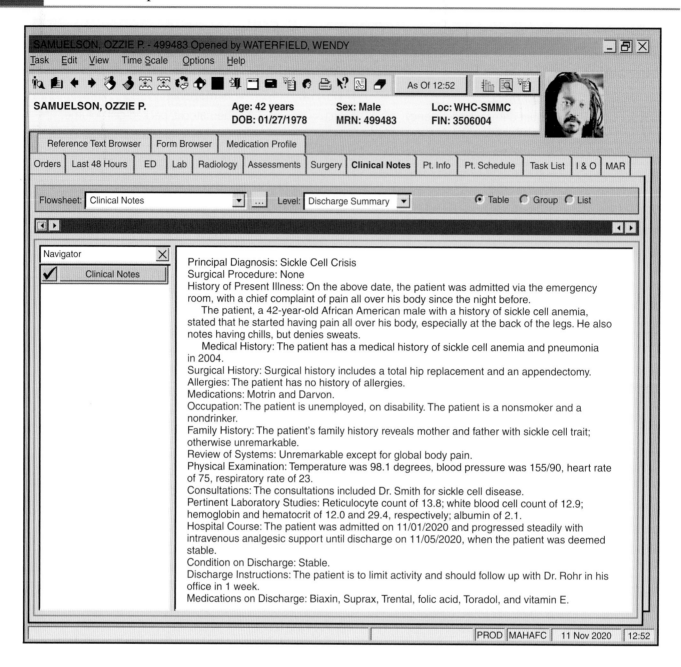

Principal Diagnosis: Sickle Cell Crisis
Surgical Procedure: None
History of Present Illness: On the above date, the patient was admitted via the emergency room, with a chief complaint of pain all over his body since the night before.
    The patient, a 42-year-old African American male with a history of sickle cell anemia, stated that he started having pain all over his body, especially at the back of the legs. He also notes having chills, but denies sweats.
    Medical History: The patient has a medical history of sickle cell anemia and pneumonia in 2004.
Surgical History: Surgical history includes a total hip replacement and an appendectomy.
Allergies: The patient has no history of allergies.
Medications: Motrin and Darvon.
Occupation: The patient is unemployed, on disability. The patient is a nonsmoker and a nondrinker.
Family History: The patient's family history reveals mother and father with sickle cell trait; otherwise unremarkable.
Review of Systems: Unremarkable except for global body pain.
Physical Examination: Temperature was 98.1 degrees, blood pressure was 155/90, heart rate of 75, respiratory rate of 23.
Consultations: The consultations included Dr. Smith for sickle cell disease.
Pertinent Laboratory Studies: Reticulocyte count of 13.8; white blood cell count of 12.9; hemoglobin and hematocrit of 12.0 and 29.4, respectively; albumin of 2.1.
Hospital Course: The patient was admitted on 11/01/2020 and progressed steadily with intravenous analgesic support until discharge on 11/05/2020, when the patient was deemed stable.
Condition on Discharge: Stable.
Discharge Instructions: The patient is to limit activity and should follow up with Dr. Rohr in his office in 1 week.
Medications on Discharge: Biaxin, Suprax, Trental, folic acid, Toradol, and vitamin E.

 Exercise 13: **Healthcare Report**

Using the healthcare report above, answer the following questions.

1. What statement in the discharge summary indicates that the patient was in sickle cell crisis?

_____

2. Did Mr. Samuelson 's parents have sickle cell anemia? How do you know?

_____

3. The patient's past healthcare history mentions a resection of his _____

Match the word parts to their definitions.

WORD PART DEFINITIONS

Suffix	Definition
-cyte	1. _____ cell
-cytosis	2. _____ producing
-emia	3. _____ condition of abnormal increase in cells
-gen	4. _____ protein substance
-globin	5. _____ formation
-penia	6. _____ wasting
-philia	7. _____ condition of attraction
-phthisis	8. _____ condition of deficiency
-poiesis	9. _____ iron substance
-siderin	10. _____ blood condition

Combining Form	Definition
cyt/o	11. _____ blood
eosin/o	12. _____ rosy-colored
erythr/o	13. _____ eat, swallow
fibrin/o	14. _____ nucleus
globin/o	15. _____ iron
granul/o	16. _____ bone marrow
hem/o	17. _____ spleen
immun/o	18. _____ fever, fire
leuk/o	19. _____ red
lymph/o	20. _____ clotting, clot
morph/o	21. _____ fiber substance
myel/o	22. _____ cell
nucle/o	23. _____ protein substance
phag/o	24. _____ safety, protection
plasm/o	25. _____ white
pyr/o	26. _____ serum
ser/o	27. _____ little grain
sider/o	28. _____ plasma
splen/o	29. _____ thymus
thromb/o	30. _____ lymph
thym/o	31. _____ shape
tonsill/o	32. _____ tonsil

WORDSHOP

Prefixes	Combining Forms	Suffixes
a-	blast/o	-ar
an-	cyt/o	-cyte
pan-	eosin/o	-cytosis
per-	erythr/o	-ectomy
poly-	globin/o	-emia
pre-	granul/o	-ia
	hem/o	-pathy
	leuk/o	-penia
	lymphaden/o	-philia
	morph/o	-phthisis
	myel/o	-siderin
	nucle/o	
	sider/o	
	splen/o	
	thromb/o	

Build blood and immune terms by combining the word parts above. Some word parts may be used more than once. Some may not be used at all. The number in parentheses indicates the number of word parts needed.

Definition	Term
1. condition of deficiency of all cells (3)	
2. condition of abnormal increase of white cells (2)	
3. condition of attraction of rosy-colored (2)	
4. deficiency of clotting cells (3)	
5. cutting out of a lymph gland (2)	
6. condition of abnormal increase of red cells (2)	
7. condition of no spleen (3)	
8. condition of deficiency of immature red blood (cells) (3)	
9. cell without little grains (3)	
10. without a blood condition (2)	
11. iron substance in the blood (2)	
12. condition of iron deficiency (2)	
13. many cell nucleus shapes (4)	
14. disease process of blood protein (3)	
15. wasting of bone marrow (2)	

Sort the terms below into the correct categories.

TERM SORTING

Anatomy and Physiology	Pathology	Procedures

adenoidectomy	erythroblastopenia	myelophthisis
agglutinogen	G6PD	phagocytosis
antigen	Hct	plasma
apheresis	hematopoiesis	prothrombin
autotransfusion	hemoglobin	purpura
BMP	hemoglobinopathy	sarcoidosis
BMT	hemophilia	Schilling test
CBC	homeostasis	septicemia
CML	interferon	sickle cell trait
CMP	interleukin	sideropenia
cytokine	lymphadenectomy	splenectomy
DIC	MCH	splenitis
diff count	monocytosis	thalassemia
ELISA	monokine	thrombocyte
eosinophil	morphology	

Replace the highlighted words with the correct terms.

TRANSLATIONS

1. Ms. Cooper was diagnosed with **inflammation of the spleen** and she was scheduled for a **removal of the spleen.**

2. Mrs. Hamilton's laboratory findings indicated **condition of deficiency of all blood cells** and she was diagnosed with **suppression of bone marrow function leading to a reduction in RBC production.**

3. Laboratory testing revealed that Marc Douglas had **a condition of abnormal increase in WBCs** and that a **blood sample submitted to propagate microorganisms that may be present** was positive for staphylococci.

4. Three weeks after the patient's kidney transplant, he was diagnosed with **a disorder occurring when donated tissue cells attack recipient cells.**

5. The patient underwent a **transplantation of bone marrow to stimulate production of normal blood cells** to treat his **rapidly progressive form of leukemia that develops from immature bone marrow stem cells.**

6. Mr. Washington was admitted with **an acute, painful exacerbation of sickle cell anemia** that was complicated by **an increased function of the spleen that results in hemolysis.**

7. **Removal of thrombocytes** from a donor was used to treat Theresa Alvarez's **deficiency of platelets that causes an inability of the blood to clot.**

8. The patient was diagnosed with **RBC deficiency caused by blood loss** and needed a/an **intravenous transfer of blood from a donor to a recipient.**

9. The cancer patient was suffering from **wasting of bone marrow.**

10. The physician suspected that Alex had **a deficiency of one of the factors necessary for the coagulation of blood** and ordered a **test of blood plasma to detect coagulation defects of the intrinsic system.**

Circulatory System

OBJECTIVES

☐ Recognize and use terms related to the anatomy and physiology of the circulatory system.

☐ Recognize and use terms related to the pathology of the circulatory system.

☐ Recognize and use terms related to the procedures for the circulatory system.

ICD-10-CM Example from Tabular

I21.Ø ST elevation (STEMI) myocardial infarction of anterior wall

Type 1 ST elevation myocardial infarction of anterior wall

I21.Ø1 ST elevation (STEMI) myocardial infarction involving left main coronary artery

I21.Ø2 ST elevation (STEMI) myocardial infarction involving left anterior descending coronary artery

ST elevation (STEMI) myocardial infarction involving diagonal coronary artery

I21.Ø9 ST elevation (STEMI) myocardial infarction

Involving other coronary artery of anterior wall

Acute transmural myocardial infarction of anterior wall

Anteroapical transmural (Q wave) infarction (acute)

Anterolateral transmural (Q wave) infarction (acute)

Anteroseptal transmural (Q wave) infarction (acute)

Transmural (Q wave) infarction (acute) (of) anterior (wall) NOS

ICD-10-PCS Example from Index

Phlebectomy

see Excision, Upper Veins **Ø5B**

see Extraction, Upper Veins **Ø5D**

see Excision, Lower Veins **Ø6B**

see Extraction, Lower Veins **Ø6D**

Phlebography

see Plain Radiography, Veins **B5Ø**

Impedance 4A04X51

Phleborrhaphy

see Repair, Upper Veins **Ø5Q**

see Repair, Lower Veins **Ø6Q**

Phlebotomy

see Drainage, Upper Veins **Ø59**

see Drainage, Lower Veins **Ø69**

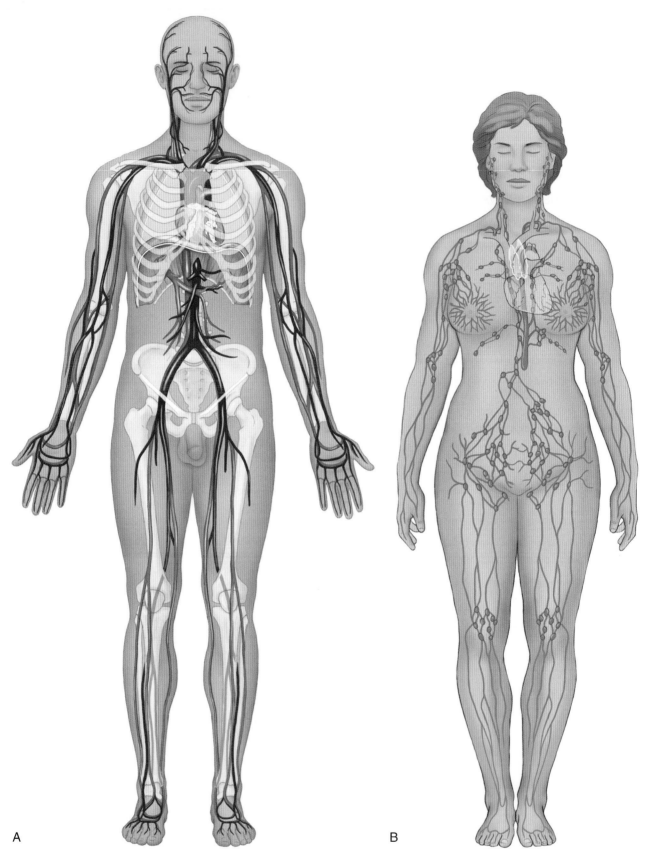

Fig. 9-1 **Circulatory system. A,** Cardiovascular system. **B,** Lymphatic system.

The circulatory system includes the body systems of the heart and vessels (the cardiovascular system) as well as that of the lymphatic organs, nodes, and their own specialized vessels (the lymphatic system) (Fig. 9-1). These subdivisions of the character for body systems comprise over a quarter of the specific body systems detailed in the Medical and Surgical section of the PCS, so as you may expect, there is a great deal of anatomy to be covered. Your knowledge of medical terminology word parts will make it much easier.

The anatomy and physiology of the system is divided into the cardiovascular structures (heart and great vessels, and upper/lower arteries and veins), followed by the lymphatic and hemic systems as detailed in the Procedural Classification System. An "upper" or "lower" vessel is defined by its position with respect to the diaphragm, with upper vessels located above the diaphragm and lower vessels located below it.

 PCS Guideline Alert

B2.1b Body systems designated as upper or lower contain body parts located above or below the diaphragm, respectively.*

*The lymphatic and hemic structures (spleen, bone marrow, and stem cells) are NOT separated into upper/lower body parts.

Terminology of the anatomy and physiology of the circulatory system is divided into the following sections:
- circulatory system functions
- pulmonary and systemic circulation
- the heart and great vessels
- blood flow through the heart
- the cardiac cycle and conductive mechanisms
- upper arteries
- lower arteries
- upper veins
- lower veins
- fetal circulation
- lymphatic and hemic structures

 Any vessel that an individual is born with is termed a "native vessel," as opposed to those that may be acquired from another individual, an animal, or made from synthetic fibers. Note that the word *native* is derived from *nat/o*, meaning "birth," and *-ive*, meaning "pertaining to".

THE CARDIOVASCULAR SYSTEM

FUNCTIONS OF THE CARDIOVASCULAR SYSTEM

The primary function of the circulatory system (Fig. 9-1) is to provide a means of transportation for nutrients, water, oxygen, hormones, and body salts (to) and wastes (from) the cells of the body. It also serves a protective role by dispatching

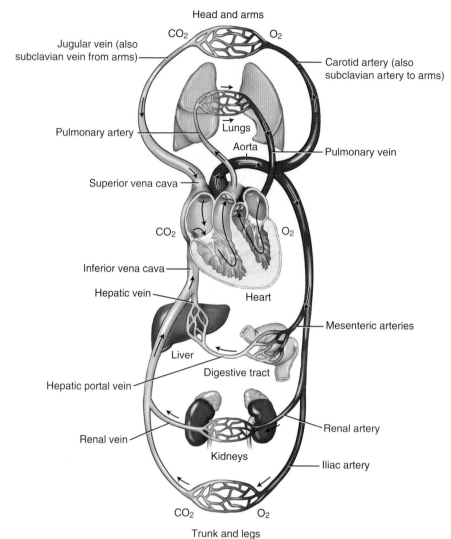

Fig. 9-2 Circulation of the blood.

specialized defensive cells through the lymphatic system. Both of these tasks require anatomical structures and mechanisms that direct these. "highways" to every cell of the body without stopping. As will be discussed, any disruption to these functions may result in a disease or disorder of the circulatory system.

Pulmonary and Systemic Circulation

Pulmonary Circulation

Pulmonary circulation begins with the right side of the heart, sending blood to the lungs to absorb **oxygen (O_2)** and to release **carbon dioxide (CO_2).** Note in Fig. 9-2 that the vessels that carry blood to the lungs from the heart are blue—to show the blood as being deoxygenated, or oxygen deficient. Once the oxygen is absorbed, the blood is considered oxygenated, or oxygen rich and is now colored red. Note also in Fig. 9-2 that the vessels traveling away from the lungs are red to show oxygenation. The blood then progresses back to the left side of the heart, where it is pumped out to begin its route through the systemic circulatory system.

Systemic Circulation

Systemic circulation carries blood from the **heart** to the cells of the body, where nutrient and waste exchange takes place. Certain organs of the body are key

oxygen = ox/i, ox/o, oxy-

carbon dioxide = capn/o

heart = cardi/o, coron/o, cordi/o

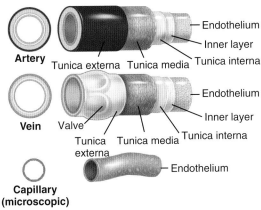

Fig. 9-3 Layers of the artery, vein and capillary.

to the process of waste removal. During systemic circulation, blood passes through the **kidneys.** This part of systemic circulation is known as **renal circulation.** In this phase, the kidneys filter much of the waste from the blood to be excreted in the urine. Blood also passes through the small intestine during systemic circulation. This phase is known as **portal circulation.** Here, the blood from the small intestine collects in the portal vein, which passes through the **liver.** The liver filters sugars from the blood and stores them for use as needed. On return to the right side of the heart, the blood is pushed out to the **lungs** to dispose of its CO_2, absorb O_2, and repeat the cycle. Fig. 9-2 shows the oxygenated/deoxygenated status of blood.

In systemic circulation, the blood traveling away from the heart first passes through the largest artery in the body, the **aorta.** From the aorta, the **vessels** branch into conducting **arteries,** then into smaller **arterioles,** and finally to the **capillaries.** Note in Fig. 9-2 that the color has changed from the red of oxygenated blood to a purple color at the capillaries. This is the site of exchange between the cells' fluids and the plasma of the circulatory system. Oxygen and other substances are supplied, and carbon dioxide is collected, along with a number of other wastes. Once the blood begins its journey back to the heart, it first goes through **venules,** then **veins,** and finally into one of the two largest veins, the **superior** or **inferior vena cava.** The great vessels commonly include the pulmonary arteries and veins, the superior and inferior venae cavae, and the aorta. In ICD-10-PCS, however, these vessels are further divided into upper and lower arteries and veins, using the diaphragm as the separation. The aorta is divided into a thoracic portion (ascending/arch and descending segment) above the diaphragm that is an upper artery, while the abdominal aorta (below the diaphragm) is a lower artery. The superior vena cava is an upper vein, while the inferior vena cava is a lower vein. All of these are great vessels, but for the reasons of coding, they need to be considered separately.

All of the vessels of the cardiovascular system (including the heart) share a lining of endothelial cells. While all carry blood, each type of vessel has a slightly different, but significant structure. Fig. 9-3 illustrates these differences. The muscular, thick arteries are composed of three tunics, or coats: the outer layer is called the **tunica externa** (adventitia), the muscle layer and elastic layer are called the **tunica media,** and the inner layer is called the **tunica interna** (intima). Compare the thickness and structure of an artery to the thinner, valvular nature of veins. Veins do not have the thick muscle coat of the arteries to propel the blood on its journey through the circulatory system but instead rely on one-way valves that prevent the backflow of blood. In addition, skeletal muscle contraction provides pumping action. The capillaries have no coats, and their diameters are so tiny that only one blood cell at a time can pass through them.

kidney = nephr/o, ren/o

renal
  ren/o = kidney
  -al = pertaining to

liver = hepat/o

lung = pulmon/o, pneum/o, pneumat/o

aorta = aort/o

vessel = vascul/o, angi/o, vas/o

artery = arteri/o

arteriole = arteriol/o

venule = venul/o

vein = ven/o, phleb/o

According to ICD-10-PCS, the inferior vena cava is classified as a lower vein. Remember, *inferior* means "lower." Most of that vein is below the diaphragm.

Exercise 1: Pulmonary and Systemic Circulation

Match the following combining forms with their meanings. More than one answer may be correct.

____ 1. vein

____ 2. artery

____ 3. heart

____ 4. venule

____ 5. lung

____ 6. aorta

____ 7. arteriole

____ 8. vessel

A. vas/o

B. pulmon/o

C. angi/o

D. phleb/o

E. arteri/o

F. ven/o

G. cardi/o

H. vascul/o

I. arteriol/o

J. aort/o

K. venul/o

Translate the terms.

9. endovascular _____

10. intravenous _____

11. pericardial _____

ANATOMY AND PHYSIOLOGY OF THE CARDIOVASCULAR SYSTEM

Heart and Great Vessels

apex = apic/o

precordium = precordi/o

atrium = atri/o

auricular = auricul/o

ventricle = ventricul/o

trabecula = trabecul/o

valve = valv/o, valvul/o

septum = sept/o

atrioventricular
  atri/o = atrium
  ventricul/o = ventricle
  -ar = pertaining to

endocardium =
  endocardi/o

myocardium =
  myocardi/o

pericardium = pericardi/o

organ, viscera = viscer/o

wall = pariet/o

epicardium = epicardi/o

transmural
  trans- = through
  mur/o = wall
  -al = pertaining to

The human heart is about the size of a fist. It is located in the mediastinum of the thoracic cavity, slightly left of the midline. Its pointed tip, the **apex,** rests just above the diaphragm. The area of the chest wall anterior to the heart and lower thorax is referred to as the **precordium** because of its location "in front of" the heart.

Inside, the heart has four chambers (Fig. 9-4). The upper chambers are called **atria** (*sing.* atrium). The ear-shaped pouch that is connected to each atrium is called the **auricular appendage** (see Fig. 9-6, *B*). Clinically, the right auricular appendage is associated with a rapid heartbeat (tachycardia), while the left auricular appendage is associated with blood clots from atrial fibrillation (an extremely rapid and irregular heartbeat). The lower chambers are called **ventricles,** which are composed of fleshy, beam-shaped structures called **trabeculae carneae** (see Fig. 9-5). Between the atria and ventricles, and between the ventricles and vessels, are **valves** that allow blood to flow through in one direction. The tissue wall between the top and bottom chambers is called the **atrioventricular septum** (*pl.* septa).

As we have already noted, the **great vessels** include the superior and inferior venae cavae, the pulmonary arteries and veins, and the aorta.

The heart wall is constructed of three distinct layers. The **endocardium** is composed of endothelial cells and connective tissue that act as a lining for each of the chambers and valves. The **myocardium** is the cardiac muscle surrounding each of these chambers. The **pericardium** is the double-folded layer of connective tissue that surrounds the heart. The pericardial cavity holds a serous fluid that protects the heart from friction. The inner layer of this double fold is called the **visceral pericardium,** and the outer membrane, closest to the body wall, is the **parietal pericardium.** Another name for the visceral pericardium is the **epicardium** because it is the structure on top of the heart. The term *transmural* is used to describe a heart disorder that is through the wall of the heart. An example would be a **transmural infarct,** which is tissue death (an infarct) that extends through the entire thickness of the heart wall from the endocardium to the epicardium.

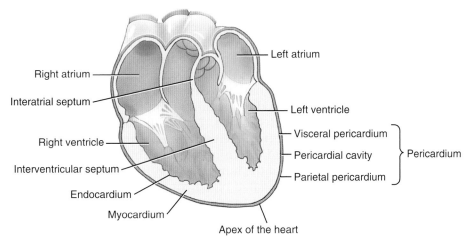

Fig. 9-4 Chambers of the heart.

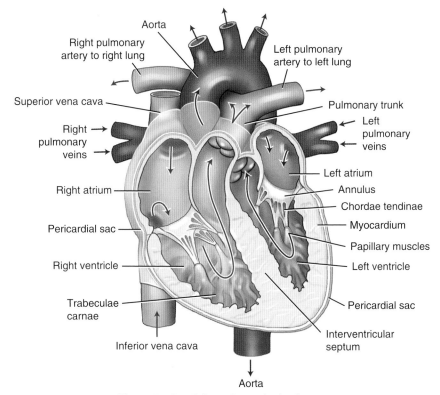

Fig. 9-5 Blood flow through the heart.

This chapter includes all the anatomy necessary to assign ICD-10 circulatory system codes, including detail on the coronary sinus, auricular appendages, and innominate artery. See Appendix H for a complete list of body parts and how they should be coded.

Coronary Circulation and Blood Flow Through the Heart

Using Fig. 9-5 as a guide, follow the route of the blood through the heart. The picture and arrows in this diagram are shaded red and blue to represent oxygenated and deoxygenated blood. Deoxygenated blood is returned to the heart through the venae cavae. The **superior vena cava** returns blood from the upper body, whereas the lower body is drained by the **inferior vena cava.** Blood is squeezed from the **right atrium (RA)** to the **right ventricle (RV)** through the **tricuspid valve (TV).** Valves are considered to be competent (capable) if they open and close properly, letting through or holding back an expected amount of blood. Once in the right ventricle the blood is squeezed out through the pulmonary semilunar valve into the **pulmonary arteries (PA),** which carry deoxygenated blood to the lungs from the heart. These are the only arteries that carry deoxygenated blood. The main pulmonary artery **(pulmonary trunk)** divides into right and left arteries to supply each lung. The **conus arteriosus** is the cone-shaped extension of the right ventricle into the pulmonary trunk. In the capillaries of the lungs, the CO_2 is passed out of the blood and O_2 is taken in. The now-oxygenated blood continues its journey back from the lungs to the left side of the heart through the **pulmonary veins (PV).** These are the only veins that carry oxygenated blood. The blood then enters the heart through the **left atrium (LA)** and has to pass the **mitral valve (MV),** also termed the **bicuspid valve,** to enter the **left ventricle (LV).** When the left ventricle contracts, the blood finally pushes out through the aortic semilunar valve into the **aorta** (the largest artery in the body) and begins yet another cycle through the body. The first part of the aorta, the **ascending aorta,** rises toward the head, then bends into the aortic arch and continues downward through the chest as the descending thoracic aorta. Once it passes the diaphragm, it is termed the **abdominal aorta.**

Each valve has a fibrous ring at its base called the **annulus.** The bicuspid valve has two leaflets (cusps) that are attached to two nipple-like papillary muscles by the **chordae tendineae,** cordlike tendons. The **papillary muscles** open and close the heart valves. The **tricuspid valve** has three leaflets attached to three papillary muscles, connected again by chordae tendineae. When a writer refers to heartstrings being tugged at in sentimental situations, he/she is referring to the chordae tendineae.

tricuspid
 tri- = three
 cusp/o = point
 -id = pertaining to

semilunar
 semi- = half
 lun/o = moon
 -ar = pertaining to

bicuspid
 bi- = two
 cusp/o = point
 -id = pertaining to

annulus, ring = annul/o

papillary = papill/o

chordae = chord/o

 CPT Coding Alert!

CPT has several codes that reference the sinus of Valsalva, a cavity in the wall of the aorta that is at the beginning of the right or left coronary artery, or which has no natural outlet at all. The first two of these sinuses are referred to as coronary sinuses because of their outlet into coronary arteries, while the third is considered a noncoronary sinus. The sinus of Valsalva is important to recognize in regard to procedures because it may be the site of an aneurysm. Synonym: aortic sinus

 CPT Coding Alert!

CPT references to the infundibulum of the heart refer to a conical structure in the anterosuperior portion of the right ventricle, at the entrance to the pulmonary trunk (arteries). Another name for the infundibulum of the heart is the conus arteriosus. The term *infundibulum* is from Latin for "funnel."

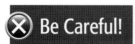 **Be Careful!**   *Don't confuse **chordae** (tendineae) with **chordee**, a disorder of the male reproductive system.*

The amount of blood expelled from the left ventricle is referred to as the **stroke volume,** while the percentage of blood expelled of the amount filling the ventricle is the **ejection fraction.** The ejection fraction is typically around 65%. Lower percentages occur in certain types of heart disease.

If a woman's heart rate is 80 beats per minute (BPM), that means her heart contracts almost 5000 times per hour and more than 100,000 times per day,

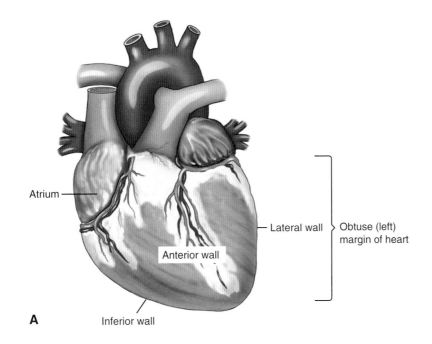

A

Atrium

Lateral wall } Obtuse (left) margin of heart

Anterior wall

Inferior wall

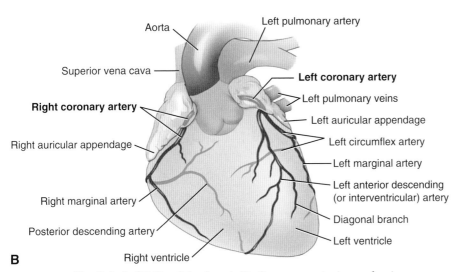

B

Aorta

Left pulmonary artery

Superior vena cava

Left coronary artery

Right coronary artery

Left pulmonary veins

Left auricular appendage

Right auricular appendage

Left circumflex artery

Left marginal artery

Right marginal artery

Left anterior descending (or interventricular) artery

Posterior descending artery

Diagonal branch

Left ventricle

Right ventricle

Fig. 9-6 A, Walls of the heart. **B,** Coronary arteries and veins.

every day, for a lifetime. Truly an amazing amount of work is accomplished by an individual's heart without a bit of conscious thought!

The heart muscle has its own dedicated system of blood supply, the **coronary arteries** (Fig. 9-6). The two main coronary arteries are called the left and right coronary arteries (LCA, RCA). The right coronary artery branches to form the posterior (interventricular) descending artery, which divides to form the atrioventricular artery and finally the posterior septal artery. The other main branch of the RCA is the marginal artery, which divides to form the acute marginal artery. The left coronary artery branches to form the anterior (interventricular) descending branch, which continues to the anterior septal artery. It also forms a circumflex branch that divides into anterior and posterior ventricular branches. They supply a constant, uninterrupted blood flow to the heart muscle. Blockage of the left anterior descending artery is referred to as the "widowmaker" due to the resultant high death rate. Table 9-1 illustrates the path of blood through the coronary arteries. The return to the circulatory system is via the coronary veins, which deposit the deoxygenated blood into the coronary sinus, a small cavity where the blood is collected before it empties into the right atrium. The shallow grooves that hold

coronary
  coron/o = heart, crown
  -ary = pertaining to

these arteries on the surface of the heart are termed the left and right coronary sulci (*sing.* sulcus). In the human embryo, the **sinus venosus** is a hollow space that holds the blood as it returns to the heart. In normal development, the right side of the space becomes part of the right atrium. On the left side it becomes the **coronary sinus** and the oblique vein. One type of heart defect, an abnormal opening between the upper chambers of the heart (termed *atrial septal defect*) can result from abnormal development of the right side of this embryonic structure. The areas of the heart wall supplied by the coronary arteries are designated as the inferior, lateral, anterior, and posterior walls. The left margin (also called the obtuse margin) is formed mainly by the left ventricle. Table 9-1 shows where the blood goes after leaving the ascending aorta.

Table 9-1 Schematic Showing Coronary Arteries

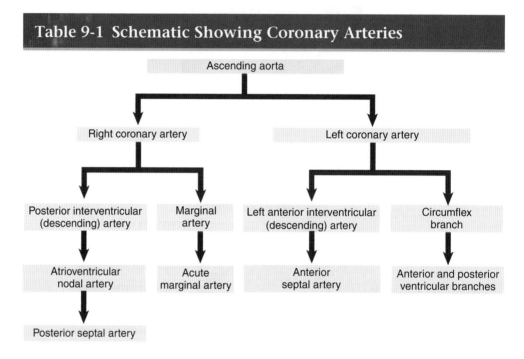

 PCS Guideline Alert

B4.4 CORONARY ARTERIES
The coronary arteries are classified as a single body part that is further specified by number of arteries treated. One procedure code specifying multiple arteries is used when the same procedure is performed, including the same device and qualifier values. Separate body part values are used to specify the number of sites treated when the same procedure is performed on multiple sites in the coronary arteries.

Conductive Mechanism System

Systemic and pulmonary circulations occur as a result of a series of coordinated, rhythmic pulsations, called *contractions* and *relaxations,* of the heart muscle. The cardiac muscle is controlled by the autonomic nervous system, so (thankfully) the heart beats involuntarily. The normal rate of these pulsations in humans is 60 to 100 bpm and is noted as a patient's heart rate. Fig. 9-7 illustrates various pulse points, places where heart rate can be measured in the body. **Blood pressure (BP)** is the resulting force of blood against the arteries. The contractive phase is **systole,** and the relaxation phase is **diastole.** Blood pressure is recorded as systolic pressure over the diastolic pressure. Optimal blood pressure is a systolic reading less than 120 and a diastolic reading less than 80. Normal blood pressure is represented by a range. See the table below for blood pressure guidelines.

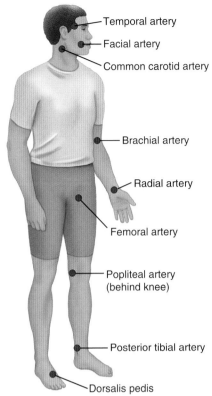

Fig. 9-7 Pulse points.

- Temporal artery
- Facial artery
- Common carotid artery
- Brachial artery
- Radial artery
- Femoral artery
- Popliteal artery (behind knee)
- Posterior tibial artery
- Dorsalis pedis

Blood Pressure Guidelines

	Systolic	Diastolic
Optimal	Under 120 and	Under 80
Normal	120-139 and	80-84
High-normal	130-139 or	85-89

The cues for the timing of the heartbeat come from the electrical pathways in the muscle tissue of the heart (Fig. 9-8) termed the **conductive mechanism.** The heartbeat begins in the right atrium at the **sinoatrial (SA) node,** called the natural pacemaker of the heart. The initial electrical signal causes the atria to undergo electrical changes that signal contraction. This electrical signal is sent to the **atrioventricular (AV) node,** specialized cardiac tissue that is located at the base of the right atrium proximal to the interatrial septum. From the AV node, the signal travels next to the **bundle of His** (also called the *atrioventricular bundle*), which carries the electrical impulse from the top to the bottom chambers. This bundle is in the interatrial septum, and its right and left bundle branches transmit the impulse to the **Purkinje fibers** in the right and left ventricles. Once the Purkinje fibers receive stimulation, they cause the ventricles to undergo electrical changes that signal contraction to force blood out to the pulmonary arteries and the aorta. If the electrical activity is normal, it is referred to as a **normal sinus rhythm (NSR)** or heart rate. Any deviation of this electrical signaling may lead to an **arrhythmia,** an abnormal heart rhythm that compromises an individual's cardiovascular functioning by pumping too much or too little blood during that segment of the cardiac cycle.

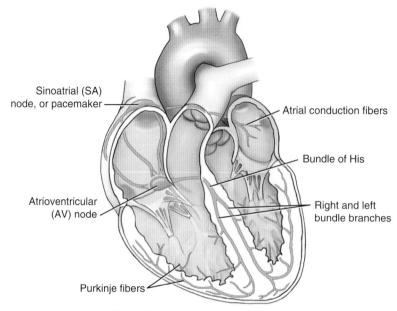

Fig. 9-8 Conductive mechanism.

ICD Note

If you see documentation for a bundle of Kent, you should realize that this is a congenital abnormal pathway between an atrium and a ventricle, not a normal anatomical structure.

electrocardiogram
  electr/o = electricity
  cardi/o = heart
  -gram = recording

Fig. 9-9 is a visual representation of the conductive mechanism of the heart through the use of an **electrocardiogram (EKG/ECG).** You can see the relationship of the electrical activity of the heart to the flow of blood through its chambers.

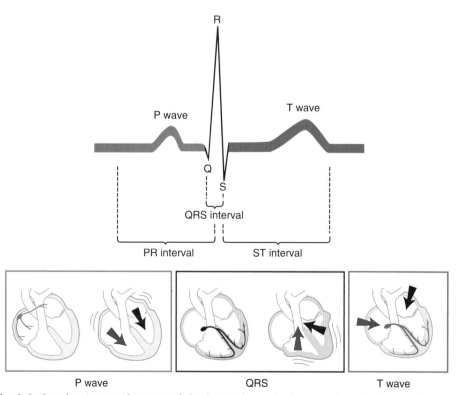

Fig. 9-9 Conductive mechanism of the heart through the use of an electrocardiogram.

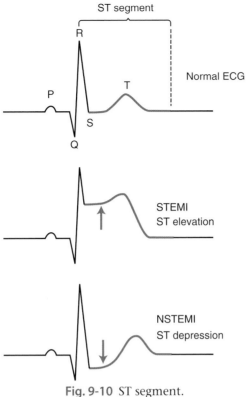

Fig. 9-10 ST segment.

When the SA node (the pacemaker of the heart) fires, the voltage of both atria decreases (referred to as *depolarization*). This drop in voltage appears as an upward tracing (termed a *deflection*) called a **P wave.** The P wave represents the atria contracting to push blood through their respective valves and into the ventricles.

The impulse next travels to the AV node, the AV bundle, and the Purkinje fibers. Once these fibers are activated, this sequence causes the ventricles to relax and contract. This depolarization appears as the **QRS segment** on an EKG.

The repolarization (the **T wave)** represents the recovery time when the atria fill with blood from the venae cavae and pulmonary veins.

The **ST segment** is an indicator of heart muscle function. Fig. 9-10 shows the comparison among the normal tracing of an ECG with the one from a STEMI (ST elevation myocardial infarction) and one from an NSTEMI (non-ST elevation myocardial infarction).

Exercise 2: **Heart and Great Vessels**

A. *Match the word parts with the meanings below.*

_____ 1. atri/o	A. heart muscle
_____ 2. endocardi/o	B. cord (used to describe the "heartstrings")
_____ 3. pericardi/o	C. point
_____ 4. ventricul/o	D. structure that allows blood to flow through in one direction
_____ 5. aort/o	E. top chamber of heart
_____ 6. myocardi/o	F. little ear (structure on atrium)
_____ 7. lun/o	G. inner lining of the heart
_____ 8. valv/o, valvul/o	H. pointed extremity
_____ 9. apic/o	I. largest artery in the body
_____ 10. sept/o	J. moon
_____ 11. auricul/o	K. little beam (used to describe fleshy tissue in ventricles)
_____ 12. trabecul/o	L. lower chamber of heart
_____ 13. chord/o	M. wall, between chambers
_____ 14. cusp/o	N. sac surrounding the heart
_____ 15. papill/o	O. nipplelike structure (supports chordae tendineae)
_____ 16. precordi/o	P. in front of the heart
_____ 17. epicardi/o	Q. structure on top of the heart
_____ 18. coron/o	R. heart, crown

B. *Match the structure in the heart and/or great vessels with its definition.*

_____ 1. chordae tendineae	A. the pacemaker of the heart
_____ 2. precordium	B. a pulmonary artery/vein, the thoracic aorta or superior vena cava
_____ 3. mitral (bicuspid) valve	C. the valve between the left ventricle and aorta
_____ 4. epicardium	D. the inner layer of the sac surrounding the heart
_____ 5. tricuspid valve	E. muscles that open/close heart valves
_____ 6. parietal pericardium	F. tissue that communicates electrical impulse from the top to the bottom chambers
_____ 7. atrioventricular septum	
_____ 8. pulmonary arteries	G. an artery/vein that an individual is born with
_____ 9. pulmonary veins	H. area anterior to the heart
_____ 10. pulmonary trunk	I. "heart strings," the cordlike tendons that connect valves
_____ 11. superior vena cava	J. valve between the right atrium and right ventricle
_____ 12. trabeculae carneae	K. valve between the right ventricle and pulmonary artery
_____ 13. papillary muscles	L. valve between the left atrium and left ventricle
_____ 14. great vessel	M. wall between the top and bottom chambers of the heart
_____ 15. native vessel	N. outer layer of the sac surrounding the heart
_____ 16. pulmonary semilunar valve	O. transmits signal to interatrial septum
_____ 17. aortic semilunar valve	P. the fleshy beamlike structure of the ventricles
_____ 18. AV node	Q. vessels that return blood from the lungs to the heart
_____ 19. SA node	R. large vein that returns blood to the heart from the upper body
_____ 20. bundle of His	S. vessels that carry blood from the heart to the lungs
	T. main pulmonary artery

To practice labeling the heart and great vessels, click on **Label It.**

Arteries

Arteries carry blood away from the heart. (Did you notice that both *arteries* and *away* start with an *A?*) For coding purposes in ICD-10-CM, the upper arteries are listed separately from the lower arteries. A quick way to remember what's upper and lower is by using the **diaphragm** to divide the body.

When we describe blood flow, we talk about first, second, and third order "branches" of vessels. If you think of the heart as the trunk of a tree, the blood flows to the different structures of the body by splitting into smaller and smaller branches (arteries). The largest of these structures are termed "first order" branches, whereas those that split off from those are called "second order" branches (and so on for third and fourth). When coding these, you may find that these third and fourth order branches are coded to their second level "parent." For example, the right lingual artery, which supplies blood to the tongue, receives its blood from the first order brachiocephalic artery, which branches into a second order right common carotid artery. From the right common carotid, a further branch (third order) is the right external carotid that then branches to a fourth order right superficial temporal artery. Finally, the lingual artery is the fifth order branch. Following it back, you can see that it is coded to the external carotid, a third order branch. For our descriptions of arteries, the listing will follow the blood flow, naming only the first and second order branches.

Upper Arteries

After leaving the aortic arch, the upper arteries (Fig. 9-11) branch toward the arms and head. The route of blood to the arms is slightly different on the right than on the left. On the right, the **innominate** (also called the **brachiocephalic**) artery is considered a first order branch.

> The word origins for *brachiocephalic* (*arms* and *head*) are helpful in understanding what body part is being supplied. ICD-10-CM, however, uses the term "innominate" for this artery. The word origin for *innominate* is literally "no name."

From it, the second order branch is the right subclavian artery, then the axillary artery, then the brachial artery, which divides into the radial and ulnar arteries, and finally those rejoin to form the palmar arches of the hand. On the left side of the body, the blood flows from the aortic arch to the left subclavian artery, on to the axillary artery, then to the brachial artery, which again divides into the radial and ulnar arteries, and then rejoins for the arteries of the hand at the palmar arch.

---

diaphragm = phren/o

lingual
  lingu/o = tongue
  -al = pertaining to

brachiocephalic
  brachi/o = arm
  cephal/o = head
  -ic = pertaining to

subclavian
  sub- = under
  clav/i = collarbone
  -an = pertaining to

axillary = axill/o

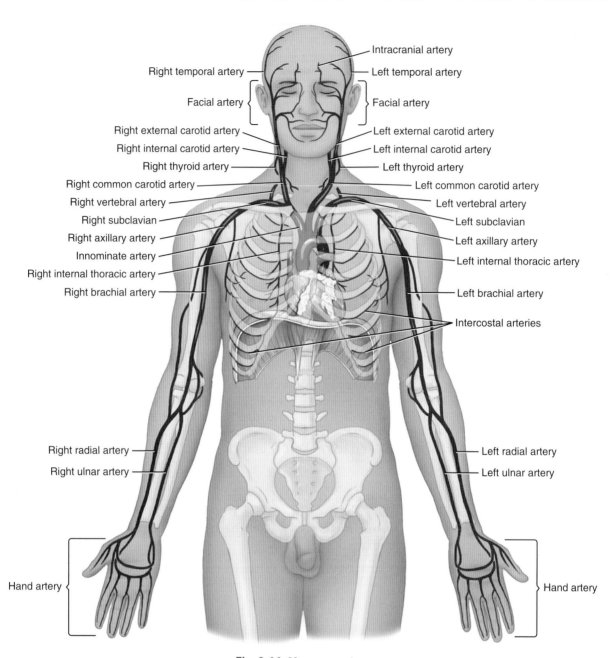

Fig. 9-11 Upper arteries.

face = faci/o

intracranial
   intra- within
   crani/o skull, cranium
   -al pertaining to

chest = thorac/o

The blood supply to the right side of the head occurs through the right common carotid to the right internal and external carotid arteries, and from the right subclavian to the right vertebral artery. On the left, blood flows to the left common carotid and branches to the left internal and external carotid arteries. The external carotids branch to supply blood to the face through the facial artery (also called the external maxillary artery). The external carotids also branch to form the superficial temporal artery and the internal maxillary artery. The right and left subclavian also carry blood to the neck through the left and right vertebral arteries. In the brain, the vertebral arteries merge to form a single basilar artery that supplies the posterior part of the **circle of Willis,** a circular formation of arteries that supply blood to the brain. These arteries in the skull are referred to as intracranial arteries.

The main blood supply to the chest is carried from the thoracic aorta to the right and left internal mammary arteries (also called the internal thoracic arteries

[ITA]) that branch from the right and left subclavian arteries. The blood supply to the thyroid is divided in two. The superior thyroid artery receives blood from the external carotid artery and supplies the upper part of the gland. The inferior thyroid artery, which supplies the lower part of the gland, receives its blood supply from the right and left subclavian arteries. The intercostal, bronchial, pericardial, esophageal, mediastinal, and superior phrenic arteries supply blood to the expected organs and structures.* Table 9-2 illustrates blood flow through the upper arteries.

rib = **cost/o**

bronchus = **bronchi/o, bronch/o**

diaphragm = **phren/o**

---

*Because the diaphragm is the dividing line between upper and lower arteries, the superior phrenic artery is included as an *upper artery* because it supplies blood flow to the upper surface of the diaphragm. The **inferior phrenic** artery, however, is categorized as a *lower artery* because its job is to supply blood to the lower surface of the same organ.

Table 9-2 Schematic Showing Upper Arteries

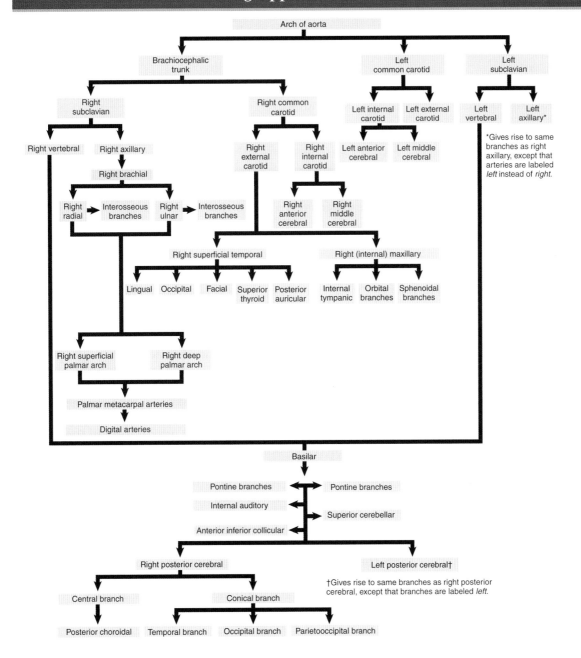

Exercise 3: Upper Arteries

A. Match the word parts with the meanings below.

____ 1. cost/o	____ 6. bronchi/o	A. armpit	F. airway
____ 2. clav/i	____ 7. cephal/o	B. chest	G. rib
____ 3. phren/o	____ 8. axill/o	C. diaphragm	H. collarbone
____ 4. brachi/o	____ 9. faci/o	D. arm	I. head
____ 5. thorac/o	___ 10. vertebr/o	E. face	J. backbone

B. Match the upper artery named with the area that it supplies blood to.

____ 1. brachial artery
____ 2. axillary artery
____ 3. superior phrenic artery
____ 4. bronchial artery
____ 5. intercostal artery
____ 6. basilar artery
____ 7. facial artery
____ 8. brachiocephalic artery
____ 9. internal thoracic artery
___ 10. left subclavian artery
___ 11. internal/external carotid artery

A. the arm and head (also called the innominate)
B. the upper aspect of the diaphragm
C. the brain
D. the face
E. shoulder, chest, and armpit
F. main blood supply to the chest
G. left side of the body
H. the airways and respiratory tract
I. muscles between ribs
J. the arm and hand
K. head

To practice labeling the upper arteries, click on **Label It.**

abdomen = celi/o

stomach = gastr/o

liver = hepat/o

kidney = ren/o

midgut = mesenter/o

ilium = ili/o

femur = femor/o

back of knee = poplite/o

tibia = tibi/o

Lower Arteries

The lower arteries (Fig. 9-12) carry blood to the abdomen, pelvis, and legs. The first order celiac artery branches from the abdominal aorta into the second order left gastric artery (supplying blood to the stomach), the hepatic artery (liver), and splenic artery (spleen, pancreas, and stomach). The superior mesenteric artery, another first order branch, supplies the small intestine and part of the large intestine, then divides into second order right, middle, and left colic arteries that supply the large intestine. The first order renal arteries supply the kidneys, while another first order artery, the inferior mesenteric, supplies the distal end of the large intestine. The suprarenal arteries supply the adrenal glands located above (supra-) each kidney. The first order common iliac arteries supply the pelvis and lower extremities, then divide into the second order right and left internal iliac arteries (that supply the urinary and reproductive organs of the pelvis) and the external iliac arteries, which supply the lower extremities. The right and left femoral arteries are branches of the external iliac arteries and supply the muscles of the thigh. The popliteal arteries branch from the femoral artery and supply the knee and leg. The anterior and posterior tibial arteries are branches from the popliteal artery that supply the front and back of the lower leg. The peroneal artery is a branch from the posterior tibial artery and serves to supply blood to the lateral leg muscles. Finally, the arteries of the foot

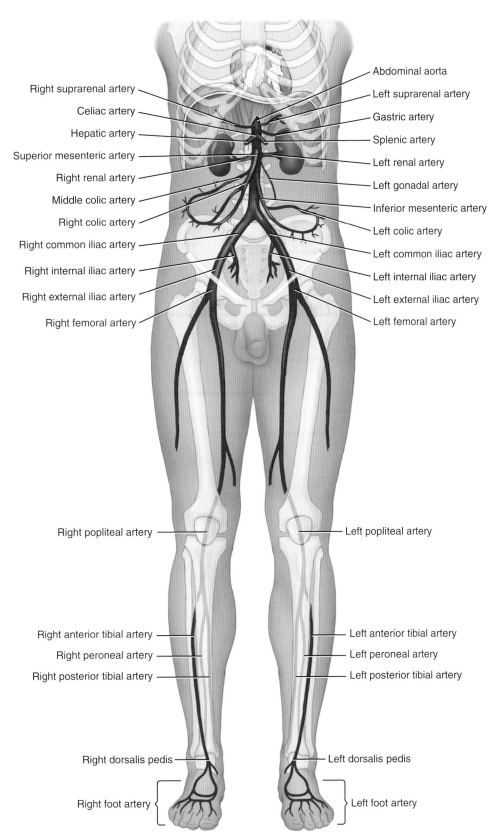

Right suprarenal artery
Celiac artery
Hepatic artery
Superior mesenteric artery
Right renal artery
Middle colic artery
Right colic artery
Right common iliac artery
Right internal iliac artery
Right external iliac artery
Right femoral artery

Abdominal aorta
Left suprarenal artery
Gastric artery
Splenic artery
Left renal artery
Left gonadal artery
Inferior mesenteric artery
Left colic artery
Left common iliac artery
Left internal iliac artery
Left external iliac artery
Left femoral artery

Right popliteal artery

Left popliteal artery

Right anterior tibial artery
Right peroneal artery
Right posterior tibial artery

Left anterior tibial artery
Left peroneal artery
Left posterior tibial artery

Right dorsalis pedis
Right foot artery

Left dorsalis pedis
Left foot artery

Fig. 9-12 Lower arteries.

| fibula = perone/o |
| foot = ped/o |
| ankle = tars/o |
| toe, finger = digit/o |

include the dorsalis pedis, which is a continuation of the anterior tibial artery and supplies blood to the ankle and dorsal part of the foot. Other arteries of the foot include the arcuate, tarsal, metatarsal, digital, and plantar arteries. Table 9-3 shows blood flow through the lower arteries. With the exception of the arcuate (meaning "bowed" or "curved") artery, the other names should be familiar from musculoskeletal anatomy.

Table 9-3 Schematic Showing Lower Arteries

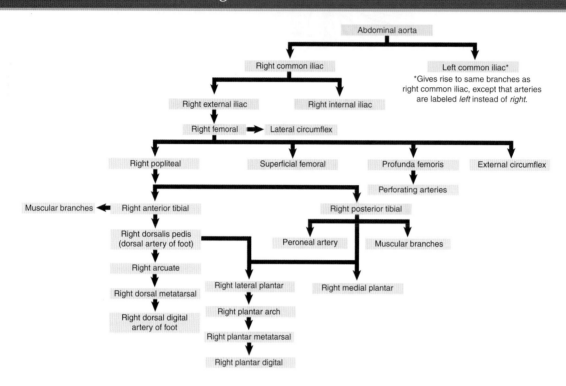

Exercise 4: Lower Arteries

A. Match the word parts with the meanings provided.

____ 1. femor/o   ____ 6. perone/o   A. midgut   F. liver

____ 2. ren/o   ____ 7. gastr/o   B. fibula   G. thighbone

____ 3. gonad/o   ____ 8. tibi/o   C. foot   H. stomach

____ 4. hepat/o   ____ 9. mesenter/o   D. sex organ   I. abdomen

____ 5. celi/o   ___ 10. ped/o   E. kidney   J. shinbone, lower leg bone

B. Match the lower artery with the area that it supplies blood to.

____ 1. peroneal artery	A. the adrenals
____ 2. dorsalis pedis artery	B. the distal part of the large intestine
____ 3. renal artery	C. the ankle and back part of the foot
____ 4. superior mesenteric artery	D. the ovaries and testes
____ 5. celiac artery	E. the knee and leg
____ 6. popliteal artery	F. the small intestine and part of large intestine
____ 7. femoral artery	G. lateral leg muscles
____ 8. gonadal artery	H. the abdominal organs
____ 9. inferior mesenteric artery	I. muscles of the thigh
____ 10. suprarenal artery	J. the kidney
____ 11. hepatic artery	K. the liver

To practice labeling the lower arteries, click on **Label It.**

Veins

Veins return blood to the heart. For coding purposes the upper and lower veins are categorized separately, in much the same way as the arteries. Fortunately, they share many of the names for the arteries, so remembering upper and lower is a bit easier than initially remembering all of those arteries. And, the same as for the arteries, the dividing line for upper and lower is the diaphragm.

vein = phleb/o, ven/o

In ICD-10-PCS the superior vena cava is classified as a great vessel of the heart, even though it is usually described as one of the two largest veins in the body. The inferior vena cava is classified as a lower vein.

In general, veins that are described as being "deep" are those that are far from the surface, while those that are "superficial" are those close to the surface.

Upper Veins

The upper veins (Fig. 9-13) return blood to the heart from the head, neck, arms, and chest cavity. If you remember that the word parts for many of the veins tell you where they are returning blood from, you just need to pay special attention to which ones drain into the larger veins that collect blood from several different ones (e.g., the jugulars, brachiocephalics, and subclavians).

In the head and neck, the facial veins drain the superficial parts of the face while the intracranial veins (e.g., ophthalmic, cerebral) drain the deeper structures of the skull. The vertebral veins drain the blood from the brain near the bones of the neck. The **external jugular veins** drain the superficial veins of

intracranial
  intra- = within
  crani/o = skull, cranium

vertebra, backbone = vertebr/o

throat, neck = jugul/o

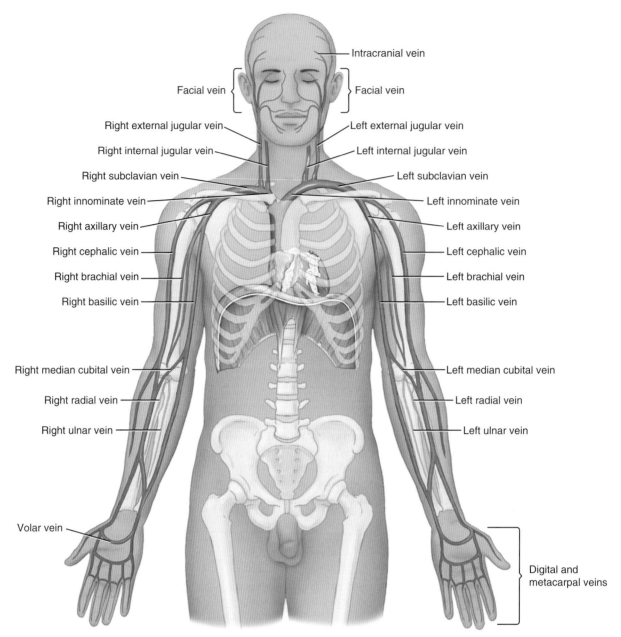

Fig. 9-13 Upper veins.

hand bone = metacarp/o

radius = radi/o

ulna = uln/o

armpit = axill/o

the head and neck, while the **internal jugular veins** drain blood from the deeper veins of the head and neck (including the intracranial veins). Both the internal and external jugular veins drain into the subclavian veins, located under the collarbones. The vertebral veins drain directly into the subclavian veins without a direct connection to one of the jugulars. The internal jugular joins the subclavian to form the brachiocephalic veins where the right and left sides merge to drain into the superior vena cava.

Blood is drained from the veins of the arms starting with the fingers and hands (e.g., palmar/volar digital and metacarpal veins). The deeper drainage of the lower arms is handled by the radial (lower lateral forearm) and ulnar (lower medial forearm) veins that anastomose (join) at the brachial vein. The brachial vein drains the upper arm, where it is eventually joined by the axillary vein, draining the area under the arm and continuing to join the subclavian, then brachiocephalic (innominate) vein, and finally the superior vena cava.

Superficial drainage of the arm is carried by the basilic veins that drain the hands and lower arm on the medial side of the arm and the cephalic veins on the lateral side. Both drain into the axillary vein and follow the same path back to the heart as the deeper veins described above. The median cubital vein (also referred to as the median basilic or antecubital vein) connects the basilic and cephalic veins and is often used as a site for blood draws. Note that the combining form *cubit/o* refers to the area of the elbow.

elbow = cubit/o

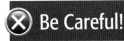 **Be Careful!** *Don't confuse the basilic vein in the arms with the basilar artery in the head.*

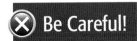 **Be Careful!** *The cephalic veins are in the arm, not in the head!*

The chest area is drained by the azygos vein *(azyg/o* means "without a yoke," meaning that it is a singular, not paired, vein), which resides in the thoracic cavity along with the hemiazygos vein and accessory hemiazygos vein that together collectively drain blood from the organs and tissues of the thoracic cavity. This includes the superior intercostal veins (draining the area between the upper ribs), the bronchial veins (draining the area around the airways of the lungs), and the pericardial veins (draining the sac surrounding the heart). The azygos vein drains the right side of the cavity, whereas the hemiazygos and accessory hemiazygos veins return blood from the left side of the same veins. These veins then drain back directly to the superior vena cava or through the brachiocephalic vein and then to the superior vena cava.

intercostal
inter- = between
cost/o = rib
-al = pertaining to

esophagus = esophag/o

Exercise 5: Upper Veins

A. Match the word parts with the meanings provided.

____ 1. azyg/o	____ 8. radi/o	A. arm
____ 2. pericardi/o	____ 9. jugul/o	B. airway, bronchus
____ 3. cephal/o	___ 10. uln/o	C. rib
____ 4. cubit/o	___ 11. vertebr/o	E. elbow
____ 5. cost/o	___ 12. clav/i	D. lower medial arm bone
____ 6. axill/o	___ 13. bronchi/o	F. sac surrounding heart
____ 7. brachi/o	___ 14. crani/o	G. armpit

H. lower lateral arm bone
I. not yoked (singular)
J. head
K. backbone
L. collarbone
M. throat, neck
N. skull

B. Match the upper veins with the areas that they drain blood from.

_____ 1. vertebral vein

_____ 2. subclavian vein

_____ 3. pericardial vein

_____ 4. external jugular vein

_____ 5. superior vena cava

_____ 6. ulnar vein

_____ 7. internal jugular vein

_____ 8. radial vein

_____ 9. brachiocephalic vein

___ 10. azygos vein

___ 11. brachial vein

___ 12. digital/metacarpal vein

___ 13. basilic vein

___ 14. cephalic vein

___ 15. axillary vein

A. superficial lateral side of lower arm and hands

B. armpit

C. thoracic cavity

D. deep vein of medial side of lower arm

E. brain, near neck bones

F. head, neck and upper extremity to superior vena cava

G. fingers and hands

H. sac surrounding the heart

I. superficial medial lower arms and hands

J. deeper veins of head and neck

K. deep vein of lateral side of lower arm

L. upper arm

M. superficial veins of head and neck

N. under the collarbone

O. upper veins of the body directly to the heart

To practice labeling the upper veins, click on **Label It.**

Lower Veins

The lower veins (Fig. 9-14) return blood to the inferior vena cava, collecting from the abdominopelvic cavity and legs.

Venous drainage for the legs begins in the toes and feet with the digital and metatarsal veins. The superficial drainage of the feet, thighs, and legs is accomplished through the **greater** and **lesser saphenous veins,** which are named for the Greek term meaning "clearly seen"—as indeed they are in their superficial location on the thigh. The greater saphenous vein is the one that is often used to furnish a short piece for coronary artery bypass grafts. Deep drainage is through the anterior and posterior tibial veins, which drain blood from the anterior and posterior lower leg and the dorsal part of the feet. The peroneal vein drains the lateral lower leg and joins the posterior tibial vein. These two veins, draining the deeper tissues of the lower leg, join to form the popliteal vein, which additionally drains the area of the knee, then continues to the femoral vein. The femoral vein drains the area of the upper thigh, where it becomes the external iliac vein.

The drainage of the abdominopelvic cavity is divided into the veins that drain within or outside of the **hepatic portal system.** The hepatic portal system drains most of the viscera in the upper abdomen, including the liver (hepatic veins), stomach (gastric veins), spleen (splenic veins), pancreas (pancreatic veins), and upper and lower midgut, which includes the small intestines, colon, and rectum (inferior and superior mesenteric veins). The esophageal veins drain the area of the esophagus. This system provides a means of detouring the blood through the liver before it is returned to the inferior vena cava. The advantages

toe = digit/o

foot bone = metatars/o

tibia = tibi/o

fibula = perone/o

back of knee = poplite/o

femur = femor/o

pelvic bone = ili/o

liver = hepat/o

gate = port/o

stomach = gastr/o

spleen = splen/o

pancreas = pancreat/o

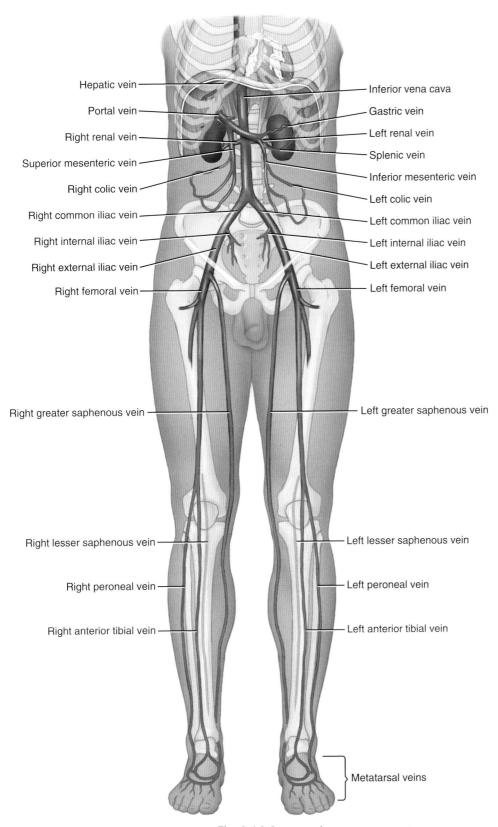

Hepatic vein

Portal vein

Right renal vein

Superior mesenteric vein

Right colic vein

Right common iliac vein

Right internal iliac vein

Right external iliac vein

Right femoral vein

Inferior vena cava

Gastric vein

Left renal vein

Splenic vein

Inferior mesenteric vein

Left colic vein

Left common iliac vein

Left internal iliac vein

Left external iliac vein

Left femoral vein

Right greater saphenous vein

Left greater saphenous vein

Right lesser saphenous vein

Right peroneal vein

Right anterior tibial vein

Left lesser saphenous vein

Left peroneal vein

Left anterior tibial vein

Metatarsal veins

Fig. 9-14 Lower veins.

mesentery = mesenter/o

adrenal gland = adren/o

kidney = ren/o

diaphragm = phren/o

include the removal and storage of glucose from the bloodstream for later use and the ability to remove toxins before they are sent back to the heart for general circulation. Outside of the hepatic portal system, the blood from the adrenal and renal veins (from the adrenal glands and kidneys), along with the inferior phrenic vein (from the lower surface of the diaphragm), empties directly into the inferior vena cava. The internal iliac vein drains the pelvic region. The internal and external iliac veins join to drain the lower extremities and pelvis through the common iliac veins, which drain into the inferior vena cava.

Exercise 6: Lower Veins

A. Match the combining form to its definition.

_____ 1. gastr/o   _____ 7. splen/o   A. toe, finger   G. shinbone

_____ 2. ren/o   _____ 8. hepat/o   B. liver   H. kidney

_____ 3. metatars/o   _____ 9. poplite/o   C. thigh   I. area behind the knee

_____ 4. port/o   ___ 10. digit/o   D. stomach   J. fibula

_____ 5. perone/o   ___ 11. mesenter/o   E. spleen   K. foot bone

_____ 6. femor/o   ___ 12. tibi/o   F. gate   L. midgut

B. Match the lower vein with the area that it drains blood from.

_____ 1. gastric   A. stomach

_____ 2. popliteal   B. groin/pelvis

_____ 3. inferior vena cava   C. kidney

_____ 4. anterior and posterior tibial   D. lower part of the body

_____ 5. hepatic   E. toes

_____ 6. splenic   F. digestive tract through the liver

_____ 7. greater and lesser saphenous   G. spleen

_____ 8. pancreatic   H. deep region of the thigh

_____ 9. hepatic portal   I. behind knee and lower leg

___ 10. renal   J. upper and lower midgut

___ 11. inferior phrenic   K. lower surface of diaphragm

___ 12. peroneal   L. anterior and posterior leg and dorsal foot

___ 13. digital   M. lateral leg

___ 14. superior and inferior mesenteric   N. superficial feet, thighs and legs

___ 15. femoral   O. liver

___ 16. internal iliac   P. pancreas

To practice labeling the lower veins, click on **Label It.**

Fetal Circulation

Because ICD-10-CM includes congenital heart defects, it is important to understand fetal circulation. Refer to Fig. 9-15 to compare the cardiovascular system before and after birth.

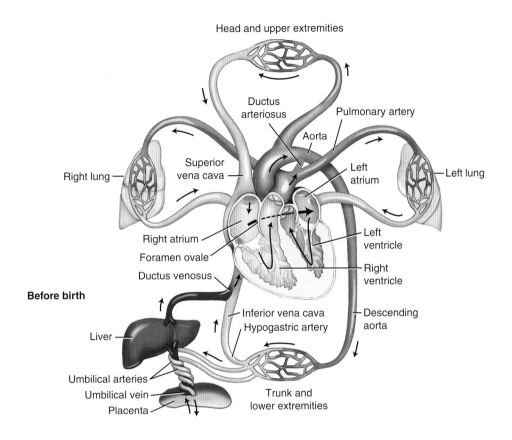

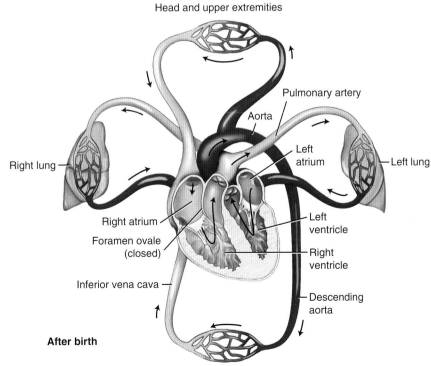

Fig. 9-15 Fetal circulation.

During gestation, the fetus shares the maternal circulatory system through the attachment of the umbilical cord to the organ of the placenta. All nutrition and oxygen are received and wastes removed through this connection.

Once the blood enters the right atrium of the fetal heart, it passes into the left atrium through a special opening named the **foramen ovale.** From the left atrium, the blood is pumped to the left ventricle, then to the aorta. From the aorta, the blood travels to the body. About one third of the blood entering the right atrium does not flow through the foramen ovale, but instead stays in the right side of the heart, eventually flowing into the pulmonary artery. Because the placenta does the work of exchanging oxygen (O_2) and carbon dioxide (CO_2) through the mother's circulation, the fetal lungs are not used for breathing. Instead of blood flowing to the lungs to pick up oxygen and then flowing to the rest of the body, the fetal circulation shunts (bypasses) most of the blood away from the lungs. In the fetus, blood is shunted from the pulmonary artery to the aorta through a connecting blood vessel called the **ductus arteriosus.** The ductus venosus is a major blood vessel that connects the left umbilical vein to the inferior vena cava and provides oxygenated blood for the fetus. After birth occurs, the foramen ovale, as well as the ductus arteriosus and ductus venosus, closes, and circulation to the lungs becomes the source of oxygen for the body. Congenital defects, including atrial septal defect and patent ductus arteriosus, occur when these structures do not close.

THE LYMPHATIC SYSTEM

FUNCTIONS OF THE LYMPHATIC SYSTEM

The **lymphatic system** is a series of organs, glands, and vessels that filter out microorganisms as the lymph passes through its various capillaries, vessels, and nodes. The lymphatic system is responsible for the following:
- Cleansing the cellular environment
- Returning proteins and tissue fluids to the blood
- Providing a pathway for the absorption of fats into the bloodstream
- Defending the body against disease

ANATOMY AND PHYSIOLOGY OF THE LYMPHATIC SYSTEM

lymph = lymph/o, lymphat/o, chyl/o

lymph vessel = lymphangi/o

lymph gland = lymphaden/o

bone marrow = myel/o

The lymphatic system (Fig. 9-16) is composed of **lymph** (or interstitial fluid), **lymph vessels, lymph glands, lymph organs** (e.g., bone marrow, tonsils, adenoids, appendix, spleen, and thymus gland), patches of tissue in the intestines called **Peyer's patches,** and **lymphoid tissue.** Lymph is the clear fluid in lymphatic vessels composed mostly of lymphocytes and monocytes. Lymph vessels are the channels that collect and carry lymph from the body tissues to the bloodstream. Lymph glands (also called lymph nodes) are lymphatic tissues that produce lymphocytes and are located along the lymphatic vessels. Lymphatic glands are named for the areas of the body they are located in.

The **hemic** and **lymphatic** systems flow through separate yet interconnected and interdependent channels. Both are systems composed of vessels and the liquids that flow through them.

Fig. 9-16 shows the relationship of the lymphatic vessels to the circulatory system. Note the close relationship between the distribution of the lymphatic vessels and the venous blood vessels. Tissue fluid is drained by the lymphatic capillaries and is transported by a series of larger lymphatic vessels toward the heart.

Bone marrow is the tissue in the center of many bones, especially the sternum (breastbone), ilium (hipbone), and vertebrae (backbones), that is responsible

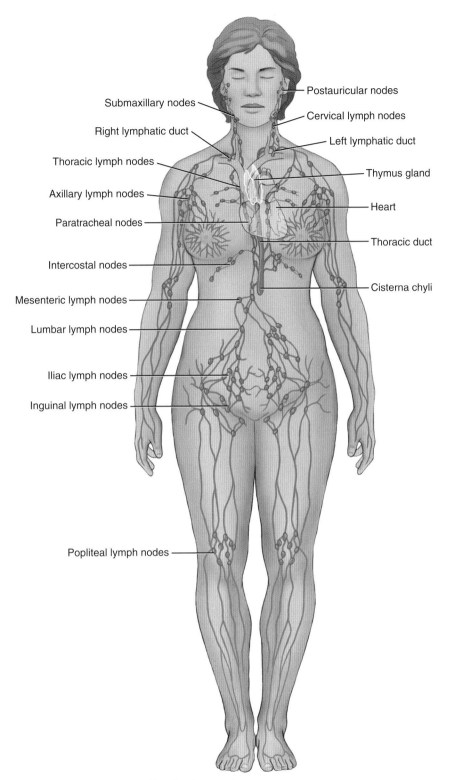

Submaxillary nodes

Postauricular nodes

Cervical lymph nodes

Right lymphatic duct

Left lymphatic duct

Thoracic lymph nodes

Thymus gland

Axillary lymph nodes

Heart

Paratracheal nodes

Thoracic duct

Intercostal nodes

Cisterna chyli

Mesenteric lymph nodes

Lumbar lymph nodes

Iliac lymph nodes

Inguinal lymph nodes

Popliteal lymph nodes

Fig. 9-16 Lymphatic system.

Circulation to lungs

Lymph capillaries

Pulmonary capillary network

Venule

Blood capillaries

Lymphatic capillaries

Arteriole

Lymph node

Lymphatic vessel

Tissue cell

Tissue space (interstitium)

Circulation to lower body

Fig. 9-16, cont'd

thymus gland = thym/o

spleen = splen/o

for the production of red and white blood cells. The white blood cells produced are either granulocytes or agranulocytes; their names come from whether they have (or lack) small grains in their appearance. The two types of agranulocytes, lymphocytes and monocytes, are key to the functioning of the immune system. Aside from the production of blood cells, the bone marrow also serves the important function of storing one of the types of lymphocytes (B cells) while they mature. B cells protect the body through the production of antibodies to antigens.

The **thymus gland,** located in the anterior superior mediastinum, is responsible for the production of T lymphocytes. T cells are a variety of further differentiated lymphocytes that are activated against specific types of pathogens.

The **spleen** is a gland located in the left upper quadrant (LUQ) of the abdomen; it is responsible for breaking down red blood cells (RBCs), storing blood, and producing lymphocytes and plasma cells.

Although part of the circulatory system, the lymphatic system does not depend on the heart muscle to force lymphatic fluid through its vessels. Instead, it depends on skeletal muscle movement, breathing, and gravity to flow. Monocytes and lymphocytes pass from the blood through the bloodstream's capillary walls into the interstitium (space between the cells in body tissue). Once there, they perform their protective/cleansing functions. Monocytes change into macrophages, destroy pathogens, and collect debris from damaged cells. Lymphocytes are much more complicated and are essential to the immune response; they are discussed in detail in Chapter 8. In brief, they function to direct their protective action toward pathogens through a variety of adaptations. Once monocytes and lymphocytes pass back into the lymphatic capillaries, the fluid is termed "lymph," or "lymphatic fluid."

Once the blood reaches the cells of the body through its capillaries, lymph travels toward the heart in the following sequence:

1. From the interstitial spaces to the lymphatic capillaries
2. From the lymphatic capillaries to the lymphatic vessels (thin, tubular-valved structures that carry lymph)

3. From the lymphatic vessels to the lymphatic nodes (also called lymph glands) that filter the debris collected through the efforts of the macrophages. These nodes can become enlarged when pathogens are present. Note the major lymph nodes in Fig. 9-16, including the cervical, axillary, and inguinal nodes.

4. From the lymph glands the lymph progresses to join the venous blood through one of two ducts. The **right lymphatic duct** empties its lymph from the right side of the upper body into the right subclavian vein, which drains into the superior vena cava. The **thoracic duct** empties its lymph from the left side and lower half of the body into the left subclavian and left internal jugular veins, which drain into the inferior vena cava. The **cisterna chyli** is a dilated sac in the lumbar area of the spine that is the origin of the thoracic duct. It is a major site of drainage from the intestines.

5. From the superior and inferior venae cavae, the venous blood with its incorporated lymph is returned to the right side of the heart to begin its journey again.

Lymph Nodes

Knowledge of terminology will help you to remember the locations of the many lymph nodes. Note that aside from the combining forms, the prefixes further describe the site.

The names and locations of the lymph nodes can be described starting with lymphatic drainage in the head. Lymph glands include the buccinators (cheeks), infraauricular (under the ears), infraparotid (under the parotid glands [near the ear]), preauricular (in front of the ear), submandibular (under the lower jawbone), submaxillary (under the upper jawbone), submental (under the chin), subparotid (under the parotid gland), and the suprahyoid (above the hyoid bone) nodes.

The main lymph nodes in the neck are the cervical nodes. Additionally, there are the jugular (named also for their location in the neck), postauricular (behind the ear), occipital (back of the head), retropharyngeal (behind the throat), and the supraclavicular (above the collarbone; also called Virchow nodes) lymph nodes. The right side of the neck has all the same nodes as the left, but also has the right jugular trunk, the right lymphatic duct, and the right subclavian (under the collarbone) trunk. Here, as in other vessels, the term "trunk" refers to the main part of the vessel before it branches into smaller vessels.

In the upper body, the axillary (armpit) lymph nodes are composed of the pectoral (chest and synonymous with anterior nodes), subclavicular (under the shoulder blade and synonymous with apical nodes), brachial (arm and also synonymous with lateral nodes), central axillary, and subscapular (under the shoulder blade and synonymous with posterior nodes) nodes.

The upper extremity lymph nodes include the cubital (elbow), infraclavicular (under the collarbone and synonymous with deltopectoral), and the epitrochlear and supratrochlear (above the trochlea of the elbow) lymph nodes.

In the thorax, there are the intercostal (between the ribs), parasternal (near the breastbone), paratracheal (near the windpipe), tracheobronchial (windpipe and the bronchi), and the mediastinal (space between the lungs) lymph nodes.

The aortic (largest artery in the body) lymph nodes include the celiac (abdominal), gastric (stomach), hepatic (liver), lumbar (loins), pancreaticosplenic (pancreas and spleen), and retroperitoneal (behind the lining of the abdominal cavity) lymph nodes.

The mesenteric (midgut) lymph nodes include the pararectal (near the rectum) and the superior and inferior mesenteric nodes.

In the pelvis, there are the suprainguinal (above the groin), subaortic (below the aorta and more commonly referred to as the common iliac), sacral (fused bone in

cheek = bucc/o

ear = auricul/o

upper jawbone = maxill/o

chin = ment/o

neck = cervic/o

pharyng/o = throat

clavicul/o = collarbone

chest = pector/o

elbow = cubit/o

ribs = cost/o

breastbone, sternum = stern/o

windpipe, trachea = trache/o

midgut = mesenter/o

groin = inguin/o

sacrum = sacr/o

sacrum = sacr/o

the lower spine, the sacrum), gluteal (the buttocks), inferior epigastric (above the stomach), and the obturator (the lateral openings in the pelvic bone) lymph nodes.
In the lower extremities, there are the femoral (thighbone) and popliteal (back of the knee) lymph nodes.

Exercise 7: Lymphatic System

A. Match the combining forms to their definitions.

____ 1. lymph/o, lymphat/o, chyl/o
____ 2. lymphangi/o
____ 3. lymphaden/o
____ 4. splen/o
____ 5. thym/o
____ 6. inguin/o
____ 7. aort/o
____ 8. occipit/o
____ 9. mesenter/o
____ 10. cost/o
____ 11. axill/o
____ 12. thorac/o
____ 13. myel/o
____ 14. cervic/o
____ 15. poplite/o
____ 16. auricul/o
____ 17. trache/o
____ 18. clavicul/o

A. largest artery in the body, aorta
B. armpit
C. groin
D. back of the head
E. chest
F. bone marrow
G. thymus gland
H. lymph vessel
I. ear
J. lymphatic fluid, lymph
K. back of knee
L. lymph gland, lymph node
M. midgut
N. rib
O. spleen
P. neck
Q. collarbone
R. windpipe, trachea

B. Match the terms to their definitions.

____ 1. lymph node
____ 2. cisterna chyli
____ 3. spleen
____ 4. thymus gland
____ 5. thoracic duct
____ 6. submaxillary nodes
____ 7. mesenteric nodes
____ 8. axillary nodes
____ 9. thoracic nodes
____ 10. postauricular nodes
____ 11. paratracheal nodes
____ 12. intercostal nodes
____ 13. right lymphatic duct
____ 14. lymph vessel
____ 15. suprainguinal nodes
____ 16. cervical nodes
____ 17. occipital nodes
____ 18. popliteal nodes

A. channels that collect and carry lymphatic fluid
B. channel that directs lymph into the right subclavian vein; drains upper right side of body
C. pertaining to the chest
D. gland in anterior superior mediastinum that produces T lymphocytes
E. pertaining to behind the ear
F. sac in the lumbar area of spine, origin of thoracic duct
G. pertaining to above the groin
H. pertaining to the back of the head
I. lymph gland, filtering tissue in lymphatic system
J. pertaining to under the upper jawbone
K. pertaining to the midgut
L. gland in LUQ, produces lymphocytes and plasma cells
M. pertaining to between the ribs
N. site of lymphatic drainage into the left subclavian and jugular veins; drains left side and lower half of body
O. pertaining to the armpit
P. pertaining to the neck
Q. pertaining to near the windpipe
R. pertaining to behind the knee

To practice labeling the lymphatic system, click on **Label It**.

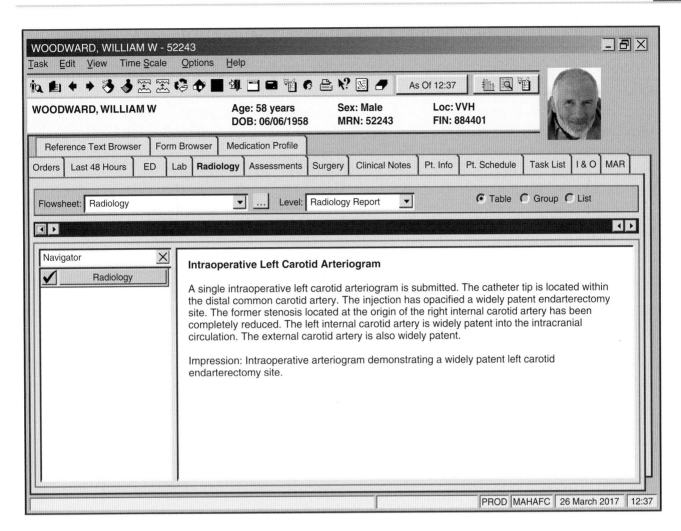

Exercise 8: Imaging Report

Underline the correct answer in the following questions using the report above.

1. "Intraoperative" tells you that the procedure was done *(before/during/after)* the operation.

2. The carotid arteries are located in the *(heart/neck/groin)* and supply blood to the *(myocardium/brain/legs)*.

3. An "endarterectomy" site would refer to an area *(within/above/near)* an artery.

4. The term "stenosis" in the report refers to a *(widening/narrowing)* of the artery.

Combining Forms for the Anatomy and Physiology of the Circulatory System

Meaning	Combining Form	Meaning	Combining Form
aorta	aort/o	carbon dioxide	capn/o
apex	apic/o	endocardium	endocardi/o
arteriole	arteriol/o	epicardium	epicardi/o
artery	arteri/o	gate	port/o
atrium	atri/o	heart	cardi/o, coron/o, cordi/o
bone marrow	myel/o	lung	pulmon/o, pneum/o, pneumat/o

Combining Forms for the Anatomy and Physiology of the Circulatory System—cont'd

Meaning	Combining Form	Meaning	Combining Form
lymph	lymph/o, lymphat/o	spleen	splen/o
lymph gland	lymphaden/o	thymus	thym/o
lymph vessel	lymphangi/o	valve	valvul/o
myocardium	myocardi/o	vein	ven/o, phleb/o
oxygen	ox/i, ox/o	ventricle	ventricul/o
pericardium	pericardi/o	venule	venul/o
precordium	precordi/o	vessel	vascul/o, angi/o, vas/o
septum, wall	sept/o		

Prefixes for Anatomy and Physiology of the Circulatory System

Prefix	Meaning
a-	without
con-	together
e-	out
infra-	under
inter-	between
intra-	within
oxy-	oxygen
para-	near
post-	behind
pre-	before
retro-	back
semi-	half
sub-	under
supra-	above

Suffixes for Anatomy and Physiology of the Circulatory System

Suffix	Meaning
-ar, -ary, -ic, -al, -id, -eal	pertaining to
-cyte	cell
-ia	condition
-ion	process of
-um	structure

You can review the anatomy of the Circulatory System by clicking on **Body Spectrum** and then **Circulatory** and **Lymphatic.**

PATHOLOGY

Terms Related to Symptoms and Signs of the Circulatory and Respiratory Systems (RØØ-R99)

Term	Word Origin	Definition
bradycardia	*brady-* slow *-cardia* heart condition	Slow heartbeat, with ventricular contractions less than 60 bpm (Fig. 9-17, B).
cardiac bruit		Abnormal sound heard on auscultation (listening with a stethoscope). Usually a blowing or swishing sound, higher pitched than a murmur. May be described as cardiac or arterial.
cardiac murmur	*cardi/o* heart *-ac* pertaining to	Abnormal heart sound heard during systole, diastole, or both, which may be described as a gentle blowing, fluttering, or humming sound.
cardialgia	*cardi/o* heart *-algia* pain	Heart pain that may be described as atypical or ischemic. Atypical pain is a stabbing or burning pain that is variable in location and intensity and unrelated to exertion. Ischemic pain is a pressing, squeezing, or weightlike cardiac pain caused by decreased blood supply that usually lasts only minutes. If specified as precordial pain, pain is in the area over the heart.
cyanosis	*cyan/o* blue *-osis* abnormal condition	Lack of oxygen in blood, seen as a bluish or grayish discoloration of skin, nail beds, and/or lips (Fig. 9-18).
diaphoresis		Profuse secretion of sweat. Also termed **hyperhidrosis** *(hidr/o* means "sweat"), although the term *diaphoresis* is more often used to describe profuse sweating when it is a symptom of a myocardial infarction.

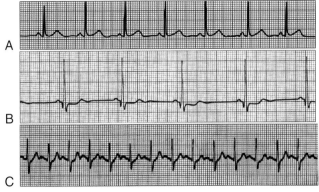

Fig. 9-17 **ECGs. A,** Normal. **B,** Bradycardia. **C,** Tachycardia.

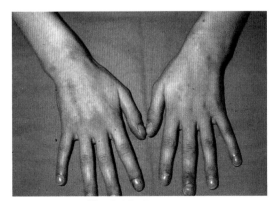

Fig. 9-18 Cyanosis.

Terms Related to Symptoms and Signs of the Circulatory and Respiratory Systems (RØØ-R99)—cont'd

Term	Word Origin	Definition
dyspnea; dyspnea on exertion (DOE)	*dys-* difficult *-pnea* breathing	Difficult and/or painful breathing; if DOE, it is experienced when effort is expended.
edema		Abnormal accumulation of fluid in interstitial spaces of tissues. Lymphedema is an accumulation of lymphatic fluid in the tissues due to inadequate drainage.
emesis	*-emesis* to vomit	The product of vomiting. The result of forcible or involuntary emptying of the stomach through the mouth.
nausea		Sensation that accompanies the urge to vomit but does not always lead to vomiting.
orthopnea	*orth/o* straight *-pnea* breathing	Difficulty with breathing relieved only when the patient is in an upright position.
pallor		Paleness of skin and/or mucous membranes. On darker-pigmented skin, it may be noted on the inner surfaces of the lower eyelids or the nail beds.
palpitations		Pounding or racing of the heart, such that the patient is aware of his/her heartbeat.
pulmonary congestion	*pulmon/o* lung *-ary* pertaining to	Excessive amount of blood in the pulmonary vessels. Usually associated with heart failure.
shortness of breath (SOB)		Breathlessness, air hunger.
syncope		Fainting, loss of consciousness.
tachycardia	*tachy-* rapid *-cardia* heart condition	Rapid heartbeat, more than 100 bpm (Fig. 9-17, C).

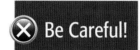 **Be Careful!**   *Do not confuse* **palpation,** *which means* examination by touch, **palpebration,** *which means* blinking, *and* **palpitation,** *which means* a pounding or racing of the heart.

Exercise 9: Cardiac Signs and Symptoms

Matching.

____ 1. syncope
____ 2. diaphoresis
____ 3. cardiac bruit
____ 4. cardiac murmur
____ 5. edema
____ 6. emesis
____ 7. palpitations
____ 8. pulmonary congestion
____ 9. cyanosis
___ 10. SOB

A. fainting
B. breathlessness, air hunger
C. accumulation of fluid in tissues
D. accumulation of blood in vessels of the lungs
E. blowing or swishing heart sound
F. gentle blowing, fluttering, or humming heart sound
G. blue color due to lack of oxygen
H. vomiting
I. profuse sweating
J. pounding of the heart

Translate the terms.

11. bradycardia_____

12. orthopnea_____

13. cardialgia_____

Terms Related to Chronic Rheumatic Heart Disease and Hypertensive Diseases (I10-I16)

Term	Word Origin	Definition
hypertension (HTN)	*hyper-* excessive, above *-tension* pressure	Excessive systemic arterial blood pressure. Can cause heart damage if persistent. Other descriptive terms include controlled/uncontrolled (whether it is or is not therapeutically corrected); primary/essential (due to unknown causes [idiopathic]); secondary (due to another disorder); transient (present for an expected, limited amount of time); or with retinopathy (literally, disease of the retina).
rheumatic heart disease (RHD)	*rheumat/o* watery flow	Damage to the heart, most often the valves, as a result of an episode of an inflammatory condition, rheumatic fever. The name is a nod to the additional fluid in the joints, which are also afflicted.

 CM Guideline Alert!

9.A HYPERTENSION

The classification presumes a causal relationship between hypertension and heart involvement and between hypertension and kidney involvement, as the two conditions are linked by the term "with" in the Alphabetic index. These conditions should be coded as related even in the absence of provider documentation explicitly linking them, unless the documentation clearly states the conditions are unrelated.

For hypertension and conditions not specifically linked by relational terms such as "with," or "due to" in the classification, provider documentation must link the conditions in order to code them as related.

*For more hypertension guidelines, see the ICD-10-CM manual.

Terms Related to Ischemic Heart Diseases (I20-I25)

Term	Word Origin	Definition
acute myocardial infarction (AMI)	*myocardi/o* heart, crown muscle *-al* pertaining to	Cardiac tissue death that occurs when the coronary arteries are occluded (blocked) by an **atheroma** (a mass of fat or lipids on the wall of an artery) or a blood clot caused by an atheroma (Fig. 9-19). AMIs are now referred to as **ST elevation myocardial infarctions (STEMI)** or **non-ST elevation myocardial infarctions (NSTEMI)** (see Fig. 9-10). Further description includes the wall of the heart affected, such as the anterior or inferior wall (see Fig. 9-6, *A*).
aneurysm (of heart)		A ballooning of the heart. A mural cardiac aneurysm refers to the heart wall, while a ventricular aneurysm refers specifically to the lower chambers of the heart.
angina pectoris	*pector/o* chest *-is* structure	Paroxysmal chest pain or discomfort occurring when the heart does not receive enough oxygen, usually when the heart rate is accelerated (Fig. 9-20). Unstable angina is a sudden chest pain that occurs regardless of activity and is indicative of a complete blockage of a coronary artery. Unstable angina may also be termed **accelerating/crescendo angina or intermediate coronary syndrome.**

⊗ Be Careful!   **Infarction** *refers to tissue death. An* **infraction** *refers to a breaking, as in an incomplete bone fracture.*

ICD Note   If a subsequent AMI occurs within 28 days of a previous AMI, a specific subsequent code is used. If a healed MI is seen on EKG, a code for "old myocardial infarction" is assigned.

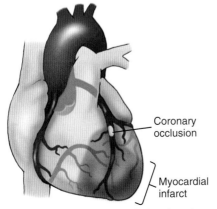

Coronary occlusion

Myocardial infarct

Fig. 9-19 Acute myocardial infarction.

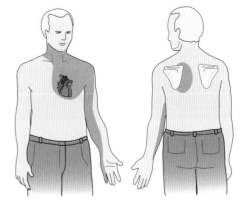

Fig. 9-20 Common sites of pain in angina pectoris.

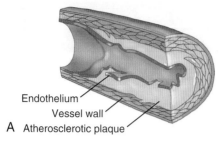
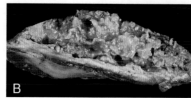
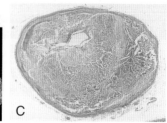

Endothelium
Vessel wall
A Atherosclerotic plaque

Fig. 9-21 Atherosclerosis.

Terms Related to Ischemic Heart Diseases (I20-I25)—cont'd

Term	Word Origin	Definition
coronary (artery) atherosclerosis	*coron/o* heart, crown *-ary* pertaining to *ather/o* fat, plaque *-sclerosis* abnormal condition of hardening	Accumulation and hardening of plaque in the coronary arteries that eventually can deprive the heart muscle of oxygen, leading to angina. Further description includes the presence or absence of angina, and the location of the plaque, whether in a native or grafted vessel. Also referred to as **coronary artery disease (CAD)** (Fig. 9-21).
ischemia	*isch/o* to hold back *-emia* blood condition	Lack of blood supply to tissues caused by a blockage or hemorrhage. Examples here relate to the heart. Acute coronary syndrome (ACS) is another term for acute ischemic heart disease.

ICD Note: ICD-10-CM provides combination codes for CAD with angina. A causal relationship can be assumed unless the angina is stated to be due to something other than CAD.

Exercise 10: Hypertension and Ischemic Heart Disease

Match the term in the first column with the meaning or synonym in the second.

____ 1. essential/primary
____ 2. transient
____ 3. infarction
____ 4. secondary
____ 5. controlled

A. due to another disorder
B. therapeutically corrected
C. idiopathic
D. limited
E. tissue death

Terms Related to Pulmonary Heart Disease and Diseases of Pulmonary Circulation (I26-I28) and Other Forms of Heart Disease (I30-I52)

Term	Word Origin	Definition
acute cor pulmonale	*cor* heart *pulmon/o* lung	Sudden right ventricular failure due to chronic pulmonary hypertension.
aortic stenosis (AS)	*aort/o* aorta *-ic* pertaining to *stenosis* narrowing	Narrowing of the aortic valve, which may be acquired or congenital (Fig. 9-22).

Continued

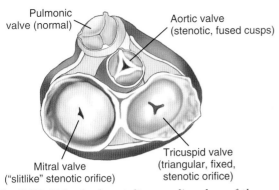

Fig. 9-22 Valvular heart disease: disorders of the aortic, mitral, and tricuspid valves.

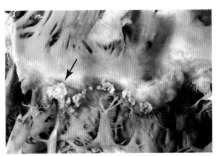

Fig. 9-23 Acute bacterial endocarditis. The valve is covered with large irregular vegetations (arrow).

Terms Related to Pulmonary Heart Disease and Diseases of Pulmonary Circulation (I26-I28) and Other Forms of Heart Disease (I3Ø-I52)—cont'd

Term	Word Origin	Definition
cardiac tamponade	*cardi/o* heart *-ac* pertaining to	Compression of heart due to buildup of fluid in pericardium.
cardiomegaly	*cardi/o* heart *-megaly* enlargement	Enlargement of the heart. May also be termed **cardiac hypertrophy** if referring to excessive development of the heart.
cardiomyopathy	*cardiomy/o* heart muscle *-pathy* disease	Disease of heart muscle. Also called **myocardiopathy**.
endocarditis	*endocardi/o* endocardium *-itis* inflammation	Inflammation of the inner lining of the heart with involvement of one or more of the valves (Fig. 9-23).
heart failure (HF)		Inability of the heart muscle to pump blood efficiently, so that it becomes overloaded. The heart enlarges with unpumped blood, and the lungs fill with fluid. Previously referred to as congestive heart failure (CHF).
mitral regurgitation (MR)		Backflow of blood from the left ventricle into the left atrium in systole across a diseased valve. It may be the result of congenital valve abnormalities, rheumatic fever, or mitral valve prolapse (MVP).
mitral stenosis (MS)	*stenosis* narrowing	Narrowing of the valve between the left atrium and left ventricle caused by adhesions on the leaflets of the valve, usually the result of recurrent episodes of rheumatic endocarditis. Left atrial hypertrophy develops and may be followed by right-sided heart failure and pulmonary edema (cor pulmonale) (see Fig. 9-22).
mitral valve prolapse (MVP)	*pro-* forward *-lapse* fall	Protrusion of one or both cusps of the mitral valve back into the left atrium during ventricular systole (Fig. 9-24).
pericarditis	*pericardi/o* pericardium *-itis* inflammation	Inflammation of the sac surrounding the heart, with the possibility of pericardial effusion (Fig. 9-25).
pulmonary embolism (PE)	*pulmon/o* lung *-ary* pertaining to	A blockage of one of the pulmonary vessels accompanied by death of lung tissue.

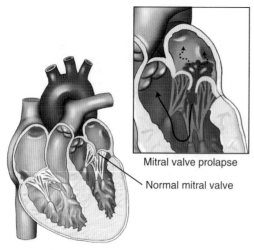

Fig. 9-24 Mitral valve prolapse.

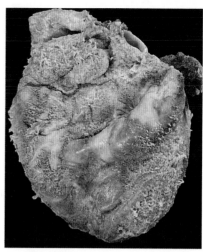

Fig. 9-25 Acute pericarditis.

Terms Related to Pulmonary Heart Disease and Diseases of Pulmonary Circulation (I26-I28) and Other Forms of Heart Disease (I3Ø-I52)—cont'd

Term	Word Origin	Definition
pulmonary hypertension	*pulmon/o* lung *-ary* pertaining to *hyper-* excessive *-tension* pressure	Excessive pulmonary arterial blood pressure. May be idiopathic (without a known cause) or as a result of other diseases such as congestive heart failure, sarcoidosis or cirrhosis of the liver.
tricuspid stenosis (TS)	*stenosis* narrowing	Relatively uncommon narrowing of the tricuspid valve associated with lesions of other valves caused by rheumatic fever. Symptoms include jugular vein distention and pulmonary congestion (see Fig. 9-22).

Terms Related to Cardiac Dysrhythmias (Arrhythmias)

Cardiac dysrhythmias fall under "Other Forms of Heart Disease" in ICD-10-CM but have been presented in a separate table for ease of learning. A dysrhythmia is an abnormal heartbeat (*dys-* means "abnormal," *rhythm/o* means "rhythm," and *-ia* means "condition"). Remember that a normal heart rate is referred to as a "normal sinus rhythm (NSR)."

Term	Word Origin	Definition
arrhythmia	*a-* no, not, without *rhythm/o* rhythm *-ia* condition	Abnormal variation from the normal heartbeat rhythm. Also called **dysrhythmia**.
atrioventricular block	*atri/o* atrium *ventricul/o* ventricle *-ar* pertaining to	Partial or complete heart block that is the result of a lack of electrical communication between the atria and the ventricles. Also termed **heart block**.

Continued

Click on **Animations** to watch a demonstration of the different types of dysrhythmias.

Terms Related to Cardiac Dysrhythmias (Arrhythmias)—cont'd

Term	Word Origin	Definition
bundle branch block (BBB)		Incomplete electrical conduction in the bundle branches, either left or right.
ectopic beats	*ec-* out of *top/o* place *-ic* pertaining to	Heartbeats that occur outside a normal rhythm.
atrial ectopic beats (AEB)	*atri/o* atrium *-al* pertaining to	Irregular contractions of the atria. Also termed **premature atrial contractions (PACs).**
ventricular ectopic beats (VEB)	*ventricul/o* ventricle *-ar* pertaining to	Irregular contractions of the ventricles. Also called **premature ventricular contractions (PVCs).** Are not always considered pathological.
fibrillation		Extremely rapid and irregular contractions (300-600/min) occurring with or without an underlying cardiovascular disorder, such as coronary artery disease.
atrial fibrillation (AF)	*atri/o* atrium *-al* pertaining to	The most common type of cardiac arrhythmia.
ventricular fibrillation	*ventricul/o* ventricle *-ar* pertaining to	Rapid, irregular ventricular contractions; may be fatal unless reversed.
flutter		Extremely rapid but regular heartbeat (250-350 bpm). **Atrial flutter** is a rapid, regular atrial rhythm.
sick sinus syndrome (SSS)		Any abnormality of the sinus node that may include the necessity of an implantable pacemaker.
ventricular tachycardia (VT)	*ventricul/o* ventricle *-ar* pertaining to *tachy-* rapid *-cardia* heart condition	Condition of ventricular contractions >100 bpm.

Exercise 11: Terms Related to Pulmonary Heart Disease, Other Forms of Heart Disease, and Cardiac Dysrhythmias

Fill in the blank.

1. Another general term for an arrhythmia_____

2. Extremely rapid and irregular contractions_____

3. An extremely rapid but regular heartbeat_____

4. The general term for a lack of electrical communication is heart or atrioventricular _____

5. Any abnormality of the sinus node_____

6. Other term for ventricular ectopic beats_____

7. The term for ventricular contractions over 100 beats per minute _____

8. The term for right ventricular heart failure due to chronic pulmonary hypertension _____

9. Narrowing of the valve between the left atrium and left ventricle _____

10. Backflow of blood from the left ventricle into the left atrium _____

Translate the following terms:

11. cardiomegaly_____

12. tachycardia_____

13. endocarditis_____

14. cardiomyopathy_____

15. pericarditis_____

16. pulmonary hypertension_____

Terms Related to Cerebrovascular Diseases (I6Ø-I69)

Term	Word Origin	Definition
aphasia	*a-* no, not, without *phas/o* speech *-ia* condition	Lack or impairment of the ability to form or understand speech. Less severe forms include dysphasia and synarthria; dysarthria refers to difficulty in the articulation (pronunciation) of speech.
apraxia	*a-* no, not, without *prax/o* purposeful movement *-ia* condition	Inability to perform purposeful movements or to use objects appropriately. This disorder is a result of damage to the cerebrum leaving the patient unable to accomplish the desired movement.
ataxia	*a-* no, not, without *tax/o* order, coordination *-ia* condition	Lack of coordination. Ataxia is a result of damage to the cerebellum that leaves the patient with the inability to coordinate muscle movements.
cerebral infarction	*cerebr/o* cerebrum, brain *-al* pertaining to	Tissue death within the brain. May be the result of a hemorrhage or a blockage (thrombosis or embolus) (Fig. 9-26). Also called **cerebrovascular accident** or **stroke**.
intracerebral hemorrhage	*intra-* within *cerebr/o* cerebrum, brain *-al* pertaining to *hem/o* blood *-rrhage* bursting forth	An escape of blood within the tissues of the brain. Can cause headache, vomiting, seizures, confusion, weakness and particularly paralysis on one side of the body.

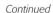

Continued

ICD-10 provides codes for late effects of stroke, such as for speech deficits and paralysis of one or more limbs. The sequelae codes in category **I69** may occur at any time after the onset of hemorrhage, infarction, or other cerebrovascular disease.

Terms Related to Cerebrovascular Diseases (I6Ø-I69)—cont'd

Term	Word Origin	Definition
monoplegia	*mono-* one *-plegia* paralysis	Paralysis of one limb on the left or right side of the body. If the prefix is replaced with *hemi-*, meaning "half," the term refers to the entire left or right side of the body. If described as *-paresis,* it is a "slight paralysis." The codes are the same for both *-plegia* and *-paresis.*
subarachnoid hemorrhage (SAH)	*sub-* under *arachnoid* (middle layer of meninges) *hem/o* blood *-rrhage* bursting forth	An escape of blood into the cavity between the arachnoid membrane and pia mater covering the CNS.

 CM Guideline Alert

9.D.1) CATEGORY I69, SEQUELAE OF CEREBROVASCULAR DISEASE

Category I69 is used to indicate conditions classifiable to categories I6Ø-67 as the causes of sequela (neurological deficits), themselves classified elsewhere. These "late effects" include neurologic deficits that persist after initial onset of conditions classifiable to categories I6Ø-67.

Codes from category I69, Sequelae of cerebrovascular disease, that specify hemiplegia, hemiparesis and monoplegia identify whether the dominant or nondominant side is affected. Should the affected side be documented, but not specified as dominant or nondominant, and the classification system does not indicate a default, code selection is as follows:
- For ambidextrous patients, the default should be dominant.
- If the left side is affected, the default is non-dominant.
- If the right side is affected, the default is dominant.

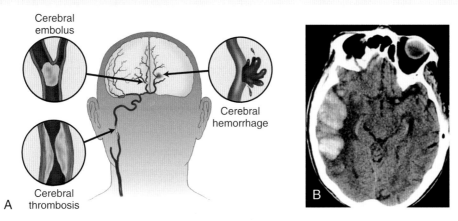

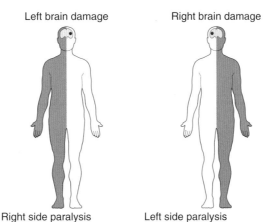

Fig. 9-26 **Cerebrovascular accident (CVA). A,** Events causing stroke. **B,** MRI showing hemorrhagic stroke in right cerebrum. **C,** Areas of the body affected by CVA.

Terms Related to Diseases of Arteries, Arterioles, and Capillaries (I7Ø-I79)

Term	Word Origin	Definition
aortic aneurysm		Localized dilation of the aorta caused by a congenital or acquired weakness in the wall of the vessel due to atherosclerosis or hypertension. May be a thoracic or an abdominal aortic aneurysm. If referred to as dissecting, the aneurysm has a tear.
arteriosclerosis	*arteri/o* artery *-sclerosis* abnormal condition of hardening	Disease in which the arterial walls become thickened and lose their elasticity, without the presence of atheromas (Fig. 9-27).
intermittent claudication		Cramplike pains in the calves resulting in limping, caused by poor circulation in the leg muscles. The term *intermittent* means that the patient experiences it at irregular intervals.
peripheral arterial occlusion	*arteri/o* artery *-al* pertaining to *occlus/o* blockage *-ion* process of	Blockage of blood flow to the extremities. Acute or chronic conditions may be present, but patients with both types of conditions are likely to have underlying atherosclerosis. Occlusion means "blockage."
peripheral vascular disease (PVD)	*vascul/o* vessel *-ar* pertaining to	Any vascular disorder limited to the extremities; may affect not only the arteries and veins but also the lymphatics.
Raynaud's syndrome	*syn-* together *-drome* to run	Idiopathic disease—that is, of unknown cause—of the peripheral vascular system that causes bilateral intermittent cyanosis/erythema/numbness of the distal ends of the fingers and toes; occurs almost exclusively in young women. Raynaud's phenomenon is secondary to rheumatoid arthritis, scleroderma, or trauma. Presentation is unilateral (Fig. 9-28).
vasculitis	*vascul/o* vessel *-itis* inflammation	Inflammation of the blood vessels. Also called **angiitis.**

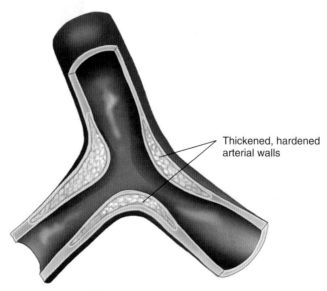

Thickened, hardened arterial walls

Fig. 9-27 Arteriosclerosis.

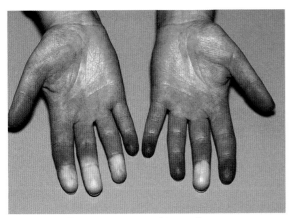

Fig. 9-28 Raynaud's syndrome.

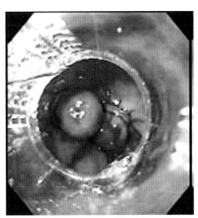

Fig. 9-29 Esophageal varices immediately after band ligation.

Terms Related to Diseases of Veins (I8Ø-I87)

Term	Word Origin	Definition
esophageal varices	*esophag/o* esophagus *-eal* pertaining to *varic/o* varices	Varicose veins that appear at the lower end of the esophagus as a result of portal hypertension; they are superficial and may cause ulceration and bleeding (Fig. 9-29).
hemorrhoid		Varicose condition of the external or internal rectal veins that causes painful swellings at the anus.
thrombophlebitis	*thromb/o* clotting, clot *phleb/o* vein *-itis* inflammation	Inflammation of either deep veins (**deep vein thrombosis,** or **DVT**) or superficial veins (**superficial vein thrombosis,** or **SVT**), with the formation of one or more blood clots. If no blood clot, termed simply **phlebitis.**
varicose veins	*varic/o* varices *-ose* pertaining to	Elongated, dilated superficial veins (varices) with incompetent valves that permit reverse blood flow. These veins may appear in various parts of the anatomy, but this particular code for varicose vein(s) has been reserved for those in the lower extremities.

Terms Related to Other and Unspecified Disorders of the Circulatory System (I95-I99)

Term	Word Origin	Definition
gangrene		Death of tissue due to a lack of blood supply.
hypotension	*hypo-* below, deficient *tens/o* stretching *-ion* process of	Condition of below-normal blood pressure. Orthostatic hypotension occurs when a patient experiences an episode of low blood pressure upon rising to a standing position. Idiopathic hypotension has no known cause.

Exercise 12: Terms Related to Cerebrovascular Diseases; Diseases of Arteries and Veins; and Unspecified Disorders of the Circulatory System

Match the term to its definition.

____ 1. peripheral arterial occlusion
____ 2. cerebral infarction
____ 3. gangrene
____ 4. hypotension
____ 5. aortic aneurysm
____ 6. varicose veins
____ 7. intracerebral hemorrhage
____ 8. Raynaud's syndrome
____ 9. esophageal varices
___ 10. hemorrhoid
___ 11. subarachnoid hemorrhage
___ 12. peripheral vascular disease
___ 13. apraxia
___ 14. ataxia
___ 15. intermittent claudication

A. death of tissue due to lack of blood supply
B. escape of blood within the tissues of the brain
C. blockage of blood flow to the extremities
D. localized dilation of the aorta caused by weakness in wall of the vessel
E. escape of blood between arachnoid membrane and pia mater
F. varicose veins in the esophagus
G. vascular disorder of the extremities; may be the arteries, veins, or lymphatics
H. elongated, dilated superficial veins
I. varicose condition of the rectal veins
J. condition of below-normal blood pressure
K. tissue death within the brain
L. idiopathic disease of peripheral vascular system of fingers and toes
M. cramplike pain in legs
N. lack of purposeful movement
O. lack of coordinated movement

Translate the following terms.

16. vasculitis_____

17. arteriosclerosis_____

18. thrombophlebitis_____

19. hypotension_____

20. aphasia_____

21. monoplegia_____

Terms Related to Diseases of Lymphatic Vessels and Lymph Nodes (I88-I89)*

Term	Word Origin	Definition
lymphadenitis	*lymphaden/o* lymph gland *-itis* inflammation	Inflammation of a lymph node.
lymphadenopathy	*lymphaden/o* lymph gland *-pathy* disease process	Disease of the lymph nodes or vessels that may be localized or generalized.
lymphangiectasis	*lymphangi/o* lymph vessel *-ectasis* expansion, dilation	A superficial dilation of lymphatic vessels.

Continued

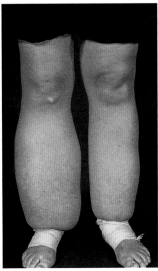

Fig. 9-30 Lymphedema. The patient had to bind her feet so that she could wear shoes.

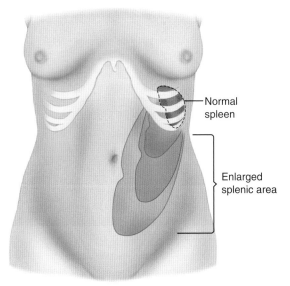

Normal spleen

Enlarged splenic area

Fig. 9-31 Splenomegaly.

Terms Related to Diseases of Lymphatic Vessels and Lymph Nodes (I88-I89)*—cont'd

Term	Word Origin	Definition
lymphangitis	*lymphangi/o* lymph vessel *-itis* inflammation	Inflammation of lymph vessels.
lymphedema	*lymph/o* lymph *-edema* swelling	Accumulation of lymphatic fluid and resultant swelling caused by obstruction, removal, or hypoplasia of lymph vessels (Fig. 9-30).
splenomegaly	*splen/o* spleen *-megaly* enlargement	Enlargement of the spleen (Fig. 9-31). Most common causes are infections, such as mononucleosis.

*Signs and symptoms are included in this table.

 ## Exercise 13: Lymphatic Disorders

Translate the terms.

1. lymphadenopathy_____

2. splenomegaly_____

3. lymphangiectasis_____

4. lymphedema_____

5. lymphangitis_____

6. lymphadenitis_____

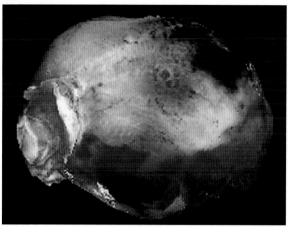

Fig. 9-32 Atrial myxoma.

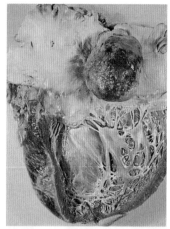

Fig. 9-33 Cardiac myxosarcoma.

Terms Related to Benign Neoplasms of the Circulatory System (D10-D36)

Term	Word Origin	Definition
atrial myxoma	*atri/o* atrium *-al* pertaining to *myx/o* mucus *-oma* tumor, mass	Benign growth usually occurring on the interatrial septum (Fig. 9-32).
hemangioma	*hemangi/o* blood vessel *-oma* tumor, mass	Noncancerous tumor of the blood vessels. May be congenital ("stork bite") or may develop later in life.
thymoma, benign	*thym/o* thymus gland *-oma* tumor, mass	Noncancerous tumor of epithelial origin that is often associated with myasthenia gravis.

Terms Related to Malignant Neoplasms of the Circulatory System (C00-C96)

Term	Word Origin	Definition
cardiac myxosarcoma	*myx/o* mucus *-sarcoma* connective tissue cancer	Rare cancer of the heart usually originating in the left atrium (Fig. 9-33).
hemangiosarcoma	*hemangi/o* blood vessel *-sarcoma* connective tissue cancer	Rare cancer of the cells that line the blood vessels.
Hodgkin lymphoma	*lymph/o* lymph *-oma* tumor	Also termed **Hodgkin disease,** this cancer is diagnosed by the detection of a type of cell specific only to this disorder: Reed-Sternberg cells.

Continued

Terms Related to Malignant Neoplasms of the Circulatory System(CØØ-C96)_cont'd

Term	Word Origin	Definition
non-Hodgkin lymphoma	*lymph/o* lymph *-oma* tumor	A collection of all other lymphatic cancers but Hodgkin lymphomas. This type is the more numerous of the two lymphomas and is the sixth most common type of cancer in the United States.
thymoma, malignant	*thym/o* thymus gland *-oma* tumor	Also termed **thymic carcinoma**, this rare malignancy of the thymus gland is particularly invasive and, unlike its benign form, is not associated with autoimmune disorders.

Exercise 14: Neoplasms of the Circulatory System

Match the neoplasms with their definitions.

____ 1. non-Hodgkin lymphoma

____ 2. thymoma

____ 3. malignant thymoma

____ 4. Hodgkin lymphoma

A. benign tumor of thymus gland
B. cancer of lymphatic system detected by presence of Reed-Sternberg cells
C. thymic carcinoma
D. a collection of all lymphatic cancers except Hodgkin lymphoma

Fill in the blank.

5. What is a benign tumor of the blood vessels?_____

6. What is a rare malignant tumor of the heart?_____

7. What is a benign tumor that originates in the atria of the heart? _____

8. What is a rare malignant tumor of the lining of the blood vessels?_____

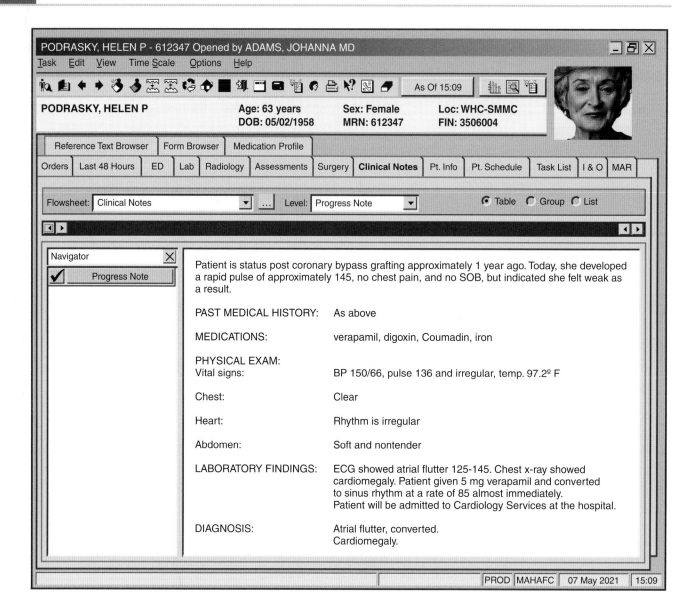

 Exercise 15: **Progress Note**

Using the report above, answer the following questions.

1. Which vessels in the cardiovascular system were operated on 1 year ago?

_____

2. "Sinus rhythm" refers to _____

3. "Flutter" is an example of a/n _____

4. "Atrial" refers to _____

5. "Cardiomegaly" means that the heart is_____

PROCEDURES

 PCS Guideline Alert

B4.4 The coronary arteries are classified as a single body part that is further specified by number of arteries treated. One procedure code specifying multiple arteries is used when the same procedure is performed, including the same device and qualifier values.

 If different procedures (e.g., angioplasty in one portion and stent placement in another portion of an artery) are performed on the coronary arteries, each must be coded. Both are dilations: one is with an intraluminal device (stent—6th character) and one is with no device.

Procedures Related to the Cardiovascular System

Terms Related to Laboratory Tests

Term	Word Origin	Definition
cardiac enzymes test		Blood test that measures the amount of cardiac enzymes characteristically released during a myocardial infarction: determines the amount of lactate dehydrogenase (LDH) and creatine phosphokinase (CK or CPK) in the blood. Troponin I and T are proteins that are released from cardiac muscle during an infarction.
C-reactive protein (CRP) test		Blood test to determine the degree of inflammation in the body. It is used to predict the risk of heart disease.
homocysteine levels		Test used to predict a patient's risk of stroke and CAD.
lipid profile		Blood test to measure the lipids (cholesterol and triglycerides) in the circulating blood.

Sample Lipid Profile

Test	Your results	Date	Normal Range
Total Cholesterol	171	11/02/2020	Under 200
HDL (high density lipoproteins)	55	11/02/2020	Over 40
Triglycerides	84	11/02/2020	Under 150
LDL (low density lipoproteins)	99	11/02/2020	Under 100

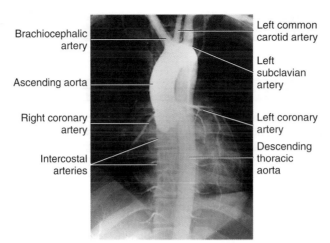

Fig. 9-34 Digital subtraction angiography (DSA).

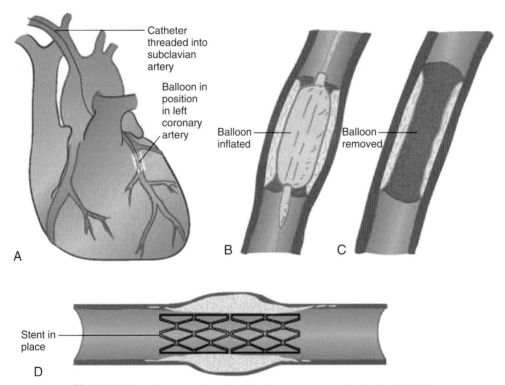

Fig. 9-35 Percutaneous transluminal coronary angioplasty (PTCA).

Terms Related to Procedures of the Great Vessels and Aorta

Term	Word Origin	Definition
angiocardiography	*angi/o* vessel *cardi/o* heart *-graphy* recording	Process of recording the vessels of the heart. Also termed coronary **angiography** (see Fig. 9-34). **Digital subtraction angiography** (DSA) takes out (subtracts) the background images to increase contrast.
angioplasty	*angi/o* vessel *-plasty* surgically forming	Forming a vessel to repair, dilate, replace, or supplement it. **Percutaneous transluminal coronary angioplasty (PTCA)** is a form of angioplasty in which a catheter is threaded into the coronary artery affected by atherosclerotic heart disease. The balloon at the tip of the catheter is inflated and deflated to compress the plaque against the wall of the artery and increase blood flow. Stents, wire mesh tubes, are placed in the arteries and used to prop them open after the angioplasty (Fig. 9-35).

Continued

Terms Related to Procedures of the Great Vessels and Aorta—cont'd

Term	Word Origin	Definition
angiotripsy	*angi/o* vessel *-tripsy* crushing	Crushing a vessel. Procedure done to control bleeding. Also called **vasotripsy**.
aortoplasty	*aort/o* aorta *-plasty* surgically forming	Forming a correction to the aorta to correct aortic defects such as aortic aneurysms.
transmyocardial revascularization (TMR)	*trans-* through *myocardi/o* myocardium *-al* pertaining to *re-* again *vascul/o* vessel *-ization* process	Procedure used to relieve severe angina in a patient who cannot tolerate a CABG or PTCA. With a laser, a series of holes is made in the heart muscle in the hope of increasing blood flow by stimulating new blood vessels to grow (angiogenesis).

Terms Related to Procedures of the Heart

Term	Word Origin	Definition
cardiac catheterization	*cardi/o* heart *-ac* pertaining to	Threading of a catheter (thin tube) into the heart to collect diagnostic information about structures in the heart, coronary arteries, and great vessels; also used as a means of access for treatment of CAD, congenital abnormalities, and heart failure (Fig. 9-36).

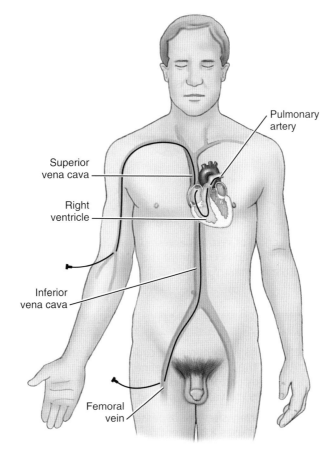

Fig. 9-36 Cardiac catheterization. The catheter is inserted into the femoral or brachial vein and advanced through the inferior vena cava through the superior vena cava, right atrium, and right ventricle and into the pulmonary artery.

CPT Coding Alert!

The CPT codes for heart and/or lung transplants can be divided into a series of codes. Codes may be for the donor cardiectomy-pneumonectomy, backbench preparation of the cadaver organs, and the actual transplantation. Note that the code for the donor cardiectomy is separate from the code for the heart transplant.

Terms Related to Procedures of the Heart—cont'd

Term	Word Origin	Definition
cardiac pacemaker		A device that is inserted into either a subcutaneous pocket on the chest or in the right ventricle to prevent the heart from beating too slowly.
cardioplegia	*cardi/o* heart *-plegia* paralysis	Immobilization of the heart in order to perform cardiac surgery. Also called asystole of the heart.
cardioversion	*cardi/o* heart *-version* turning	Changing an abnormal heart rhythm to a normal one using either chemicals or electricity.
coronary artery bypass graft (CABG)	*coron/o* heart, crown *-ary* pertaining to	Open-heart surgery in which a piece of a blood vessel from another location is grafted onto one of the coronary arteries to reroute blood around a blockage (Fig. 9-37).

Continued

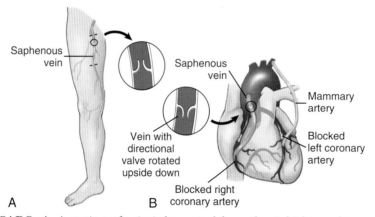

Fig. 9-37 CABG. A, A section of vein is harvested from the right leg and is anastomosed to a coronary artery to bypass an occlusion of the right coronary artery. **B,** Bypass of the left coronary artery with a mammary artery.

 PCS Guideline Alert

B3.6b Coronary artery bypass procedures are coded differently from other bypass procedures as described in the previous guideline. Rather than identifying the body part bypassed from, the body part identifies the number of coronary arteries bypassed to, and the qualifier specifies the vessel bypassed from.

B3.6c If multiple coronary artery sites are bypassed, a separate procedure is coded for each coronary artery site that uses a different device and/or qualifier.

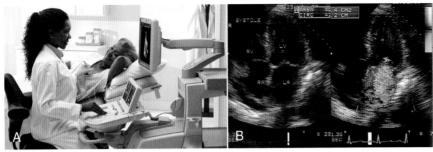

Fig. 9-38 **A,** Person undergoing echocardiography. **B,** Color Doppler image of the heart.

Terms Related to Procedures of the Heart—cont'd

Term	Word Origin	Definition
echocardiography (ECHO)	*echo-* sound *cardi/o* heart *-graphy* recording	Use of ultrasonic waves directed through the heart to study the structure and motion of the heart (Fig. 9-38). **Transesophageal echocardiography (TEE)** images the heart through a transducer introduced into the esophagus.
electrocardiography (ECG, EKG)	*electr/o* electricity *cardi/o* heart *-graphy* recording	Recording of electrical impulses of the heart as wave deflections of a needle on an instrument called an electrocardiograph. A **Holter monitor** is a portable EKG device with electrodes, which is worn on a belt for measurement of cardiac activity during daily activities (usually 24 hours) (Fig. 9-39).
heart transplant		The replacement of a failing, defective heart with a healthy donor heart. May or may not include lungs.
left ventricular assist device (LVAD)	*ventricul/o* ventricle *-ar* pertaining to	A mechanical pump device that assists a patient's weakened heart by pulling blood from the left ventricle into the pump and then ejecting it out into the aorta. LVADs may be used on patients awaiting a transplant.
minimally invasive direct coronary artery bypass (MIDCAB)	*coron/o* heart, crown *-ary* pertaining to	Surgical procedure in which the heart is still beating while a minimal incision is made over the blocked coronary artery and an artery from the chest wall is used as the bypass.
pericardiocentesis	*pericardi/o* sac surrounding the heart *-centesis* surgical puncture	Surgical puncture of the pericardium to remove fluid from the pericardial sac for emergency treatment (cardiac tamponade) or for diagnostic purposes. Also called a **pericardial tap**.
pericardiolysis	*pericardi/o* sac surrounding the heart *-lysis* releasing, destroying, breaking down	Release of adhesions of the pericardium. May be done to treat a sequela of a pericardial inflammation.
radiofrequency ablation (RFA)		Used to correct arrhythmias by destroying aberrant electrical pathways with heat. (The term ablation means to destroy.)
septoplasty	*sept/o* wall, partition *-plasty* surgically forming	The process of forming a closure of an abnormal opening in an interatrial or interventricular wall.
valvuloplasty	*valvul/o* valve *-plasty* surgically forming	Repair of a heart valve damaged in disorders such as tricuspid stenosis or rheumatic heart disease.

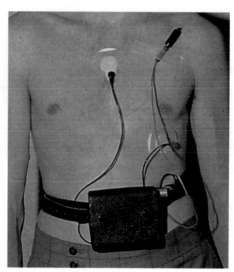

Fig. 9-39 Holter monitor.

Click on **Animations** to watch a demonstration of pericardiocentesis.

Terms Related to Procedures of the Arteries and Veins

Term	Word Origin	Definition
arteriorrhaphy	*arteri/o* artery *-rrhaphy* suturing	Suture of an artery.
endarterectomy	*end-* within *arteri/o* artery *-ectomy* cutting out	Removal of the atheromatous plaque from the inner lining of an artery (see Fig. 9-40).
phlebectomy	*phleb/o* vein *-ectomy* cutting out	Removal of a vein. If termed **ambulatory**, it is a procedure to remove superficial varicose veins.
phlebography	*phleb/o* vein *-graphy* recording	Process of x-ray recording a vein after injection of a contrast medium.
phlebotomy	*phleb/o* vein *-tomy* cutting	Literally cutting of a vein for the purpose of collecting blood. Also called **venipuncture.**
sclerotherapy	*scler/o* hard *-therapy* treatment	Intravenous injection of a chemical substance to treat varicose veins.
venotripsy	*ven/o* vein *-tripsy* crushing	Process of crushing a vein to control bleeding.

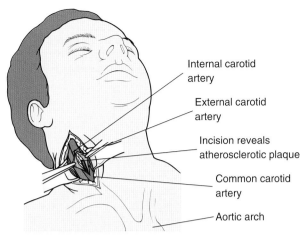

Internal carotid artery

External carotid artery

Incision reveals atherosclerotic plaque

Common carotid artery

Aortic arch

Fig. 9-40 Carotid endarterectomy.

Terms Related to Procedures of the Lymph Glands, Spleen and Thymus

Term	Word Origin	Definition
lymphadenectomy	*lymphaden/o* lymph gland/node *-ectomy* cutting out	To cut out part or all of a lymph gland. Usually performed as part of treatment for a malignant neoplasm.
lymphangiography	*lymphangi/o* lymph vessel *-graphy* recording	Imaging of lymph vessels and glands after the injection of a contrast medium to increase the visibility of the area being studied. May be done in conjunction with a lymph node biopsy to determine the possible spread of cancer (Fig. 9-41).
splenectomy	*splen/o* spleen *-ectomy* cutting out	To cut out part or all of the spleen to treat splenomegaly or a ruptured spleen.
splenopexy	*splen/o* spleen *-pexy* suspension	Fixing a spleen that is out of place because of trauma or a congenital condition.
thymectomy	*thym/o* thymus gland *-ectomy* cutting out	To cut out part or all of the thymus gland to treat cancer or myasthenia gravis.

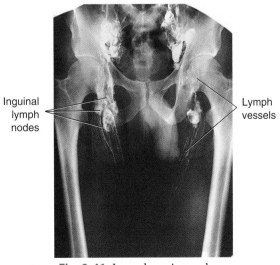

Inguinal lymph nodes

Lymph vessels

Fig. 9-41 Lymphangiography.

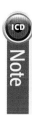

 A sentinel node biopsy is a surgical procedure used to help diagnose and treat breast cancer and melanoma. Sentinel nodes are the first lymph glands that a tumor drains into, so if cancer cells are not found in this gland, indicating spread to the lymphatic system from the primary tumor, removing subsequent nodes for biopsy is unnecessary.

Exercise 16: Procedures of the Heart, Vessels, Arteries, Veins, and Lymph System

Match the terms to their definitions.

_____ 1. septoplasty
_____ 2. TMR
_____ 3. cardioplegia
_____ 4. CABG
_____ 5. MIDCAB
_____ 6. ECHO
_____ 7. ECG
_____ 8. LVAD
_____ 9. phlebotomy
_____ 10. thymectomy

A. a series of holes is made in the heart muscle in the hope of increasing blood flow
B. recording of electrical impulses of the heart
C. to cut out part or all of the thymus gland
D. sonography of the heart
E. surgical procedure in which the heart is still beating while an artery from the chest wall is used as the bypass
F. immobilization of the heart
G. cutting of a vein
H. pump that pulls blood from the left ventricle into the pump and then ejects it out into the aorta
I. grafting an artery onto a coronary artery to reroute blood around a blockage
J. process of forming a closure of an abnormal opening in wall

Build the terms.

11. fixing/suspending the spleen in place _____
12. turning (an abnormal) heart (rhythm from abnormal to normal) _____
13. crushing a vein _____
14. recording a lymph vessel _____
15. suturing an artery _____
16. forming a vessel _____
17. releasing the sac surrounding the heart _____
18. surgically forming part or all of a valve _____

PHARMACOLOGY

As in other body systems, medications may be available over the counter (OTC) or require a prescription (Rx). An example of an OTC drug used in this system is chewable "baby" aspirin (81 mg), sometimes given to patients at high risk for having a myocardial infarction. Rx drugs used to treat the cardiovascular system may be grouped as follows:

angiotensin-converting enzyme (ACE) inhibitors: Relax blood vessels by preventing the formation of the vasoconstrictor angiotensin II. This inhibition causes a decrease in water retention and blood pressure and an improvement in cardiac output. ACE inhibitors are commonly used to treat hypertension and heart failure. Examples are lisinopril (Prinivil), enalapril (Vasotec), and quinapril (Accupril).

angiotension II receptor blockers (ARBs): Lower blood pressure by inhibiting the vasoconstrictor angiotension II from binding its action sites. Examples include irbesartan (Avapro) and valsartan (Diovan).

antiarrhythmic drugs: Restore normal sinus rhythm via various mechanisms to treat cardiac arrhythmias. Examples are digoxin (Lanoxin), amiodarone (Pacerone), and flecainide (Tambocor).

anticoagulants: Prevent the formation of blood clots. Examples are warfarin (Coumadin) and heparin.

antihyperlipidemics: Lower LDL and/or raise HDL cholesterol levels to reduce the risk of heart attack or stroke. Subtypes include fibrates, HMG-CoA reductase inhibitors or "statins", bile acid sequestrants, niacin, and other miscellaneous types. Examples are gemfibrozil (Lopid), atorvastatin (Lipitor), cholestyramine (Questran), niacin (Niaspan), and ezetimibe (Zetia).

antihypertensives: Lower blood pressure. Types include ACE inhibitors, ARBs, beta-blockers, CCBs, and renin inhibitors.

beta-blockers: Depress the heart rate and force of heart contractions by decreasing the effectiveness of the nerve impulses to the cardiovascular system. They typically are prescribed to treat angina pectoris, hypertension, and cardiac arrhythmias. Examples are propranolol (Inderal), atenolol (Tenormin), and metoprolol (Lopressor).

calcium channel blockers (CCBs): Decrease myocardial oxygen demand by inhibiting the flow of calcium to smooth muscle cells of the heart, which causes arterial relaxation. CCBs are used to treat angina, hypertension, and heart failure. Examples are diltiazem (Cardizem), verapamil (Calan), amlodipine (Norvasc), and nifedipine (Procardia).

diuretics: Promote the excretion of sodium and water as urine; they are used in the treatment of hypertension and heart failure. Examples of diuretics are furosemide (Lasix), hydrochlorothiazide (Hydrodiuril), and triamterene (Maxzide, combo with hydrochlorothiazide).

nitrates (antianginals): Relax blood vessels and reduce myocardial oxygen consumption to lessen the pain of angina pectoris; also used to treat hypertension and heart failure. Examples include isosorbide dinitrate (Isordil) and nitroglycerin (Nitro, Nitro-Dur).

renin inhibitors: Relax blood vessels by decreasing renin conversion of angiotensinogen to angiotensin I. The first agent approved in this class is aliskiren (Tekturna).

thrombolytics: Aid in the dissolution of blood clots. "Clot busters" are used to treat obstructing coronary thrombi (clots). Examples are alteplase (Activase), reteplase (Retevase), and tenecteplase (TNKase).

vasodilators: Dilate blood vessels to treat hypertension, heart failure, or angina. Examples include riociguat (Adempas), hydralazine (Dralzine), and nitrates.

Exercise 17: **Pharmacology**

Match the type of drug with the disease(s) it treats. There may be more than one answer.

____ 1. antiarrhythmic	____ 6. diuretic
____ 2. beta-blocker	____ 7. thrombolytic
____ 3. ACE inhibitor	____ 8. anticoagulant
____ 4. antianginal	____ 9. statin
____ 5. calcium channel blocker	

A. hypertension
B. existing thrombosis
C. dysrhythmia
D. angina
E. heart failure
F. formation of thromboses
G. high LDL cholesterol

RECOGNIZING SUFFIXES FOR PCS

Now that you've finished reading about the procedures for the circulatory system, take a look at this review of the *suffixes* used in their terminology. Each of these suffixes is associated with one or more root operations in the medical surgical section or one of the other categories in PCS.

Suffixes and Root Operations for the Circulatory System

Suffix	Root Operation
-centesis	Drainage
-ectomy	Excision, resection
-lysis	Release
-plasty	Dilation, repair, replacement, supplement
-pexy	Repair, reposition
-rrhaphy	Repair
-tomy	Drainage
-tripsy	Occlusion

Abbreviations (Anatomy)

Abbreviation	Meaning	Abbreviation	Meaning
AV	atrioventricular	MV	mitral valve
BP	blood pressure	NSR	normal sinus rhythm
BPM	beats per minute	O_2	oxygen
CO_2	carbon dioxide	PA	pulmonary artery
CRP	C-reactive protein	PV	pulmonary vein
CV	cardiovascular	RA	right atrium
ITA	internal thoracic artery	RCA	right coronary artery
LA	left atrium	RV	right ventricle
LCA	left coronary artery	SA	sinoatrial
LV	left ventricle	TV	tricuspid valve

Abbreviations (Pathology)

Abbreviation	Meaning
AEB	atrial ectopic beat
ACS	acute coronary syndrome
AF	atrial fibrillation
AMI	acute myocardial infarction
AS	aortic stenosis
BBB	bundle branch block
CAD	coronary artery disease
CHF	congestive heart failure
CVA	cerebrovascular accident
DOE	dyspnea on exertion
DVT	deep vein thrombosis
HF	heart failure
HTN	hypertension
MR	mitral regurgitation
MS	mitral stenosis
MVP	mitral valve prolapse
NSTEMI	non-ST elevation myocardial infarction
PAC	premature atrial contraction
PDA	patent ductus arteriosus
PE	pulmonary embolism
PVC	premature ventricular contraction
PVD	peripheral vascular disease
RHD	rheumatic heart disease
RFA	radiofrequency ablation
SAH	subarachnoid hemorrhage
SOB	shortness of breath
SSS	sick sinus syndrome
STEMI	ST elevation myocardial infarction
SVT	superficial vein thrombosis
TS	tricuspid stenosis
VEB	ventricular ectopic beat
VT	ventricular tachycardia

Abbreviations (Procedures)

Abbreviation	Meaning
CABG	coronary artery bypass graft
CK, CPK	creatine phosphokinase
CRP	C-reactive protein
DSA	digital subtraction angiography
ECHO	echocardiography
ECG, EKG	electrocardiography
HDL	high-density lipoproteins
LDH	lactate dehydrogenase
LDL	low-density lipoproteins
LVAD	left ventricular assist device
MIDCAB	minimally invasive direct coronary artery bypass
PTCA	percutaneous transluminal coronary angioplasty
TEE	transesophageal echocardiogram
TMR	transmyocardial revascularization
VT	ventricular tachycardia

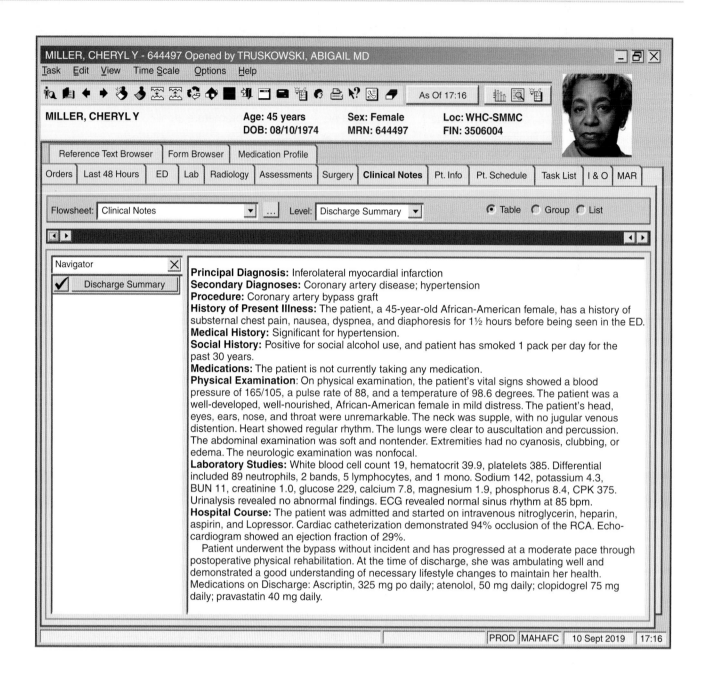

MILLER, CHERYL Y - 644497 Opened by TRUSKOWSKI, ABIGAIL MD

Task   Edit   View   Time Scale   Options   Help

MILLER, CHERYL Y

	Age: 45 years	Sex: Female	Loc: WHC-SMMC
	DOB: 08/10/1974	MRN: 644497	FIN: 3506004

Reference Text Browser   Form Browser   Medication Profile

Orders | Last 48 Hours | ED | Lab | Radiology | Assessments | Surgery | **Clinical Notes** | Pt. Info | Pt. Schedule | Task List | I & O | MAR

Flowsheet: Clinical Notes   Level: Discharge Summary   ● Table   ○ Group   ○ List

Navigator

✓ Discharge Summary

Principal Diagnosis: Inferolateral myocardial infarction
Secondary Diagnoses: Coronary artery disease; hypertension
Procedure: Coronary artery bypass graft
History of Present Illness: The patient, a 45-year-old African-American female, has a history of substernal chest pain, nausea, dyspnea, and diaphoresis for 1½ hours before being seen in the ED.
Medical History: Significant for hypertension.
Social History: Positive for social alcohol use, and patient has smoked 1 pack per day for the past 30 years.
Medications: The patient is not currently taking any medication.
Physical Examination: On physical examination, the patient's vital signs showed a blood pressure of 165/105, a pulse rate of 88, and a temperature of 98.6 degrees. The patient was a well-developed, well-nourished, African-American female in mild distress. The patient's head, eyes, ears, nose, and throat were unremarkable. The neck was supple, with no jugular venous distention. Heart showed regular rhythm. The lungs were clear to auscultation and percussion. The abdominal examination was soft and nontender. Extremities had no cyanosis, clubbing, or edema. The neurologic examination was nonfocal.
Laboratory Studies: White blood cell count 19, hematocrit 39.9, platelets 385. Differential included 89 neutrophils, 2 bands, 5 lymphocytes, and 1 mono. Sodium 142, potassium 4.3, BUN 11, creatinine 1.0, glucose 229, calcium 7.8, magnesium 1.9, phosphorus 8.4, CPK 375. Urinalysis revealed no abnormal findings. ECG revealed normal sinus rhythm at 85 bpm.
Hospital Course: The patient was admitted and started on intravenous nitroglycerin, heparin, aspirin, and Lopressor. Cardiac catheterization demonstrated 94% occlusion of the RCA. Echocardiogram showed an ejection fraction of 29%.
   Patient underwent the bypass without incident and has progressed at a moderate pace through postoperative physical rehabilitation. At the time of discharge, she was ambulating well and demonstrated a good understanding of necessary lifestyle changes to maintain her health. Medications on Discharge: Ascriptin, 325 mg po daily; atenolol, 50 mg daily; clopidogrel 75 mg daily; pravastatin 40 mg daily.

PROD MAHAFC 10 Sept 2019 17:16

Exercise 18: Discharge Summary

1. Define the signs and symptoms presented by Ms. Miller in the report above.

   A. dyspnea_____

   B. diaphoresis_____

   C. hypertension_____

2. Where was the chest pain perceived?_____

3. How do you know that Ms. Miller did not lack oxygen in her extremities? _____

4. What was the name of the ultrasound procedure performed to assess her cardiac function? _____

_____

5. What procedure was done to treat her CAD?_____

6. Which structures were evaluated by tapping and listening? _____

Go to the Evolve website to interactively build terms, label images, memorize word parts, and practice using circulatory terms in context.

Match the word parts to their definitions.

WORD PART DEFINITION

Prefix/Suffix		Definition
brady-	1.	_____ heart condition
-cardia	2.	_____ expansion, dilation
echo-	3.	_____ disease
-ectasis	4.	_____ slow
-graphy	5.	_____ abnormal condition of hardening
-megaly	6.	_____ sound
-pathy	7.	_____ rapid
-sclerosis	8.	_____ recording
tachy-	9.	_____ structure
-um	10.	_____ enlargement

Combining Form		Definition
angi/o	11.	_____ artery
aort/o	12.	_____ heart
arteri/o	13.	_____ lung
ather/o	14.	_____ clotting, clot
atri/o	15.	_____ blood
cardi/o	16.	_____ endocardium
coron/o	17.	_____ vessel
cyan/o	18.	_____ midgut
endocardi/o	19.	_____ myocardium
epicardi/o	20.	_____ vein
hem/o	21.	_____ lymph gland
lymph/o	22.	_____ aorta
lymphaden/o	23.	_____ lymph vessel
lymphangi/o	24.	_____ heart
mesenter/o	25.	_____ fat, plaque
myocardi/o	26.	_____ epicardium
pericardi/o	27.	_____ lymph
phleb/o	28.	_____ atrium
pulmon/o	29.	_____ wall, septum
sept/o	30.	_____ vessel
thromb/o	31.	_____ blue
vascul/o	32.	_____ pericardium

WORDSHOP

Prefixes	Combining Forms	Suffixes
a-	angi/o	-algia
brady-	arteri/o	-ar
dys-	atri/o	-cardia
echo-	cardi/o	-centesis
end-	cardiomy/o	-ectasis
tachy-	endocardi/o	-ectomy
	lymphangi/o	-graphy
	pericardi/o	-ia
	phleb/o	-itis
	rhythm/o	-pathy
	thromb/o	-plasty
	ven/o	-sclerosis
	ventricul/o	-tripsy

Build circulatory terms by combining the word parts above. Some word parts may be used more than once. Some may not be used at all. The number in parentheses indicates the number of word parts needed.

Definition	Term
1. disease of heart muscle (2)	
2. inflammation of clot in a vein (3)	
3. rapid heart condition (2)	
4. recording heart sound (3)	
5. dilation of a lymph vessel (2)	
6. surgically forming a vessel (2)	
7. condition of abnormal rhythm (3)	
8. inflammation of the endocardium (2)	
9. heart pain (2)	
10. surgical puncture of the sac surrounding the heart (2)	
11. pertaining to the atrium and ventricle (3)	
12. removal of a vein (2)	
13. abnormal condition of hardening of an artery (2)	
14. cutting out within an artery (3)	
15. crushing a vein (2)	

Sort the terms into the correct categories.

TERM SORTING

Anatomy and Physiology	Pathology	Procedures

angiocardiography	cardioversion	pericardiocentesis
angiotripsy	cyanosis	pericardiolysis
angina pectoris	diastole	phlebography
annulus	ECG	phlebotomy
aorta	electrocardiogram	Purkinje fibers
arrhythmia	endarterectomy	septoplasty
arteriosclerosis	endocarditis	septum
atrium	endocardium	SOB
BBB	hemorrhoid	spleen
bradycardia	hypertension	splenomegaly
bundle of His	ischemia	splenopexy
CABG	lymphadenitis	systole
capillary	mesentery	tricuspid valve
cardiomegaly	MIDCAB	ventricle
cardioplegia	MVP	venule

Replace the highlighted words with the correct terms.

TRANSLATIONS

1. After being admitted for **cardiac tissue death that occurred when the coronary arteries are occluded**, the patient had **open heart surgery in which a piece of a blood vessel is grafted onto one of the coronary arteries**.

2. After experiencing **tissue death within the brain**, the patient was left with **paralysis of one limb on the left or right side of his body**.

3. Mrs. Williams had **abnormal accumulation of fluid in interstitial tissue spaces** and was diagnosed with **the inability of the heart muscle to pump blood efficiently**.

4. The 72-year-old man had an advanced case of **accumulation and hardening of plaque in the coronary arteries.** He had a history of cigarette smoking and **heart pain.**

5. The patient underwent **x-ray imaging of a vein after the introduction of a contrast medium** to diagnose his **inflammation of veins.**

6. Mr. Singh was admitted with **profuse secretion of sweat** and **rapid heartbeat.**

7. The patient was diagnosed with **paroxysmal chest pain or discomfort** and **lack of blood supply to tissues caused by a blockage.**

8. The cardiologist ordered **surgical puncture of the pericardium to remove fluid** to treat Hugo's **compression of the heart caused by fluid in the pericardium.**

9. Malcolm's **narrowing of the tricuspid valve caused by rheumatic fever** was treated with a **repair of a heart valve.**

10. Because the patient's **disease of heart muscle** had worsened, she was put on a **mechanical pump device that assists a patient's weakened heart.**

ICD-10-CM Example from Tabular

J31 Chronic rhinitis, nasopharyngitis and pharyngitis

Use additional code to identify:

exposure to tobacco smoke (**Z77.22**)

exposure to tobacco smoke in the perinatal period (**P96.81**)

history of tobacco use (**Z87.891**)

occupational exposure to environmental tobacco smoke (**Z57.31**)

tobacco dependence (**F17.-**)

tobacco use (**Z72.0**)

ICD-10-PCS Example from Index

Rhinoplasty

see Alteration, Nasal mucosa and soft tissue **090K**

see Repair, Nasal mucosa and soft tissue **09QK**

Replacement, Nasal mucosa and soft tissue **09RK**

see Supplement, Nasal mucosa and soft tissue **09UK**

Rhinorrhaphy—*see* **Repair, Nose 09QK**

Rhinoscopy 09JKXZZ

CHAPTER OUTLINE

FUNCTIONS OF THE RESPIRATORY SYSTEM

ANATOMY AND PHYSIOLOGY

PATHOLOGY

PROCEDURES

PHARMACOLOGY

RECOGNIZING SUFFIXES FOR PCS

ABBREVIATIONS

OBJECTIVES

☐ Recognize and use terms related to the anatomy and physiology of the respiratory system.

☐ Recognize and use terms related to the pathology of the respiratory system.

☐ Recognize and use terms related to procedures for the respiratory system.

FUNCTIONS OF THE RESPIRATORY SYSTEM

- Delivering oxygen (O_2) to the blood for transport to cells in the body.
- Excreting the waste product of cellular respiration, carbon dioxide (CO_2).
- Filtering, cleansing, warming, and humidifying air taken into the lungs.
- Regulating the pH of the blood.
- Helping the production of sound for speech and singing.
- Providing the tissue that receives the stimulus for the sense of smell, olfaction.

The respiratory system (Fig. 10-1) partners with the circulatory system to deliver oxygen to and remove carbon dioxide from the cells of the body. The process of breathing in and out is called **respiration.** Breathing in (**inspiration** or

respiratory
  re- = again
  spir/o = to breathe
  -atory = pertaining to

inspiration
  in- = in
  spir/o = to breathe
  -ation = process of

air = pneum/o, aer/o

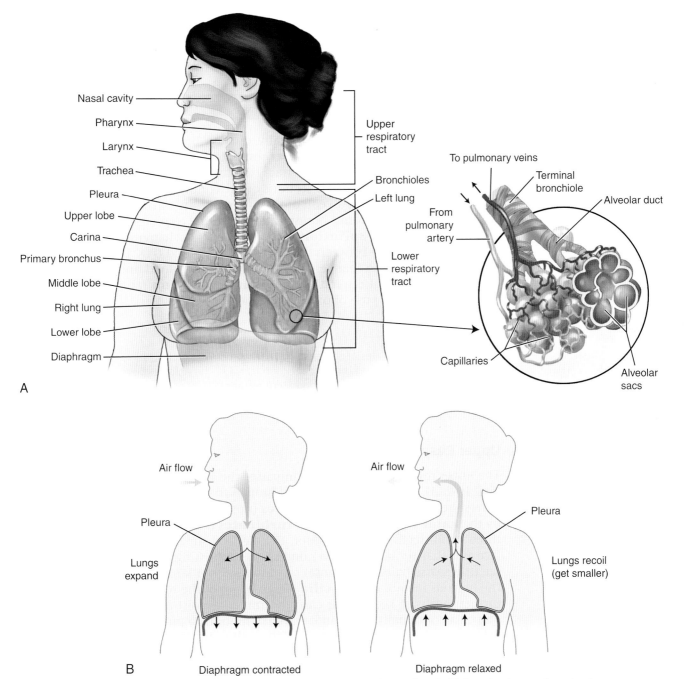

Fig. 10-1 A, The respiratory system showing a bronchial tree *(inset)* . **B,** Inspiration and expiration.

inhalation) pulls air containing oxygen into the lungs, where it passes into the circulatory system. Carbon dioxide is released when air is pushed out of the lungs (**expiration** or **exhalation**). When one dies, one breathes out and no longer breathes in again—hence the expression the patient has "expired." Using the combining form *spir/o,* meaning "to breathe," we can see that respiration means to breathe again (and again). The term *ventilation* is used to describe the movement of air into the lungs, whether it is a natural or an artificial activity.

Filtering, cleansing, warming, and humidifying air are important processes that protect the lungs from disease and allow for an optimal environment for gas exchange. The acidity and alkalinity (pH) of the blood are accomplished through mechanisms that control the rate of breathing to keep the blood pH within a narrow range. The function of producing sound (**phonation**) for speech and singing is accomplished by the interaction of air and the structures of the voice box, the larynx, and the hollow cavities, the sinuses, connected to the nasal passages.

Finally, although the sense of smell, **olfaction,** is not strictly a function of respiration, it is accomplished by the tissue in the nasal cavity, which receives the stimulus for smell and routes it to the brain through the nervous system.

ANATOMY AND PHYSIOLOGY

The respiratory system is anatomically divided into conduction passageways and gas exchange surfaces. The upper respiratory tract (the nose, pharynx, and larynx) and the lower respiratory tract (the trachea, bronchial tree, and lungs) (Fig. 10-1, *A*) make up the two sections of the conduction passageways. The gas exchange surfaces are the alveoli of the lungs and the cells of the body.

There are two main forms of respiration: external respiration and internal respiration. **External respiration** is the process of exchanging oxygen (O_2) and carbon dioxide (CO_2) between the lungs and the blood (Fig. 10-1, *B*). **Internal respiration** is the exchange of gases between the blood and the cells of the body. A third type of respiration, **cellular respiration** (also called **cellular metabolism**), is the use of oxygen to generate energy.

This chapter includes all the anatomy necessary to assign ICD-10 respiratory system codes, including detail on the cuneiform cartilage, the antrum of Highmore, and the vestibular folds. See Appendix H for a complete list of body parts and how they should be coded.

Upper Respiratory Tract

The upper respiratory system encompasses the area from the nose to the larynx (Fig. 10-2, *A*). Air can enter the body through the mouth, but for the most part it enters the body through the two **nares** (nostrils) of the nose that are separated by the **nasal septum.** The **nasal turbinates** (also called **nasal conchae**) are three scroll-shaped bones (inferior, middle, and superior) that increase the surface area that air must pass over on its way to the lungs (Fig. 10-2, *B*). The vibrissae (the coarse hairs in the nose) serve to filter out large particulate matter, and the mucous membrane and **cilia** (small hairs) of the respiratory tract provide a further means of keeping air clean, warm, and moist as it travels to the lungs. The cilia continually move in a wavelike motion to push the sticky mucus and debris out of the respiratory tract. The air then travels up and backward, where it is filtered, warmed, and humidified by the environment in the upper portion of the nasal cavity. Damage to the cilia keeps the germ-laden mucus from leaving the body and consequently provides a hospitable environment for infection.

exhalation
  ex- = out
  hal/o = to breathe
  -ation = process of

phonation
  phon/o = sound
  -ation = process of

oxygen = ox/i, ox/o, oxy-

carbon dioxide = capn/o

mouth = or/o, stomat/o

nose = nas/o, rhin/o

septum
  sept/o = wall
  -um = structure

mucus = muc/o

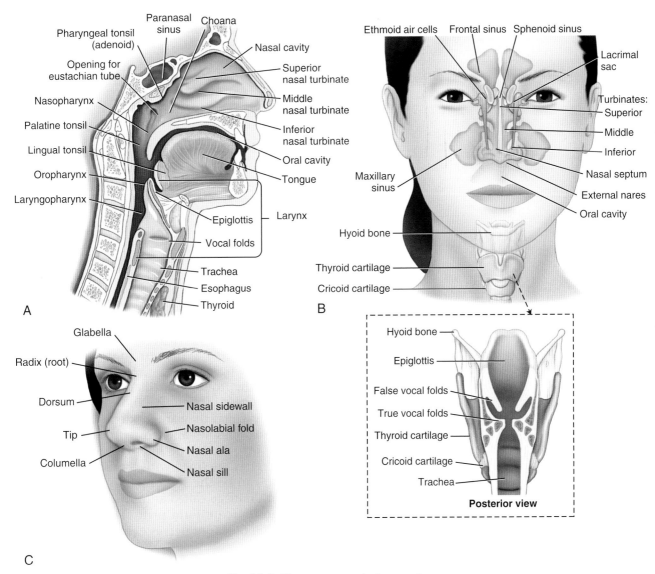

Fig. 10-2 The upper respiratory system.

CPT Coding Alert!

CPT uses terminology that describes the different landmarks of the nose. (See Fig. 10-2, C.) The columella is the area of the nose between the tip and the nasal base. Surgeries of this area of the nose are termed columelloplasties, usually to lengthen the tip of the nose.

Click on **Animations** to see how the respiratory cycle works.

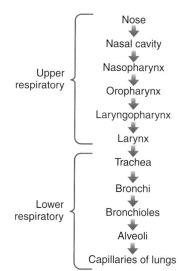

Fig. 10-3 Schematic of the order in which air passes through the upper respiratory system and into the lower respiratory system.

Fig. 10-3 illustrates the route of air into the body. The receptors for olfaction are located in the nasal cavity, which is connected to the **paranasal sinuses,** collectively named for their proximity to the nose.

The paranasal sinuses, divided into the frontal, maxillary (the largest sinus, also referred to as the *antrum of Highmore*), sphenoid, and ethmoid cavities, acquire their names from the bones in which they are located. The paired ethmoid sinuses are divided into anterior, middle, and posterior **air cells.** The function of sinus cavities in the skull is to warm and filter the air taken in and to assist in the production of sound. They are lined with a mucous membrane that drains into the nasal cavity and can be the site of painful inflammation. Each sinus has a natural opening for drainage called an **ostium.** The ethmoid bone cradles the **olfactory bulb** in the cribriform plate. This sievelike bone has numerous openings through which olfactory nerves descend into the nasal cavity.

Air continues to travel from the back of the nasal cavity to the **nasopharynx,** a part of the throat (**pharynx**) behind the nasal cavity. The nasal choanae are the paired openings (left and right) to the nostrils posterior to the nasopharynx. The **eustachian tubes** (also called the **auditory** or **pharyngotympanic tubes**) connect the ears with the throat at this point and serve to equalize pressure between the ears and the throat. The nasopharynx is the site of the pharyngeal tonsils (**adenoids**), which are made of lymphatic tissue and help to protect the respiratory system from pathogens. The next structure, the **oropharynx,** is the part of the throat posterior to the oral cavity. It is the location of more lymphatic tissue, the palatine tonsils, so named because they are continuous with the roof of the mouth (the palate). The lingual tonsils, located on the posterior aspect of the tongue, also serve a protective function. Note that the oropharynx is part of the digestive system as well as the respiratory system; both food and air pass through it. Below the oropharynx is the part of the throat referred to as the **laryngopharynx** because it adjoins the opening of the larynx.

The **larynx,** commonly referred to as the **voice box,** is the main organ of sound production. It is a short tube that is composed of nine sets of supportive, protective cartilaginous structures and two sets of vocal folds, one true and one false. The **false vocal folds,** also called the **vestibular folds** for their location at the entrance to the larynx, do not function in the production of speech. Speaking and singing are controlled by the **true vocal folds** (also termed **vocal cords**), which are composed of the glottis, two muscular folds, and the space between them (the rima glottidis). The pitch of one's voice is determined by the

---

paranasal
   para- = near
   nas/o = nose
   -al = pertaining to

sinus = sinus/o, sin/o

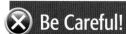 **Be Careful!**

Do not confuse the **ost/i** *in* ostium *with the combining form for bone,* **oste/o.**

nasopharynx
   nas/o = nose
   pharyng/o = throat, pharynx

eustachian tube = salping/o

pharynx = pharyng/o

adenoid = adenoid/o

oropharynx
   or/o = mouth
   pharyng/o = throat, pharynx

lingual
   lingu/o = tongue
   -al = pertaining to

tonsil = tonsill/o

laryngopharynx
   laryng/o = larynx, voice box
   pharyng/o = pharynx

larynx = laryng/o

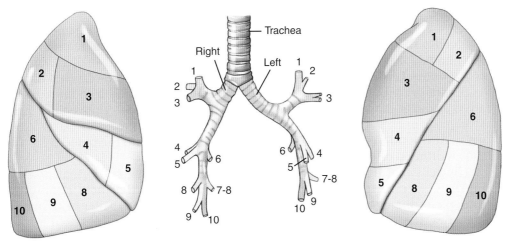

Fig. 10-4 Primary, second, and tertiary bronchi that correspond to lung, lobe, and segment.

degree to which the vocal cords are stretched as they vibrate. Loudness of speech is determined by the force of the exhaled air that travels out through the larynx. One of the cartilages, the **epiglottis,** is an oval-shaped structure that covers the trachea (windpipe) when an individual swallows to prevent food from being pulled into the windpipe instead of the esophagus. When looking at the anatomy of the neck, it is useful to note the proximity of the thyroid gland, which is anterior and inferior to the larynx. Although the thyroid gland will be described more fully in the chapter on the endocrine system, one can see that its location allows for a shared connection, the thyroid cartilage. Normally larger and more angular in the male than in the female, the thyroid cartilage consists of a pair of thin plates called *laminae.* These plates cover the anterior surface of the larynx, and are attached to the hyoid bone on either side with the thyrohyoid ligament. The area where the two plates join is the **laryngeal prominence,** commonly called the **Adam's apple.** The cricoid cartilage, named for its ring-like appearance, forms the lower part of the larynx, attaching it to the trachea. The paired arytenoid cartilages, located in the back upper border of the cricoid cartilage, are attached to the vocal folds and function to close them. The corniculate cartilages are located at the tip of the cricoid cartilage, while the cuneiform (wedge-shaped) cartilages are in front of the corniculate cartilage.

Lower Respiratory Tract

The lower respiratory tract begins with the **trachea** (or windpipe), which extends from the larynx into the chest cavity. The trachea is composed of several C-shaped rings, which prevent the airway from collapsing. The trachea lies within the space between the lungs called the **mediastinum.** Air travels into the lungs as the trachea bifurcates (branches) at the carina, a keel-shaped cartilage where the right and left airways, called **bronchi** (*sing.* bronchus), divide into smaller branches. The metaphor of an upside-down tree makes sense here, as one can imagine the trachea as the trunk and the bronchi and bronchioles as branches

Each **lung** is composed of sections called **lobes,** which correspond to the secondary bronchi that supply these areas within each lung. The right lung is made up of three lobes, whereas the left has only two (see Fig. 10-1, *A*). The abbreviations for the lobes of the lungs are RUL (right upper lobe), RML (right middle lobe), RLL (right lower lobe), LUL (left upper lobe), and LLL (left lower lobe). Within each of these lobes, the secondary bronchi branch out to tertiary bronchi, and the areas that each supplies are referred to as **segments** (Fig. 10-4). Each segment is supplied with blood from a segmental artery that branches off the pulmonary arteries. The segments are named by their location (e.g., anterior,

epiglottis = epiglott/o

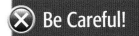

Do not confuse the nasal conchae with the nasal choanae.

trachea, windpipe = trache/o

chest = thorac/o, steth/o, pector/o

mediastinum = mediastin/o

bronchus = bronch/o, bronchi/o

lung = pulmon/o, pneum/o, pneumon/o

lobe = lob/o, lobul/o

apex, tip, point = apic/o

base = bas/o

bronchiole = bronchiol/o

alveolus = alveol/o

posterior, apical, basal, medial, or lateral). The **lingula** is the area where the superior and inferior segments appear on the left lung. Although named for its tonguelike shape, it has been postulated that it may represent the remnants of a left middle lobe. At the end of the segmental bronchi are still smaller branches called **bronchioles.** These bronchioles end in terminal bronchioles that branch to respiratory bronchioles. The respiratory bronchioles extend into microscopic alveolar ducts capped by delicate air sacs called **alveoli** (*sing.* alveolus). Each alveolus is in contact with a blood capillary to provide a means of exchange of gases. At this point O_2 is diffused across cell membranes into the blood cells, and CO_2 is diffused out to be expired.

The cells that line the respiratory tract include **goblet cells** (that produce mucus) and **ciliated basal** (also termed **stem) cells** (that help cleanse the lining). As the bronchial tree progressively divides into smaller and smaller branches, the shapes of the cells that line it change from a thicker to a thinner appearance. Tall, simple columnar cells in the primary bronchi give way to squat, simple cuboidal cells in the terminal bronchioles. The cells in the terminal bronchioles are still equipped with ciliated cells to remove debris from the airways, but the presence of goblet cells (with their secretion of mucus) is missing. As gas exchange becomes the most important function, simple squamous (scaly, flat) cells appear in the alveoli. The epithelial lining of the alveoli is composed of type I and type II cells. Type I cells are responsible for gas exchange, while type II cells produce a substance called *surfactant* that keeps the lung from collapsing.

As mentioned earlier, the respiratory system is important in the maintenance of the acidity and alkalinity of the blood through regulation of the pH. Because blood pH is measured by the concentration of hydrogen ions (H^+), one needs to understand how oxygen and carbon dioxide are involved.

When O_2 passes from the alveoli through the capillaries of the lung to begin its journey to the cells of the body, it binds to red blood cells (RBCs) and dissolves in the liquid portion of the blood, the plasma. The RBCs contain a protein called **hemoglobin** that increases the potential amount of oxygen that can be carried by the blood. The oxygen binds with this protein (now called **oxyhemoglobin)** and continues its ride to the cells, where it is given off to be used in cellular respiration by the power plants of the cell, the **mitochondria.** Without oxygen, energy needed for cellular functions cannot be generated. This is why an anemic person feels tired—oxygen is in short supply because there is a diminished number of RBCs.

oxyhemogobin

 oxy- = oxygen
 hem/o = blood
 -globin = protein
   substance

The mitochondria use oxygen for the energy transformation that results in the formation of carbon dioxide. CO_2 then travels back to the lungs to be excreted, catching a ride again on the RBCs as carbonic acid (H_2CO_3), which is made up of carbon dioxide and water. If the pH is too high, the carbonic acid will split to form bicarbonate (HCO_3) and a hydrogen ion that will increase the concentration of hydrogen ions and cause the pH to fall. If the pH is too low, the bicarbonate ions will bond with unattached hydrogen ions, lowering the concentration of hydrogen ions and causing the pH to rise. Once at the capillaries, it converts back to carbon dioxide and water, where it is exhaled as warm, moist breath.

Blood pH decreases (becomes more acidic) as carbon dioxide levels increase. To compensate, we breathe faster and deeper (**hyperventilation**) to move the CO_2 out of our bodies. The carbonic acid that is carried back to the lungs can also act as a buffer, a ready donor/receiver of hydrogen ions to adjust the pH as needed. Receptors in the carotid arteries and the aorta sense the pH level and provide stimulation for its adjustment.

Ketoacidosis, a complication of diabetes mellitus, is a drop in pH caused by the excessive breakdown of fats. The resulting **Kussmaul's respirations,** characterized by rapid, deep breathing, are an effort by the body to decrease the amount of CO_2 and raise the blood's pH.

It should be noted that the lungs are assisted by the urinary system in the regulation of blood pH. The kidneys are responsible for monitoring and adjusting the concentration of bicarbonate ions, recycling them back into the bloodstream as needed and excreting excess hydrogen ions into the urine.

Each lung is also enclosed by a double-folded, serous membrane called the **pleura** (*pl.* pleurae). The side of the membrane that coats the lungs is the **visceral pleura**; the side that lines the inner surface of the rib cage is the **parietal pleura.** The two sides of the pleural membrane contain a serous (watery) fluid that facilitates the expansion and contraction of the lungs with each breath.

The muscles responsible for normal, quiet respiration are the dome-shaped **diaphragm** and the muscles between the ribs **(intercostal muscles).** On inspiration, the diaphragm is pulled down as it contracts and the intercostal muscles expand, pulling air into the lungs because of the resulting negative pressure (see Fig. 10-1, *B*). On expiration the diaphragm and intercostal muscles relax, pushing air out of the lungs.

pleura = pleur/o
viscera, organ = viscer/o
wall = pariet/o, sept/o
diaphragm = diaphragmat/o, diaphragm/o, phren/o
intercostal   inter- = between   cost/o = rib   -al = pertaining to

 Be Careful!   **Salping/o** *means both* eustachian tubes *and* fallopian tubes.

 Be Careful!   *Don't confuse* **bronchi/o,** *which means* bronchial tubes, *with* **brachi/o,** *which means the* arm.

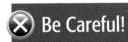 Exercise 1: **Anatomy and Physiology of the Respiratory System**

Match the respiratory structure with its combining form or prefix.

____ 1. pleura
____ 2. lobe
____ 3. tonsil
____ 4. mucus
____ 5. diaphragm
____ 6. windpipe
____ 7. adenoids
____ 8. eustachian tube
____ 9. bronchiole
____ 10. rib
____ 11. to breathe
____ 12. throat
____ 13. alveolus
____ 14. lung
____ 15. sinus
____ 16. bronchus

____ 17. voice box
____ 18. mouth
____ 19. nose
____ 20. mediastinum
____ 21. in
____ 22. air
____ 23. out
____ 24. epiglottis
____ 25. wall
____ 26. carbon dioxide
____ 27. oxygen
____ 28. point, tip
____ 29. tongue
____ 30. base
____ 31. chest

A. ox/i
B. bronch/o, bronchi/o
C. salping/o
D. pneum/o, pneumon/o, pulmon/o
E. hal/o, spir/o
F. pharyng/o
G. adenoid/o
H. pariet/o
I. rhin/o, nas/o
J. pneum/o, aer/o
K. capn/o
L. lob/o, lobul/o
M. diaphragm/o, phren/o
N. thorac/o, pector/o, steth/o

O. trache/o
P. alveol/o
Q. tonsill/o
R. pleur/o
S. sin/o, sinus/o
T. muc/o
U. epiglott/o
V. laryng/o
W. in-
X. bronchiol/o
Y. cost/o
Z. mediastin/o
AA. ex-
BB. or/o, stomat/o
CC. apic/o
DD. bas/o
EE. lingu/o

To practice labeling the respiratory system, click on **Label It.**

You can review the anatomy of the respiratory system by clicking on **Body Spectrum Electronic Anatomy Coloring Book, then Respiratory.**

Combining Forms for the Anatomy and Physiology of the Respiratory System

Meaning	Combining Form	Meaning	Combining Form
adenoid	adenoid/o	mediastinum	mediastin/o
air	pneum/o, aer/o	mouth	or/o, stomat/o
alveolus	alveol/o	mucus	muc/o
base	bas/o	nose	nas/o, rhin/o
bronchiole	bronchiol/o	oxygen	ox/i, ox/o
bronchus	bronch/o, bronchi/o	pharynx (throat)	pharyng/o
carbon dioxide	capn/o	pleura	pleur/o
chest	steth/o, thorac/o, pector/o	point, tip, apex	apic/o
columella	columell/o	rib	cost/o
diaphragm	diaphragm/o, diaphragmat/o, phren/o	septum, wall	sept/o, pariet/o
		sinus	sinus/o, sin/o
epiglottis	epiglott/o	sound	phon/o
eustachian tube	salping/o	to breathe	spir/o, hal/o
larynx (voice box)	laryng/o	tongue	lingu/o
lobe	lob/o, lobul/o	tonsil	tonsill/o
lung	pulmon/o, pneumon/o, pneum/o	trachea (windpipe)	trache/o
		viscera	viscer/o

Prefixes for Anatomy and Physiology of the Respiratory System

Prefix	Meaning
ex-	out
in-	in
inter-	between
oxy-	oxygen
para-	near
re-	again

PATHOLOGY

Terms Related to Symptoms and Signs Involving the Respiratory System (R00-R99)

Term	Word Origin	Definition
aphonia	*a-* no, not, without *phon/o* sound *-ia* condition	Loss of ability to produce sounds. **Dysphonia** is difficulty making sounds.
apnea	*a-* no, not, without *-pnea* breathing	Abnormal, periodic cessation of breathing.
bradypnea	*brady-* slow *-pnea* breathing	Abnormally slow breathing.

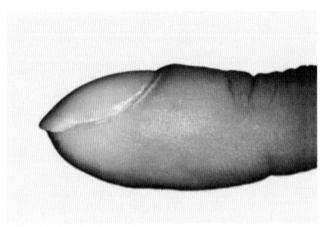

Fig. 10-5 Clubbing.

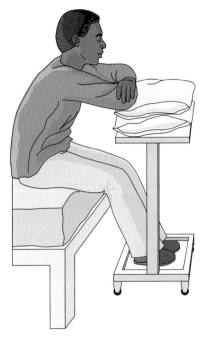

Sitting on the edge of a bed with the arms folded and placed on two or three pillows positioned over a nightstand.

Fig. 10-6 Orthopnea position that clients with chronic obstructive pulmonary disease can assume to ease the work of breathing.

Terms Related to Symptoms and Signs Involving the Respiratory System (R00-R99)—cont'd

Term	Word Origin	Definition
Cheyne-Stokes respiration		Deep, rapid breathing followed by a period of apnea.
clubbing		Abnormal enlargement of the distal phalanges as a result of diminished O_2 in the blood (Fig. 10-5).
cyanosis	*cyan/o* blue *-osis* abnormal condition	Lack of oxygen in blood seen as bluish or grayish discoloration of the skin, nail beds, and/or lips.
dyspnea	*dys-* difficult *-pnea* breathing	Difficult and/or painful breathing. **DOE is dyspnea on exertion. Eupnea** is good, normal breathing. (eu- means healthy, normal.)
epistaxis		Nosebleed. Also called **rhinorrhagia**.
hemoptysis	*hem/o* blood *-ptysis* spitting	Coughing up blood or blood-stained sputum.
hypercapnia	*hyper-* excessive *capn/o* carbon dioxide *-ia* condition	Condition of excessive CO_2 in the blood.

Continued

Terms Related to Symptoms and Signs Involving the Respiratory System (R00-R99)—cont'd

Term	Word Origin	Definition
hyperpnea	*hyper-* excessive *-pnea* breathing	Excessively deep breathing. Hypopnea is extremely shallow breathing.
hyperventilation	*hyper-* excessive	Abnormally increased breathing.
hypoxemia	*hypo-* deficient *ox/o* oxygen *-emia* blood condition	Condition of deficient O_2 in the blood. **Hypoxia** is the condition of deficient oxygen in the tissues.
orthopnea	*orth/o* straight *-pnea* breathing	Condition of difficult breathing unless in an upright position (Fig. 10-6).
pleurodynia	*pleur/o* pleura *-dynia* pain	Pain in the chest caused by inflammation of the intercostal muscles.
pyrexia	*pyr/o* fire *-exia* condition	Fever. Technically, any temperature above 98.6°F (37°C) is considered a fever, but above 100.4°F (38°C) is considered a significant fever. **SARS-Covid-19** is an amalgamation of an acronym (**SARS**) and a portmanteau (**co** = corona + **vi** = virus + **d** = disease + **19** for the year it was first named). The term for the virus itself, is SARS-CoV-2.
shortness of breath (SOB)		Breathlessness; air hunger.
sputum, abnormal		Mucus coughed up from the lungs and expectorated through the mouth. If abnormal, may be described as to its amount, color, or odor.
tachypnea	*tachy-* fast *-pnea* breathing	Rapid, shallow breathing.
thoracodynia	*thorac/o* chest *-dynia* pain	Chest pain.

Terms Related to Abnormal Breath Sounds (R06-R09)

An important part of the diagnostic process is the evaluation of breath sounds, usually through the use of a **stethoscope**. This "listening" is termed **auscultation**, and the "tapping" is called **percussion**. Normal breath sounds are termed **vesicular**, misnamed by the inventor of the stethoscope, Laennec. He interpreted the sound as originating from the tiny sacs of the alveoli, instead of the trachea and bronchi, where they actually occur. Abnormal breath sounds are collectively referred to as **adventitious sounds**.

Term	Word Origin	Definition
friction sounds		Sounds made by dry surfaces rubbing together. Characteristic of inflamed pleurae; may also have a grating or creaking sound.
hiccough		Sound produced by the involuntary contraction of the diaphragm, followed by rapid closure of the glottis. Also called **hiccup, singultus**.
rales		Also called **crackles** or **crepitations**, an abnormal lung sound heard on inspiration, characterized by discontinuous bubbling, clicking, or rattling noises. May be associated with pneumonia or congestive heart failure and are characterized as moist, dry, fine, and/or coarse.
rhonchi		If used as a term without further description (see *wheezing*), rhonchi are continuous abnormal rumbling sounds heard on expiration, caused by airways blocked with secretions.
stridor		Continuous, high-pitched inspiratory sound from the larynx; a sign of upper airway obstruction or epiglottitis.
wheezing		Continuous sounds heard during inspiration and/or expiration. If high pitched and having a whistling sound (as in an asthma attack), they may also be referred to as **sibilant rhonchi. Sonorous rhonchi** are wheezes that are lower in pitch and that have a snoring or rumbling sound (as in bronchitis). The sibilant rhonchi are caused by airways narrowed from constriction or swelling, while the sonorous rhonchi are caused by secretions in the bronchi.

Exercise 2: Respiratory Symptoms and Signs and Abnormal Chest Sounds

Match the term to its definition.

____ 1. apnea	A. coughing up blood or blood-stained sputum
____ 2. Cheyne-Stokes respiration	B. crackles
____ 3. SOB	C. high-pitched whistling sound made during breathing
____ 4. cyanosis	D. lack of oxygen in blood seen as bluish discoloration of skin, nails, and/or lips
____ 5. hemoptysis	
____ 6. bradypnea	E. pain in the chest caused by inflammation of intercostal muscles
____ 7. orthopnea	F. abnormally slow breathing
____ 8. pleurodynia	G. fever
____ 9. pyrexia	H. abnormal rumbling sound heard on auscultation
____ 10. hyperventilation	I. chest pain
____ 11. tachypnea	J. deep, rapid breathing followed by a period of apnea
____ 12. thoracodynia	K. abnormal, periodic cessation of breathing
____ 13. rales	L. nosebleed
____ 14. rhonchi	M. rapid, shallow breathing
____ 15. stridor	N. high-pitched inspiratory sound from the larynx
____ 16. wheezing	O. air hunger
____ 17. sputum	P. mucus coughed up from the lungs
____ 18. clubbing	Q. difficult and/or painful breathing
____ 19. epistaxis	R. abnormal enlargement of the distal phalanges as a result of decreased oxygen in the blood
____ 20. dyspnea	
	S. abnormally increased breathing
	T. condition of difficult breathing unless upright

Build the term.

21. condition of excessive carbon dioxide_____

22. blood condition of deficient oxygen_____

23. condition of without sound_____

24. chest pain_____

25. fast breathing_____

Terms Related to Acute Upper Respiratory Infections (J00-J06)

Term	Word Origin	Definition
epiglottitis	*epiglott/o* epiglottis *-itis* inflammation	Inflammation of the epiglottis (Fig. 10-7). **Supraglottitis** is an inflammation of the area immediately above the glottis that includes the epiglottis.
laryngitis	*laryng/o* larynx, voice box *-itis* inflammation	Inflammation of the voice box.
nasopharyngitis	*nas/o* nose *pharyng/o* pharynx, throat *-itis* inflammation	The common cold. Also referred to as **coryza**.
obstructive laryngitis		Acute viral infection of early childhood, marked by stridor caused by spasms of the larynx, trachea, and bronchi. Also called **croup**.
pharyngitis	*pharyng/o* pharynx, throat *-itis* inflammation	Inflammation or infection of the pharynx, usually causing symptoms of a sore throat.
sinusitis	*sinus/o* sinus *-itis* inflammation	Inflammation of one or more of the paranasal sinuses. **Pansinusitis** refers to an inflammation of all of the sinuses (*pan-* means *all*).
tracheitis	*trache/o* trachea, windpipe *-itis* inflammation	Inflammation of the windpipe.

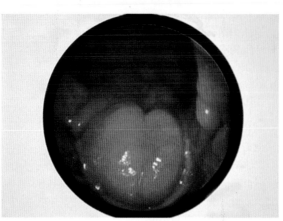

Fig. 10-7 Epiglottitis. The epiglottis is red and swollen.

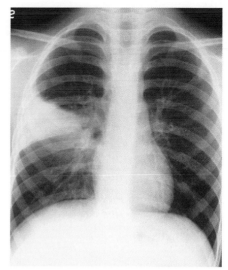

Fig. 10-8 Right upper lobe (RUL) pneumonia.

Terms Related to Influenza and Pneumonia (J09-J18)

Term	Word Origin	Definition
influenza		Also known as the **flu**. Acute infectious disease of the respiratory tract caused by a virus. Avian (bird) flu is caused by type A influenza virus. The latest bird flu is caused by H7N9 virus. Swine flu is caused by H1N1 virus.
pneumonia	*pneumon/o* lung *-ia* condition	Inflammation of the lungs caused by a variety of pathogens. If infectious, it is termed **pneumonia**; if noninfectious, **pneumonitis**. The name(s) of the lobes are used to describe the extent of the disease (e.g., **RUL pneumonia** is pneumonia of the right upper lobe) (Fig. 10-8). If both lungs are affected, it is termed **double pneumonia**.
severe acute respiratory syndrome (SARS)	*syn-* together, with *-drome* to run	Viral respiratory disorder caused by a coronavirus. Usually results in pneumonia. Note that this is NOT the same as influenza.

CM Guideline Alert

10.D Ventilator Associated Pneumonia
1) Documentation of Ventilator Associated Pneumonia
As with all procedural or postprocedural complications, code assignment is based on the provider's documentation of the relationship between the condition and the procedure.

Code J95.851, Ventilator associated pneumonia, should be assigned only when the provider has documented ventilator associated pneumonia (VAP). An additional code to identify the organism (e.g., Pseudomonas aeruginosa, code B96.5) should also be assigned. Do not assign an additional code from categories J12-J18 to identify the type of pneumonia.

Code J95.851 should not be assigned for cases where the patient has pneumonia and is on a mechanical ventilator and the provider has not specifically stated that the pneumonia is a complication attributable to the mechanical ventilator; query the provider.

2) Ventilator Associated Pneumonia Develops After Admission
A patient may be admitted with one type of pneumonia (e.g., code J13, Pneumonia due to Streptococcus pneumonia) and subsequently develops VAP. In this instance, the principal diagnosis would be the appropriate code from categories J12-J18 for the pneumonia diagnosed at the time of admission. Code J95.851, Ventilator associated pneumonia, would be assigned as an additional diagnosis when the provider has also documented the presence of ventilator associated pneumonia.

CM Guideline Alert

10.C INFLUENZA DUE TO CERTAIN IDENTIFIED INFLUENZA VIRUSES

Code only confirmed cases of influenza due to certain identified influenza viruses (category J09), and due to other identified influenza virus (category J10). This is an exception to the hospital inpatient guideline Section II, H. (Uncertain Diagnosis)

In this context, "confirmation" does not require documentation of positive laboratory testing specific for avian or other novel influenza A or other identified influenza virus. However, coding should be based on the provider's diagnostic statement that the patient has avian influenza, or other novel influenza A, for category J09, or has another particular identified strain of influenza, such as HINI or H3N2, but not identified as novel or variant, for category J10.

If the provider records "suspected" or "possible" or "probable avian influenza, or novel influenza, or other identified influenza, then the appropriate influenza code from category J11, Influenza due to unidentified influenza virus, should be assigned. A code from category J09, Influenza due to certain identified influenza viruses, should not be assigned nor should a code from category J10, Influenza due to other identified influenza virus.

Terms Related to Other Acute Lower Respiratory Infections (J20-J22)

Term	Word Origin	Definition
bronchiolitis	*bronchiol/o* bronchiole *-itis* inflammation	Viral inflammation of the bronchioles; more common in children younger than 18 months.
bronchitis	*bronch/o* bronchus *-itis* inflammation	Inflammation of the bronchi. May be acute or chronic.

Exercise 3: Congenital Disorders, Acute Upper Respiratory Infections, Influenza and Pneumonia, and Other Acute Lower Respiratory Infections

Match the term to its definition.

____ 1. sinusitis
____ 2. pharyngitis
____ 3. obstructive laryngitis
____ 4. epiglottitis
____ 5. influenza
____ 6. pneumonia

A. inflammation of the epiglottis
B. inflammation or infection of the throat
C. inflammation of the lungs caused by a variety of pathogens
D. inflammation of one or more sinuses
E. acute infectious disease of the respiratory tract caused by a virus
F. croup

Translate the terms.

7. nasolaryngitis_____

8. tracheitis_____

9. bronchiolitis_____

Terms Related to Other Diseases of Upper Respiratory Tract (J30-J39)

Term	Word Origin	Definition
deviated septum	*sept/o* wall, septum *-um* structure	Deflection of the nasal septum that may obstruct the nasal passages, resulting in infection, sinusitis, shortness of breath, headache, or recurring epistaxis.
hypertrophy of nasal turbinates	*hyper-* excessive *-trophy* development	Excessive development (enlargement) of the scroll-like bones within the nasal cavity.
laryngismus	*laryng/o* larynx, voice box *-ismus* spasm condition	A spasm of the larynx. Also called **stridulus**.
nasal mucositis (ulcerative)	*mucos/o* mucus *-itis* inflammation	Inflammation of the mucous membrane within the nose. *Ulcerative* indicates that there is erosion of the mucous membrane.
polyps, nasal and vocal cord		Small tumorlike growths that project from a mucous membrane surface, including the inside of the nose, the paranasal sinuses, and the vocal cords (Fig. 10-9).
rhinorrhea	*rhin/o* nose *-rrhea* discharge, flow	Discharge from the nose.

Terms Related to Specific Infections of the Respiratory System (A15-B97)

Term	Word Origin	Definition
diphtheria		Bacterial respiratory infection characterized by a sore throat, fever, and headache.
pertussis		Bacterial infection of the respiratory tract with a characteristic high-pitched "whoop." Also called **whooping cough.**
respiratory syncytial virus (RSV)		Acute respiratory disorder usually occurring in the lower respiratory tract in children and the upper respiratory tract in adults. Most common cause of bronchiolitis and pneumonia in infants and highly contagious in young children.
rhinomycosis	*rhin/o* nose *myc/o* fungus *-osis* abnormal condition	Abnormal condition of fungus in the in the nasal membranes.
tuberculosis (TB)		Chronic infectious disorder caused by an acid-fast bacillus, *Mycobacterium tuberculosis* (Fig. 10-10). Transmission is normally by inhalation or ingestion of infected droplets. Multidrug-resistant tuberculosis (MDR TB) is fatal in 80% of cases.

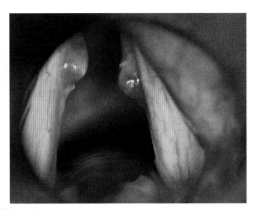

Fig. 10-9 Polypoid nodules of the vocal cords.

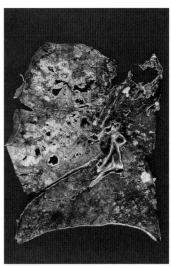

Fig. 10-10 Massive destruction of lung parenchyma by tuberculosis.

Terms Related to Chronic Lower Respiratory Diseases (J40-J47)

Term	Word Origin	Definition
asthma		Respiratory disorder characterized by recurring episodes of paroxysmal (sudden, episodic) dyspnea. Patients exhibit coughing, wheezing, and shortness of breath. If the attack becomes continuous (termed **status asthmaticus**), it may be fatal (Fig. 10-11). If described as extrinsic, the cause is from an allergic reaction to an inhaled substance. If intrinsic, the cause is unknown (idiopathic). **Intermittent asthma** is less than 2× a week, while **persistent asthma** is more than 2× per week.
bronchiectasis	*bronchi/o* bronchus *-ectasis* dilation	Chronic dilation of the bronchi. Symptoms include dyspnea, expectoration of foul-smelling sputum, and coughing.
chronic obstructive pulmonary disease (COPD)	*pulmon/o* lung *-ary* pertaining to	Respiratory disorder characterized by a progressive and irreversible diminishment in inspiratory and expiratory capacity of the lungs. Patient experiences dyspnea on exertion (DOE), difficulty inhaling or exhaling, and a chronic cough.
emphysema (including panlobular)		Abnormal condition of the pulmonary system characterized by distention and destructive changes of the alveoli. The most common cause is tobacco smoking, but exposure to environmental particulate matter may also cause the disease (Fig. 10-12).

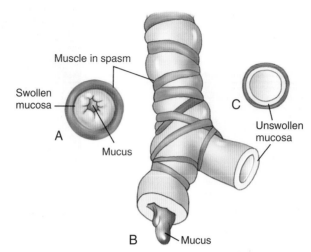

Fig. 10-11 Factors causing expiratory obstruction in asthma. A, Cross section of a bronchiole occluded by muscle spasm, swollen mucosa, and mucus. **B**, Longitudinal section of an obstructed bronchiole. **C**, Cross section of a clear bronchiole.

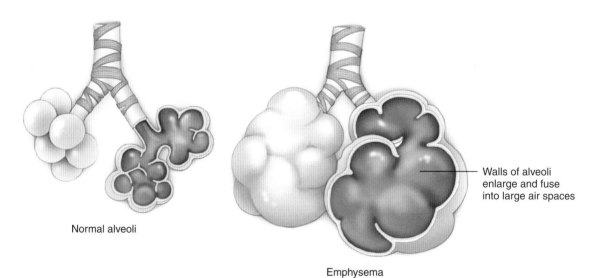

Fig. 10-12 Emphysema.

CM Guideline Alert

10A. Chronic Obstructive Pulmonary Disease (COPD) and Asthma
1) Acute Exacerbation of Chronic Obstructive Bronchitis and Asthma
The codes in categories J44 and J45 distinguish between uncomplicated cases and those in acute exacerbation. An acute exacerbation is a worsening or a decompensation of a chronic condition. An acute exacerbation is not equivalent to an infection superimposed on a chronic condition, although an exacerbation may be triggered by an infection.

Terms Related to Lung Disease Due to External Agents (J60-J70)

Term	Word Origin	Definition
pneumoconiosis	*pneum/o* lung *coni/o* dust *-osis* abnormal condition	Loss of lung capacity caused by an accumulation of dust in the lungs. Types may include **asbestosis** (abnormal condition of asbestos in the lungs) (Fig. 10-13), **silicosis** (abnormal accumulation of glass dust in the lungs), and **coal workers' pneumoconiosis (CWP)** (Fig. 10-14).

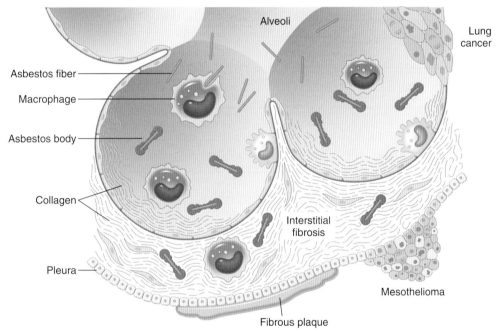

Fig. 10-13 Asbestosis. Note the asbestos bodies, the fibrous plaque on the pleural surface, and the development of mesothelioma.

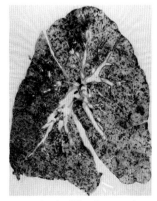

Fig. 10-14 Coal workers' pneumoconiosis. The lungs show increased black pigmentation.

Exercise 4: Other Diseases of Upper Respiratory Tract; Specific Infections of the Respiratory System; Chronic Lower Respiratory Diseases; Lung Diseases Due to External Agents

Match the terms to their definitions.

____ 1. diphtheria
____ 2. pertussis
____ 3. tuberculosis
____ 4. RSV
____ 5. deviated septum
____ 6. COPD
____ 7. emphysema
____ 8. nasal mucositis
____ 9. hypertrophy of nasal turbinates

A. chronic infectious disorder caused by *Mycobacterium tuberculosis*
B. inflammation of the mucous membrane within the nose
C. whooping cough
D. respiratory disorder characterized by a progressive diminishment in lung capacity
E. acute respiratory disorder that can cause bronchiolitis in infants
F. excessive development (enlargement) of the scroll-like bones within the nasal cavity
G. abnormal pulmonary condition characterized by distention and destructive changes of the alveoli
H. bacterial respiratory infection characterized by sore throat, fever, and headache
I. deflection of the nasal septum

Build the terms.

10. spasm of the larynx_____

11. abnormal condition of fungus in the nose_____

12. dilation of the bronchus_____

13. abnormal condition of dust in the lung_____

Terms Related to Other Respiratory Diseases Principally Affecting the Interstitium (J80-J84)		
Term	**Word Origin**	**Definition**
acute respiratory distress syndrome (ARDS)		Sudden, severe lung dysfunction due to a number of different disorders (e.g., pneumonia, trauma). Patients have extreme difficulty with breathing and may need mechanical ventilation.
pulmonary edema	*pulmon/o* lung *-ary* pertaining to	Accumulation of fluid in the lung tissue. Often present in congestive heart failure, it is caused by the inability of the heart to pump blood.
pulmonary fibrosis	*fibr/o* fiber *-osis* abnormal condition	A stiffening of the lungs as a result of the formation of fibrous tissue. Idiopathic in origin.

Terms Related to Suppurative and Necrotic Conditions of the Lower Respiratory Tract (J85-J86)

Term	Word Origin	Definition
abscess of lung		Localized accumulation of pus in the lung.
pyothorax	*py/o* pus *-thorax* chest (pleural cavity)	Pus in the pleural cavity. Also called **empyema**.

Terms Related to Other Diseases of the Pleura (J90-J94)

Term	Word Origin	Definition
hemothorax	*hem/o* blood *-thorax* chest (pleural cavity)	Blood in the pleural cavity (Fig. 10-15).
hydrothorax	*hydr/o* water *-thorax* chest (pleural cavity)	An accumulation of serous fluid in the pleural cavity
pleural effusion	*pleur/o* pleura *-al* pertaining to	Abnormal accumulation of fluid in the intrapleural space.
pneumothorax	*pneum/o* air *-thorax* chest (pleural cavity)	Air or gas in the pleural space causing the lung to collapse (Fig. 10-16).

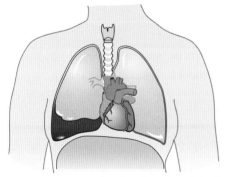

Fig. 10-15 Hemothorax. Blood below the right lung causes the lung to collapse.

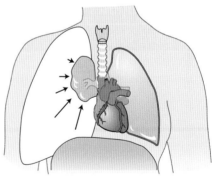

Fig. 10-16 Pneumothorax. The lung collapses as air gathers in the pleural space.

Terms Related to Intraoperative and Postprocedural Complications and Disorders of the Respiratory System, Not Elsewhere Classified (J95)

Term	Word Origin	Definition
pneumonia, ventilator-associated	*pneum/o* lung *-ia* abnormal condition	An inflammation of the lungs that is the documented result of ventilator usage.

Terms Related to Other Diseases of the Respiratory System (J96-J99)

Term	Word Origin	Definition
acute respiratory failure (ARF)		A sudden inability of the respiratory system to provide oxygen and/or remove CO_2 from the blood. May be caused by cardiac or pulmonary dysfunction or drug intoxication.
atelectasis	*a-* not *tel/e* complete *-ectasis* dilation	Collapse of lung tissue or an entire lung.
bronchospasm	*bronch/o* bronchus *-spasm* sudden, involuntary contraction	A sudden involuntary contraction of the bronchi, as in an asthma attack.

 CM Guideline Alert

10.C ACUTE RESPIRATORY FAILURE
1) Acute respiratory failure as principal diagnosis
A code from subcategory J96.0, Acute respiratory failure, or subcategory J96.2, Acute and chronic respiratory failure, may be assigned as a principal diagnosis when it is the condition established after study to be chiefly responsible for occasioning the admission to the hospital, and the selection is supported by the Alphabetic Index and Tabular List. However, chapter-specific coding guidelines (such as obstetrics, poisoning, HIV, newborn) that provide sequencing direction take precedence.

Terms Related to Injuries to the Thorax (S20-S29)

Term	Word Origin	Definition
flail chest		A condition in which multiple rib fractures cause instability in part of the chest wall and in which the lung under the injured area contracts on inspiration and bulges out on expiration (Fig. 10-17).

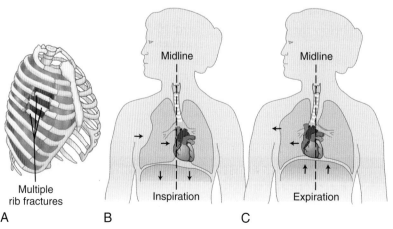

Fig. 10-17 Flail chest. A, Fractured rib sections are unattached to the rest of the chest wall. **B,** On inspiration, the flail segment of ribs is sucked inward, causing the lung to shift inward. **C,** On expiration, the flail segment of ribs bellows outward, causing the lung to shift outward. Air moves back and forth between the lungs instead of through the upper airway.

Exercise 5: Other Respiratory Diseases Principally Affecting the Interstitium; Suppurative and Necrotic Conditions of the Lower Respiratory Tract; Other Diseases of the Pleura and Respiratory System; Injuries to the Thorax

Match the terms to their definitions.

_____ 1. ARDS
_____ 2. pulmonary edema
_____ 3. pulmonary fibrosis
_____ 4. abscess of lung
_____ 5. hemothorax
_____ 6. pleural effusion
_____ 7. pneumothorax
_____ 8. flail chest
_____ 9. ARF

A. localized accumulation of pus in the lung
B. accumulation of fluid in lung tissue
C. sudden inability of the respiratory system to provide oxygen and remove carbon dioxide from the blood
D. stiffening of the lungs as a result of formation of fibrous tissue
E. injury to the chest wall caused by multiple rib fractures that allow the lung to bulge out on expiration
F. blood in the pleural cavity
G. air or gas in the pleural space that causes the lung to collapse
H. abnormal accumulation of fluid in the intrapleural space
I. sudden severe lung dysfunction due to pneumonia, trauma, etc.

Translate the terms.

10. bronchospasm_____

11. atelectasis_____

12. pyothorax_____

13. hydrothorax_____

Respiratory Neoplasms

Because organs are composed of tissues and tissues are constructed from a variety of cell types, cancer of an organ can occur in a number of different varieties, depending on which types of cells mutate. Fig. 10-18 shows the three main categories of lung cancer along with the types of cells from which they originate.

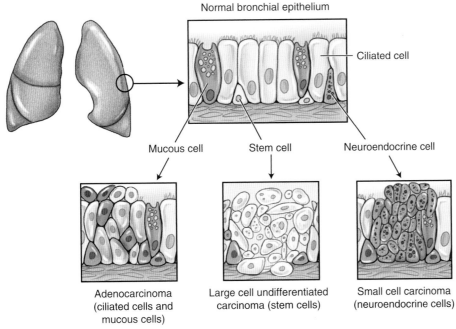

Fig. 10-18 Types of lung cancer.

Terms Related to Benign Neoplasms

Term	Word Origin	Definition
mucous gland adenoma	*muc/o* mucus *-ous* pertaining to *aden/o* gland *-oma* tumor, mass	A benign tumor of the mucous glands of the respiratory system (Fig. 10-19).
papilloma	*papill/o* nipple *-oma* tumor, mass	A benign tumor of epithelial origin named for its nipplelike appearance.

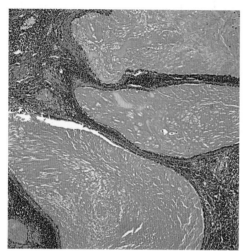

Fig. 10-19 Micrograph of a mucous gland adenoma.

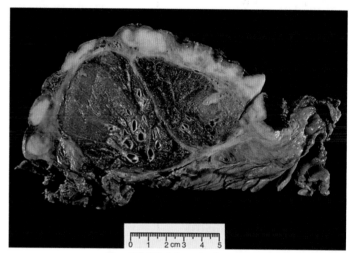

Fig. 10-20 Mesothelioma.

Terms Related to Malignant Neoplasms

Term	Word Origin	Definition
mesothelioma	*-oma* tumor, mass	A rare malignancy of the pleura or other protective tissues that cover the internal organs of the body. Often caused by exposure to asbestos (Fig. 10-20).

Terms Related to Malignant Neoplasms—cont'd

Term	Word Origin	Definition
non–small cell lung cancer (NSCLC)		Group of cancers that arise from cells that line the bronchi (squamous and adenocarcinoma) or are on or near the surface of the lung (large cell).
adenocarcinoma	*aden/o* gland *-carcinoma* cancer of epithelial origin	NSCLC derived from the mucus-secreting glands in the lungs (see Fig. 10-18).
large cell carcinoma	*carcinoma* cancer of epithelial origin	NSCLC originating in the lining of the smaller bronchi (see Fig. 10-18).
squamous cell carcinoma	*squam/o* scaly *-ous* pertaining to *carcinoma* cancer of epithelial origin	NSCLC originating in the squamous epithelium of the larger bronchi.
pulmonary sulcus tumor		A malignant tumor of the superior sulcus in the apex of the upper lobe of the right or left lung. Usually a non–small cell tumor, these tumors are linked to tobacco smoke or asbestos exposure. Also known as **superior sulcus tumor** or **Pancoast tumor.**
small cell lung cancer (carcinoma) (SCLC)	*carcinoma* cancer of epithelial origin	Second most common type of lung cancer. Associated with smoking. Derived from neuroendocrine cells in the bronchi (see Fig. 10-18). Also called **oat cell carcinoma.**

Exercise 6: Benign and Malignant Neoplasms

Fill in the blanks.

1. A benign tumor named for its nipplelike appearance is a/an _____.

2. A malignant neoplasm often caused by exposure to asbestos is _____.

3. Another name for small cell lung cancer is _____.

4. A non–small cell lung cancer derived from mucus-secreting glands in the lungs is called a/an _____.

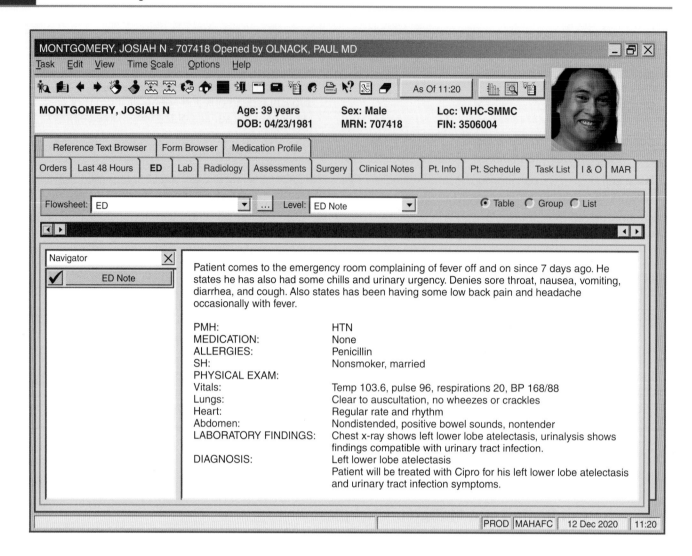

Patient comes to the emergency room complaining of fever off and on since 7 days ago. He states he has also had some chills and urinary urgency. Denies sore throat, nausea, vomiting, diarrhea, and cough. Also states has been having some low back pain and headache occasionally with fever.

PMH:	HTN
MEDICATION:	None
ALLERGIES:	Penicillin
SH:	Nonsmoker, married
PHYSICAL EXAM:	
Vitals:	Temp 103.6, pulse 96, respirations 20, BP 168/88
Lungs:	Clear to auscultation, no wheezes or crackles
Heart:	Regular rate and rhythm
Abdomen:	Nondistended, positive bowel sounds, nontender
LABORATORY FINDINGS:	Chest x-ray shows left lower lobe atelectasis, urinalysis shows findings compatible with urinary tract infection.
DIAGNOSIS:	Left lower lobe atelectasis
	Patient will be treated with Cipro for his left lower lobe atelectasis and urinary tract infection symptoms.

 Exercise 7: Emergency Room Note

Using the emergency room note above, answer the following questions.

1. What phrase in the emergency room note tells you that the patient's chest is free of fluid or exudates?

    _____.

2. What term tells you that the patient has not exhibited a whistling sound made during breathing?

    _____.

3. What term tells you that the patient has not exhibited any discontinuous bubbling noises in his chest?

    _____.

4. What was the diagnostic imaging procedure used?_____.

5. What term tells you that the patient has a collapsed lung?_____.

PROCEDURES

Terms Related to Procedures

Term	Word Origin	Definition
arterial blood gases (ABG)	*arteri/o* artery *-al* pertaining to	Blood test that measures the amount of oxygen and carbon dioxide in the blood.
adenoidectomy	*adenoid/o* adenoid *-ectomy* cutting out	Removal of the adenoids (also called the **pharyngeal tonsils**).
antrotomy	*antr/o* antrum *-tomy* cutting	Cutting one of the sinuses for the purpose of drainage. Also called **sinusotomy.** CPT references a radical sinusotomy (Caldwell-Luc) that is performed with or without removal of antrochoanal polyps.
bronchography	*bronch/o* bronchus *-graphy* recording	Recording the bronchi through imaging techniques using a contrast medium (Fig. 10-21).
bronchoscopy	*bronch/o* bronchus *-scopy* viewing	Viewing a bronchus using an instrument (Fig. 10-22).
columelloplasty of the nose	*columell/o* little column *-plasty* surgically forming	A surgical repair of the area of the nose between the nasal base and the tip.

Continued

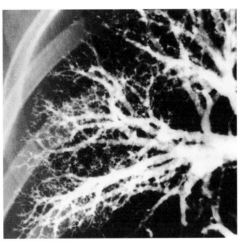

Fig. 10-21 Bronchography.

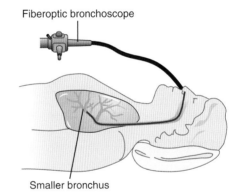

Fig. 10-22 Bronchoscopy.

If a bronchoscopy is done for the purpose of a biopsy, it is not coded as an inspection, but as an excision.

CPT Coding Alert!

Lysis of intranasal synechia(e)—an intranasal synechia is an adhesion or scarring that has formed within the nose after nasal surgery, trauma, or nasal packing. The synechiae cause a discharge, sinusitis, and/or a nasal obstruction. While an "Unspecified disorder of nose and nasal sinuses" works in ICD-10-PCS, it has its own specific code in CPT.

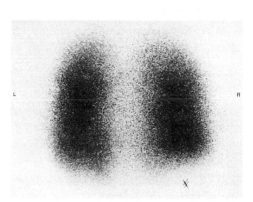

Fig. 10-23 Lung ventilation image of normal lungs.

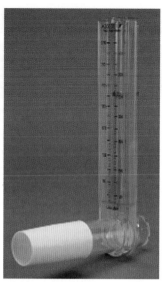

Fig. 10-24 Peak flow meter.

Terms Related to Procedures—cont'd

Term	Word Origin	Definition
endotracheal airway	*endo-* within *trache/o* trachea, windpipe *-al* pertaining to	A device that is positioned in the trachea for the purposes of establishing an airway.
ethmoidectomy	*ethmoid/o* ethmoid *-ectomy* cutting out	Cutting out part or all of the ethmoid bone. Usually done to treat a chronic sinus infection.
laryngoplasty	*laryng/o* larynx, voice box *-plasty* surgically forming	Surgically forming the larynx for the purpose of improving the voice for patients with hoarseness.
lung VQ scan		An imaging technique used to assess the areas of the lungs that are receiving air, but are not perfused with blood, possibly as a result of a blood clot (Fig. 10-23).
Mantoux skin test		Intradermal injection of purified protein derivative (PPD) used to detect the presence of tuberculosis antibodies.
metered dose inhaler (MDI)		A portable device that delivers a measured dose of an aerosol medication for inhalation. An additional device, a spacer, is an add-on chamber that holds the dispensed dose of medication, allowing the user to inhale it more slowly.
nebulizer		A battery- or electric-powered device/machine used to turn a liquid medication into a fine mist for inhalation through a mouthpiece or face mask. A hand-held nebulizer (HHN) is the portable form.
peak flow meter		Instrument used in a pulmonary function test (PFT) to measure breathing capacity (Fig. 10-24).

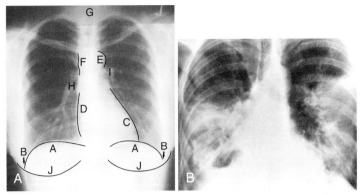

Fig. 10-25 **A**, Normal PA chest x-ray. The backward "L" in the upper right corner is placed on the film to indicate the left side of the patient's chest. *A*, Diaphragm. *B*, Costophrenic angle. *C*, Left ventricle. *D*, Right atrium. *E*, Aortic arch. *F*, Superior vena cava. *G*, Trachea. *H*, Right bronchus. *I*, Left bronchus. *J*, Breast shadows. **B**, X-ray of lung with pneumonia.

Terms Related to Procedures—cont'd

Term	Word Origin	Definition
plain radiography, chest (CXR)	*radi/o* rays *-graphy* recording	One of the most common imaging techniques; used to visualize abnormalities of the respiratory system (Fig. 10-25). X-rays may also include the use of a contrast medium, as in a **pulmonary angiography**, which uses a dye injected into the blood vessels of the lung, followed by subsequent x-ray imaging to demonstrate the flow of blood through these vessels.
pleurocentesis	*pleur/o* pleura *-centesis* surgical puncture	Surgical puncture to remove fluid or air from the pleural cavity.
pleurodesis	*pleur/o* pleura *-desis* fixation	The mechanical fixation of the two pleural membranes in order to prevent pleural effusions. If the fixation is done surgically (not chemically), it is called **pleurosclerosis.**
pleurolysis	*pleur/o* pleura *-lysis* breaking down	The surgical separation of pleural adhesions through the use of an endoscope and electrical cauterization. The adhesions are often caused by scarring from repeated pleural inflammation.
positive end expiratory pressure (PEEP)		A method of providing assistance in exhalation through the use of an endotracheal tube, a tracheostomy, a face mask, or nasal prongs.
pressure support ventilation (PSV)		A method of breathing assistance to increase a patient's ability to inhale through an endotracheal tube.
pulmonary function tests (PFTs)	*pulmon/o* lung *-ary* pertaining to	Procedures for determining the capacity of the lungs to exchange O_2 and CO_2 efficiently. See the table on the following page for examples of PFTs.
pulmonary resections and excisions		Excision of a segment or a lobe of the lung or the entire lung. Called a **lobectomy** when an entire lobe is resected and a **pneumonectomy** when the entire lung is resected (Fig. 10-26).

Continued

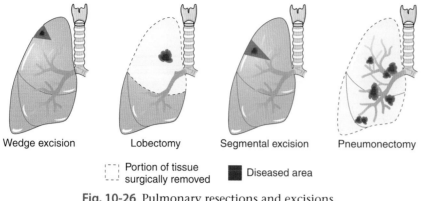

Wedge excision   Lobectomy   Segmental excision   Pneumonectomy

 Portion of tissue surgically removed   ▮ Diseased area

Fig. 10-26 Pulmonary resections and excisions.

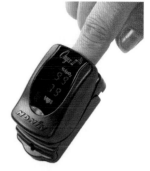

Fig. 10-27 Pulse oximetry.

ℯ

Click on **Animations** to see how pulse oximetry is performed

Terms Related to Procedures—cont'd

Term	Word Origin	Definition
pulse oximetry	*ox/i* oxygen *-metry* measuring	Measuring the oxygen level of the blood using a pulse oximeter. A noninvasive cliplike device is attached to either the earlobe or fingertip (Fig. 10-27).
quantiFERON®-TB Gold test (QFT)		Definitive blood test used to diagnose tuberculosis.

Examples of Pulmonary Function Tests

Function	Abbreviation	Description
Forced expiratory volume	FEV	Amount of air that can be exhaled with force in one breath.
Forced residual capacity	FRC	Amount of air remaining after a normal exhalation.
Forced vital capacity	FVC	Amount of air that can be exhaled with force after one inhales as deeply as possible.
Inspiratory capacity	IC	Amount of air that can be inspired after a normal expiration.
Tidal volume	TV	Amount of air normally inspired and expired in one respiration.
Total lung capacity	TLC	Amount of air in the lungs after one inhales as deeply as possible.

PCS Guideline Alert

B3.8 PCS contains specific body parts for anatomical subdivisions of a body part, such as lobes of the lungs or liver and regions of the intestine. Resection of the specific body part is coded whenever all of the body part is cut out or off, rather than coding Excision of less specific body part.

Example: Left upper lung lobectomy is coded to Resection of Upper Lung Lobe, Left rather than Excision of Lung, Left.

Terms Related to Procedures—cont'd

Term	Word Origin	Definition
rhinoplasty	*rhin/o* nose *-plasty* surgically forming	Surgically forming by correcting, altering, supplementing, or replacing the nose.
septoplasty	*sept/o* septum, wall *-plasty* surgically forming	Surgically straightening the wall between the nares to correct a deviation.
spirometry	*spir/o* to breathe *-metry* measuring	Test to measure the air capacity of the lungs. A **spirometer** is an instrument to measure breathing.
sputum culture and sensitivity		Cultivation of microorganisms from sputum that has been collected from expectoration (spitting).
tracheoesophageal fistulization (TEF)	*trache/o* trachea, windpipe *esophag/o* esophagus *-eal* pertaining to	The creation of a new opening between the trachea and the esophagus after a laryngectomy to preserve the ability to speak.
tracheostomy	*trache/o* trachea, windpipe *-stomy* making a new opening	New opening of the trachea. A tracheostomy device is an instrument used to facilitate the maintenance of an opening in the trachea (Fig. 10-28).
tracheotomy	*trache/o* trachea, windpipe *-tomy* cutting	Cutting the trachea to establish an airway.
turbinectomy	*turbin/o* turbinate bone *-ectomy* cutting out	Cutting out part or all of a turbinate bone, usually the inferior turbinate, to allow for greater air flow.

Continued

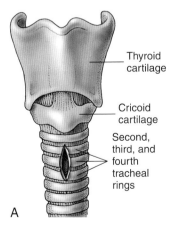
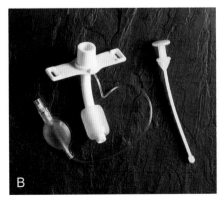
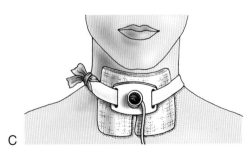

Thyroid cartilage

Cricoid cartilage

Second, third, and fourth tracheal rings

A   B   C

Fig. 10-28 A, Vertical tracheal incision for a tracheostomy. **B,** Tracheostomy tube. **C,** Placement of gauze and tie around a tracheostomy tube.

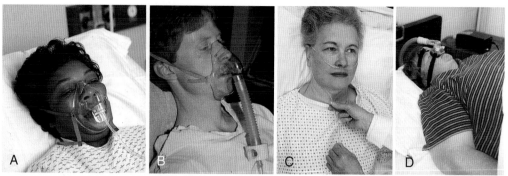

Fig. 10-29 Routes of oxygen therapy. A, Simple face mask. **B**, Venturi mask. **C**, Nasal cannula. **D**, CPAP.

Terms Related to Procedures—cont'd

Term	Word Origin	Definition
ventilation		A general term for devices that assist the breathing process.
		Patients who need assistance in attaining adequate O_2 levels may need a mechanical device called a **ventilator** to provide positive-pressure breathing. The device delivers the O_2 in different ways. If a low level of O_2 is required, a nasal cannula (tube) may be adequate. Face masks are another option. The amount of O_2 may be monitored more accurately with a Venturi mask. If high O_2 concentrations are necessary, a nonrebreathing or partial rebreathing mask may be used.
		Positive-pressure breathing (PPB) is a respiratory therapy technique designed to deliver air at greater than atmospheric pressure to the lungs. **Pressure support ventilation (PSV)** is a patient-moderated ventilation support, in which the patient initiates each breath. **Continuous positive airway pressure (CPAP)** may be delivered through a ventilator and endotracheal tube or a nasal cannula, face mask, or hood over the patient's head. Fig. 10-29 presents several examples of oxygenation therapy.
		Mechanical ventilation is an artificial means of providing breathing to a patient who cannot breathe adequately on his/her own. An endotracheal airway (tube) connects the patient's lungs to the machine. Because this tube passes between the vocal cords on its route through the trachea, the patient cannot speak while it is in place (Fig. 10-30). The use of mechanical ventilation may facilitate the transmission of pathogens into the lungs, and as a result, various types of pneumonia may be a complication of ventilator use.

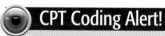

CPT Coding Alert!

Ventilation Management Services are documented in CPT for hospital inpatient/observation, nursing facilities, and home ventilator management.

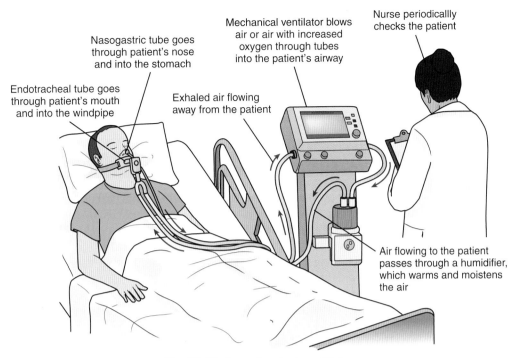

Nasogastric tube goes through patient's nose and into the stomach

Mechanical ventilator blows air or air with increased oxygen through tubes into the patient's airway

Nurse periodicallly checks the patient

Endotracheal tube goes through patient's mouth and into the windpipe

Exhaled air flowing away from the patient

Air flowing to the patient passes through a humidifier, which warms and moistens the air

Fig. 10-30 A mechanical ventilator.

 Exercise 8: **Procedures**

Match the terms to their definitions.

_____ 1. antrotomy
_____ 2. bronchoscopy
_____ 3. endotracheal airway
_____ 4. laryngoplasty
_____ 5. lung VQ scan
_____ 6. peak flow meter
_____ 7. PEEP
_____ 8. pleurolysis
_____ 9. PSV
_____ 10. septoplasty
_____ 11. MDI
_____ 12. tracheoesophageal fistulization
_____ 13. lobectomy
_____ 14. pneumonectomy
_____ 15. ventilation

A. viewing a bronchus
B. creation of a new opening between the trachea and esophagus
C. cutting one of the sinuses for drainage
D. general term for devices that assist the breathing process
E. surgical release of pleural adhesions
F. excision of a lobe of the lung
G. device inserted in the trachea to establish an airway
H. surgically forming the larynx
I. portable device that delivers a measured dose of aerosol medication for inhalation
J. method of breathing assistance to aid a patient's ability to inhale through an endotracheal tube
K. excision of an entire lung
L. surgically forming the wall between the nares to correct a defect
M. instrument used to measure breathing capacity
N. imaging technique used to assess areas of lungs that are receiving air, but are not perfused with blood
O. method of providing assistance in exhalation

Build the term.

16. recording the bronchi

_____.

17. cutting out the ethmoid bone_____.

18. fixation of the pleura_____.

19. making a new opening of the trachea_____.

20. cutting out a turbinate_____.

21. surgically forming the nose_____.

22. surgical puncture of the pleura_____.

PHARMACOLOGY

One route of administration for respiratory pharmaceuticals is a **ventilator**, a device that assists respiration and provides intensive positive-pressure breathing. A **hand-held nebulizer (HHN)** is a powered device that converts liquids into a fine spray, such as for inhaled medications. An **inhaler** is a non mechanical device for administering medications that are inhaled, such as vapors or fine powders. A **spacer**, a device connected to the inhaler that contains the mist expelled from the inhaler until the user can breathe it, usually is used for children and individuals who have difficulty using the inhaler device alone.

antihistamines: Block histamine receptors to manage allergies associated with allergic rhinitis or allergy-induced asthma. Examples are clemastine (Tavist), diphenhydramine (Benadryl), loratadine (Claritin), and fexofenadine (Allegra).
antitussives: Suppress the cough reflex. Examples include dextromethorphan (Delsym), codeine (Robitussin AC), and benzonatate (Tessalon).
bronchodilators: Relax bronchi to improve ventilation to the lungs. Examples include theophylline (Theo-Dur), umeclidinium (Incruse Ellipta), and albuterol (Proventil, Ventolin). Bronchodilators are often administered via inhalation.
decongestants: Reduce congestion or swelling of mucous membranes. Examples are pseudoephedrine (Sudafed) and phenylephrine (Sudafed PE).
expectorants: Promote the expulsion of mucus from the respiratory tract. An example is guaifenesin (Mucinex).
inhaled corticosteroids: Reduce airway inflammation to improve ventilation or reduce nasal congestion. Administered via oral or nasal inhalation accordingly. Examples include fluticasone (Flovent, Flonase), mometasone (Nasonex), and beclomethasone (Qvar).
mucolytics: Break up thick mucus in the respiratory tract. An example is N-acetyl-cysteine (Mucomyst).

Exercise 9: Pharmacology

Matching.

_____ 1. relaxes the bronchi

_____ 2. expels mucus

_____ 3. reduces congestion

_____ 4. blocks histamine receptors to manage allergies

_____ 5. suppresses coughs

A. antihistamine

B. antitussive

C. bronchodilator

D. decongestant

E. expectorant

6. What type of mechanical device is used to produce a fine spray for inhaled medications?_____
_____.

7. What type of nonmechanical device is used to administer medications that are inhaled, such as fine powders or vapors?_____

8. A/An_____ is a device designed to assist in respiration and intensive positive-pressure breathing.

RECOGNIZING SUFFIXES FOR PCS

Now that you've finished reading about the procedures for the respiratory system, take a look at this review of the *suffixes* used in their terminology. Each of these suffixes is associated with one or more root operations in the medical surgical section or one of the other categories in PCS.

Suffixes and Root Operations for the Respiratory System

Suffix	Root Operation
-centesis	Drainage
-desis	Destruction
-ectomy	Excision, resection
-lysis	Release
-plasty	Alteration, reposition, repair, replacement, supplement
-rrhaphy	Repair
-tomy	Drainage

Abbreviations

Abbreviation	Meaning
ABG	arterial blood gases
ARDS	acute respiratory distress syndrome
ARF	acute respiratory failure
CO_2	carbon dioxide
COPD	chronic obstructive pulmonary disease
CPAP	continuous positive airway pressure
CWP	coal workers' pneumoconiosis
CXR	chest x-ray
DOE	dyspnea on exertion
HHN	hand-held nebulizer
LLL	left lower lobe
LUL	left upper lobe
MDI	metered dose inhaler
MDRTB	multidrug-resistant tuberculosis

Abbreviation	Meaning
NSCLC	non–small cell lung cancer
O_2	oxygen
PEEP	positive end expiratory pressure
PFT	pulmonary function test
PSV	pressure support ventilation
QFT	quantiferon–TB Gold test
RLL	right lower lobe
RML	right middle lobe
RSV	respiratory syncytial virus
RUL	right upper lobe
SARS	severe acute respiratory syndrome
SCLC	small cell lung cancer
SOB	shortness of breath
TB	tuberculosis
TEF	tracheoesophageal fistulization
VAP	ventilator-associated pneumonia

Go to the Evolve website to interactively build terms, label images, memorize word parts, and practice using respiratory terms in context.

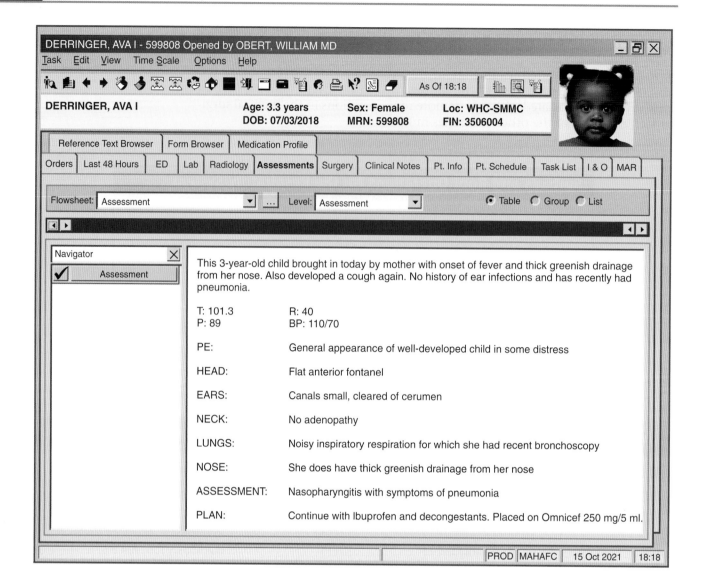

 Exercise 10: **Progress Note**

Using the progress note above, answer the following questions.

1. The patient has a history of infection of which organs?_____

2. The term "inspiratory" refers to what?_____

3. What was the recent endoscopic procedure that the patient had undergone?_____

4. What are the sites of the current infection?_____

5. What are the respiratory disorders that have been diagnosed in this patient?_____

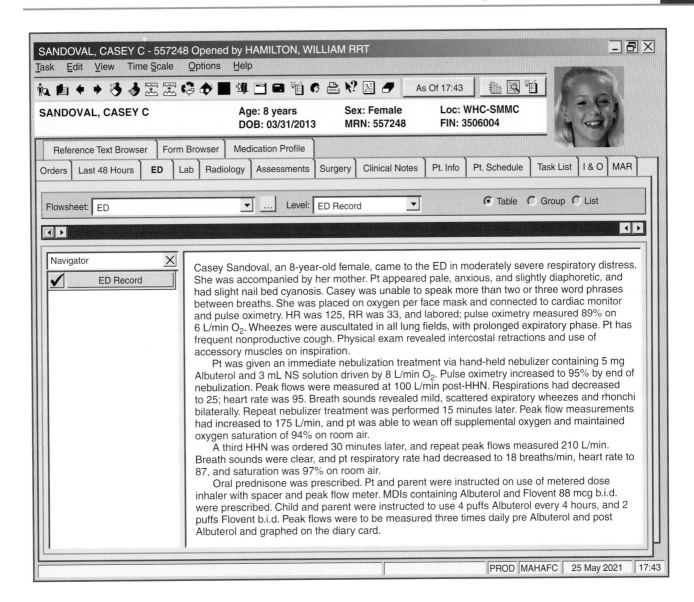

SANDOVAL, CASEY C - 557248 Opened by HAMILTON, WILLIAM RRT

Task   Edit   View   Time Scale   Options   Help

As Of 17:43

SANDOVAL, CASEY C

	Age: 8 years	Sex: Female	Loc: WHC-SMMC
	DOB: 03/31/2013	MRN: 557248	FIN: 3506004

Reference Text Browser | Form Browser | Medication Profile

Orders | Last 48 Hours | **ED** | Lab | Radiology | Assessments | Surgery | Clinical Notes | Pt. Info | Pt. Schedule | Task List | I & O | MAR

Flowsheet: ED   Level: ED Record   ● Table   ○ Group   ○ List

Navigator
✓ ED Record

Casey Sandoval, an 8-year-old female, came to the ED in moderately severe respiratory distress. She was accompanied by her mother. Pt appeared pale, anxious, and slightly diaphoretic, and had slight nail bed cyanosis. Casey was unable to speak more than two or three word phrases between breaths. She was placed on oxygen per face mask and connected to cardiac monitor and pulse oximetry. HR was 125, RR was 33, and labored; pulse oximetry measured 89% on 6 L/min O_2. Wheezes were auscultated in all lung fields, with prolonged expiratory phase. Pt has frequent nonproductive cough. Physical exam revealed intercostal retractions and use of accessory muscles on inspiration.

   Pt was given an immediate nebulization treatment via hand-held nebulizer containing 5 mg Albuterol and 3 mL NS solution driven by 8 L/min O_2. Pulse oximetry increased to 95% by end of nebulization. Peak flows were measured at 100 L/min post-HHN. Respirations had decreased to 25; heart rate was 95. Breath sounds revealed mild, scattered expiratory wheezes and rhonchi bilaterally. Repeat nebulizer treatment was performed 15 minutes later. Peak flow measurements had increased to 175 L/min, and pt was able to wean off supplemental oxygen and maintained oxygen saturation of 94% on room air.

   A third HHN was ordered 30 minutes later, and repeat peak flows measured 210 L/min. Breath sounds were clear, and pt respiratory rate had decreased to 18 breaths/min, heart rate to 87, and saturation was 97% on room air.

   Oral prednisone was prescribed. Pt and parent were instructed on use of metered dose inhaler with spacer and peak flow meter. MDIs containing Albuterol and Flovent 88 mcg b.i.d. were prescribed. Child and parent were instructed to use 4 puffs Albuterol every 4 hours, and 2 puffs Flovent b.i.d. Peak flows were to be measured three times daily pre Albuterol and post Albuterol and graphed on the diary card.

PROD | MAHAFC | 25 May 2021 | 17:43

 Exercise 11: Emergency Department Report

Using the ED report above, answer the following questions.

1. In your own words, explain the meaning of the symptoms "slightly diaphoretic" and "slight nail bed cyanosis."_____.

2. How is oxygen measured in pulse oximetry?_____
_____.

3. Name and define the two abnormal chest sounds heard on auscultation in this report._____
_____.

4. What is the purpose of a peak flow meter?_____.

Match the word parts to their definitions.

WORD PART DEFINITIONS

Prefix/Suffix
brady-
dys-
-ectasis
hyper-
hypo-
-ismus
-pnea
-ptysis
tachy-
-thorax

Definition

1. _____ fast
2. _____ excessive
3. _____ deficient
4. _____ slow
5. _____ breathing
6. _____ spitting
7. _____ chest (pleural cavity)
8. _____ difficult
9. _____ spasm condition
10. _____ dilation

Combining Form
apic/o
capn/o
coni/o
cost/o
laryng/o
muc/o
myc/o
nas/o
ox/i
pector/o
pharyng/o
phren/o
pleur/o
pneum/o
py/o
rhin/o
salping/o
sept/o
sin/o
spir/o
tonsill/o
trache/o

Definition

11. _____ carbon dioxide
12. _____ lung
13. _____ chest
14. _____ to breathe
15. _____ apex
16. _____ pleura
17. _____ nose
18. _____ septum, wall
19. _____ dust
20. _____ fungus
21. _____ throat
22. _____ mucus
23. _____ oxygen
24. _____ diaphragm
25. _____ windpipe
26. _____ pus
27. _____ rib
28. _____ sinus
29. _____ tonsil
30. _____ eustachian tube
31. _____ voice box
32. _____ nose

WORDSHOP

Prefixes	Combining Forms	Suffixes
dys-	bronch/o	-al
endo-	capn/o	-ation
ex-	coni/o	-desis
hyper-	cost/o	-dynia
inter-	esophag/o	-eal
tachy-	hal/o	-ia
	myc/o	-itis
	nas/o	-metry
	ox/i	-osis
	pharyng/o	-plasty
	pleur/o	-pnea
	pneum/o	-scopy
	py/o	-stomy
	rhin/o	-thorax
	sept/o	-tomy
	trache/o	

Build respiratory terms by combining the word parts above. Some word parts may be used more than once. Some may not be used at all. The number in parentheses indicates the number of word parts needed.

Definition	Term
1. condition of excessive carbon dioxide (3)	
2. abnormal condition of fungus in the nose (3)	
3. abnormal condition of dust in the lung (3)	
4. pertaining to the windpipe and esophagus (3)	
5. process of breathing out (3)	
6. pain in the pleura (2)	
7. inflammation of the nose and throat (3)	
8. surgically forming the septum (2)	
9. pus in the chest (pleural cavity) (2)	
10. inflammation of the trachea (2)	
11. fixation of the pleura (2)	
12. pertaining to between the ribs (3)	
13. measuring oxygen (2)	
14. viewing the bronchus (2)	

Sort the terms into the correct categories.

TERM SORTING

Anatomy and Physiology	Pathology	Procedures

alveolus	eustachian tube	pleurolysis
aphonia	exhalation	pneumonia
apnea	hyperpnea	PSV
ARDS	laryngismus	pulmonary resection
atelectasis	mediastinum	pulse oximetry
bronchiectasis	mucus	rhinomycosis
bronchoscopy	nebulizer	rhonchi
COPD	olfaction	septoplasty
CPAP	oropharynx	sinus
CXR	oxygen	sinusitis
diaphragm	oxyhemoglobin	sinusotomy
diphtheria	PEEP	tracheotomy
emphysema	phonation	trachea
epiglottis	pleura	tracheostomy
epistaxis	pleurocentesis	ventilation

Replace the highlighted words with the correct terms.

TRANSLATIONS

1. **Difficult breathing** and **air hunger** were signs that Sari had asthma.

2. The patient's **difficulty making sounds** and **inflammation of the voice box** were associated with an upper respiratory infection.

3. The baby had **a continuous, high-pitched inspiratory sound from the larynx**, which was a sign of **inflammation of the epiglottis**.

4. Dr. Hollander told Ryan's mother that her son's fever and **chest pain** were symptoms of **abnormal accumulation of fluid in the intrapleural space**.

5. The patient underwent a **CXR** to see if she had **an infectious inflammation of the lungs**.

6. After 3 days of severe **inflammation or infection of the pharynx**, Abby also developed **inflammation of the voice box**.

7. **A noninvasive test to measure the oxygen level of the blood** and **a test to measure the air capacity of the lungs** were performed on the patient.

8. Marketta's **deflection of the nasal septum** was treated with **a surgical straightening of the wall between the nares**.

9. **Surgical puncture to remove fluid or air from the pleural cavity** was necessary to treat the patient's **blood in the pleural cavity**.

10. The pulmonologist diagnosed Mr. Borasky with chronic **dilation of the bronchi** and **respiratory disorder characterized by a progressive and irreversible diminishment in capacity of the lungs**.

11. After the patient's treatment for **pertaining to the larynx** cancer, she had a temporary **new opening of the trachea**.

ICD-10-CM Example from Tabular

G82 Paraplegia (paraparesis) and quadriplegia (quadriparesis)

Note: This category is to be used only when the listed conditions are reported without further specification, or are stated to be old or longstanding, but of unspecified cause. The category is also for use in multiple coding to identify these conditions resulting from any cause.

Excludes1

congenital cerebral palsy (**C80.-**)

functional quadriplegia (**R53.2**)

hysterical paralysis (**F44.4**)

G82.2 Paraplegia

Paralysis of both lower limbs NOS

Paraparesis (lower) NOS

Paraplegia (lower) NOS

G82.20 Paraplegia, unspecified

G82.21 Paraplegia, complete

G82.22 Paraplegia, incomplete

G82.5 Quadriplegia

G82.50 Quadriplegia, unspecified

G82.51 Quadriplegia, C1-C4 complete

G82.52 Quadriplegia, C1-C4 incomplete

G82.53 Quadriplegia, C5-C7 complete

G82.54 Quadriplegia, C5-C7 incomplete

ICD-10-PCS Example from Index

Neuroplasty

see Repair, Central Nervous System and Cranial Nerves **00Q**

see Supplement, Central Nervous System and Cranial Nerves **00U**

see Repair, Peripheral Nervous System **01U**

Neurorrhaphy

see Repair, Central Nervous System **00Q**

see Repair, Peripheral Nervous System **01Q**

CHAPTER OUTLINE

FUNCTIONS OF THE NERVOUS SYSTEM

ANATOMY AND PHYSIOLOGY

PATHOLOGY

PROCEDURES

PHARMACOLOGY

RECOGNIZING SUFFIXES FOR PCS

ABBREVIATIONS

OBJECTIVES

☐ Recognize and use terms related to the anatomy and physiology of the nervous system.

☐ Recognize and use terms related to the pathology of the nervous system.

☐ Recognize and use terms related to the procedures for the nervous system.

FUNCTIONS OF THE NERVOUS SYSTEM

The nervous system (Fig. 11-1) plays a major role in **homeostasis**, keeping the other body systems coordinated and regulated to achieve optimal performance. It accomplishes this goal by helping the individual respond to his or her internal and external environments.

The nervous and endocrine systems are responsible for communication and control throughout the body. There are three main **neural** functions:
1. Collecting information about the external and internal environment *(sensing)*.
2. Processing this information and making decisions about action *(interpreting)*.
3. Directing the body to put into play the decisions made *(acting)*.

homeostasis
  home/o = same
  -stasis = stopping, controlling

nerve = neur/o

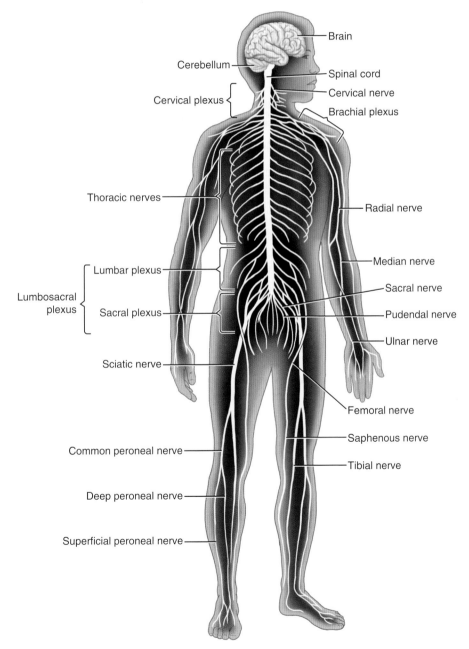

Fig. 11-1 The nervous system.

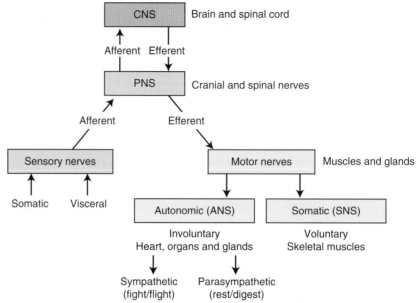

Fig. 11-2 Schematic of the nervous system into the CNS and PNS.

ANATOMY AND PHYSIOLOGY

Organization of the Nervous System

Nerves are composed of several neurons, or nerve cells. Although neurons cannot be seen without a microscope, some nerves are easily visible. The nerves that extend from the foot to the brain can be over 2 meters long. Neural **tracts** are pathways between different parts of the nervous system. An example is the pyramidal tract (corticospinal tract), which is named for its triangular shape and which joins the two hemispheres of the cerebral cortex and the spinal cord.

The nervous system is divided into two main systems. (See Fig. 11-2 for a schematic of the divisions). **The central nervous system (CNS)** is composed of the brain and the spinal cord. It is the only site of nerve cells called *interneurons,* which connect sensory and motor neurons. **The peripheral nervous system (PNS)** is composed of the nerves that extend from the brain and spinal cord to the tissues of the body. These are organized into 12 pairs of cranial nerves and 31 pairs of spinal nerves. The PNS is further divided into sensory and motor nerves. **Sensory (afferent) nerves** carry impulses to the brain and spinal cord, whereas **motor (efferent) nerves** carry impulses away from the brain and spinal cord.

PNS nerves are further categorized into two subsystems:

body = somat/o

Somatic nervous system (SNS): this system is *voluntary* in nature. These nerves collect information from and return instructions to the skin, muscles, and joints.

Autonomic nervous system (ANS): mostly *involuntary* functions are controlled by this system as sensory information from the internal environment is sent to the CNS, and, in return, motor impulses from the CNS are sent to involuntary muscles: the heart, glands, and organs.

This chapter includes all the anatomy necessary to assign ICD-10 nervous system codes, including detail on the basal ganglia, corpus callosum, and the choroid plexus. See Appendix H for a complete list of body parts and how they should be coded.

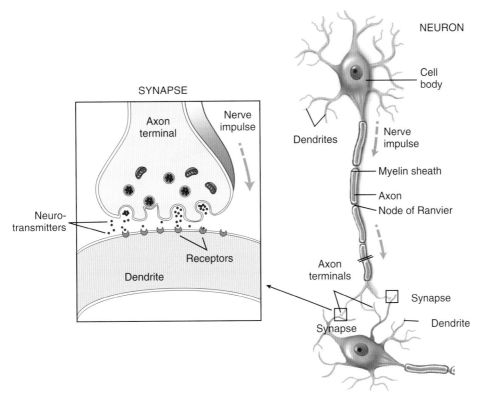

Fig. 11-3 The nerve cell (neuron) with an inset of a synapse.

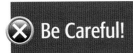 **Be Careful!** *Remember that* **efferent** *means to carry away, whereas* **afferent** *means to carry toward. In the nervous system, these terms are used to refer to away from and toward the brain.*

Cells of the Nervous System

The nervous system is made up of the following two types of cells:
1. Parenchymal cells, or **neurons,** the cells that carry out the work of the system.
2. Stromal cells, or **glia**, the cells that provide a supportive function.

Neurons
The basic unit of the nervous system is the nerve cell, or **neuron** (Fig. 11-3). Not all neurons are the same, but all have features in common. **Dendrites**, projections from the cell body, receive neural impulses, also called *action potentials*, from a stimulus of some kind. This impulse travels along the dendrite and into the cell body, which is the control center of the cell. This cell body contains the nucleus and surrounding cytoplasm.

From the cell body, the neural impulse moves out along the **axon**, a slender, elongated projection that carries the neural impulse toward the next neuron. The **terminal fibers** result from the final branching of the axon and are the site of the **axon terminals**, which store the chemical **neurotransmitters** like dopamine (responsible for affecting voluntary movement regulation) and serotonin (responsible for mood, sleep, and appetite). Many axons are covered by a **myelin sheath**, which is a substance produced by the Schwann cells that coats the axons in the peripheral nervous system. This coating gives the cells a whitish appearance, as opposed to the gray appearance of unmyelinated axons and cell bodies. The nodes of Ranvier are areas of neurons not covered by Schwann cells. The outer cell membrane of the Schwann cell is the **neurilemma**. Because the CNS is mostly unmyelinated, it is associated with the phrase "using your gray matter."

neuron
 neur/o = nerve
 -on = structure

dendrite = dendr/o

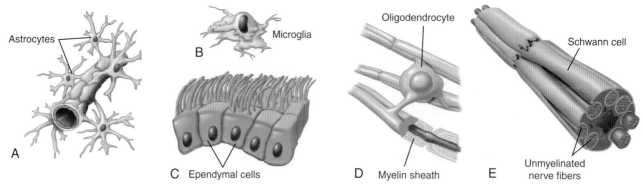

Fig. 11-4 Types of neuroglia. **A,** Astrocyte. **B,** Microglia. **C,** Ependymal cells. **D,** Oligodendrocyte. **E,** Schwann cell.

From the axon's terminal fibers, the neurotransmitter is released from the cell to travel across the space between these terminal fibers and the dendrites of the next cell. This space is called the **synapse** (see Fig. 11-3). The impulse continues in this manner until its destination is reached. A nerve is a group of bundled axons in the PNS. Most nerves contain both sensory and motor fibers.

Glia

The supportive, or stromal, glia are also called **neuroglia** (Fig. 11-4). They accomplish their supportive function by physically holding the neurons together and also protecting them. There are different kinds of neuroglia, including astrocytes, ependymal cells, oligodendroglia, microglia, and Schwann cells. **Astrocytes** connect neurons and blood vessels and form a structure called the **blood-brain barrier (BBB),** which prevents or slows the passage of some drugs and disease-causing organisms to the CNS. **Ependymal cells** line the ventricles of the brain and produce cerebrospinal fluid. **Oligodendroglia** cover the axons of neurons in the central nervous system, forming their myelin sheath. **Microglia** perform an active protective function by engulfing and ingesting infectious organisms.

neuroglia
    neur/o = nerve
    -glia = glue

astrocyte
    astr/o = star
    -cyte = cell

oligodendroglia
    olig/o = scanty
    dendr/o = dendrite
    -glia = glue

microglia
    micro- = tiny
    -glia = glue

> ⊗ **Be Careful!**   *The abbreviation* **BBB** *can stand for either* blood-brain barrier *or* bundle branch block, *a cardiac condition.*

 ## Exercise 1: Organization of the Nervous System

Fill in the blanks.

1. The two main divisions of the nervous system are the _____ and the _____.

Underline the correct answer.

2. Sensory neurons (*transmit, receive*) information (*to, from*) the CNS.

3. Motor neurons, also called (*efferent, afferent*) neurons, transmit information (*to, from*) the CNS.

4. The (*somatic, autonomic*) nervous system is voluntary in nature, whereas the (*somatic, autonomic*) nervous system is largely involuntary.

Exercise 2: Cells of the Nervous System

Match the terms with their word parts.

___ 1. star   ___ 4. glue   A. -glia   D. astr/o
___ 2. body   ___ 5. dendrite   B. somat/o   E. neur/o
___ 3. nerve   C. dendr/o

Translate the terms.

6. perineural _____

7. oligodendritic _____

8. microglial _____

The Central Nervous System

As stated previously, the CNS is composed of the **brain** and the **spinal cord**.

brain = encephal/o

Brain (Encephalon)

The brain is one of the most complex organs of the body. It is divided into four parts: the **cerebrum**, the **diencephalon**, the **brainstem**, and the **cerebellum** (Fig. 11-5).

cerebrum = cerebr/o

cerebellum = cerebell/o

Cerebrum

The largest portion of the brain, the cerebrum, is divided into two halves, or **hemispheres** (Fig. 11-6). It is responsible for thinking, reasoning, and memory. The surfaces of the hemispheres are covered with gray matter and are called the **cerebral cortex**. Arranged into folds, the valleys are referred to as **sulci** (*sing.* sulcus), and the ridges are called the **gyri** (*sing.* gyrus). The cerebrum is further divided into sections called **lobes**, each of which has its own functions:

cortex = cortic/o

lobe = lob/o

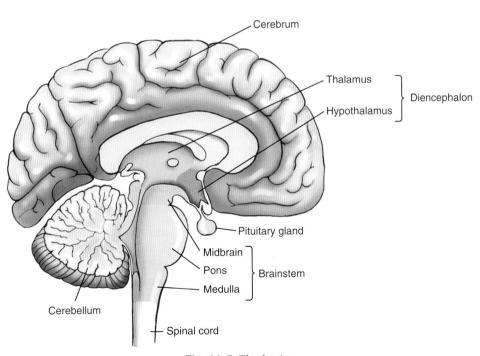

Fig. 11-5 The brain.

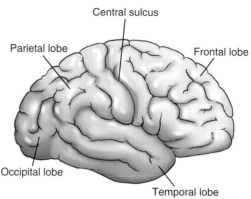

Fig. 11-6 The cerebrum.

1. The **frontal lobe** contains the function of speech and the motor area that controls voluntary movement on the contralateral side of the body. It also is in charge of personality, emotions, and problem solving.
2. The **temporal lobes** contain the auditory and olfactory areas, and are where sequencing and memory occur.
3. The **parietal lobes** control the sensations of touch and taste, and also control spatial perception.
4. The **occipital lobe** is responsible for vision.
5. The **insular lobes**, located under the frontal and temporal lobes, are responsible for empathy, interceptive (internal sensing) awareness, and cognition. The term **insula** is derived from the Latin word meaning "island," probably because it is not obviously continuous with the other lobes. Synonyms for the insular lobe are *the island of Reil* and *insular cortex*.

The **corpus callosum** is the thick band of nerve fibers that joins the two hemispheres of the cerebrum. The **septum pellucidum** is a membrane inferior to the corpus callosum that separates parts of the lateral ventricles. The lack of this membrane is associated with a variety of developmental disorders.

The **basal ganglia**, located under the cerebrum, are a collection of structures responsible for a number of different functions. The corpus striatum functions as a reception area that actuates the **globus pallidum** to perform an inhibitory action on motor function areas. The **substantia nigra** has a function in the release of dopamine. The subthalamic nucleus influences the globus pallidum after receiving stimulus from either the cerebral cortex or the striatum. The claustrum is a thin layer of gray matter with poorly understood functioning, although it is considered to be part of the basal ganglia. Collectively, damage to the basal ganglia plays a role in several neurological disorders, including Parkinson's disease and Huntington's disease.

globus pallidum = pallid/o

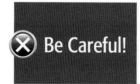 **Be Careful!**   **Basal ganglia** *is a misnomer because ganglia only appear in the PNS.* **Basal nuclei** *is the more technically correct name, although "basal ganglia" is more commonly used. Collections of cell bodies in the CNS are termed "nuclei," whereas in the PNS, they are called "ganglia." ICD-10 uses the term "basal ganglia."*

Diencephalon

The diencephalon is composed of the **thalamus** and the structure inferior to it, the **hypothalamus**. The thalamus is responsible for relaying sensory information (with the exception of smell) and translating it into sensations of pain, temperature, and touch. The **epithalamus**, which includes the pineal gland, is named for its location above the thalamus. It connects the limbic system to the rest of the brain. The limbic system is responsible for motivated behavior and arousal and influences the endocrine and autonomic motor systems. The medial and lateral **geniculate nuclei** are sensory relays within the thalamus that receive and send visual and auditory information. Together they are termed the **metathalamus**. The **pulvinar** are nuclei located in the medial posterior thalamus with functions involving visual attention.

The hypothalamus activates, integrates, and controls the peripheral autonomic nervous system, along with many functions such as body temperature, sleep, and appetite. The **mammillary bodies** are small rounded structures that participate in the ability to recognize people, places, and objects that are stored in memory.

Brainstem

The brainstem connects the cerebral hemispheres to the spinal cord. It is composed of three main parts: the midbrain, pons, and medulla oblongata. The **midbrain** connects the pons and cerebellum with the hemispheres of the cerebrum. It is the site of reflex centers for eye and head movements in response to visual and auditory stimuli. The **superior and inferior colliculi** of the midbrain are composed of sensory visual and auditory nerve fibers. The **cerebral peduncles** of the midbrain are motor nerve fibers that connect to the spinal cord and cerebellum. The **pons** serves as a bridge between the medulla oblongata and the cerebrum. The **pneumotaxic** and **apneustic centers** are networks of neurons that regulate respiration. The anterior part of the pons is the **basis pontis,** which has a role in motor function. The **locus ceruleus** (Latin for "blue spot") functions in the physiological response to stress. The **superior olivary nucleus** is involved in hearing. Finally, the lowest part of the brainstem, the **medulla oblongata**, regulates heart rate, blood pressure, and breathing.

Cerebellum

Located inferior to the occipital lobe of the cerebrum, the **cerebrum** coordinates voluntary movement but is involuntary in its function. For example, walking is a voluntary movement. The coordination needed for the muscles and other body parts to walk smoothly is involuntary and is controlled by the cerebellum.

Spinal Cord

The **spinal cord** extends from the medulla oblongata to the first lumbar vertebra (Fig. 11-7). It then extends into a structure called the **cauda equina** (which means "horse's tail" in Latin). The **conus medullaris** is the end of the spinal cord, whereas the cauda equina is the collection of nerve roots that extends from it.

The spinal cord is protected by the bony vertebrae surrounding the spinal, or vertebral, canal and the coverings unique to the CNS, called **meninges**. The spinal cord is composed of gray matter, the cell bodies of motor neurons, and **white matter**, the myelin-covered axons or nerve fibers that extend from the nerve cell bodies. The 31 pairs of spinal nerves emerge from the spinal cord at the **nerve roots**.

Meninges

The **meninges** act as protective coverings for the CNS and are composed of three layers separated by spaces (Fig. 11-8). The **dura mater** is the tough, fibrous outer covering of the meninges. Its literal meaning is "hard mother." The falx cerebri is the sickle-shaped fold between the hemispheres. The dura mater is classified as **cranial dura mater** and **spinal dura mater**. The **tentorium cerebella** is an extension of the dura mater that separates the cerebellum from the lower part of the occipital lobes. The **diaphragm sellae** is a small dural fold that covers the sella turcica; it has a small opening for the infundibulum of the pituitary. The space between the dura mater and arachnoid membrane is called the **subdural space**. If in the skull, it is the *cranial subdural*

 Be Careful!

Myel/o *can mean* bone marrow *or* spinal cord; *memorization and context will be the student's only methods to determine which is which.*

spinal cord = cord/o, chord/o, myel/o

meninges = mening/o, meningi/o

nerve root = rhiz/o, radicul/o

dura mater = dur/o

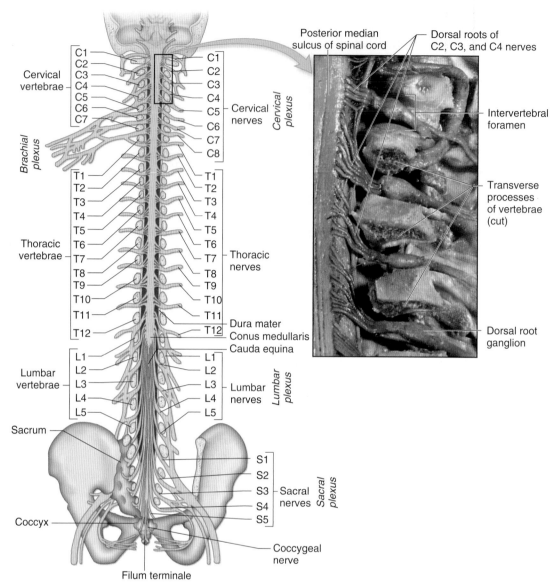

Fig. 11-7 The spinal cord with an inset of a cervical segment showing emerging cervical nerves.

To see a demonstration of the vertebral column and spinal nerves, click on **Animations.**

space; if in the spine, it is referred to as the *spinal subdural space*. Likewise, the subarachnoid space is further categorized as *cranial subarachnoid* and *spinal sub-arachnoid* spaces. The next layer is the **arachnoid membrane**, a thin, delicate membrane that takes its name from its spidery appearance. The **subarachnoid space** is the space between the arachnoid membrane and the pia mater. It contains **cerebrospinal fluid (CSF)**, a clear fluid that protects the brain and spinal cord and removes waste products and monitors for internal changes. CSF is also present in cavities in the brain called **ventricles**. Finally, the **pia mater** is the thin, vascular membrane that is the innermost of the three meninges; its literal meaning is "soft mother." The arachnoid and pia mater are referred to as **lepto-meninges** for their slender appearance as opposed to the thick, tough nature of the dura mater.

ventricle = ventricul/o

slim, delicate = lept/o

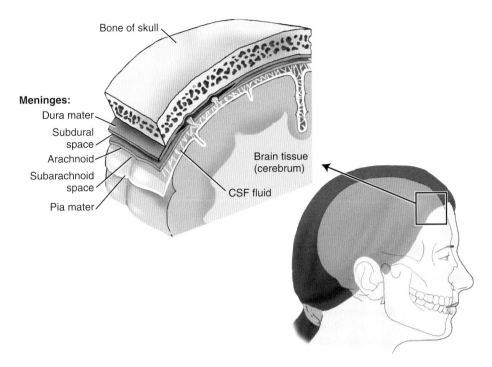

Fig. 11-8 The meninges.

To see the function of brain ventricles, click on **Animations.**

There are four ventricles in the brain: two lateral ventricles (left and right), the third ventricle, and the fourth ventricle. Each is connected by foramina (openings). The lateral ventricles are connected by the **foramen of Monro** and the third and fourth by the **aqueduct of Sylvius**. The **choroid plexus** is the membrane within the ventricles of the brain and spinal cord that is lined with ependymal cells that produce CSF. **Cisterns** are dilations of the subarachnoid space that contain CSF. The **cisterna magna** is between the dorsal surface of the medulla oblongata and the cerebellum and receives its CSF from the fourth ventricle.

magna = large

The Peripheral Nervous System

The peripheral nervous system is divided into:
- 12 pairs of cranial nerves that conduct impulses between the brain and head, neck, thoracic, and abdominal areas, and
- 31 pairs of spinal nerves that closely mimic the organization of the vertebrae and provide innervations to the rest of the body.

The peripheral nerves are a combination of **afferent (sensory) nerves** and efferent **(motor) nerves.** The motor nerves are either voluntary or involuntary. The **autonomic nervous system (ANS)** consists of nerves that regulate involuntary function such as cardiac or smooth muscle. The ANS is further divided into the sympathetic and parasympathetic nervous systems, two opposing mechanisms that provide balance in the body:
- The **sympathetic nervous system** is capable of producing a "fight-or-flight" response. This is the part of the nervous system that helps the individual respond to perceived stress. The heart rate and blood pressure increase, digestive processes slow, and sweat and adrenal glands increase their secretions.

- The **parasympathetic nervous system** tends to do the opposite of the sympathetic nervous system—slowing the heart rate, lowering blood pressure, increasing digestive functions, and decreasing adrenal and sweat gland activity. This is sometimes called the "rest and digest" system. An example of a sensory response follows:

"Eight-year-old Joey is hungry. He decides to sneak some cookies before dinner. Afraid his mother will see him, he surreptitiously takes a handful into the hall closet and shuts the door. As he begins to eat, the closet door flies open. Joey's heart begins to race as he whips the cookies out of sight. When he sees it's only his sister, he relaxes and offers her a cookie as a bribe not to tell on him."

Joey's afferent (sensory) somatic neurons carried the message to his brain that he was hungry. This message was interpreted by his brain as a concern, and the response was to sneak cookies from the jar and hide himself as he ate them. When the closet door flew open, his sensory neurons perceived a danger and triggered a sympathetic "fight-or-flight" response, which raised his heart rate and blood pressure and stimulated his sweat glands. When the intruder was perceived to be harmless, his parasympathetic nervous system took over and reduced his heart rate, bringing it back to normal. The same afferent fibers perceived the intruder in two different ways, with two different sets of autonomic motor responses (sympathetic and parasympathetic).

Cranial Nerves

Cranial nerves are named by their number and also their function or distribution. See Fig. 11-9 and the table on the next page.

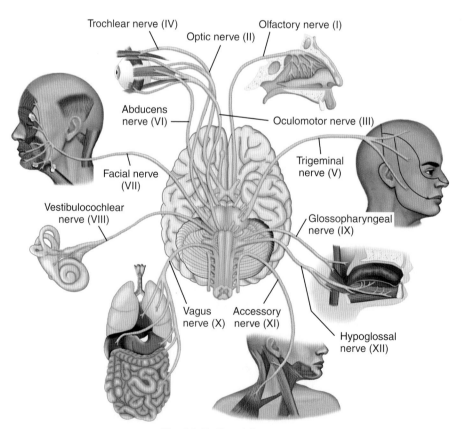

Fig. 11-9 Cranial nerves.

The Cranial Nerves

Number	Name	Origin of Sensory Fibers	Effector Innervated by Motor Fibers
I	Olfactory	Olfactory epithelium of nose (smell)	None
II	Optic	Retina of eye (vision)	None
III	Oculomotor	Proprioceptors* of eyeball muscles	Muscles that move eyeball; muscles that change shape of lens; muscles that constrict pupil
IV	Trochlear	Proprioceptors* of eyeball muscles	Muscles that move eyeball
V	Trigeminal	Teeth and skin of face	Some muscles used in chewing
VI	Abducens	Proprioceptors* of eyeball muscles	Muscles that move eyeball
VII	Facial	Taste buds of anterior part of tongue	Muscles used for facial expression; submaxillary and sublingual salivary glands
VIII	Vestibulocochlear (auditory)		None
	Vestibular branch	Semicircular canals of inner ear (senses of movement, balance, and rotation)	
	Cochlear branch	Cochlea of inner ear (hearing)	
IX	Glossopharyngeal	Taste buds of posterior third of tongue and lining of pharynx	Parotid salivary gland; muscles of pharynx used in swallowing
X	Vagus	Nerve endings in many of the internal organs (e.g., lungs, stomach, aorta, larynx)	Parasympathetic fibers to heart, stomach, small intestine, larynx, esophagus, and other organs
XI	Spinal accessory	Muscles of shoulder	Muscles of neck and shoulder
XII	Hypoglossal	Muscles of tongue	Muscles of tongue

*Proprioceptors are receptors located in muscles, tendons, or joints that provide information about body position and movement.

Note that PCS requires certain ganglia, neural branches and structures be coded to specific nerves. In the cranial nerves, they are as follows:

- The **olfactory bulb**, the structure responsible for our sense of smell, is coded to the first cranial nerve, the **olfactory nerve.**
- The **optic chiasma** is the area of the brain where the optic nerve fibers partially cross and is coded to the second cranial nerve, the **optic nerve**. If damage to the optic nerve fibers occurs before (proximal to) the chiasma, the patient will exhibit loss of vision on the same side of the lesion. If the damage occurs after (distal to) the chiasma, the vision in the opposite eye is affected because of the crossing. The optic chiasma is coded to the optic nerve.

ophthalmic
  ophthalm/o = eye
  -ic = pertaining to

mandibular
  mandibul/o = lower jaw
  -ar = pertaining to

maxillary
  maxill/o = upper jaw
  -ary = pertaining to

- The fifth cranial nerve, the **trigeminal nerve**, has three main branches: the **ophthalmic nerve**, the **mandibular nerve**, and the **maxillary nerve.** The ophthalmic nerve receives sensory information from several structures of the eye (except the retina) and the skin of the forehead and nose. The maxillary nerve receives information from the teeth of the upper jaw and the sinuses and skin of the midface. The mandibular nerve has both sensory and motor functions for the lower jaw. Each of these nerves arises from the **Gasserian ganglion**, also referred to as the *trigeminal ganglion*, which is a sensory ganglion. This collection of nerves is significant in that it is the site of a dormant herpesvirus after a primary herpes infection.

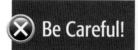 **Be Careful!** *Don't confuse the* **optic nerve**, *the second cranial nerve, with the* **ophthalmic nerve**, *which is coded to the trigeminal nerve, the fifth cranial nerve.*

vestibulocochlear
  vestibul/o = vestibule
  cochle/o = cochlea
  -ar = pertaining to

- The **facial nerve** (cranial nerve VII) has five structures coded to it that have word parts associated with the ear. The chorda tympani is named for its path through the middle ear, but is actually involved in the perception of taste. The greater superficial petrosal nerve innervates the lacrimal glands. The nerve to the stapes innervates the muscle of one of the ossicles of the ear. The parotid plexus is the location of branching of the facial nerve at one of the salivary glands near the ear. Finally, the posterior auricular nerve provides sensation from and innervation to the external ear and occipital region of the head. Also coded to the facial nerve are the geniculate and submandibular ganglia. The **geniculate ganglion**, named for its bent knee appearance, is a mix of sensory, motor, and parasympathetic nerves that provide a sense of taste and innervates several glands in the head and neck. The submandibular ganglion is part of the autonomic nervous system as one of the four parasympathetic ganglia of the head and neck.

- The **vestibulocochlear nerve**, cranial nerve VIII, is termed the **acoustic nerve** in PCS. Because its primary functions are balance and hearing, it's not surprising that the vestibular (sensing positional information) and cochlear (carrying information about sound) nerves are coded to it. The vestibular ganglion (also called *Scarpa's ganglion*) connects the vestibular nerve and semicircular canals of the inner ear. The spiral ganglion, a collection of nerve cells in the cochlea that sends sound to the cochlear nerve, is also coded to cranial nerve VIII.

glossopharyngeal
  gloss/o = tongue
  pharyng/o = throat
  -eal = pertaining to

- The **glossopharyngeal nerve**, cranial nerve IX, is used to code the carotid sinus nerve and the tympanic nerve. The carotid sinus nerve supplies the area that is the small cavity at the beginning of the internal carotid artery, the carotid sinus, along with the structure of the carotid body. This nerve carries impulses that detect pressure and changes in pH in the carotid body. The tympanic nerve (also called *Jacobson's nerve*) is a mix of sensory, parasympathetic, and sympathetic nerve fibers that serve the middle ear, the parotid gland, and the carotid plexus.

laryngeal
  laryng/o = voice box
  -eal = pertaining to

pulmonary
  pulmon/o = lung
  -ary = pertaining to

- The last of the cranial nerves that require extra detail is the tenth cranial nerve, the **vagus nerve.** Coded to this nerve are the anterior and posterior vagal trunks that direct nerves to organs in the front and back of the body, along with the superior and recurrent (inferior) **laryngeal nerves** (serving the voice box) and the **pharyngeal** and **pulmonary plexuses.** The pharyngeal plexus has sensory and motor fibers for parts of the throat, whereas the pulmonary plexus supplies the lungs.

Spinal Nerves

If the nerve fibers from several spinal nerves form a network, it is termed a **plexus.** Collections of cell bodies in the PNS are referred to as **ganglia** (*sing.* ganglion). Spinal nerves are named by their location (cervical, thoracic, lumbar, sacral, and coccygeal) and by number. These nerves are either sensory (often referred to as *cutaneous*) or muscular. **Dermatomes** are skin surface areas supplied by a single afferent spinal nerve. These areas are so specific that it is actually possible to map the body by dermatomes (Fig. 11-10, *A*). This specificity can be demonstrated in patients with shingles, who show similar patterns as specific peripheral nerves are affected (Fig. 11-10, *B*). **Myotomes** are the areas of muscles that are supplied by a single efferent spinal nerve (Fig. 11-10, *C*).

- **Occipital nerves** (greater, third, and sub-) are coded to **cervical nerves** that supply the skin and muscles of the head and neck.
- **Head and neck sympathetic nerves** are used to code the ciliary, otic, sphenopalatine (also referred to as *pterygopalatine*), and submandibular (formerly called *submaxillary*) ganglia. The internal carotid plexus and the cavernous plexus are located near the internal carotid artery. The internal carotid plexus is lateral to it, whereas the cavernous plexus is inferior and medial to it. The stellate ganglion, named for its starlike appearance

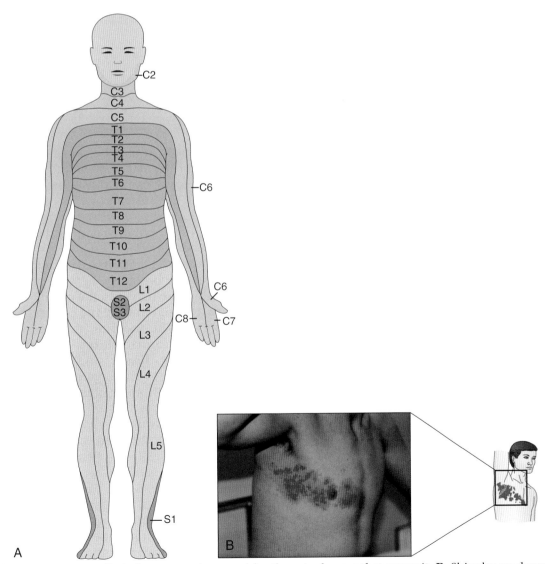

Fig. 11-10 A, Dermatomes. Each dermatome is named for the spinal nerve that serves it. **B,** Shingles on dermatome T4.

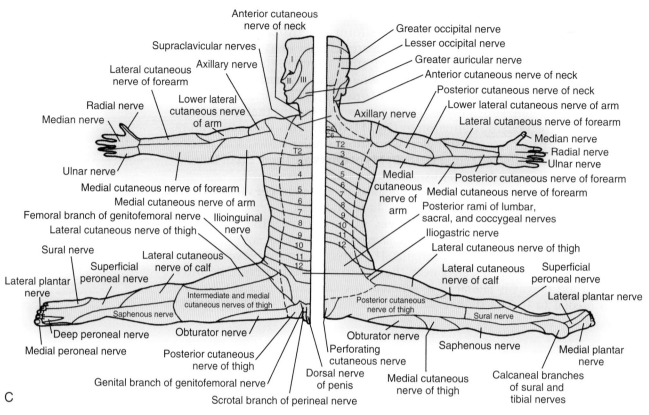

Anterior cutaneous
nerve of neck
Supraclavicular nerves
Axillary nerve
Lateral cutaneous
nerve of forearm
Radial nerve
Median nerve
Lower lateral
cutaneous nerve
of arm
Ulnar nerve
Medial cutaneous nerve of forearm
Medial cutaneous nerve of arm
Femoral branch of genitofemoral nerve
Lateral cutaneous nerve of thigh
Ilioinguinal
nerve
Sural nerve
Superficial
peroneal nerve
Lateral cutaneous
nerve of calf
Lateral plantar
nerve
Intermediate and medial
cutaneous nerves of thigh
Saphenous nerve
Deep peroneal nerve
Obturator nerve
Medial peroneal nerve
Posterior cutaneous
nerve of thigh
Genital branch of genitofemoral nerve
Dorsal nerve
of penis
Perforating
cutaneous nerve
Scrotal branch of perineal nerve

Greater occipital nerve
Lesser occipital nerve
Greater auricular nerve
Anterior cutaneous nerve of neck
Posterior cutaneous nerve of neck
Lower lateral cutaneous nerve of arm
Axillary nerve
Lateral cutaneous nerve of forearm
Median nerve
Radial nerve
Ulnar nerve
Medial
cutaneous
nerve of
arm
Posterior cutaneous nerve of forearm
Medial cutaneous nerve of forearm
Posterior rami of lumbar,
sacral, and coccygeal nerves
Iliogastric nerve
Lateral cutaneous nerve of thigh
Lateral cutaneous
nerve of calf
Superficial
peroneal nerve
Lateral plantar nerve
Posterior cutaneous
nerve of thigh
Sural nerve
Obturator nerve
Saphenous nerve
Medial plantar
nerve
Medial cutaneous
nerve of thigh
Calcaneal branches
of sural and
tibial nerves

C

Fig. 11-10 cont'd C, Myotomes.

intercostal
  inter- = between
  cost/o = rib
  -al = pertaining to

intercostobrachial
  inter- = between
  cost/o = rib
  brachi/o = arm
  -ial = pertaining to

subcostal
  sub- = under, below
  cost/o = rib
  -al = pertaining to

thoracic
  thorac/o = chest
  -ic = pertaining to

is located in the lower part of the neck; it may be cut in order to control hyperhidrosis (excessive sweating) or Raynaud's phenomenon. The **cervical ganglia** (inferior and superior) are sympathetic nerves in the neck area.

- The **median nerve** is used to code the anterior interosseous and the palmar cutaneous nerve.
- The **radial nerve** is used to code the dorsal digital, musculospiral, palmar cutaneous, and posterior interosseous nerves.
- The **intercostal**, **intercostobrachial**, and **subcostal nerves** are coded to the thoracic nerve. Note that each incorporates the word part for the ribs *(cost/o)*, which will help you locate these nerves to the chest.
- **Thoracic autonomic nerves** are used to code the cardiac, esophageal, thoracic, and pulmonary plexuses. The superior, middle, and inferior cardiac nerves, which are part of the cardiac plexus, are coded as a thoracic sympathetic nerve. The **greater, lesser**, and **least splanchnic** nerves, which are sympathetic nerves to the organs within the thorax and the thoracic ganglion, part of the thoracic plexus, are also coded as a thoracic sympathetic nerve.
- The **abdominal sympathetic nerve** is used to code a large number of plexuses, ganglia, and nerves. Fortunately, the word parts should be familiar to students who have completed the digestive system chapter. The celiac plexus (also called the *solar plexus*) and ganglion serve the belly, whereas the hepatic, gastric, renal, splenic, suprarenal, and pancreatic plexuses serve the liver, stomach, kidneys, spleen, adrenals, and pancreas respectively. The inferior and superior mesenteric plexuses and ganglia serve the mesentery, whereas the superior and inferior hypogastric plexuses serve the pelvic cavity. The myenteric plexus (also called Auerbach's plexus) is the primary nervous supply to the digestive system and is responsible for gastric motility. The pelvic splanchnic nerves regulate the evacuation of the bowels and bladder. The

submucous plexus, also called *Meissner's plexus*, innervates smooth muscle, whereas the **abdominal aortic plexus** surrounds the abdominal aorta.

- The **superior clunic** and the **lumbosacral trunk** are coded to the lumbar nerve.
- The **lumbar sympathetic nerve** is used to code the lumbar ganglion and the lumbar splanchnic nerve.
- The **pudendal nerve** is used to code the posterior labial or posterior scrotal nerves.
- The **sacral sympathetic nerve** is used to code the ganglion impar (also called the ganglion of Walther), the pelvic and sacral splanchnic nerve, and the sacral ganglion.
- The **saphenous nerve** is coded to the entry of the femoral nerve.
- The **tibial nerve** is used to code the medial popliteal, medial sural cutaneous, and medial and lateral plantar nerves.
- The **peroneal nerve** is used to code the lateral sural cutaneous nerve.

lumbosacral
lumb/o = lower back
sacr/o = sacrum
-al = pertaining to

tibial
tibi/o = shinbone
-al = pertaining to

peroneal
perone/o = lower, lateral leg bone
-al = pertaining to

⊗ Be Careful! The term **dermatome** *can be used to describe an instrument that cuts thin slices of skin for grafting, and the term also signifies a mesodermal layer in early development, which becomes the dermal layers of the skin.*

Exercise 3: Central and Peripheral Nervous System

A. Match the following parts of the brain with their functions.

____ 1. pons
____ 2. parietal cerebral lobe
____ 3. hypothalamus
____ 4. temporal cerebral lobe
____ 5. midbrain
____ 6. cerebellum
____ 7. occipital cerebral lobe
____ 8. thalamus
____ 9. frontal cerebral lobe
____ 10. medulla oblongata

A. auditory and olfactory activity
B. relays sensory information
C. reflex center for eye and head movements
D. sensation of vision
E. regulates heart rate, blood pressure, and breathing
F. regulates temperature, sleep, and appetite
G. speech and motor activity
H. connects medulla oblongata with cerebrum
I. coordinates voluntary movement
J. sensation of touch and taste

B. Match the CNS part with its combining form.

____ 1. cerebellum   ____ 6. cerebrum
____ 2. spinal cord   ____ 7. brain
____ 3. meninges   ____ 8. skin
____ 4. nerve root   ____ 9. spine
____ 5. dura mater   ____ 10. ventricle

A. meningi/o, mening/o   F. cerebr/o
B. myel/o, cord/o, chord/o G. spin/o
C. dur/o   H. cerebell/o
D. rhiz/o, radicul/o   I. encephal/o
E. dermat/o   J. ventricul/o

Translate the terms.

11. intraventricular _____.

12. epidural _____.

13. paraspinal _____.

14. infracerebellar _____.

To practice labeling the nervous system, click on **Label it.**

Combining Forms for the Anatomy and Physiology of the Nervous System

Meaning	Combining Form	Meaning	Combining Form
body	somat/o	meninges	mening/o, meningi/o
brain	encephal/o	nerve	neur/o
cerebellum	cerebell/o	nerve root	rhiz/o, radicul/o
cerebrum	cerebr/o	same	home/o
cortex	cortic/o	skin	dermat/o
dendrite	dendr/o	spinal cord	cord/o, chord/o, myel/o
dura mater	dur/o	star	astr/o
globus pallidum	pallid/o	ventricle	ventricul/o
lobe	lob/o	vestibule	vestibul/o

Suffixes for the Anatomy and Physiology of the Nervous System

Suffix	Meaning
-cyte	cell
-glia	glue
-on	structure
-stasis	stopping, controlling
-tome	instrument used to cut

You can review the anatomy of the nervous system by clicking on **Body Spectrum Electronic Anatomy Coloring Book,** then **Nervous.**

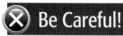

*Don't confuse **dysarthria** (difficulty with speech) with **dysarthrosis** (any disorder of a joint).*

PATHOLOGY

The signs and symptoms for this system encompass many systems because of the nature of the neural function: communicating, or failing to communicate, with other parts of the body.

Terms Related to Symptoms and Signs of the Nervous System (R13-R56)

Term	Word Origin	Definition
amnesia		Loss of memory caused by brain damage or severe emotional trauma.
anomia	*a-* no, not, without *nom/o* name *-ia* condition	The inability to name everyday objects. A type of aphasia.
aphasia	*a-* no, not, without *phas/o* speech *-ia* condition	Lack or impairment of the ability to form or understand speech. Less severe forms include **dysphasia** and **dysarthria**; dysarthria refers to difficulty in the articulation (pronunciation) of speech.
asthenia	*a-* no, not, without *-sthenia* condition of strength	Weakness.
ataxia	*a-* no, not, without *tax/o* order, coordination *-ia* condition	A condition of a lack of coordination.
athetosis		Continuous involuntary slow, writhing movement of the extremities.
coma		Deep, prolonged unconsciousness from which the patient cannot be aroused; usually the result of a head injury, neurological disease, acute hydrocephalus, intoxication, or metabolic abnormalities.
convulsion		Neuromuscular reaction to abnormal electrical activity within the brain. Causes include fever or epilepsy, a recurring seizure disorder; also called a **seizure.**
dysphagia	*dys-* difficult, bad *phag/o* eat, swallow *-ia* condition	Condition of difficulty with swallowing.
fasciculation		Involuntary contraction of small local muscles.
paresthesia	*para-* abnormal *esthesi/o* feeling *-ia* condition	Feeling of prickling, burning, or numbness.
spasm		Involuntary muscle contraction of sudden onset. Examples are hiccoughs, tics, and stuttering.
syncope		Fainting. A **vasovagal attack** is a form of syncope that results from abrupt emotional stress involving the vagus nerve's effect on blood vessels.
tremors		Rhythmic, quivering, purposeless skeletal muscle movements seen in some elderly individuals and in patients with various neurodegenerative disorders.
vertigo		Dizziness; abnormal sensation of movement when there is none, either of oneself moving or of objects moving around oneself.

Terms Related to Traumatic Conditions (S06)

Term	Word Origin	Definition
concussion		Serious head injury characterized by one or more of the following: loss of consciousness, amnesia, seizures, or a change in mental status.
contusion, cerebral		Head injury of sufficient force to bruise the brain. Bruising of the brain often involves the brain surface and causes extravasation of blood without rupture of the pia arachnoid; often associated with a concussion.
hematoma	*hemat/o* blood *-oma* tumor, mass	Localized collection of blood, usually clotted, in an organ, tissue, or space, due to a break in the wall of a blood vessel (Fig. 11-11). Epidural hematomas occur above the dura mater. Subdural hematomas occur between the dura mater and arachnoid meninges. May be the result of a traumatic brain injury (TBI).

 Be Careful!

Although the word origin of the term **hematoma** *means a blood tumor, this is a misnomer. A hematoma is a mass of blood that has leaked out of a vessel and pooled.*

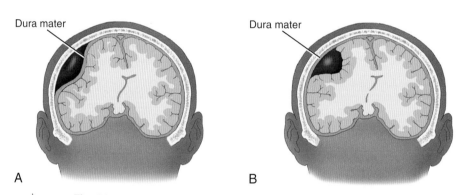

Fig. 11-11 **A,** Epidural hematoma. **B,** Subdural hematoma.

 ICD Note

The Glasgow Coma Scale (GCS) is an objective, neurological measurement of a patient's level of consciousness. The scale uses a composite score of 3 to indicate deep unconsciousness with gradations up to 15 to indicate full consciousness. The GCS is used with traumatic brain injury or sequelae of cerebrovascular accident codes. It is composed of three separate codes that individually report a patient's visual, verbal, and motor status. The 7th digit refers to when the score was recorded: in the field, at arrival to the emergency department, on hospital admission, or 24 hours or more after admission.

Exercise 4: Signs and Symptoms, Congenital Disorders, and Trauma

Match the terms to their definitions.

____	1.	syncope
____	2.	tremors
____	3.	vertigo
____	4.	spasm
____	5.	paresthesia
____	6.	athetosis
____	7.	convulsion
____	8.	amnesia
____	9.	ataxia
____	10.	fasciculation
____	11.	asthenia
____	12.	coma
____	13.	concussion
____	14.	cerebral contusion

A. head injury of sufficient force to bruise the brain

B. involuntary contraction of small local muscles

C. serious head injury characterized by loss of consciousness, amnesia, or change in mental status

D. dizziness

E. loss of memory caused by brain damage or severe emotional trauma

F. involuntary muscle contraction of sudden onset

G. lack of muscular coordination

H. continuous slow, writhing movement of the extremities

I. rhythmic, purposeless skeletal muscle movements

J. neuromuscular reaction to abnormal electrical activity in the brain

K. weakness

L. feeling of prickling, burning, or numbness

M. fainting

N. deep, prolonged unconsciousness from which the patient cannot be aroused

Translate the terms.

15. aphasia _____

16. dysphagia _____

17. hematoma _____

Terms Related to Inflammatory Diseases of the Central Nervous System (G00-G09)

Term	Word Origin	Definition
encephalitis	*encephal/o* brain *-itis* inflammation	Inflammation of the brain, most frequently caused by a virus transmitted by the bite of an infected mosquito.
meningitis	*mening/o* meninges *-itis* inflammation	Any infection or inflammation of the membranes covering the brain and spinal cord, most commonly due to viral infection, although more severe strains are bacterial or fungal.

Terms Related to Systemic Atrophies Primarily Affecting the Central Nervous System (G10-G14)

Term	Word Origin	Definition
amyotrophic lateral sclerosis (ALS)	*a-* no, not, without *my/o* muscle *troph/o* development *-ic* pertaining to *later/o* side *-al* pertaining to *sclerosis* condition of hardening	Degenerative, fatal disease of the motor neurons, in which patients exhibit progressive muscle weakness and atrophy; also called **Lou Gehrig's disease.**
Huntington's disease		Inherited disorder that manifests itself in adulthood as a progressive loss of neural control, uncontrollable jerking movements, and dementia. Also called **Huntington's chorea.** Chorea is derived from the Latin word for "dance."
postpolio syndrome (PPS)	*post-* after *poli/o* gray *syn-* together *-drome* run	Although **poliomyelitis** (an inflammation of the gray matter of the spinal cord) has been virtually eradicated, some patients who have had polio report symptoms of exhaustion and muscle and joint pain decades after their initial illness.

Terms Related to Extrapyramidal and Movement Disorders (G20-G26)

Term	Word Origin	Definition
Parkinson's disease (PD)		Progressive neurodegenerative disease characterized by tremors, fasciculations, slow shuffling gait, bradykinesia (slow movement), dysphasia, and dysphagia. Its cause is unknown (Fig. 11-12).

Terms Related to Other Degenerative Disorders of the Central Nervous System (G30-G32)

Term	Word Origin	Definition
Alzheimer's disease (AD)		Progressive neurodegenerative disease in which patients exhibit an impairment of cognitive functioning. The cause of disease is unknown. Alzheimer's is the most common cause of dementia (Fig. 11-13).
mild cognitive impairment (MCI)		Loss or impairment of cognitive abilities, although not as severe as AD. Also called **incipient dementia**.

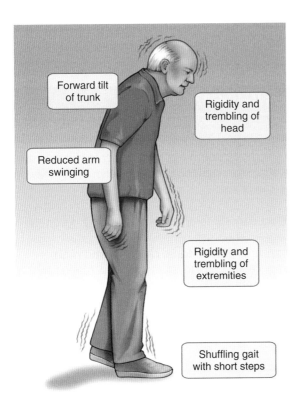

Forward tilt of trunk

Rigidity and trembling of head

Reduced arm swinging

Rigidity and trembling of extremities

Shuffling gait with short steps

Fig. 11-12 Signs of Parkinson's disease.

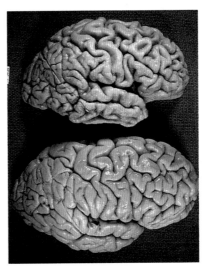

Fig. 11-13 Alzheimer's disease. The affected brain *(top)* is smaller and shows narrow gyri and widened sulci compared with the normal, age-matched brain *(bottom)*.

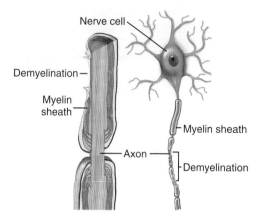

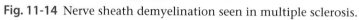
Fig. 11-14 Nerve sheath demyelination seen in multiple sclerosis.

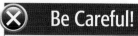

Be Careful!

MS *stands for* musculoskeletal system, mitral stenosis, *and* multiple sclerosis.

Terms Related to Demyelinating Diseases of the Central Nervous System (G35-G37)

Term	Word Origin	Definition
multiple sclerosis (MS)	*sclerosis* condition of hardening	Neurodegenerative disease characterized by destruction of the myelin sheaths on the CNS neurons (demyelination) and their abnormal replacement by the gradual accumulation of hardened plaques. The disease may be progressive or characterized by remissions and relapses. Cause is unknown (Fig. 11-14).

Terms Related to Episodic and Paroxysmal Disorders (G40-G47)

Term	Word Origin	Definition
dyssomnia	*dys-* difficult *somn/o* sleep *-ia* condition	Disorders of the sleep-wake cycles. **Insomnia** is the inability to sleep or stay asleep. **Hypersomnia** is excessive depth or length of sleep, which may be accompanied by daytime sleepiness.
epilepsy	*epi-* above *-lepsy* seizure	Group of disorders characterized by some or all of the following: recurrent seizures, sensory disturbances, abnormal behavior, and/or loss of consciousness. Types of seizures include **tonic clonic (grand mal)**, accompanied by temporary loss of consciousness and severe muscle spasms; **absence seizures (petit mal)**, accompanied by loss of consciousness exhibited by unresponsiveness for short periods without muscle involvement. **Status epilepticus** is a condition of intense, unrelenting, life-threatening seizures. **Pseudoseizures** are false seizures. Causes may be trauma, tumor, intoxication, chemical imbalance, or vascular disturbances.

Continued

Terms Related to Episodic and Paroxysmal Disorders (G40-G47)—cont'd

Term	Word Origin	Definition
migraine		Headache of vascular origin. The onset of a migraine may be preceded by an **aura**, a sensation of light or warmth. Migraines are further classified as intractable (difficult to treat) and with/without **status migrainosus** (lasting longer than 72 hours).
narcolepsy	*narc/o* sleep *-lepsy* seizure	Disorder characterized by sudden attacks of sleep. **Cataplexy** is a loss of muscle tone that results in collapse without loss of consciousness (*cata-* means "down"; *-plexy* means "seizure").
transient ischemic attack (TIA)		Temporary ischemia of cerebral tissue due to an occlusion (blockage) from a thrombus (*pl.* thrombi) or embolus (*pl.* emboli), or as a result of a cerebral hemorrhage. Results of a TIA depend on the duration and location of the ischemia. These sequelae may include paralysis, weakness, speech defects, and sensory changes that last less than 24 hours.

Exercise 5: Diseases that Primarily Affect the CNS

Fill in the blank.

1. What progressive neurodegenerative disease is characterized by tremors, bradykinesia, and a slow, shuffling gait? _____

2. What progressive neurodegenerative disease causes impairment of cognitive functions? _____

3. What headache of vascular origin may be preceded by an aura? _____

4. What group of disorders is characterized by recurrent seizures, sensory disturbances, abnormal behavior, and/or loss of consciousness? _____

5. What temporary ischemia of cerebral tissue is due to an occlusion or a cerebral hemorrhage?_____

6. What neurodegenerative disease is characterized by demyelination of the CNS neurons? _____

Build the terms.

7. seizure of sleep _____

8. difficult sleep condition _____

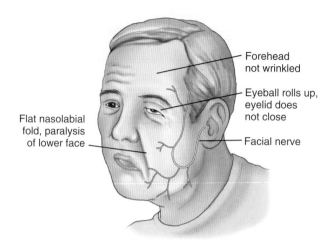

Fig. 11-15 The facial characteristics of Bell's palsy.

Forehead
not wrinkled

Eyeball rolls up,
eyelid does
not close

Facial nerve

Flat nasolabial
fold, paralysis
of lower face

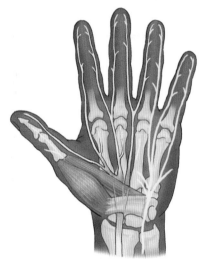

Fig. 11-16 Carpal tunnel syndrome.

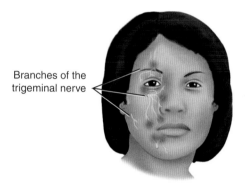

Branches of the
trigeminal nerve

Fig. 11-17 Trigeminal neuralgia: distribution of trigger zones.

Terms Related to Nerve, Nerve Root, and Plexus Disorders (G50-G59)

Term	Word Origin	Definition
Bell's palsy		Paralysis of the facial nerve. Unknown in cause, the condition usually resolves on its own within 6 months (Fig. 11-15).
carpal tunnel syndrome (CTS)	*carp/o* wrist bone *-al* pertaining to *syn-* joined together *-drome* to run	Compression injury that manifests itself as fluctuating pain, numbness, and paresthesias of the hand caused by compression of the median nerve at the wrist (Fig. 11-16).
causalgia	*caus/o* burning *-algia* pain	Nerve pain, described by patients as a "burning pain."
meralgia paresthetica	*mer/o* thigh *-algia* pain *par-* abnormal *-esthetica* feeling, sensation	Condition of a burning, tingling sensation in the thigh caused by injury to one of the femoral nerves.
trigeminal neuralgia	*neur/o* nerve *-algia* pain	Chronic facial pain that affects the fifth cranial nerve (Fig. 11-17). Usually experienced on one side of the face. The pain is episodic and intense. Also known as **tic douloureux**.

Terms Related to Polyneuropathies and Other Disorders of the PNS (G60-G65)

Term	Word Origin	Definition
Guillain-Barré syndrome		Autoimmune disorder of acute polyneuritis producing profound myasthenia that may lead to paralysis.
polyneuropathy	*poly-* many *neur/o* nerve *-pathy* disease condition	A general term describing a disorder of several peripheral nerves.

Terms Related to Diseases of Myoneural Junction and Muscle (G70-G73)

Term	Word Origin	Definition
muscular dystrophy (MD)	*muscul/o* muscle *-ar* pertaining to *dys-* bad, abnormal *troph/o* development *-y* condition, process of	Group of disorders characterized as an inherited progressive atrophy of skeletal muscle without neural involvement (Fig. 11-18).
myasthenia gravis	*my/o* muscle *a-* without, no *-sthenia* condition of strength *gravis* severe	Usually severe condition characterized by fatigue and progressive muscle weakness, especially of the face and throat (Fig. 11-19).

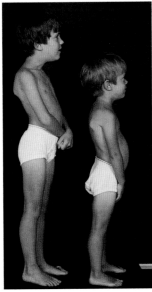

Fig. 11-18 Muscular dystrophy. These brothers show typical stance, lumbar lordosis and forward thrusting of the abdomen.

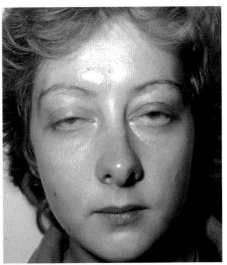

Fig. 11-19 Facial muscular weakness in myasthenia gravis.

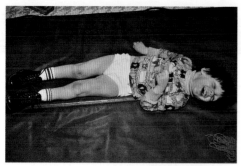

Fig. 11-20 A child with spastic quadriplegic cerebral palsy.

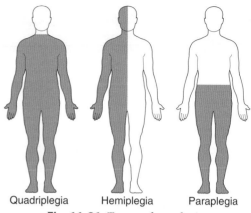

Quadriplegia   Hemiplegia   Paraplegia

Fig. 11-21 Types of paralysis.

Terms Related to Cerebral Palsy, Other Paralytic Syndromes, and Other Disorders of the Nervous System (G80-G99)

Term	Word Origin	Definition
cerebral palsy (CP)	*cerebr/o* cerebrum *-al* pertaining to	Motor function disorder as a result of permanent, nonprogressive brain defect or lesion caused perinatally. Neural deficits may include paralysis, ataxia, athetosis, seizures, and/or impairment of sensory functions (Fig. 11-20).
diplegia	*di-* two *-plegia* paralysis	Paralysis of the same body part on both sides of the body.
hemiparesis	*hemi-* half *-paresis* slight paralysis	Muscular weakness or slight paralysis on the left or right side of the body.
hemiplegia	*hemi-* half *-plegia* paralysis	Paralysis on the left or right side of the body (Fig. 11-21).
hydrocephalus	*hydr/o* water *-cephalus* head	Condition of abnormal accumulation of fluid in the ventricles of the brain. Usually diagnosed in babies; may also occur in adults as a result of stroke, trauma, or infection.
locked-in state		Damage to the upper brainstem that leaves the patient paralyzed and mute.
monoplegia	*mono-* one *-plegia* paralysis	Paralysis of one limb on the left or right side of the body.
paraplegia	*para-* abnormal *-plegia* paralysis	Paralysis of the lower limbs and trunk (Fig. 11-21).
quadriplegia	*quadri-* four *-plegia* paralysis	Paralysis of arms, legs, and trunk (Fig. 11-21).

ICD Note

Paralysis is the loss of muscle function. Paralysis may be complete (no movement/function below the level of injury) or incomplete (some movement/function possible below the level of injury). Flaccid paralysis, characterized by weakening or loss of muscle tone, is associated with lower motor neuron damage. Examples are polio and ALS. Spastic paralysis is characterized by involuntary muscle contractions and lack of tendon reflexes and is the result of upper motor neuron damage. Multiple sclerosis is an example.

Be Careful! *If the suffix **-paresis** is used, it indicates a weakness of the body parts affected, not a total loss of muscle tone.*

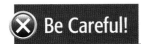 **CM Guideline Alert**

6A. DOMINANT/NONDOMINANT SIDE

Codes from category G81, Hemiplegia and hemiparesis, and subcategories, G83.1, Monoplegia of lower limb, G83.2, Monoplegia of upper limb, and G83.3, Monoplegia, unspecified, identify whether the dominant or nondominant side is affected. Should the affected side be documented, but not specified as dominant or nondominant, and the classification system does not indicate a default, code selection is as follows:
- For ambidextrous patients, the default should be dominant.
- If the left side is affected, the default is non-dominant.
- If the right side is affected, the default is dominant.

 As mentioned in Chapter 1, some diseases have manifestations and sequelae. ICD-10-CM has expanded cerebrovascular disease codes to include both the sequelae and the manifestations. For example hemiplegia and hemiparesis following cerebral infarction affecting the right dominant side would be coded as I69.351.

 ## Exercise 6: Diseases that Primarily Affect the PNS

Match the terms to their definitions.

___ 1. trigeminal neuralgia

___ 2. carpal tunnel syndrome

___ 3. Guillain-Barré syndrome

___ 4. MD

___ 5. myasthenia gravis

___ 6. cerebral palsy

___ 7. hemiparesis

___ 8. paraplegia

___ 9. quadriplegia

___ 10. monoplegia

___ 11. locked-in state

___ 12. Bell's palsy

A. compression injury that manifests itself as pain, numbness, and paresthesia of the hand

B. paralysis of arms, legs, and trunk

C. severe condition characterized by fatigue and progressive muscle weakness of the face and throat

D. slight paralysis on one side of the body

E. damage to the upper brainstem that leaves the patient paralyzed and mute

F. chronic facial pain that affects the fifth cranial nerve

G. paralysis of the facial nerve

H. paralysis of one limb

I. motor function disorder resulting from nonprogressive brain defect or lesion caused perinatally

J. paralysis of the lower limbs and trunk

K. autoimmune disorder that produces myasthenia that may lead to paralysis

L. group of disorders characterized as an inherited progressive atrophy of skeletal muscle without neural involvement

Translate the terms.

13. causalgia _____

14. meralgia paresthetica _____

15. polyneuropathy _____

16. hemiplegia _____

17. diplegia _____

Terms Related to Neoplasms of the CNS*

Term	Word Origin	Definition
astrocytoma	*astr/o* star *cyt/o* cell *-oma* tumor, mass	Tumor arising from star-shaped glial cells that is malignant in higher grades. A grade IV astrocytoma is referred to as a glioblastoma multiforme, the most common primary brain cancer (Fig. 11-22).
ependymoma		Tumors of the cells that line the ventricles of the brain. In children, ependymomas are usually intracranial; in adults they are most often intraspinal.
medulloblastoma	*medull/o* medulla *blast/o* embryonic *-oma* tumor, mass	Tumor that arises from embryonic tissue in the cerebellum. Most commonly seen in children.
meningioma	*meningi/o* meninges *-oma* tumor, mass	Slow-growing, usually benign tumor of the meninges. Although benign, may cause problems because of its size and location (Fig. 11-23).
neuroblastoma	*neur/o* nerve *blast/o* embryonic *-oma* tumor, mass	Highly malignant tumor arising from either the autonomic nervous system or the adrenal medulla. Usually affects children younger than 10 years of age.

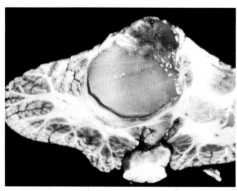

Fig. 11-22 Pilocytic astrocytoma in the cerebellum with a nodule of tumor in a cyst.

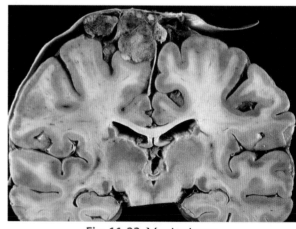

Fig. 11-23 Meningioma.

Terms Related to Neoplasms of the PNS*

Term	Word Origin	Definition
ganglioneuroma	*gangli/o* ganglia *neur/o* nerve *-oma* tumor, mass	Usually benign, slow-growing tumor that originates in the autonomic nervous system cells.
neurofibroma	*neur/o* nerve *fibr/o* fiber *-oma* tumor, mass	Benign fibrous tumors of tissue surrounding the nerve sheath.
schwannoma		A type of tumor, benign or malignant, that is most commonly found in the inner ear (vestibular schwannoma).

*Most neoplasms that are related to the nervous system arise from the supportive glial cells, although a few others do occur. It is important to note the difference between primary brain cancers (those that originate in the brain) and metastatic cancers that have spread to the brain from another location.

Exercise 7: Neoplasms of the CNS and PNS

Build the terms.

1. ganglia nerve tumor _____.

2. tumor of the meninges _____

3. star cell tumor _____.

4. nerve fiber tumor _____.

5. embryonic tumor of the medulla _____

6. embryonic nerve tumor _____

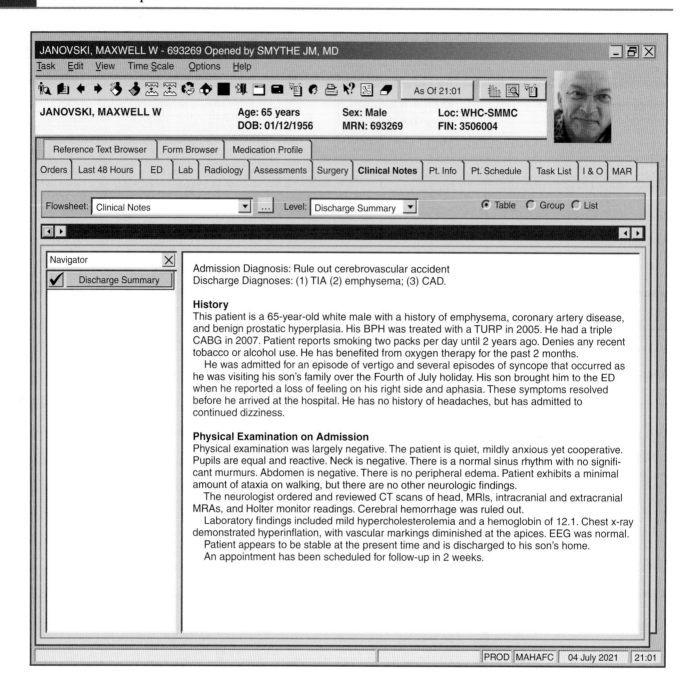

Admission Diagnosis: Rule out cerebrovascular accident
Discharge Diagnoses: (1) TIA (2) emphysema; (3) CAD.

History
This patient is a 65-year-old white male with a history of emphysema, coronary artery disease, and benign prostatic hyperplasia. His BPH was treated with a TURP in 2005. He had a triple CABG in 2007. Patient reports smoking two packs per day until 2 years ago. Denies any recent tobacco or alcohol use. He has benefited from oxygen therapy for the past 2 months.

He was admitted for an episode of vertigo and several episodes of syncope that occurred as he was visiting his son's family over the Fourth of July holiday. His son brought him to the ED when he reported a loss of feeling on his right side and aphasia. These symptoms resolved before he arrived at the hospital. He has no history of headaches, but has admitted to continued dizziness.

Physical Examination on Admission
Physical examination was largely negative. The patient is quiet, mildly anxious yet cooperative. Pupils are equal and reactive. Neck is negative. There is a normal sinus rhythm with no significant murmurs. Abdomen is negative. There is no peripheral edema. Patient exhibits a minimal amount of ataxia on walking, but there are no other neurologic findings.

The neurologist ordered and reviewed CT scans of head, MRIs, intracranial and extracranial MRAs, and Holter monitor readings. Cerebral hemorrhage was ruled out.

Laboratory findings included mild hypercholesterolemia and a hemoglobin of 12.1. Chest x-ray demonstrated hyperinflation, with vascular markings diminished at the apices. EEG was normal.

Patient appears to be stable at the present time and is discharged to his son's home.

An appointment has been scheduled for follow-up in 2 weeks.

Exercise 8: Discharge Summary

Using the discharge summary above, answer the following questions.

1. Patient was admitted for vertigo and syncope. Define each. _____.

2. What is a TIA? _____.

3. Aphasia refers to_____.

4. Ataxia refers to _____.

PROCEDURES

Terms Related to Procedures

Term	Word Origin	Definition
cerebral angiography	*cerebr/o* cerebrum *-al* pertaining to *angi/o* vessel *-graphy* recording	X-ray of the cerebral arteries, including the internal carotids, taken after the injection of a contrast medium (Fig. 11-24); also called **cerebral arteriography**.
chemothalamectomy	*chem/o* chemical, drug *thalam/o* thalamus *-ectomy* cutting out	Injection of chemical substance to destroy part of the thalamus. Used to treat Parkinson's and Huntington's diseases.
cordotomy	*cord/o* spinal cord *-tomy* cutting	Incision of the spinal cord to relieve pain. Also spelled **chordotomy**.
craniotomy	*crani/o* skull, cranium *-tomy* cutting	Incision into the skull as a surgical approach or to relieve intracranial pressure; also called **trephination.**
deep tendon reflexes (DTR)		Assessment of an automatic motor response by striking a tendon. Useful in diagnosis of TIA and CVA. Babinski's sign is the loss or diminution of the Achilles tendon reflex seen in sciatica.

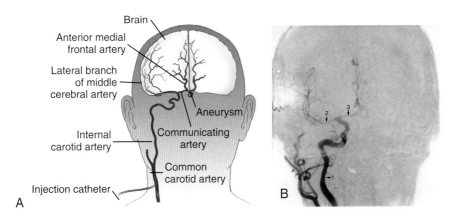

Fig. 11-24 Cerebral angiography. A, Insertion of dye through a catheter in the common carotid artery outlines the vessels of the brain. **B,** Angiogram showing vessels. 1, internal carotid artery; 2, middle cerebral artery; 3, middle meningeal artery.

CPT Coding Alert!

Decompression of the spinal cord (to relieve pressure) can be done by partially or completely removing the vertebral body through a variety of approaches. CPT has a code for each of these, each listed as a vertebral corpectomy. *Corp/o* here refers to the vertebral body, the anterior oval segment of an individual backbone.

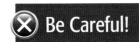 **Be Careful!** *Don't confuse a cordotomy, which is an incision of the spinal cord, with a vertebral corpectomy, an excision of a vertebral body.*

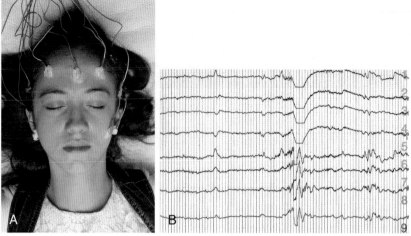

Fig. 11-25 EEG. A, Photograph of person with electrodes attached. **B,** EEG tracing showing selection of readings of brain activity.

Terms Related to Procedures—cont'd

Term	Word Origin	Definition
echoencephalography	*echo* -sound *encephal/o* brain *-graphy* recording	Ultrasound exam of the brain, usually done only on newborns because sound waves do not readily penetrate bone.
electroencephalography (EEG)	*electr/o* electricity *encephal/o* brain *-graphy* recording	Record of the electrical activity of the brain. May be used in the diagnosis of epilepsy, infection, and coma (Fig. 11-25).
ganglionectomy of the dorsal root	*ganglion/o* ganglion *-ectomy* cutting out	Removal of the dorsal root ganglia to treat pain.
hemispherectomy	*hemi-* half *spher/o* sphere, round *-ectomy* cutting out	Removal of a cerebral hemisphere to treat intractable epilepsy.
lumbar puncture (LP)	*lumb/o* lower back *-ar* pertaining to	Procedure to aspirate CSF from the lumbar subarachnoid space. A needle is inserted between two lumbar vertebrae to withdraw the fluid for diagnostic purposes. Once removed, the CSF is analyzed to detect pathogens and abnormalities. Also called a **spinal tap** (Fig. 11-26).
myelography	*myel/o* spinal cord *-graphy* recording	X-ray of the spinal canal after the introduction of a radiopaque contrast.

Continued

 CPT Coding Alert!

CPT has a code for a neuroendoscopic procedure that involves fenestration of the septum pellucidum. Fenestration means "to make a new opening," from the Latin word for a window.

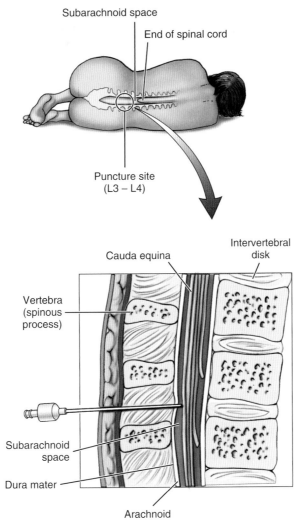

Fig. 11-26 Lumbar puncture.

Terms Related to Procedures—cont'd

Term	Word Origin	Definition
nerve block		Use of anesthesia to prevent sensory nerve impulses from reaching the CNS.
nerve conduction test		Test of the functioning of CNS or peripheral nerves. Conduction time (impulse travel) through a nerve is measured after a stimulus is applied; used to diagnose polyneuropathies.
neurectomy	*neur/o* nerve *-ectomy* cutting out	Excision of part or all of a nerve to alleviate pain.
neurexeresis	*neur/o* nerve *-exeresis* tearing out	Removal of the fifth cranial nerve to treat trigeminal neuralgia.
neuroplasty	*neur/o* nerve *-plasty* surgically forming	Surgical repair of a nerve.

Terms Related to Procedures—cont'd

Term	Word Origin	Definition
neurotomy	*neur/o* nerve *-tomy* cutting	Incision of a nerve. Radiofrequency ablation is used to treat facet joint pain in the neck and back.
pallidotomy	*pallid/o* globus pallidum *-tomy* cutting	Destruction of the globus pallidum to treat Parkinson's disease. The procedure relieves muscular rigidity and tremors.
phrenemphraxis	*phren/o* diaphragm, phrenic nerve *-emphraxis* obstructing, crushing	Crushing of the phrenic nerve to cause its paralysis. Also called **phrenicotripsy** and **phreniclasis**.
polysomnography (PSG)	*poly-* many *somn/o* sleep *-graphy* recording	Measurement and record of a number of functions while the patient is asleep (e.g., cardiac, muscular, brain, ocular, and respiratory functions). Most often used to diagnose sleep apnea (Fig. 11-27).
rhizotomy	*rhiz/o* spinal nerve root *-tomy* cutting	Resection of the dorsal root of a spinal nerve to relieve pain.
sympathectomy	*sympath/o* to feel with *-ectomy* cutting out	Surgical interruption of part of the sympathetic pathways for the relief of chronic pain or to promote vasodilation.
tractotomy	*tract/o* tract, pathway *-tomy* cutting	Cutting of a nerve tract to alleviate pain.
transcutaneous electrical nerve stimulation (TENS)	*trans-* through *cutane/o* skin *-ous* pertaining to	Method of pain control effected by the application of electrical impulses through the skin (Fig. 11-28).
vagotomy	*vag/o* vagus nerve *-tomy* cutting	Cutting of a branch of the vagus nerve to reduce the secretion of gastric acid (Fig. 11-29).

Continued

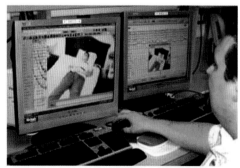

Fig. 11-27 Polysomnography.

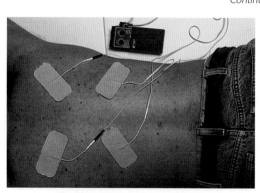

Fig. 11-28 TENS treatment.

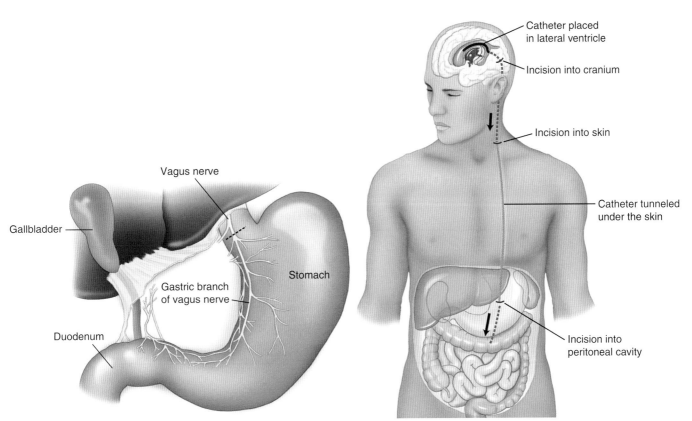

Fig. 11-29 Vagotomy.

Fig. 11-30 Ventriculoperitoneostomy.

Terms Related to Procedures—cont'd		
Term	**Word Origin**	**Definition**
ventriculocisternostomy	*ventricul/o* ventricle *cistern/o* box, cistern *-stomy* making a new opening	The creation of a new opening between a blocked ventricle and a cerebral cistern. Used to treat hydrocephalus.
ventriculoperitoneostomy	*ventricul/o* ventricle *peritone/o* peritoneum *-stomy* making a new opening	Procedure to drain fluid from brain ventricles through a shunt, catheter, and valve that leads to the abdominal cavity (Fig. 11-30). **Neuroendoscopy**, a procedure that uses a fiberoptic camera to visualize neural structures, is used to place the shunt.
ventriculostomy, endoscopic	*endo-* within *-scopic* pertaining to viewing *ventricul/o* ventricle *-stomy* making a new opening	A new opening between the third ventricle and the subarachnoid space; used to treat one type of hydrocephalus.

⊗ **Be Careful!**   *A ventriculoatriostomy is a new opening between a ventricle of the **brain** and an upper chamber of the heart.*

RECOGNIZING SUFFIXES FOR PCS

Now that you've finished reading about the procedures for the nervous system, take a look at this review of the *suffixes* used in their terminology. Each of these suffixes is associated with one or more root operations in the medical surgical section or one of the other categories in PCS.

Suffixes and Root Operations for the Nervous System

Suffix	Root Operation
-ectomy	Excision, resection, destruction
-emphraxis	Destruction
-exeresis	Extraction
-plasty	Repair, supplement
-stomy	Bypass, drainage
-tomy	Drainage, division, destruction

Exercise 9: Procedures

Match the terms to their definitions.

____1. neurexeresis
____2. hemispherectomy
____3. tractotomy
____4. ventriculocisternostomy
____5. pallidotomy
____6. EEG
____7. cordotomy
____8. rhizotomy
____9. nerve conduction test
___10. TENS
___11. PSG
___12. LP
___13. craniotomy
___14. myelography

A. record of the electrical activity of the brain
B. removal of a cerebral hemisphere to treat epilepsy
C. test of the functioning CNS or peripheral nerves
D. incision of the spinal cord to relieve pain
E. procedure to aspirate CSF from the lumbar subarachnoid space
F. removal of the fifth cranial nerve to treat trigeminal neuralgia
G. destruction of the globus pallidum to treat Parkinson's disease
H. method of pain control effected by the application of electrical impulses to the skin
I. incision into the skull to relieve intracranial pressure
J. creation of a new opening between a blocked ventricle and a cerebral cistern
K. x-ray of the spinal canal using radiopaque contrast
L. resection of a dorsal root of a spinal nerve to relieve pain
M. measurement and record of body functions while a patient is asleep
N. cutting of a nerve tract to relieve pain

Translate the terms.

15. chemothalamectomy _____

16. phrenemphraxis _____

17. echoencephalography _____

18. vagotomy _____

19. neuroplasty _____

20. ventriculoperitoneostomy _____

PHARMACOLOGY

analgesics: Reduce pain. NSAIDs (nonsteroidal antiinflammatory drugs) and opioids (narcotic analgesics) are commonly used types. Examples include morphine (MS Contin), hydrocodone (Vicodin in combination with acetaminophen), sumatriptan (Imitrex), acetaminophen (Tylenol), and naproxen (Aleve).

anesthetics: Cause a loss of feeling or sensation. They can act either locally (local anesthetic) or systemically (general anesthetic), and a general anesthetic can induce unconsciousness. Examples include propofol (Diprivan) and lidocaine (Xylocaine).

anticonvulsants: Reduce the frequency and severity of epileptic or other convulsive seizures. Examples include clonazepam (Klonopin), carbamazepine (Tegretol), and phenytoin (Dilantin).

antiparkinsonian drugs: Increase levels of dopamine to treat Parkinson's disease. Examples include levodopa and carbidopa (Sinemet), bromocriptine (Parlodel), and tolcapone (Tasmar).

antipyretics: Reduce fever. Examples include aspirin (Bayer), acetaminophen (Tylenol), and ibuprofen (Advil).

hypnotics: Promote sleep. They may also be referred to as *soporifics* or *somnifacients*. Many hypnotics have a sedative effect also. Examples include temazepam (Restoril), zolpidem (Ambien), and eszopiclone (Lunesta).

neuromuscular blockers: Inhibit the action of acetylcholine at the motor nerve end plate to cause paralysis. May be used in surgery to minimize patient movement. Examples include pancuronium (Pavulon), vecuronium (Norcuron), and succinylcholine (Anectine).

sedatives: Inhibit neuronal activity to calm and relax. Many sedatives also have hypnotic effects. Examples include alprazolam (Xanax), lorazepam (Ativan), and phenobarbital (Luminal).

stimulants: Increase synaptic activity of targeted neurons in the CNS to treat narcolepsy, attention-deficit/hyperactivity disorder, and fatigue, and to suppress the appetite. Examples include dextroamphetamine (Dexedrine), methylphenidate (Ritalin), caffeine, and phentermine (Adipex-P).

Exercise 10: **Pharmacology**

Match the drug type with its effect.

____ 1. treats PD
____ 2. relieves pain
____ 3. calms and relaxes
____ 4. induces sleep
____ 5. reduces fever
____ 6. reduces severity of seizures
____ 7. causes paralysis
____ 8. causes loss of sensation

A. anesthetic
B. antipyretic
C. soporific
D. anticonvulsant
E. sedative
F. neuromuscular blocker
G. analgesic
H. antiparkinsonian drug

Abbreviations

Abbreviation	Meaning	Abbreviation	Meaning
AD	Alzheimer's disease	MD	muscular dystrophy
ALS	amyotrophic lateral sclerosis	MS	multiple sclerosis
ANS	autonomic nervous system	PD	Parkinson's disease
BBB	blood-brain barrier	PNS	peripheral nervous system
C1-C8	cervical nerves	PPS	postpolio syndrome
CNS	central nervous system	PSG	polysomnography
CP	cerebral palsy	S1-S5	sacral nerves
CSF	cerebrospinal fluid	SNS	somatic nervous system
CTS	carpal tunnel syndrome	T1-T12	thoracic nerves
EEG	electroencephalogram	TBI	traumatic brain injury
L1-L5	lumbar nerves	TENS	transcutaneous electrical nerve stimulation
LP	lumbar puncture		
MCI	mild cognitive impairment	TIA	transient ischemic attack

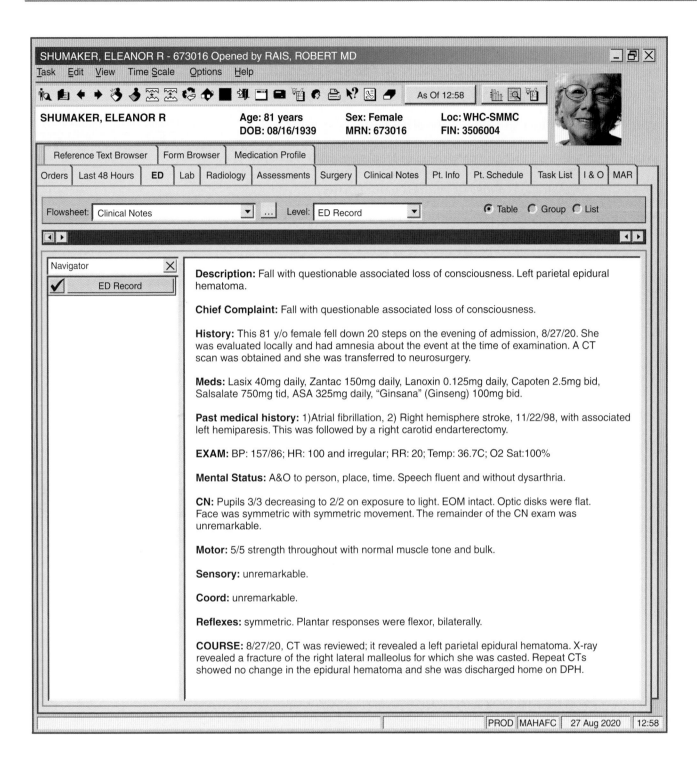

SHUMAKER, ELEANOR R - 673016 Opened by RAIS, ROBERT MD

Task   Edit   View   Time Scale   Options   Help

SHUMAKER, ELEANOR R   Age: 81 years   Sex: Female   Loc: WHC-SMMC
                             DOB: 08/16/1939   MRN: 673016   FIN: 3506004

Reference Text Browser | Form Browser | Medication Profile

Orders | Last 48 Hours | **ED** | Lab | Radiology | Assessments | Surgery | Clinical Notes | Pt. Info | Pt. Schedule | Task List | I & O | MAR

Flowsheet: Clinical Notes   Level: ED Record   Table   Group   List

Navigator

ED Record

Description: Fall with questionable associated loss of consciousness. Left parietal epidural hematoma.

Chief Complaint: Fall with questionable associated loss of consciousness.

History: This 81 y/o female fell down 20 steps on the evening of admission, 8/27/20. She was evaluated locally and had amnesia about the event at the time of examination. A CT scan was obtained and she was transferred to neurosurgery.

Meds: Lasix 40mg daily, Zantac 150mg daily, Lanoxin 0.125mg daily, Capoten 2.5mg bid, Salsalate 750mg tid, ASA 325mg daily, "Ginsana" (Ginseng) 100mg bid.

Past medical history: 1)Atrial fibrillation, 2) Right hemisphere stroke, 11/22/98, with associated left hemiparesis. This was followed by a right carotid endarterectomy.

EXAM: BP: 157/86; HR: 100 and irregular; RR: 20; Temp: 36.7C; O2 Sat:100%

Mental Status: A&O to person, place, time. Speech fluent and without dysarthria.

CN: Pupils 3/3 decreasing to 2/2 on exposure to light. EOM intact. Optic disks were flat. Face was symmetric with symmetric movement. The remainder of the CN exam was unremarkable.

Motor: 5/5 strength throughout with normal muscle tone and bulk.

Sensory: unremarkable.

Coord: unremarkable.

Reflexes: symmetric. Plantar responses were flexor, bilaterally.

COURSE: 8/27/20, CT was reviewed; it revealed a left parietal epidural hematoma. X-ray revealed a fracture of the right lateral malleolus for which she was casted. Repeat CTs showed no change in the epidural hematoma and she was discharged home on DPH.

PROD | MAHAFC | 27 Aug 2020 | 12:58

Exercise 11: ED Record

Using the ED record on the previous page, answer the following questions.

1. Which term means a "weakness or slight paralysis on one side of the body" ?_____

2. Which term refers to a difficulty in the articulation of speech? _____

3. Which term tells you that the patient had bleeding within her skull? _____

4. An epidural hematoma is above or below the dura mater? _____

Go to the Evolve website to interactively build terms, label images, memorize word parts, and practice using nervous system terms in context.

WORD PART DEFINITIONS

Prefix/Suffix
-emphraxis
hemi-
-lepsy
mono-
-oma
para-
-paresis
-plegia
poly-
quadri-

Definition

1. _____ four
2. _____ slight paralysis
3. _____ half
4. _____ many
5. _____ one
6. _____ seizure
7. _____ tumor, mass
8. _____ abnormal
9. _____ obstructing, crushing
10. _____ paralysis

Combining Form
astr/o
blast/o
cerebell/o
cerebr/o
cord/o
cortic/o
dendr/o
dur/o
encephal/o
esthesi/o
mening/o
myel/o
narc/o
neur/o
pallid/o
phag/o
phas/o
radicul/o
rhiz/o
somn/o
tax/o
ventricul/o

Definition

11. _____ cortex
12. _____ eat
13. _____ order, coordination
14. _____ nerve root
15. _____ cerebellum
16. _____ feeling
17. _____ embryonic
18. _____ spinal cord
19. _____ dura mater
20. _____ speech
21. _____ ventricle
22. _____ brain
23. _____ spinal cord
24. _____ dendrite
25. _____ sleep
26. _____ nerve
27. _____ cerebrum
28. _____ star
29. _____ nerve root
30. _____ sleep
31. _____ globus pallidum
32. _____ meninges

WORDSHOP

Prefixes	Combining Forms	Suffixes
a-	blast/o	-exeresis
dys-	crani/o	-graphy
echo-	encephal/o	-ia
epi-	esthesi/o	-itis
hemi-	medull/o	-lepsy
mono-	neur/o	-oma
para-	phag/o	-paresis
peri-	phas/o	-pathy
poly-	rach/i	-plegia
quadri-	rhiz/o	-sthenia
	somn/o	-stomy
	spin/o	-tomy

Build nervous system terms by combining the word parts above. Some word parts may be used more than once. Some may not be used at all. The number in parentheses indicates the number of word parts needed.

Definition	Term
1. disease condition of many nerves (3)	
2. inflammation of the brain (2)	
3. paralysis of four (2)	
4. sound recording of the brain (3)	
5. cutting the nerve (2)	
6. condition of without speech (3)	
7. condition of difficult eating (3)	
8. seizure above (the body) (2)	
9. condition of abnormal feeling (3)	
10. recording of (many) sleep (3)	
11. cutting the spinal nerve root (2)	
12. tearing out a nerve (2)	
13. embryonic tumor of the medulla (3)	
14. condition of difficult sleep (3)	
15. slight paralysis of half (the body) (2)	

Sort the terms into the categories.

TERM SORTING

Anatomy and Physiology	Pathology	Procedures

amnesia
aphasia
BBB
cauda equina
causalgia
cerebellum
chemothalamectomy
CNS
cordotomy
craniotomy
CSF
dendrite
diplegia
dura mater
EEG

epilepsy
fasciculation
ganglia
glia
hematoma
meninges
meningioma
meningitis
MS
myelography
nerve block
neurectomy
neurexeresis
neuron
neuroplasty

neurotransmitter
phrenemphraxis
polyneuropathy
PPS
rhizotomy
spasm
sympathectomy
synapse
syncope
TENS
thalamus
TIA
vagotomy
ventricle
ventriculoperitoneostomy

Replace the highlighted words with the correct terms.

TRANSLATIONS

1. Mr. Sharif had a right-sided **temporary ischemia of cerebral tissue due to an occlusion or a cerebral hemorrhage** that temporarily affected the **pertaining to the opposite side** side.

2. After Roberto's TIA, he suffered temporary **slight paralysis on the left or right side of the body** and **condition of lack of the ability to form or understand speech.**

3. As a result of a blow to the head, the patient sustained an epidural **localized collection of blood** and **resultant loss of memory caused by brain damage.**

4. Ms. C reported **dizziness** and **fainting** before her arrival at the emergency department.

5. The patient presented with a recurring **headache of vascular origin.**

6. As a result of a stroke, Ben suffered a **condition of abnormal accumulation of fluid in the ventricles of the brain.** He was treated with **the creation of a new opening between a blocked ventricle and a cerebral cistern.**

7. Mrs. Aubrum was experiencing **rhythmic, quivering, purposeless skeletal muscle movements** and **condition of difficulty with swallowing** and was ultimately diagnosed with Parkinson's disease.

8. The neurosurgeon performed a **removal of a cerebral hemisphere** to treat the patient's **group of disorders characterized by seizures and/or loss of consciousness.**

9. A **procedure to aspirate CSF from the lumbar subarachnoid space** was done to rule out any **infection or inflammation of the membranes covering the brain and spinal cord.**

10. Helen O'Neal underwent **measurement and record of a number of functions while patient is asleep** to determine why she was experiencing **disorders of the sleep-wake cycles.**

Mental and Behavioral Disorder

OBJECTIVES

☐ Recognize and use terms related to the pathology of mental and behavioral health.

☐ Recognize and use terms related to the procedures for mental and behavioral health.

ICD-10-CM Example from Tabular
F40 Phobic anxiety disorders
   F40.0 Agoraphobia
      F40.00 Agoraphobia, unspecified
      F40.01 Panic disorder with agoraphobia
      Excludes1 panic disorder without agoraphobia **(F41.0)**
      F40.02 Agoraphobia without panic disorder
   F40.1 Social phobias
      Anthropophobia
      Social anxiety disorder
      Social anxiety disorder of childhood
      Social neurosis
   F40.10 Social phobia, unspecified
   F40.11 Social phobia, generalized

ICD-10-PCS Example from Index
Psychological Tests
   Cognitive Status **GZ14ZZZ**
   Developmental **GZ10ZZZ**
   Intellectual and Psychoeducational **GZ12ZZZ**
   Neurobehavioral Status **GZ14ZZZ**
   Neuropsychological **GZ13ZZZ**
   Personality and Behavioral **GZ11ZZZ**

INTRODUCTION TO MENTAL AND BEHAVIORAL HEALTH

Although many body system disorders are described by their abnormal laboratory, physical, or clinical findings, mental and behavioral disorders are not as easily defined. In the United States, the *Diagnostic and Statistical Manual of Mental Disorders* (DSM), currently a multi-axial classification developed by the American Psychiatric Association (APA), is in its fifth edition (DSM-5). This revision will eventually result in a closer alignment to ICD-10 and its single axis format. Consider the following:

- One of every five American adults and children has been diagnosed with a mental condition (HCUPnet 2015).
- The most common DRG for inpatient admissions is psychosis (Definitive HealthCare.com).
- Approximately 40 million Americans are diagnosed with anxiety (NAMI).
- Approximately 6.5 million Americans are classified as intellectually disabled.

Given these statistics, the terminology related to mental and behavioral disorders is content that cannot be ignored (Special Olympics).

The term **behavioral health** reflects an integration of the outdated concept of the separate nature of the body (physical health/illness) and the mind (mental health/illness). Advances in research continually acknowledge the roles of culture, environment and spirituality in influencing physical and behavioral health. The use of the term *behavior* refers to observable, measurable activities that may be used to evaluate the progress of treatment.

Similar to previous chapters, this chapter examines disorders that result when an individual has a maladaptive response to his or her environment (internal or external). (See Chapter 11 for an explanation of the anatomy and physiology of the brain and nervous system.) However, even though some mental illnesses have organic causes in which neurotransmitters and other known brain functions play a role, there is no mental "anatomy" per se. Instead, behavioral health is a complex interaction among an individual's emotional, physical, mental and behavioral processes in an environment that includes cultural and spiritual influences.

Mental health may be defined as a relative state of mind in which a person who is healthy is able to cope with and adjust to the recurrent stresses of everyday living in a culturally acceptable way. Thus mental illness may be generally defined as a functional impairment that substantially interferes with or limits one or more major life activities for a significant duration.

PATHOLOGY

Terms Related to Signs and Symptoms Involving Cognition, Perception, Emotional State and Behavior and Speech and Voice (R40-R49)

Affect is observable demonstration of emotion that can be described in terms of quality, range and appropriateness. The following list defines the most significant types of affect encountered in behavioral health:

- **Blunted**: moderately reduced range of affect.
- **Flat**: the diminishment or loss of emotional expression sometimes observed in individuals with schizophrenia, mental retardation and some depressive disorders.
- **Labile**: multiple, abrupt changes in affect seen in certain types of schizophrenia and bipolar disorder.
- **Full/wide range of affect**: generally appropriate emotional response.

Term	Word Origin	Definition
amnesia		Inability to remember either isolated parts of the past or one 's entire past; may be caused by brain damage or severe emotional trauma.
anhedonia	*an-* no, not, without *hedon/o* pleasure *-ia* condition	Absence of the ability to experience either pleasure or joy, even in the face of causative events.
confabulation		Effort to conceal a gap in memory by fabricating detailed, often believable stories. Associated with alcohol abuse.
dyscalculia	*dys-* difficult *calcul/o* stone *-ia* condition	Abnormal difficulty with performing mathematical calculations.
dysphoria	*dys-* abnormal *phor/o* to carry, to bear *-ia* condition	Generalized negative mood characterized by depression.
echolalia	*echo-* severberation *-lalia* condition of babbling	Repetition of words or phrases spoken by others.
euphoria	*eu-* good, well *phor/o* to carry, to bear *-ia* condition	Exaggerated sense of physical and emotional well-being not based on reality, disproportionate to the cause, or inappropriate to the situation.
hallucination		Any unreal sensory perception that occurs with no external cause.
hyperkinesis	*hyper-* excessive *-kinesis* movement	Excessive movement and activity.
stupor		From the Latin term for "numbness," a stupor is a state of near unconsciousness.

Exercise 1: Signs and Symptoms of Mental Illness

Match the term to the definition.

___ 1. amnesia
___ 2. confabulation
___ 3. dysphoria
___ 4. echolalia
___ 5. euphoria
___ 6. hallucination
___ 7. stupor

A. inability to remember the past
B. repetition of word or phrases spoken by others
C. an effort to conceal a memory gap by fabrication
D. any unreal sensory perception that occurs with no external cause
E. exaggerated sense of well-being not based on reality
F. a state of near unconsciousness
G. generalized negative mood characterized by depression

Build the following terms.

8. condition of without pleasure _____

9. excessive movement _____

Terms Related to Mental Disorders Due to Known Physiological Conditions (FØ1-FØ9)

Term	Word Origin	Definition
dementia	*de-* down, lack of *ment/o* mind *-ia* condition	Lack of normal mental functioning due to injury or disease. May include changes to personality as well as memory and reasoning.
postconcussional syndrome		A degenerative brain disease associated with repeated blows to the skull. Recently discovered in professional athletes whose sports involve frequent traumatic brain injuries. Also known as **chronic traumatic encephalopathy (CTE)**.

Terms Related to Mental and Behavioral Disorders Due to Psychoactive Substance Use (F1Ø-F19)

Substance-related disorders are the most rapidly increasing group of disorders in the mental health chapter. These include abuse of a number of substances, including alcohol, opioids, cannabinoids, sedatives, hypnotics or anxiolytics, cocaine, stimulants (including caffeine), hallucinogens, nicotine and volatile solvents (inhalants). Classifications for **substance abuse** include psychotic, amnesiac, and late-onset disorders. It is important to be aware that addiction is not a character flaw. Rather, addiction has a neurological basis; the effects of specific drugs are localized to equally specific areas of the brain.

An individual is considered an "abuser" if he or she uses substances in ways that threaten health or impair social or economic functioning. The term *harmful use* indicates a pattern of drug use that causes damage to health. If the term *tolerance* is used to describe someone's usage, it means a state in which the body becomes accustomed to the substances ingested; hence the user requires greater amounts to create the desired effect. Individuals who exhibit a lessening or disappearance of a disease or disorder are said to be in *remission.* ICD-10-CM uses "in remission" codes instead of "history" codes.

Term	Word Origin	Definition
delirium tremens (DTs)		Acute and sometimes fatal delirium induced by the cessation of ingesting excessive amounts of alcohol over a long period.
dependence		Difficulty in controlling use of a drug.

Continued

Terms Related to Mental and Behavioral Disorders Due to Psychoactive Substance Use (F10-F19)—cont'd

Term	Word Origin	Definition
intoxication	*in-* in *toxic/o* poison *-ation* process of	Episode of behavioral disturbance following ingestion of alcohol or psychotropic drugs. ICD-10-CM provides a code for blood alcohol level.
withdrawal state		Group of symptoms that occur during cessation of the use of a regularly taken drug.

Terms Related to Schizophrenia, Schizotypal, Delusional and Other Non-Mood Psychotic Disorders (F20-F29)

Term	Word Origin	Definition
catatonia	*cata-* down *ton/o* tension *-ia* condition	Paralysis or immobility from psychological or emotional, rather than physical, causes.
catatonic schizophrenia	*cata-* down *ton/o* tension *-ic* pertaining to *schiz/o* split *phren/o* mind *-ia* condition	Also called **schizophrenic catalepsy.** This form of schizophrenia is dominated by prominent psychomotor disturbances that may alternate between extremes, such as hyperkinesis and stupor, and may be accompanied by a dreamlike (oneiric) state and hallucinations.
delirium		Condition of confused, unfocused, irrational agitation. In mental disorders, agitation and confusion may also be accompanied by a more intense disorientation, incoherence, or fear, and illusions, hallucinations, and delusions.
hebephrenia	*hebe* goddess of youth *phren/o* mind *-ia* condition	Although more often referred to as **disorganized schizophrenia,** hebephrenia was named for its original association with initial occurrence at the time of puberty. It is characterized by prominent affective changes, fleeting and fragmentary delusions and hallucinations, and irresponsible and unpredictable behaviors. Shallow, inappropriate mood, flighty thoughts, social isolation, and incoherent speech are also present.
oneirism	*oneir/o* dream *-ism* state	A state of a dreamlike hallucination.
paranoia	*para-* abnormal *-noia* condition of the mind	A type of delusional disorder, paranoia includes the inaccurate perception of suspicious thinking. Also called **delusional disorder,** or late **paraphrenia.**
psychosis	*psych/o* mind *-osis* abnormal condition	Disassociation with or impaired perception of reality; may be accompanied by hallucinations, delusions, incoherence, akathisia (the inability to sit still), and/or disorganized behavior.

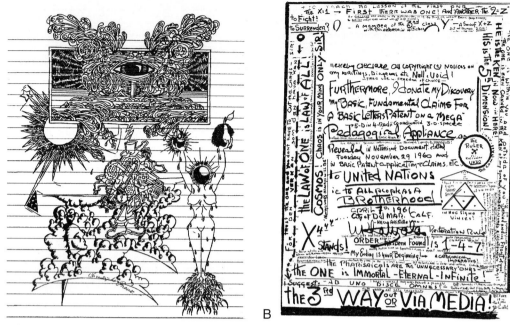

Fig. 12-1 A, This drawing by a patient with schizophrenia demonstrates thought disorder. **B,** Drawing by a delusional patient with schizophrenia.

Terms Related to Schizophrenia, Schizotypal, Delusional and Other Non-Mood Psychotic Disorders (F2Ø-F29)—cont'd

Term	Word Origin	Definition
schizophrenia	*schiz/o* split *phren/o* mind *-ia* condition	A group of disorders characterized by fundamental distortions of thinking and perception, coupled with affect that is inappropriate or blunted. The patient exhibits characteristic inability to recognize an appropriate perception of reality, although his/her intellectual capacity is usually intact (Fig. 12-1).
schizotypal disorder		Unlike the other forms of schizophrenia, patient exhibits anhedonia, eccentric behavior, cold affect, and social isolation. Also called **borderline schizophrenia, latent schizophrenia,** and **prodromal schizophrenia.**

Terms Related to Mood [Affective] Disorders (F3Ø-F39)

Term	Word Origin	Definition
bipolar disorder (BP, BD)	*bi-* two *pol/o* pole *-ar* pertaining to	Disorder characterized by swings between an elevation of mood, increased energy and activity (**hypomania** and **mania**), and a lowering of mood and decreased energy and activity (depression). Formerly referred to as manic depression.
cyclothymia	*cycl/o* recurring *-thymia* condition of the mind	Disorder characterized by recurring episodes of mild elation and depression that are not severe enough to warrant a diagnosis of bipolar disorder.

Continued

Terms Related to Mood [Affective] Disorders (F3Ø-F39)—cont'd

Term	Word Origin	Definition
dysthymia	*dys-* difficult *-thymia* condition of the mind	Mild, chronic depression of mood that lasts for years but is not severe enough to justify a diagnosis of depression. **Euthymia** is a normal range of moods and emotions.
major depressive disorder		Depression typically characterized by its degree (minimal, moderate, severe) or number of occurrences (single or recurrent, persistent). Patient exhibits dysphoria, reduction of energy, and decrease in activity. Symptoms include anhedonia, lack of ability to concentrate, and fatigue. Patient may experience parasomnias (abnormal sleep patterns), diminished appetite, and loss of self-esteem. **SAD (seasonal affective disorder)** is caused by decreased exposure to sunlight in autumn and winter.
mania	*mania* from the Greek term for "madness"	A state of an unstable, inappropriate mood.
premenstrual dysphoric disorder (PMDD)		PMDD is a more serious form of PMS that is classified as a type of major depressive disorder. See Chapter 6 for the definition of PMS.

 Exercise 2: Mental and Behavioral Disorders Due to Known Physiological Conditions; Psychoactive Substance Use; Schizophrenia, Schizotypal, Delusional, and Other Non-Mood Psychotic Disorders; and Mood Disorders

Match the terms with their definitions.

___ 1. intoxication
___ 2. DTs
___ 3. dependence
___ 4. harmful use
___ 5. tolerance
___ 6. withdrawal state
___ 7. remission
___ 8. hebephrenia
___ 9. catatonic schizophrenia
___ 10. schizotypal disorder
___ 11. mania
___ 12. BP
___ 13. major depressive disorder
___ 14. dysthymia
___ 15. catatonia
___ 16. delirium

A. acute delirium induced by cessation of ingesting excessive amounts of alcohol over an extended period.

B. state of unstable, inappropriate mood

C. disorganized schizophrenia

D. difficulty in controlling drug use

E. group of symptoms that occur during cessation of the use of a regularly ingested drug

F. episode of behavioral disturbance following ingestion of alcohol or psychotropic drugs

G. disorder characterized by swings between an elevation and a lowering of mood, energy and activity

H. mild, chronic depression of mood that lasts for years

I. form of schizophrenia dominated by prominent psychomotor disturbances that may alternate between extremes

J. depression characterized by its degree or number of occurrences

K. the lessening or disappearance of a disease/disorder

L. form of schizophrenia in which patient exhibits anhedonia, cold affect, and social isolation

M. pattern of drug use that damages health

N. state in which the body becomes accustomed to ingested substances

O. paralysis/immobility caused by psychological causes

P. condition of confused, irrational agitation

Translate the terms.

17. schizophrenia_____

18. paranoia_____

19. psychosis _____

20. cyclothymia_____

21. oneirism_____

Terms Related to Anxiety, Dissociative, Stress-Related, Somatoform and Other Nonpsychotic Mental Disorders (F40-F48)

Term	Word Origin	Definition
acrophobia	*acro-* heights, extremes *-phobia* condition of fear, sensitivity	Fear of heights.
agoraphobia	*agora-* marketplace *-phobia* condition of fear, sensitivity	Fear of leaving home and entering crowded spaces.
androphobia	*andr/o* man, men *-phobia* condition of fear, sensitivity	Fear of men.
anthropophobia	*anthrop/o* man *-phobia* condition of fear, sensitivity	Fear of scrutiny by other people; also called **social phobia.**
anxiety		Anticipation of impending danger and dread accompanied by restlessness, tension, tachycardia, and breathing difficulty not associated with an apparent stimulus.
claustrophobia	*claustr/o* a closing *-phobia* condition of fear, sensitivity	Fear of enclosed spaces.
delusion		Persistent belief in a demonstrable untruth or a provable, inaccurate perception despite clear evidence to the contrary.
dissociative identity disorder		Maladaptive coping with severe stress by developing one or more separate personalities. A less severe form, **dissociative disorder or dissociative reaction,** results in identity confusion accompanied by amnesia, oneirism, and somnambulism. Formerly termed **multiple personality disorder.**
dyslexia	*dys-* difficult *lex/o* word *-ia* condition	Inability or difficulty with reading and/or writing.

Continued

Terms Related to Anxiety, Dissociative, Stress-Related, Somatoform and Other Nonpsychotic Mental Disorders (F40-F48)—cont'd

Term	Word Origin	Definition
generalized anxiety disorder (GAD)		Anxiety disorder characterized by excessive, uncontrollable, and often irrational worry about everyday things that is disproportionate to the actual source of worry.
gynephobia	*gyn/e* female, women *-phobia* condition of fear, sensitivity	Fear of women.
illusion		Inaccurate sensory perception based on a real stimulus; examples include mirages and interpreting music or wind as voices.
obsessive- compulsive disorder (OCD)		Disorder characterized by recurrent, distressing, and unavoidable preoccupations or irresistible drives to perform specific rituals (e.g., constantly checking locks, excessive handwashing) that the patient feels will prevent some harmful event.
panic disorder (PD)		Anxiety disorder characterized by recurring, severe panic attacks. Common symptoms of an attack include rapid heartbeat, perspiration, dizziness, dyspnea, uncontrollable fear, and hyperventilation.
post-traumatic stress disorder (PTSD)		Extended emotional response to a traumatic event. Symptoms may include flashbacks, recurring nightmares, anhedonia, insomnia, hypervigilance, anxiety, depression, suicidal thoughts, and emotional blunting.
somatoform disorder	*somat/o* body *-form* shape	Any disorder that has unfounded physical complaints by the patient, despite medical assurance that no physiological problem exists. One type of somatoform disorder, hypochondriacal disorder, is a preoccupation with the possibility of having one or more serious and progressive physical disorders.

Terms Related to Behavioral Syndromes Associated With Physiological Disturbances and Physical Factors (F50-F59)

Term	Word Origin	Definition
anorexia nervosa	*an-* without *orex/o* appetite *-ia* condition *nervos/o* nervous *-a* noun ending	Prolonged refusal to eat adequate amounts of food and an altered perception of what constitutes a normal minimum body weight caused by an intense fear of becoming obese. Primarily affects adolescent females; emaciation and amenorrhea result (Fig. 12-2).

Terms Related to Behavioral Syndromes Associated With Physiological Disturbances and Physical Factors (F50-F59)—cont'd

Term	Word Origin	Definition
bulimia nervosa		Eating disorder in which the individual repetitively eats large quantities of food and then purges the body through self-induced vomiting or inappropriate use of laxatives.
hypersomnia	*hyper-* excessive *somn/o* sleep *-ia* condition	Excessive length or depth of sleep, especially during daytime.
hypoactive sexual desire disorder	*hypo-* under, deficient	Indifference or unresponsiveness to sexual stimuli; inability to achieve orgasm during intercourse. Formerly called **frigidity.**
idiopathic insomnia	*in-* not, without *somn/o* sleep *-ia* condition	An inability to fall (or stay) asleep without a known cause.
nymphomania	*nymph/o* woman *-mania* condition of madness	Relentless drive to achieve sexual orgasm in the female. In the male, the condition is called **satyriasis.**
postpartum depression (PPD) disorder	*post-* after *part/o* birth *-um* noun ending	Disorder in which symptoms of depression occur within one year after the birth of a child. May be due to hormonal change and/or stress.
somnambulism	*somn/o* sleep *ambul/o* to walk *-ism* condition	Sleepwalking.

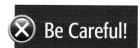 **Be Careful!** *Do not confuse PPD for* postpartum depression *with PPD for* purified protein derivative, *a substance used in the detection of tuberculosis.*

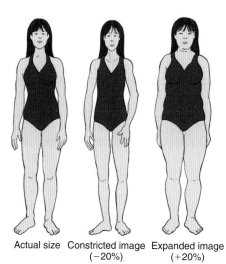

Actual size   Constricted image   Expanded image
(−20%)   (+20%)

Fig. 12-2 The perception of body shape and size can be evaluated with the use of special computer drawing programs that allow a subject to distort (increase or decrease) the width of an actual picture of a person's body by as much as 20%. Subjects with anorexia consistently adjusted their own body picture to a size 20% larger than its true form, which suggests that they have a major problem with the perception of self-image.

Exercise 3: Anxiety, Dissociative, Stress-Related, Somatoform, and Other Nonpsychotic Mental Disorders; Behavioral Syndromes Associated with Physiological Disturbances and Physical Factors

Match the terms with their definitions.

___ 1. anthropophobia
___ 2. hypersomnia
___ 3. claustrophobia
___ 4. illusion
___ 5. androphobia
___ 6. GAD
___ 7. PD
___ 8. OCD
___ 9. PTSD
___ 10. dissociative identity disorder
___ 11. somatoform disorder
___ 12. hypochondriacal disorder
___ 13. anorexia nervosa
___ 14. bulimia nervosa
___ 15. PPD
___ 16. delusion
___ 17. hypoactive sexual desire disorder

A. fear of enclosed spaces
B. maladaptive coping with severe stress by developing one or more separate personalities
C. disorder characterized by recurrent and unavoidable preoccupation or drive to perform specific rituals
D. eating disorder in which an individual repetitively eats a large amount of food and then purges
E. a type of somatoform disorder
F. persistent belief in a demonstrable untruth
G. excessive sleep
H. disorder characterized by excessive, uncontrollable, and often irrational worry about everyday things that is disproportionate to the actual source of worry
I. depression occurring after childbirth due to hormonal changes and/or stress
J. any disorder that has unfounded physical complaints by the patient
K. indifference or unresponsiveness to sexual stimuli
L. fear of scrutiny by other people
M. extended emotional response to a traumatic event
N. prolonged refusal to eat adequate amounts of food because of the fear of becoming obese
O. anxiety disorder characterized by recurring severe panic attacks.
P. inaccurate sensory perception based on a real stimulus
Q. fear of men

Build the terms.

18. condition of fear of the marketplace_____

19. condition of fear of females_____

20. condition of without sleep_____

21. condition of woman madness_____

22. condition of fear of heights_____

23. condition of walking in sleep_____

Terms Related to Disorders of Adult Personality and Behavior (F60-F69)

Term	Word Origin	Definition
antisocial personality disorder		Disorder in which the patient shows a complete lack of interest in social obligations, to the extreme of showing antipathy for other individuals. Patients frustrate easily, are quick to display aggression, show a tendency to blame others, and do not change their behavior even after punishment. Also called **dissocial personality disorder.**

Terms Related to Disorders of Adult Personality and Behavior (F60-F69)—cont'd

Term	Word Origin	Definition
borderline personality disorder (BPD)		Disorder characterized by impulsive, unpredictable mood and self-image, resulting in unstable interpersonal relationships and a tendency to see and respond to others as unwaveringly good or evil.
factitious disorder		Also known as **Munchhausen's syndrome**, this is a disorder in which the individual intentionally fakes or causes a physical or mental illness in him/herself. If the falsified illness is imposed on another individual (for example, a child), it is termed **factitious disorder by proxy (Munchhausen's by proxy)**. Factitious disorder is different from a somatoform disorder in that the individual is aware that the illness is not genuine.
fetishism	*fetish/o* charm *-ism* condition	Reliance on an object as a stimulus for sexual arousal and pleasure.
kleptomania	*klept/o* to steal *-mania* condition of madness	Uncontrollable impulse to steal.
necrophilia	*necr/o* death *phil/o* attraction *-ia* condition	Abnormal sexual attraction to dead bodies.
obsessive-compulsive personality disorder (OCPD)		Characterized by recurrent and unavoidable preoccupations or irresistible drives to perform specific rituals (e.g., constantly checking locks, excessive handwashing) that the patient feels will prevent some harmful event. OCD differs from OCPD in that OCD patients find their preoccupations distressing, while those with OCPD consider them natural and normal.
paranoid personality disorder	*para-* abnormal *-oid* resembling, like	State in which the individual exhibits inappropriate suspicious thinking, self-importance, a lack of ability to forgive perceived insults, and an extreme sense of personal rights.
paraphilia	*para-* abnormal *phil/o* attraction *-ia* condition	An abnormal sexual attraction to objects, situations, or individuals that is not part of normal stimulation.
pedophilia	*ped/o* child *phil/o* attraction *-ia* condition	Sexual preference, either in fantasy or actuality, for children as a means of achieving sexual excitement and gratification.
pyromania	*pyr/o* fire *-mania* condition of madness	Uncontrollable impulse to set fires.
schizoid personality disorder	*schiz/o* split *-oid* resembling, like	Condition in which the patient withdraws into a fantasy world, with little need for social interaction. Most patients have little capacity to experience pleasure or to express their feelings.
trichotillomania	*trich/o* hair *till/o* to pull *-mania* condition of madness	Uncontrollable impulse to pull one's hair out by the roots.

CM Guideline Alert for Factitious Disorder by Proxy C.5.c.

Munchausen's syndrome by proxy (MSBP) is a disorder in which a caregiver (perpetrator) falsely reports or causes an illness or injury in another person (victim) under his or her care, such as a child, an elderly adult, or a person who has a disability. The condition is also referred to as "factitious disorder imposed on another" or "factitious disorder by proxy." The perpetrator, not the victim, receives this diagnosis. Assign code F68.A, Factitious disorder imposed on another, to the perpetrator's record. For the victim of a patient suffering from MSBP, assign the appropriate code from categories T74, Adult and child abuse, neglect and other maltreatment, confirmed, or T76, Adult and child abuse, neglect and other maltreatment, suspected.

Terms Related to Intellectual Disabilities (F70-F79)

Condition of subaverage intellectual ability, with impairments in social and education functioning. The intelligence quotient (IQ) is a measure of an individual's intellectual functioning compared with the general population.

Term	Word Origin	Definition
mild intellectual disabilities		IQ range of 50-55 to 70; learning difficulties result.
moderate intellectual disabilities		IQ range of 35-40 to 50-55; support needed to function in society.
severe intellectual disabilities		IQ range of 20-25 to 35-40; continuous need for support to live in society.
profound intellectual disabilities		IQ less than 20-25; severe self-care limitations.

Terms Related to Pervasive and Specific Developmental Disorders (F80-F89)

Term	Word Origin	Definition
pervasive developmental disorders (PDD)		A group of disorders characterized by impaired communication and social interaction that includes autism, and Rett's and Asperger's syndromes. Not to be confused with specific developmental disorders (SDD) such as dyslexia and dyscalculia.
Asperger's syndrome		Disorder characterized by impairment of social interaction and repetitive patterns of inappropriate behavior. Often considered a high-functioning form of autism.
autistic disorder		Condition of abnormal development of social interaction, impaired communication, and repetitive behaviors. Also known as **autism.**
Rett's syndrome		Condition characterized by initial normal functioning followed by loss of social and intellectual functioning. Usually diagnosed only in girls.

Terms Related To Behavioral and Emotional Disorders with Onset Usually Occurring in Childhood and Adolescence (F90-F98)

Term	Word Origin	Definition
attention-deficit/hyperactivity disorder (ADHD)		Series of syndromes that includes impulsiveness, inability to concentrate, and short attention span.
conduct disorder		Any of a number of disorders characterized by patterns of persistent aggressive and defiant behaviors.
oppositional defiant disorder (ODD)		A type of conduct disorder that is characterized by hostile, disobedient behavior.

Exercise 4: Disorders of Adult Personality and Behavior; Pervasive and Specific Developmental Disorders; Mental Retardation; Behavioral and Emotional Disorders with Onset Usually Occurring in Childhood and Adolescence

A. Match the terms with their definitions.

___ 1. paranoid personality disorder
___ 2. schizoid personality disorder
___ 3. antisocial personality disorder
___ 4. borderline personality disorder
___ 5. OCPD
___ 6. kleptomania
___ 7. paraphilia
___ 8. fetishism
___ 9. pedophilia
___ 10. PDD
___ 11. autistic disorder
___ 12. Rett's syndrome
___ 13. Asperger's syndrome
___ 14. factitious disorder

A. condition in which the patient withdraws into a fantasy world, with little need for social interaction
B. disorder in which patient shows a complete lack of interest in social obligations and antipathy toward others
C. the uncontrollable urge to steal
D. reliance on an object as a stimulus for sexual arousal and pleasure
E. condition of abnormal development of social interaction, impaired communication, and repetitive behaviors
F. disorder characterized by impulsive, unpredictable mood and self-image, resulting in unstable interpersonal relationships
G. an abnormal sexual attraction to objects, situations, or individuals that is not part of normal stimulation
H. group of disorders characterized by impaired communication and social interaction
I. disorder characterized by recurrent and unavoidable preoccupations or irresistible drive to perform specific rituals
J. high-functioning form of autism
K. sexual preference for children
L. state in which the individual is suspicious, self-important, unforgiving, and has an extreme sense of personal rights
M. disorder characterized by initial normal functioning
N. disorder in which an individual intentionally fakes an illness

B. Match the terms with their definitions.

___ 1. mild intellectual disabilities
___ 2. moderate intellectual disabilities
___ 3. severe intellectual disabilities
___ 4. profound intellectual disabilities
___ 5. ADHD
___ 6. conduct disorder
___ 7. ODD

A. IQ range of 20-40
B. series of syndromes that includes impulsiveness, inability to concentrate, and short attention span
C. IQ range of 50-70
D. type of conduct disorder characterized by hostile, disobedient behavior
E. IQ range of 35-55
F. IQ less than 20
G. disorder characterized by patterns of persistent aggressive and defiant behaviors.

Translate the terms.

8. pyromania_____

9. trichotillomania_____

10. necrophilia_____

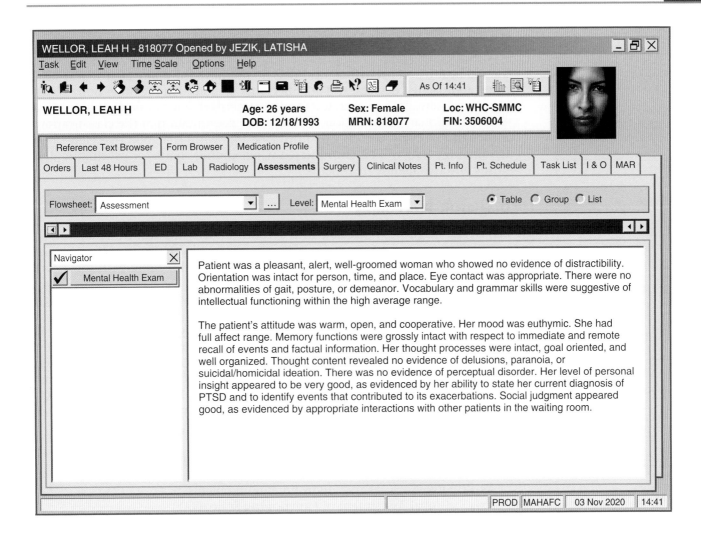

WELLOR, LEAH H - 818077 Opened by JEZIK, LATISHA

Task Edit View Time Scale Options Help

WELLOR, LEAH H

Age: 26 years
DOB: 12/18/1993

Sex: Female
MRN: 818077

Loc: WHC-SMMC
FIN: 3506004

Reference Text Browser | Form Browser | Medication Profile

Orders | Last 48 Hours | ED | Lab | Radiology | **Assessments** | Surgery | Clinical Notes | Pt. Info | Pt. Schedule | Task List | I & O | MAR

Flowsheet: Assessment   Level: Mental Health Exam   ⦿ Table ○ Group ○ List

Navigator
✓ Mental Health Exam

Patient was a pleasant, alert, well-groomed woman who showed no evidence of distractibility. Orientation was intact for person, time, and place. Eye contact was appropriate. There were no abnormalities of gait, posture, or demeanor. Vocabulary and grammar skills were suggestive of intellectual functioning within the high average range.

The patient's attitude was warm, open, and cooperative. Her mood was euthymic. She had full affect range. Memory functions were grossly intact with respect to immediate and remote recall of events and factual information. Her thought processes were intact, goal oriented, and well organized. Thought content revealed no evidence of delusions, paranoia, or suicidal/homicidal ideation. There was no evidence of perceptual disorder. Her level of personal insight appeared to be very good, as evidenced by her ability to state her current diagnosis of PTSD and to identify events that contributed to its exacerbations. Social judgment appeared good, as evidenced by appropriate interactions with other patients in the waiting room.

PROD | MAHAFC | 03 Nov 2020 | 14:41

 Exercise 5: **Mental Status Report**

Using the mental status report above, answer the following questions:

1. What term indicates that the patient exhibited a normal range of emotions? _____

_____

2. What term indicates that the patient exhibited generally appropriate emotional response? _____

_____

3. How do you know that the patient did not exhibit any persistent beliefs in things that are untrue?

_____

4. What is her current diagnosis? _____

PROCEDURES

Mental health and behavioral disorders do not have the many anatomical structures, approaches, devices, and qualifiers that are found in the other body system chapters. There are, however, tests and treatments that are important to study, as well as cautionary information regarding the coordination of the classifications. Although not every term is explained, the following is a good overview of the terminology that will be encountered when coding charts for psychiatric diagnostic and therapeutic treatments.

Diagnostic Procedures

Behavioral diagnoses must take into account underlying healthcare abnormalities that may cause or influence a patient's mental health. Some of the common laboratory and imaging procedures are mentioned here, along with procedures that are traditionally considered to be psychological.

Diagnostic Criteria

The adoption of ICD-10 and DSM-5 will change how mental and behavioral disorders are diagnosed and billed. DSM-IV was based on a multi-axial assessment diagnostic tool measuring mental health of the individual across five axes. The first three (if present) were stated as diagnostic codes, whereas Axis IV was a statement of factors influencing the patient's mental health (e.g., lack of social supports, unemployment), and Axis V was a numerical score that summarized a patient's overall functioning.

Axis I: Clinical Disorders
Axis II: Personality Disorders and/or Mental Retardation
Axis III: General Medical Conditions
Axis IV: Psychosocial and Environmental Problems
Axis V: Global Assessment of Functioning Scale (GAF)

DSM-5 has moved to a nonaxial documentation of diagnosis, which combines the Axis I, Axis II, and Axis III with notations for Axis IV and Axis V.

Mental Status Examination (MSE)

A mental status examination (MSE) is a diagnostic procedure used to determine a patient's current mental state. It includes assessment of the patient's appearance, affect, thought processes, cognitive function, insight, and judgment.

Laboratory Tests

There are several laboratory tests that help establish a mental health diagnosis. Patients may have blood counts (complete blood cell count [CBC] with differential), blood chemistry, thyroid function panels, screening tests for syphilis (rapid plasma reagin [RPR] or microhemagglutination assay for *Treponema pallidum* [MHA-TP]), urinalyses with drug screen, urine pregnancy checks for females with childbearing potential, blood alcohol levels, serum levels of medications, and human immunodeficiency virus (HIV) tests in high-risk patients.

Imaging

Imaging is most helpful in ruling out neurologic disorders and in research; it is less helpful in diagnosing or treating psychiatric problems. Computed tomography (CT) scans and magnetic resonance imaging (MRI) can be used to screen for brain lesions. A **functional magnetic resonance image (fMRI)** is one that uses the magnetic properties of hydrogen molecules to map three-dimensional neuronal activity in the brain. It is a noninvasive technique, like a regular MRI, that is performed with similar equipment, but is performed after a specific task

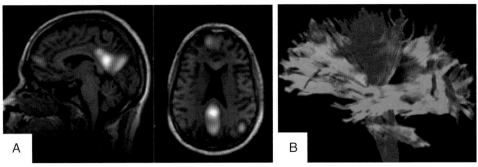

Fig. 12-3 Example of fMRI related to a working memory experiment.

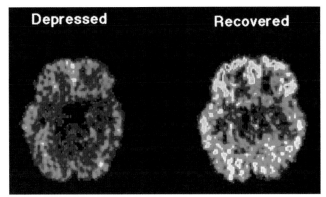

Fig. 12-4 PET scans of a depressed individual's brain when depressed *(left)* and after recovery through treatment with medication *(right)*. Several brain areas, particularly the prefrontal cortex *(at top)*, show diminished activity (darker colors) during depression.

is completed. It is used in diagnosis and presurgical planning of a variety of neurological and mental health–related disorders such as brain tumors, depression, epilepsy, Alzheimer's disease and stroke (Fig. 12-3). **Positron emission tomography (PET)** scans can be used to examine and map the metabolic activity of the brain (Fig. 12-4). Central nervous system imaging in ICD-10-PCS is coded as plain radiography, fluoroscopy CT scans, MRIs, or ultrasonography. The body part characters will be familiar from coverage of the nervous system, while the detail includes the type of contrast and whether it is unenhanced or enhanced.

Psychological Testing and Treatment
In ICD-10 psychological tests are divided into categories of developmental, personality and behavioral, intellectual and psychoeducational, neuropsycho- logical and neurobehavioral, and cognitive status. Some of these many tests are listed below.

Bender Gestalt test: a test of visuomotor and spatial abilities; useful for children and adults.
Cognistat: also called the **Neurobehavioral Cognitive Status Examination (NCSE),** this is a test to measure a patient's abilities in five areas to test their cognitive abilities. It is used to measure disability in patients with substance abuse, strokes, and traumatic brain injuries.
Draw-a-Person (DAP) Test: analysis of patient's drawings of male and female individuals. Used to assess personality.
Minnesota Multiphasic Personality Inventory (MMPI): assessment of personality characteristics through a battery of forced-choice questions.
Rorschach: a projective test using inkblots to determine the patient's ability to integrate intellectual and emotional factors into his or her perception of the environment.

Thematic Apperception Test (TAT): a test in which patients are asked to make up stories about the pictures they are shown. This test may provide information about a patient's interpersonal relationships, fantasies, needs, conflicts, and defenses.

Wechsler Adult Intelligence Scale (WAIS): a measure of verbal IQ, performance IQ, and full-scale IQ.

Wechsler Intelligence Scale for Children (WISC): a measure of intellectual development in children.

 Exercise 6: **Diagnostic Procedures**

Match the diagnostic procedures with their definitions.

___ 1. WAIS
___ 2. TAT
___ 3. PET scan
___ 4. MMPI
___ 5. Rorschach
___ 6. GAF
___ 7. Bender Gestalt
___ 8. fMRI

A. numerical measure of overall mental health
B. provides information about needs, fantasies, and interpersonal relationships
C. measures personality characteristics
D. IQ test
E. test of visuomotor and spatial skills
F. imaging of metabolic activity (in brain)
G. examines integration of emotional and intellectual factors
H. an imaging technique using magnetic properties of molecules to image the brain

Terms Related to Psychotherapy

Term	Word Origin	Definition
adaptive behavioral therapy		A treatment that focuses on reducing repetitive and unwanted behaviors. Most often used to treat children and adults on the autism spectrum.
behavioral therapy		Therapeutic attempt to alter an undesired behavior by substituting a new response or set of responses to a given stimulus.
cognitive therapy		Wide variety of treatment techniques that attempts to help the individual alter inaccurate or unhealthy perceptions and patterns of thinking.
psychoanalysis	*psych/o* mind *ana-* up, apart *-lysis* breaking down	Behavioral treatment developed initially by Sigmund Freud to analyze and treat any dysfunctional effects of unconscious factors on a patient's mental state. This therapy uses techniques that include analysis of defense mechanisms and dream interpretation.
psychodynamic therapy	*psych/o* mind *dynam/o* power *-ic* pertaining to	Treatment that is based on revealing the motivations of behavior from past emotional experience and using the knowledge to effect change.

 CPT Coding Alert!

Biofeedback has one code and no qualifiers in ICD-10-PCS, while CPT-4 has codes for "any modality" as well as for muscular control.

Terms Related to Substance Abuse Treatment

Term	Word Origin	Definition
detoxification		Removal of a chemical substance (drug or alcohol) as an initial step in treatment of a chemically dependent patient.
pharmacotherapy	*pharmac/o* drug *-therapy* treatment	The use of medication to affect behavior and/or emotions. Medications used and coded are: nicotine replacement, methadone maintenance, levo-alpha-acetyl-methadol (LAAM), Antabuse, naltrexone, naloxone, clonidine, bupropion.

Terms Related to Other Therapeutic Methods

Term	Word Origin	Definition
biofeedback		A technique used to acquire a greater awareness of physiological functions through the use of sensors with the goal of changing dysfunctional responses to more appropriate ones. Biofeedback is used to treat anxiety and ADHD.
electroconvulsive therapy (ECT)	*electr/o* electricity *con-* together *vuls/o* to pull *-ive* pertaining to *therapy* treatment	Method of inducing convulsions to treat affective disorders in patients who have been resistant or unresponsive to drug therapy. Treatment may include one or both hemispheres of the brain.
hypnosis	*hypn/o* sleep *-sis* state of, condition	The induction of an altered state of consciousness to change an unwanted behavior or emotional response. Also called **hypnotherapy.**
light therapy		Exposure of the body to light waves to treat patients with depression due to seasonal fluctuations (SAD) (Fig. 12-5). Sometimes called **phototherapy.**
narcosynthesis	*narc/o* sleep, stupor *-synthesis* bring together	The use of intravenous barbiturates to elicit repressed memories or thoughts.

CPT Coding Alert!

CPT-4 has one code for ECT (90870), while ICD-10-PCS has qualifiers for whether the treatment was on one or both sides and whether single or multiple seizures were induced.

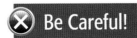

Be Careful! *Phototherapy can also be used to describe procedures to treat jaundice and psoriasis.*

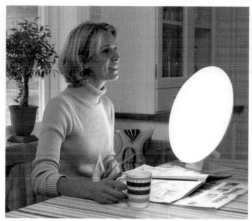

Fig. 12-5 Broad-spectrum fluorescent lamps, such as this one, are used in daily therapy sessions from autumn into spring for individuals with SAD. Patients report that they feel less depressed within 3 to 7 days. (Courtesy Apollo Light Systems.)

 Exercise 7: Procedures

Fill in the blanks with the following terms.

cognitive therapy	**light therapy**
ECT	**psychoanalysis**
behavioral therapy	**narcosynthesis**
adaptive behavioral therapy	**biofeedback**

1. Patients are treated with _____ when an attempt is made to replace maladjusted patterns with a new response to a given stimulus.

2. What type of therapy uses exposure of the body to light waves to treat patients with depression caused by seasonal flctuations?_____

3. What is a method of inducing convulsions to treat affective disorders in patients who have been resistant or unresponsive to drug therapy? _____

4. What therapy is used to analyze and treat any dysfunctional effects of unconscious factors on a patient's mental state?_____

5. What are any of the various methods of treating mental and emotional disorders that help a person change attitudes, perceptions, and patterns of thinking? _____
_____

6. What is the use of intravenous barbiturates to elicit repressed memories or thoughts called? _____
_____

7. What is a treatment that focuses on reducing repetitive and unwanted behaviors? _____

8. What is the treatment that uses sensors to increase awareness of maladaptive body functions and help individuals correct them? _____

Build the term.

9. treatment with drugs_____

10. process of removal of poison_____

11. pertaining to power of the mind_____

12. state of sleep_____

PHARMACOLOGY

A major part of treatment for behavioral disorders is the use of drug therapy. Various neurotransmitters may be out of balance in the brain, causing mental disorders. Many drugs have been developed to improve this balance and minimize symptoms of these disorders. Examples include the following:

antialcoholics: Discourage use of alcohol. Naltrexone (ReVia) can be used for alcohol and narcotic withdrawal. Disulfiram (Antabuse) is used to deter alcohol consumption.

antidepressants: Alter neurotransmitter balance in the brain to improve mood, calm anxiety, relieve symptoms of neuropathic pain, or treat a variety of other disorders. Many drug classes are available, including selective serotonin reuptake inhibitors (SSRIs), tricyclic antidepressants (TCAs), monoamine oxidase inhibitors (MAOIs), and some newer unclassified agents. Examples include fluoxetine (Prozac), sertraline (Zoloft), mirtazapine (Remeron), bupropion (Wellbutrin), and venlafaxine (Effexor).

antipsychotics or neuroleptics: Control psychotic symptoms such as hallucinations and delusions. Haloperidol (Haldol) and chlorpromazine (Thorazine) are examples of typical antipsychotics; olanzapine (Zyprexa) and risperidone (Risperdal) are examples of the newer atypical antipsychotics.

anxiolytics: Relieve symptoms of anxiety. These drugs are often used as sedatives or sedative-hypnotics as well. Examples are lorazepam (Ativan), buspirone (BuSpar), and alprazolam (Xanax).

cholinesterase inhibitors: Combat the cognitive deterioration seen in disorders characterized by dementia, such as Alzheimer's disease. Also known as **acetylcholinesterase inhibitors (AChEIs).** Examples are donepezil (Aricept) and galantamine (Razadyne).

hypnotics: Promote sleep. Hypnotics, sedatives, sedative-hypnotics, and anxiolytics are often similar in effect and may be used interchangeably. Zolpidem (Ambien), zaleplon (Sonata), and flurazepam (Dalmane) are examples of hypnotics.

mood stabilizers: Balance neurotransmitters in the brain to reduce or prevent acute mood swings (mania or depression). Lithium (Lithobid) is the most well-known mood stabilizer. Some anticonvulsants such as divalproex sodium (Depakote) and lamotrigine (Lamictal) are also considered mood stabilizers. Some antipsychotics may also have mood-stabilizing effects.

NMDA receptor antagonists: Preserve cognitive function in patients suffering from progressive memory loss by blocking glutamate activity. Memantine (Namenda) is the only drug of this class currently used for this purpose.

sedatives and sedative-hypnotics: Exert a calming effect with or without inducing sleep. The most commonly used agents are benzodiazepines such as diazepam (Valium) and barbiturates such as phenobarbital (Luminal).

stimulants: Generally increase synaptic activity of targeted neurons to increase alertness. Examples include methylphenidate (Ritalin) and caffeine.

 Exercise 8: **Pharmacology**

Match the drug class with the drug action.

___ 1. mood stabilizer
___ 2. antidepressant
___ 3. cholinesterase inhibitor
___ 4. sedative

___ 5. anxiolytic
___ 6. stimulant
___ 7. antialcoholic
___ 8. hypnotic

A. discourages use of alcohol
B. increases CNS synaptic activity
C. balances neurotransmitters in the brain
D. reduces anxiety
E. improves cognition from effects of dementia
F. controls psychotic symptoms
G. prevents acute mood swings
H. calms and relaxes

Abbreviations

Abbreviation	Meaning
ADHD	attention-deficit/hyperactivity disorder
APA	American Psychiatric Association
BP, BD	bipolar disorder
BPD	borderline personality disorder
CBC	complete blood count
CT	computed tomography
DAP	Draw-a-Person Test
DSM	*Diagnostic and Statistical Manual of Mental Disorders*
DTs	delirium tremens
ECT	electroconvulsive therapy
fMRI	functional magnetic resonance imaging
GAD	generalized anxiety disorder
GAF	Global Assessment of Functioning Scale
HIV	human immunodeficiency virus
IQ	intelligence quotient
MHA-TP	microhemagglutination assay for *Treponema pallidum*
MMPI	Minnesota Multiphasic Personality Inventory
MR	mental retardation

Abbreviation	Meaning
MRI	magnetic resonance imaging
MSBP	Munchausen's syndrome by proxy
MSE	mental status examination
NCSE	Neurobehavioral Cognitive Status Examination
OCD	obsessive-compulsive disorder
OCPD	obsessive-compulsive personality disorder
ODD	oppositional defiant disorder
PD	panic disorder
PDD	pervasive developmental disorder
PET	positron emission tomography
PPMD	premenstrual dysphoric disorder
PPD	postpartum depression
PTSD	post-traumatic stress disorder
RPR	rapid plasma reagin
SAD	seasonal affective disorder
SDD	specific developmental disorders
TAT	Thematic Apperception Test
WAIS	Wechsler Adult Intelligence Scale
WISC	Wechsler Intelligence Scale for Children

Go to Evolve to interactively build terms, memorize word parts, and practice using mental and behavioral health terms in context.

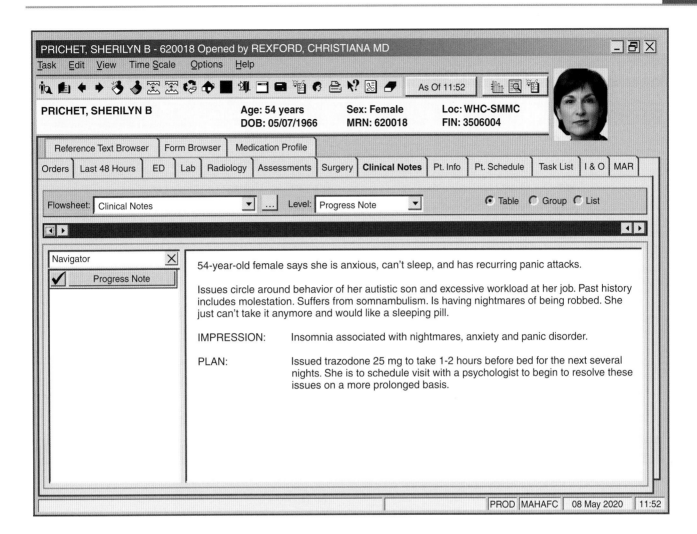

PRICHET, SHERILYN B - 620018 Opened by REXFORD, CHRISTIANA MD

Task   Edit   View   Time Scale   Options   Help

As Of 11:52

PRICHET, SHERILYN B

Age: 54 years   Sex: Female   Loc: WHC-SMMC
DOB: 05/07/1966   MRN: 620018   FIN: 3506004

Reference Text Browser   Form Browser   Medication Profile

Orders | Last 48 Hours | ED | Lab | Radiology | Assessments | Surgery | **Clinical Notes** | Pt. Info | Pt. Schedule | Task List | I & O | MAR

Flowsheet: Clinical Notes   Level: Progress Note   ⦿ Table   ○ Group   ○ List

Navigator

✓   Progress Note

54-year-old female says she is anxious, can't sleep, and has recurring panic attacks.

Issues circle around behavior of her autistic son and excessive workload at her job. Past history includes molestation. Suffers from somnambulism. Is having nightmares of being robbed. She just can't take it anymore and would like a sleeping pill.

IMPRESSION: Insomnia associated with nightmares, anxiety and panic disorder.

PLAN: Issued trazodone 25 mg to take 1-2 hours before bed for the next several nights. She is to schedule visit with a psychologist to begin to resolve these issues on a more prolonged basis.

PROD   MAHAFC   08 May 2020   11:52

 Exercise 9: **Progress Note**

Using the progress note above, answer the following questions:

1. The Impression section notes that the patient has panic disorder. What is the meaning of the term?_____
   _____

2. What disorder does her son have? What are its manifestations? _____
   _____

3. Sherilyn is diagnosed with a disorder in which the mood may be described as an "anticipation of impending danger and dread accompanied by restlessness, tension, tachycardia, and breathing difficulty not associated with an apparent stimulus." What is it? _____

4. What is somnambulism?_____

Match the word parts to their definitions.

WORD PART DEFINITIONS

Prefix/Suffix
acro-
agora-
an-
cata-
eu-
-ism
-kinesis
-lalia
-mania
-oid
para-
-phobia
-thymia

Definition

1. _____ condition of babbling
2. _____ condition of madness
3. _____ no, not, without
4. _____ condition of sensitivity, fear
5. _____ condition of mind
6. _____ marketplace
7. _____ good, well
8. _____ resembling, like
9. _____ down
10. _____ condition
11. _____ heights
12. _____ movement
13. _____ abnormal

Combining Form
anthrop/o
calcul/o
claustr/o
cycl/o
hedon/o
hypn/o
klept/o
ment/o
nymph/o
oneir/o
orex/o
ped/o
phil/o
phor/o
phren/o
pol/o
psych/o
pyr/o
somat/o
somn/o

Definition

14. _____ pleasure
15. _____ recurring
16. _____ appetite
17. _____ mind
18. _____ body
19. _____ man
20. _____ woman
21. _____ dream
22. _____ pole
23. _____ mind
24. _____ to steal
25. _____ stone
26. _____ sleep
27. _____ sleep
28. _____ mind
29. _____ attraction
30. _____ fire
31. _____ a closing
32. _____ to carry, to bear
33. _____ child

WORDSHOP

Prefixes	Combining Forms	Suffixes
acro-	ambul/o	-ia
agora-	calcul/o	-ism
an-	cycl/o	-kinesis
dys-	gyn/e	-lalia
echo-	hedon/o	-mania
hyper-	hypn/o	-osis
	oneir/o	-phobia
	phren/o	-sis
	psych/o	-thymia
	pyr/o	
	schiz/o	
	somn/o	
	till/o	
	trich/o	

Build mental and behavioral terms by combining the word parts above. Some word parts may be used more than once. Some may not be used at all. The number in parentheses indicates the number of word parts needed.

Definition	Term
1. condition of no pleasure (3)	
2. condition of difficult stone (3)	
3. condition of fear or sensitivity to women (2)	
4. abnormal condition of mind (2)	
5. condition of fire madness (2)	
6. excessive movement (2)	
7. dream state (2)	
8. condition of fear of heights or extremes (2)	
9. state of sleep (2)	
10. condition of sleepwalking (3)	
11. condition of hair-pulling madness (3)	
12. condition of excessive sleep (3)	
13. condition of recurring mind (2)	
14. condition of babbling (2)	
15. condition of split mind (3)	

Replace the highlighted words with the correct terms.

TRANSLATIONS

1. The patient had **a moderately reduced range of affect** and **anxiety disorder characterized by recurring severe panic attacks.**

   _____
   _____

2. Amy was admitted with a diagnosis of **prolonged refusal to eat adequate amounts of food** and **disorder characterized by recurring episodes of mild elation and depression.**

   _____
   _____

3. The patient was referred to a sleep therapist for **excessive length or depth of sleep** and **sleepwalking.**

   _____
   _____

4. Marielle underwent **exposure of the body to light waves** after telling her doctor that she had **absence of the ability to experience pleasure or joy** and SAD.

   _____
   _____

5. Because Mr. Ballestero was experiencing **generalized negative mood characterized by depression** and **an exaggerated sense of well-being not based on reality,** he was diagnosed with **a disorder characterized by swings between elevation and lowering of mood.**

   _____
   _____

6. After Andrew McKlin returned home from Iraq, he suffered from **anticipation of impending danger and dread** and **extended emotional response to a traumatic event.**

   _____
   _____

7. Cho Ling told her psychologist that she thought she had **extreme fear of heights** and **fear of enclosed spaces.**

   _____
   _____

8. Adam was washing his hands 40 times a day, and his psychiatrist diagnosed **recurrent, distressing, and unavoidable preoccupation to perform specific rituals.**

   _____
   _____

9. The patient's **disassociation with or impaired perception of reality** was accompanied by **unreal sensory perceptions that occur with no external cause.**

   _____
   _____

10. Tiffany showed signs of **a syndrome that includes impulsiveness, inability to concentrate, and short attention span.**

   _____
   _____

Eye and Adnexa

13

OBJECTIVES

☐ Recognize and use terms related to the anatomy and physiology of the eye.

☐ Recognize and use terms related to the pathology of the eye.

☐ Recognize and use terms related to procedures for the eye.

CM Example from Tabular
H20.1 Chronic iridocyclitis
> Use additional code for any associated cataract **(H26.21-)**
> Excludes2 posterior cyclitis **(H30.2-)**
> **H20.10** Chronic iridocyclitis, unspecified eye
> **H20.11** Chronic iridocyclitis, right eye
> **H20.12** Chronic iridocyclitis, left eye
> **H20.13** Chronic iridocyclitis, bilateral

PCS Example from Index
Keratectomy, kerectomy
> *see* Excision, Eye **08B**
> *see* Resection, Eye **08T**
Keratocentesis
> *see* Drainage, Eye **089**
Keratoplasty
> *see* Repair, Eye **08Q**
> *see* Replacement, Eye **08R**
> *see* Supplement, Eye **08U**
Keratotomy
> *see* Drainage, Eye **089**
> *see* Repair, Eye **08Q**

vision = opt/o, optic/o

FUNCTION OF THE EYE

The function of the eyes and adnexa (accessory structures) is to provide an individual with the sense of **vision** by capturing light rays and focusing them on the retina to produce an image. The *interpretation* of these images is the function of the nervous system. With certain visual disorders, the image may be correctly imaged by the eye, but misinterpreted by the brain.

ANATOMY AND PHYSIOLOGY

eye = ocul/o, ophthalm/o

The eye can be divided into the **ocular adnexa**—the structures that surround and support the function of the eyeball—and the structures of the globe of the eye itself: the **eyeball.** Our binocular vision sends two slightly different images to the brain in order to produce depth of vision. The Latin term for the right eye is **oculus dextra (OD),** with the left eye termed **oculus sinistra (OS).** Please note that the combining forms *dextr/o* and *sinistr/o* refer to right and left; not right and evil! The term for "each eye" is **oculus uterque (OU).**

 CM Guideline Alert

B13. LATERALITY
Some ICD-10-SM codes indicate laterality, specifying whether the condition occurs on the left, right or is bilateral. If no bilateral code is provided and the condition is bilateral, assign separate codes for both the left and right side. If the side is not identified in the medical record, assign the code for the unspecified side.

When a patient has a bilateral condition and each side is treated during separate encounters, assign the "bilateral" code (as the condition still exists on both sides), including for the encounter to treat the first side. For the second encounter for treatment after one side has previously been treated and the condition no longer exists on that side, assign the appropriate unilateral code for the side where the condition still exists (e.g., cataract surgery performed on each eye in separate encounters). The bilateral code would not be assigned for the subsequent encounter, as the patient no longer has the condition in the previously treated site. If the treatment on the first side did not completely resolve the condition, then the bilateral code would still be appropriate.

Ocular Adnexa

orbit = orbit/o

Each of our paired eyes is encased in a protective, bony socket called the **orbit** or **orbital cavity.**

Within the orbit, the eyeball is protected by a cushion of fatty tissue. The eyebrows mark the supraorbital area and provide a modest amount of protection from perspiration and sun glare. Further protection is provided by the upper and lower eyelids and the eyelashes that line their edges (Fig. 13-1).

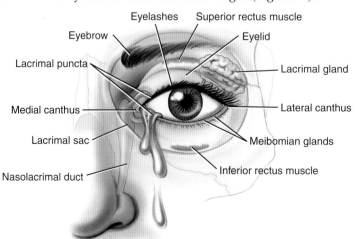

Fig. 13-1 Ocular adnexa.

This chapter includes all the anatomy necessary to assign ICD-10 eye and adnexa codes, including detail on the zonule of Zinn, the pars plana, and the scleral venous sinus. See Appendix H for a complete list of body parts and how they should be coded.

The corners of the eyes are referred to as the **canthi** *(sing.* canthus); the inner canthus is termed *medial* (toward the middle of the body), and the outer canthus is *lateral* (toward the side of the body). The area where the upper and lower eyelids meet is referred to as the **palpebral fissure.** This term is related to the function of blinking, called **palpebration** through the combining form *palpebr/o,* meaning "eyelid." Note the ***Be Careful*** box for another potentially confusing combining form that is also used for the dense connective tissue within the eyelids, the tarsal plates.

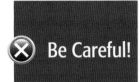

Be Careful! **Tars/o** *can refer to a flat structure that gives shape to the eyelid (the tarsal plate) or to bones in the ankle. From the Greek word* **tarsus,** *meaning a flat surface, it refers to the horizontal level appearance of each eyelid and also the bones that make up the instep of the foot. Let context be your guide when a medical term incorporates this combining form!*

The eyelids are lined with a thin, protective mucous membrane called the **conjunctiva** *(pl.* conjunctivae) that spreads to coat the anterior surface of the eyeball as well. The conjunctival sacs (also referred to as the upper and lower fornix of the eye) are the folded extensions of this membrane that provide the looseness necessary for movement of the eye.

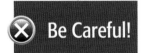

Be Careful! The term **palpebrate** *means to blink or wink. Do not confuse this with the terms* **palpate** *(meaning to touch) or* **palpitate** *(meaning to throb).*

Also surrounding the eye are two types of glands. Sebaceous glands in the eyelids called **meibomian glands,** or tarsal glands, secrete oil to lubricate the eyelashes, and **lacrimal glands** above the eyes produce tears to keep the eyes moist. These glands can become blocked or infected. The lacrimal gland, or tear gland, provides a constant source of cleansing and lubrication for the eye. The process of producing tears is termed **lacrimation.** The lacrimal glands are located in the upper outer corners of the orbit. The constant blinking of the eyelids spreads the tears across the eyeball. The tears then drain into two small holes called the *lacrimal punctum* (plural *puncta)* in the upper and lower eyelids in the medial canthus, then into the **lacrimal ducts** (also called the *lacrimal canals* or *canaliculi [tiny canals]),* next into the **lacrimal sacs,** and finally into the **nasolacrimal ducts,** which carry the tears to the nasal cavity. Normally, there are few tears that need draining, but when an individual cries, the excess tears exit down the cheeks and through the nose.

The **extraocular muscles** attach the eyeball to the orbit and, on impulse from the cranial nerves, move the eyes (Fig. 13-2). These six voluntary (skeletal) muscles are made up of four rectus (straight) and two oblique (diagonal) muscles. The origin of five of these muscles is in a ringlike structure surrounding the optic nerve behind the eyeball called the **annulus of Zinn** (also referred to as the *annular tendon).* This is mentioned only because later, when the lens of the eye is described, another structure in the lens called a **zonule of Zinn** will be named. Note that the muscle to raise the eyelids, the **levator palpebrae superior muscle,** is also labeled. "Levator" is used for any muscles whose function it is to elevate a structure. When this muscle is dysfunctional, it can result in an eyelid that droops (ptosis). The **orbicularis oculi** are the sphincter (ringlike) muscles that close the eye.

---

canthus = canth/o

eyelid = blephar/o, palpebr/o

conjunctiva = conjunctiv/o

lacrimal (tear) glands = dacryoaden/o

tears = lacrim/o, dacry/o

lacrimal (tear) sac = dacryocyst/o

nasolacrimal
    nas/o = nose
    lacrim/o = tears
    -al = pertaining to

extraocular
    extra- = outside
    ocul/o = eye
    -ar = pertaining to

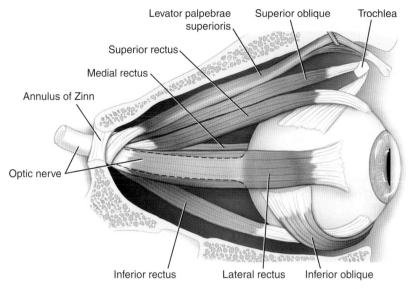

Fig. 13-2 Extraocular muscles.

 Exercise 1: Ocular Adnexa

A. Match the term with its correct combining form or prefix.

_____ 1. membrane that lines eyelids and covers the surface of the eyes

_____ 2. eyelid

_____ 3. tear

_____ 4. vision

_____ 5. eye

_____ 6. bony socket of the eye

_____ 7. nose

_____ 8. tear gland

_____ 9. tear sac

A. nas/o

B. conjunctiv/o

C. optic/o, opt/o

D. ophthalm/o, ocul/o

E. dacryoaden/o

F. blephar/o, palpebr/o

G. dacryocyst/o

H. dacry/o, lacrim/o

I. orbit/o

B. Match the structure to its definition or function.

_____ 1. lacrimal gland

_____ 2. meibomian gland

_____ 3. palpebral fissure

_____ 4. levator palpebrae superior muscle

_____ 5. canthi

_____ 6. conjunctiva

_____ 7. lacrimal punctum

_____ 8. extraocular muscles

_____ 9. nasolacrimal duct

A. where the upper and lower eyelids meet

B. corners of the eye

C. mucous membrane that coats the anterior surface of the eyeball

D. produces tears to keep eyes moist

E. secretes oil to lubricate eyelashes

F. two small holes into which tears drain

G. muscle that raises the eyelid

H. attach the eyeball to the orbit

I. carries tears to the nasal cavity

To practice labeling the structures of the eye, click on **Label It.**

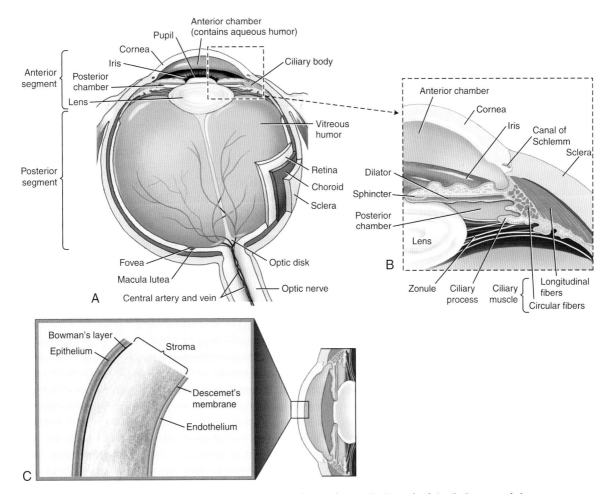

Fig. 13-3 A, Cross section of an eyeball viewed from above. **B,** Detail of **A. C,** Layers of the cornea.

The Eyeball

The anatomy of the eyeball itself is traditionally explained in three layers or tunics. The outer layer, or **fibrous tunic,** consists of the sclera and cornea. The middle layer, or **vascular tunic,** is composed of the choroid, ciliary body, and iris. The inner layer, or **nervous tunic,** consists of the retina (Fig. 13-3). CPT, however, differentiates coding of some of its procedures depending on whether they are in the anterior segment (the forward most third of the eyeball) or the posterior segment (the remaining back two thirds of the eyeball). To be specific, the anterior segment includes the structures in front of the vitreous humor: the cornea, the iris, the ciliary body, and the lens. The posterior segment includes the vitreous humor, the retina, the choroid, and the optic nerve. Because the sclera does have segments in both the anterior and posterior locations, it will be important to note the area of the sclera that is treated (See Fig. 13-3, inset).

The Outer/Fibrous Layer (Sclera)

The outermost lateral and posterior portion of the eye, the white of the eye, is called the **sclera,** which means "hard." Its three sections are the episcleral layer (literally the layer on top of the sclera), **Schlemm's canal** (also called the *scleral venous sinus),* which is a ringlike tube that returns excess fluid to the bloodstream collected from the final layer of the sclera, and the **trabecular** network. The deepest layer of the sclera, the trabecular network is spongy, porous tissue that serves to drain fluid from the eye in order to maintain healthy intraocular pressure.

sclera = scler/o

trabecula = trabecul/o

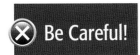

Be Careful!

*The combining form **kerat/o** refers to the structure of the cornea, but also to the condition of a body part having a hard or horny appearance, such as a seborrheic keratosis.*

cornea = corne/o, kerat/o

Cornea

The **cornea** is the anterior transparent continuation of the sclera. There are 5 layers of the cornea. From outer layer to inner they are as follows:
1. epithelium
2. Bowman's layer
3. stroma
4. Desemet's membrane
5. endothelium

The combining forms for the cornea *(corne/o* and *kerat/o)* refer to the tough nature of this part of the outer layer of the eye. The border of the cornea, between it and the sclera, is called the **limbus.** The combining form *limb/o* refers to an edge, as in the margin between two structures. The cornea is where refraction (the bending of light) begins as light enters the eye.

limbus = limb/o

 CPT Coding Alert!

CPT requires knowledge of the layers of the cornea in order to correctly code certain corneal surgeries.

The Middle/Vascular Layer (Uvea)

The **uvea** is the middle, highly vascular layer of the eye. It includes the iris, the ciliary body, and the choroid. The **choroid membrane** is the network of blood vessels that lies between the outer coat, the sclera, and the inner layer, the retina, and provides oxygen and nourishment for the internal structures of the eye. The **ciliary body** is a thin vascular structure with two distinct functions. The first function involves the capillaries of the ciliary body that produce a fluid called the **aqueous humor.** It nourishes the cornea, gives shape to the anterior eye, and maintains an optimum intraocular pressure. The aqueous humor circulates in both the anterior chamber, between the cornea and the iris, and the posterior chamber, behind the iris and in front of the lens. The second function of the ciliary body involves the ciliary muscles and processes that attach to the lens of the eye and contract when needed to help the eye focus on an object (the process of **accommodation).** The **pars plana,** also called the *ciliary disk,* is the flat part (pars) of the ciliary body. The ciliary muscles extend into ciliary processes that extend to the **zonules of Zinn,** and form a ring of tiny strands that complete the attachment of the muscles of the ciliary body to the lens.

uvea = uve/o
choroid = choroid/o
ciliary body = cycl/o

Iris

The **iris** *(pl.* irides) is a smooth muscle that contracts and relaxes to moderate the amount of light that enters the eye. In most individuals, this is the colored part of the eye (brown, gray, hazel, blue) because of its pigmentation. Individuals with albinism, however, have reddish-pink irides because a lack of pigment makes the blood cells visible as they travel through the vessels supplying the iris.

iris = irid/o, ir/o

Pupil

The **pupil** is the opening in the center of the iris (that appears as a dark area) where the light continues its progress through to the lens.

pupil = pupill/o, core/o, cor/o

 PCS Guideline Alert

B2.1 Body systems contain body part values that include contiguous body parts. These general body part values are used:
  a. When a procedure is performed on the general body part as a whole
  b. When the specific body part cannot be determined
  c. In the root operations change, removal and revision, when the specific body part value is not in the table.

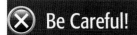 **Be Careful!**

Core/o *and* **cor/o** *are combining forms for the pupil of the eye, and* **corne/o** *is a combining form for the cornea.*

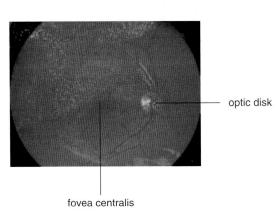

fovea centralis

Fig. 13-4 The retina.

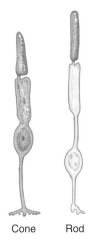

Cone   Rod

Fig. 13-5 Rod and cone.

Between the lens and the inner layer, the retina, is a transparent jellylike substance called the vitreous humor (also called the **vitreous body**), which holds the choroid membrane against the retina to ensure an adequate blood supply. The combining form *vitre/o* means "glass" or "glassy," which may refer to its appearance, although it is not especially helpful to define the term.

The Inner/Nervous Layer (Retina)

The inner layer of the eye, called the **retina,** is composed of several parts. The pars optica retinae contain the sensory receptors (rods and cones), the optic disk, the ora serrata, the macula lutea, and the fovea centralis. This layer is nourished by the retinal vessels that radiate from the optic nerve (Fig. 13-4).

The sensory receptors for the images carried by the light rays are named for their appearance. They are the **rods,** which appear throughout the retina and are responsible for vision in dim light, and the **cones,** which are concentrated in the central area of the retina and are responsible for color vision (Fig. 13-5). Three types of cones, termed L, M, and S (for long, medium, and short) cones, are endowed with photopigments that react to different wavelengths of light that produce the perception of red, green, and blue vision. Those individuals who have difficulty with their color vision (through inheritance or trauma) have deficiencies in one or more of these cones.

The **optic disk** is the small area in the retina where the optic nerve enters the eye. Also called the *optic papilla* for its nipplelike appearance, it is referred to as the "blind spot" of the eye because of its lack of light receptors. The **ora serrata** (*ora* is the plural of *os,* meaning "an opening," whereas *serrata* refers to its "notched" appearance) is the jagged border between the retina and the ciliary body of the choroid. The **macula lutea** (literally meaning a "yellow spot") is the area of central vision in the retina, whereas the **fovea centralis,** or simply *fovea,* is the depression in the middle of the macula that is the area of sharpest vision because of its high density of cones (color receptors). The term *fovea* means a "small pit," so the fovea centralis is literally a small pit in the middle of a yellow spot. The **crystalline lens** is a biconvex, transparent, avascular structure made of protein and covered by an elastic capsule.

vitreous humor = vitre/o

retina = retin/o

optic disk = papill/o

macula lutea = macul/o

lens = phak/o, phac/o

CPT Coding Alert!

CPT's surgical section divides intraocular procedures into anterior and posterior segments. Coders need to be careful to note, for example, whether the anterior or posterior segment of the sclera is being treated.

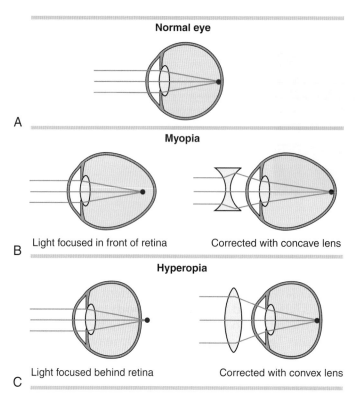

Fig. 13-6 Refraction in **A**, normal vision; **B**, myopia; and **C**, hypermetropia.

Vision

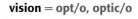

vision = opt/o, optic/o

The ocular adnexa and the fibrous, vascular, and nervous layers, or tunics, are essential to vision. All parts work together with impressive harmony. The eye muscles coordinate their movements with one another; the cornea and pupil control the amount of light that enters the eye; the lens focuses the image on the retina; and the optic nerve transmits the image to the brain through an opening within the skull termed the *optic foramen*.

Two important mechanisms contribute to the ability to see. As light hits the eye, it passes first through the cornea, which bends the rays of light (refraction) so that they are projected properly onto the receptor cells in the eye. The muscles in the ciliary body adjust the shape of the lens to aid in this refraction. The lens flattens to adjust to something seen at a distance or thickens for close vision (a process called **accommodation).** Errors of refraction are the most common reason for lens prescriptions. See Fig. 13-6 for an example of refraction in normal vision, as well as in nearsightedness (myopia) and farsightedness (hypermetropia), and how they are corrected through the use of corrective lenses.

Exercise 2: The Eyeball

A. Match the parts of the eye with the correct combining forms. More than one answer may be correct.

_____ 1. ir/o, irid/o

_____ 2. papill/o

_____ 3. canth/o

_____ 4. cor/o, core/o, pupill/o

_____ 5. phac/o, phak/o

_____ 6. cycl/o

_____ 7. kerat/o

A. cornea

B. ciliary body

C. iris

D. corner of the eye

E. pupil

F. lens

G. optic disk

B. Match the structure with its definition or function.

____ 1. sclera
____ 2. trabecular network
____ 3. cornea
____ 4. limbus
____ 5. choroid membrane
____ 6. macula lutea
____ 7. aqueous humor
____ 8. iris
____ 9. pupil
____ 10. vitreous humor
____ 11. retina
____ 12. rod
____ 13. cone
____ 14. optic disk
____ 15. uvea

A. provides oxygen and nourishment for internal structures of the eye

B. nourishes the cornea, gives shape to the eye, and maintains optimal intraocular pressure

C. holds the choroid membrane against the retina to ensure an adequate blood supply

D. smooth muscle that contracts and relaxes to moderate the amount of light that enters the eye

E. area in the retina where the optic nerve enters the eye

F. sensory receptor responsible for vision in dim light

G. inner layer of the eye

H. white of the eye

I. drains fluid from the eye to maintain healthy intraocular pressure

J. opening in iris that allows light to progress to the lens

K. sensory receptor responsible for color vision

L. border of the cornea and sclera

M. area of central vision in the retina

N. middle, highly vascular area of the eye

O. anterior continuation of the sclera

Combining Forms for the Anatomy and Physiology of the Eye

Meaning	Combining Form	Meaning	Combining Form
choroid	choroid/o	macula lutea	macul/o
ciliary body	cycl/o	notched	serrat/o
conjunctiva	conjunctiv/o	optic disk	papill/o
cornea	corne/o, kerat/o	orbit	orbit/o
corner (of eye)	canth/o	pupil	pupill/o, core/o, cor/o
eye	ophthalm/o, ocul/o	retina	retin/o
eyelid	blephar/o, palpebr/o	sclera	scler/o
iris	irid/o, ir/o	tarsal plate (of the eyelid)	tars/o
lacrimal (tear) gland	dacryoaden/o	tears	lacrim/o, dacry/o
lacrimal (tear) sac	dacryocyst/o	uvea	uve/o
lens	phak/o, phac/o	vision	opt/o, optic/o
limbus	limb/o	vitreous humor	vitre/o, vitr/o

You can review the anatomy of the eye by clicking on **Body Spectrum Electronic Anatomy Coloring Book,** then **Senses.**

PATHOLOGY

Terms Related to Disorders of the Eyelid, Lacrimal System, and Orbit (H00-H05)

Term	Word Origin	Definition
blepharitis	*blephar/o* eyelid *-itis* inflammation	Inflammation of an eyelid.
blepharochalasis	*blephar/o* eyelid *-chalasis* relaxation, slackening	Hypertrophy of the skin of the eyelid.
blepharoptosis	*blephar/o* eyelid *-ptosis* drooping, prolapse, falling	Drooping of the upper eyelid. Also called **ptosis of the eyelid**.
chalazion		Hardened swelling of a meibomian gland resulting from a blockage. Also called **meibomian cyst** (Fig. 13-7).
dacryoadenitis	*dacroaden/o* lacrimal gland *-itis* inflammation	Inflammation of a lacrimal gland.
dacryocystitis	*dacryocyst/o* lacrimal sac *-itis* inflammation	Inflammation of a lacrimal sac.
ectropion	*ec-* out *trop/o* turning *-ion* process of	Turning outward (eversion) of the eyelid, exposing the conjunctiva (Fig. 13-8).
entropion	*en-* in *trop/o* turning *-ion* process	Turning inward of the eyelid toward the eye (Fig. 13-9).
epiphora		Overflow of tears; excessive lacrimation.
exophthalmos	*ex-* out *ophthalm/o* eye *-os* condition	Protrusion of the eyeball from its orbit; may be congenital or the result of an endocrine disorder (Fig. 13-10).
hordeolum		Infection of one of the sebaceous glands of an eyelash (Fig. 13-11). Also called a **stye**.

Continued

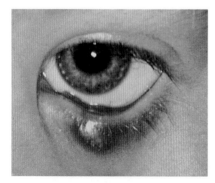

Fig. 13-7 Chalazion.

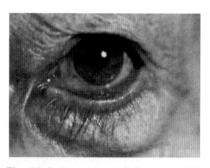

Fig. 13-8 Ectropion of the lower lid.

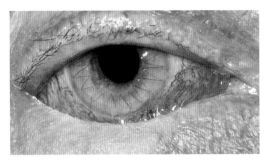

Fig. 13-9 Entropion of the lower lid. Note that this patient has undergone corneal transplantation.

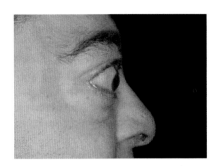

Fig. 13-10 Exophthalmos.

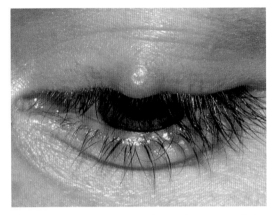

Fig. 13-11 Acute hordeolum of upper eyelid.

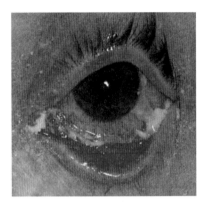

Fig. 13-12 Acute purulent conjunctivitis.

Terms Related to Disorders of the Eyelid, Lacrimal System, and Orbit (H00-H05)—cont'd

Term	Word Origin	Definition
lacrimal canaliculitis	*lacrim/o* tear *-al* pertaining to *canalicul/o* little canal *-itis* inflammation	Inflammation of the tear ducts, especially the lacrimal canaliculi.

Terms Related to Conjunctiva Disorders (H10-H11)

Term	Word Origin	Definition
conjunctivitis	*conjunctiv/o* conjunctiva *-itis* inflammation	Inflammation of the conjunctiva, commonly known as pinkeye, a highly contagious disorder (Fig. 13-12).
pinguecula		A yellowish noncancerous growth on the conjunctiva covering the eyeball in the area of the palpebral fissure. Usually asymptomatic; if irritated is termed pingueculitis.
pterygium	*pteryg/o* wing *-ium* structure	A winglike growth of the conjunctiva at the medial canthus of the eye, usually as a result of excessive exposure to wind/weather.

Terms Related to Disorders of Sclera, Cornea, Iris, and Ciliary Body (H15-H22)

Term	Word Origin	Definition
hyphema	*hypo-* under *hem/o* blood *-a* noun ending	Blood in the anterior chamber of the eye as a result of hemorrhage due to trauma.
iridocyclitis	*irid/o* iris *cycl/o* ciliary body *-itis* inflammation	Inflammation of the anterior uvea, specifically the iris and ciliary body. Symptoms include photophobia (sensitivity to light), miosis (constriction of the pupil), and synechia (adhesion of the cornea to the lens).
keratitis	*kerat/o* cornea *-itis* inflammation	Inflammation of the cornea.
keratomalacia	*kerat/o* cornea *-malacia* softening	Literally a softening of the cornea, this condition is the result of a vitamin A deficiency and malnutrition. Often leads to xerophthalmia (dry eye) and nyctalopia (night blindness).
scleritis	*scler/o* sclera *-itis* inflammation	Inflammation of the sclera (white of the eye); usually associated with autoimmune disorders.
synechia	*syn-* together	Adhesion of the lens to the cornea.
uveitis	*uve/o* uvea *-itis* inflammation	Inflammation of the uvea (iris, ciliary body, and choroid).

Exercise 3: Disorders of the Eyelid, Lacrimal System, Orbit, Conjunctiva, Sclera, Cornea, Iris, and Ciliary Body

Match the terms to their definitions.

_____ 1. chalazion
_____ 2. hordeolum
_____ 3. ectropion
_____ 4. entropion
_____ 5. dacryocystitis
_____ 6. epiphora
_____ 7. lacrimal canaliculitis
_____ 8. conjunctivitis
_____ 9. pinguecula
_____ 10. pterygium
_____ 11. keratitis
_____ 12. hyphema
_____ 13. uveitis
_____ 14. scleritis
_____ 15. iridocyclitis
_____ 16. synechia

A. infection of a sebaceous gland of an eyelash
B. inflammation of the conjunctiva
C. blood in the anterior chamber of the eye due to trauma
D. hardened swelling of a meibomian gland due to blockage
E. inflammation of the sclera
F. yellowish noncancerous growth on the conjunctiva in the palpebral fissure area
G. inflammation of the lacrimal sac
H. inflammation of the anterior uvea, specifically the iris and ciliary body
I. inflammation of the uvea
J. excessive lacrimation
K. turning outward of the eyelid
L. inflammation of the cornea
M. inflammation of the tear ducts
N. adhesion of the lens to the cornea
O. winglike growth of the conjunctiva at the medial canthus
P. turning inward of the eyelid

Build the terms.

17. drooping of the upper eyelid_____

18. inflammation of a tear gland_____

19. softening of the cornea _____

20. slackening of the eyelid_____

Terms Related to Disorders of the Lens (H25-H28)

Term	Word Origin	Definition
aphakia	*a-* no, not, without *phak/o* lens *-ia* condition	Condition of no lens, either congenital or acquired.
cataract		Progressive loss of transparency of the lens of the eye (Fig. 13-13). Age-related (senile) cataracts can be classified as opacities of the lens in the center (nuclear) or on the periphery (cortical). "Incipient" cataracts are those that are immature and only partially block vision as opposed to mature cataracts that are opaque.

Terms Related to Disorders of Choroid and Retina (H30-H36)

Term	Word Origin	Definition
age-related macular degeneration (ARMD or AMD)		Progressive destruction of the macula, resulting in a loss of central vision. This is the most common visual disorder after the age of 75 (Fig. 13-14). Appears as "wet" (exudative) or "dry" (nonexudative) form depending on whether there is bleeding and leaking under the macula.
posterior cyclitis	*cycl/o* ciliary body *-itis* inflammation	Inflammation of the ciliary body. Note that iridocyclitis is categorized with disorders of the ciliary body, whereas posterior cyclitis is with the choroid and retina. Also referred to as pars planitis because the pars plana is a structure within the ciliary body.

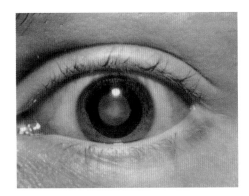

Fig. 13-13 The cloudy appearance of a lens affected by a cataract.

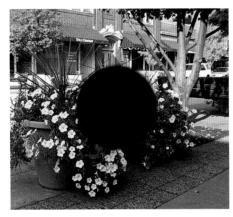

Fig. 13-14 Macular degeneration.

Terms Related to Disorders of Choroid and Retina (H30-H36)—cont'd

Term	Word Origin	Definition
retinal ischemia	*retin/o* retina *-al* pertaining to *isch/o* hold back, suppress *-emia* blood condition	Lack of blood flow to the retina.
retinal tear, retinal detachment	*retin/o* retina *-al* pertaining to	Separation of the retina from the choroid layer. May be due to trauma, inflammation of the interior of the eye, or aging. A hole in the retina allows fluid from the vitreous humor to leak between the two layers.
retinitis pigmentosa	*retin/o* retina *-itis* inflammation	Hereditary, degenerative disease marked by nyctalopia and a progressive loss of the visual field (Fig. 13-15).

Terms Related to Glaucoma (H40-H42)

Term	Word Origin	Definition
glaucoma	*glauc/o* gray, bluish green *-oma* mass, tumor	Group of disorders characterized by abnormal intraocular pressure due to obstruction of the outflow of the aqueous humor. Chronic or primary open-angle glaucoma (Fig. 13-16) is characterized by an open anterior chamber angle. Angle-closure or narrow-angle glaucoma is characterized by an abnormally narrowed anterior chamber angle.

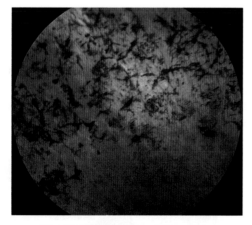

Fig. 13-15 Retinitis pigmentosa.

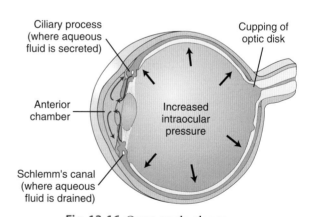

Ciliary process (where aqueous fluid is secreted)

Cupping of optic disk

Anterior chamber

Increased intraocular pressure

Schlemm's canal (where aqueous fluid is drained)

Fig. 13-16 Open-angle glaucoma.

Terms Related to Disorders of Vitreous Body and Globe (H43-H44)

Term	Word Origin	Definition
panophthalmitis	*pan-* all *ophthalm/o* eye *-itis* inflammation	Inflammation of the entire eye.
purulent endophthalmitis	*endo-* within *ophthalm/o* eye *-itis* inflammation	Infection within the eyeball usually caused by a bacterial infection. Purulent means "pertaining to pus."

Terms Related to Disorders of Optic Nerve and Visual Pathways (H46-H47)

Term	Word Origin	Definition
optic neuritis	*opt/o* vision *-ic* pertaining to *neur/o* nerve *-itis* inflammation	Inflammation of the optic nerve; often mentioned as a predecessor to the development of multiple sclerosis.
optic papillitis	*opt/o* vision *-ic* pertaining to *papill/o* optic disk *-itis* inflammation	Inflammation of the optic disk usually accompanied by varying degrees of visual deficiencies.
papilledema	*papill/o* optic disk *-edema* swelling	A swelling of the optic disk, usually secondary to intracranial pressure.
retrobulbar neuritis	*retro-* behind *bulb/o* globe *-ar* pertaining to	Inflammation of the optic nerve behind the eyeball. A type of optic neuritis, the etiology is unknown.

 Exercise 4: **Disorders of Choroid, Retina, Lens, Glaucoma, Vitreous Body, Globe, Optic Nerve, and Visual Pathways**

Match the terms to their definitions.

____ 1. retinal ischemia
____ 2. ARMD
____ 3. posterior cyclitis
____ 4. retinitis pigmentosa
____ 5. cataract
____ 6. glaucoma
____ 7. purulent endophthalmitis
____ 8. retinal detachment
____ 9. optic neuritis
____ 10. optic papillitis
____ 11. retrobulbar neuritis

A. progressive destruction of the macula, resulting in a loss of central vision
B. hereditary, degenerative disease resulting in nyctalopia and progressive visual field loss
C. group of disorders characterized by abnormal intraocular pressure due to obstruction of outflow of aqueous humor
D. inflammation of the optic disk
E. separation of the retina from the choroid layer
F. bacterial infection within the eyeball
G. inflammation of the optic nerve behind the eyeball
H. inflammation of the optic nerve
I. progressive loss of transparency of the lens of the eye
J. inflammation of the ciliary body
K. lack of blood flow to the retina

Translate the terms.

12. condition of no lens_____

13. swelling of the optic disk_____

14. inflammation of all the eye_____

Terms Related to Disorders of Ocular Muscles, Binocular Movement, Accommodation, and Refraction (H49-H52)

Term	Word Origin	Definition
astigmatism (Astig, As, Ast)		Malcurvature of the cornea leading to blurred vision. If uncorrected, asthenopia (muscle weakness or fatigue) may result.
esotropia	*eso-* inward *trop/o* turning *-ia* condition	Turning inward of one or both eyes (Fig. 13-17).
exotropia	*exo-* outward *trop/o* turning *-ia* condition	Turning outward of one or both eyes (Fig. 13-18).
hypermetropia	*hyper-* excessive *metr/o* measure *-opia* vision condition	Farsightedness; refractive error that does not allow the eye to focus on nearby objects (also termed hyperopia) (see Fig. 13-6).
myopia (MY)	*my/o* to shut *-opia* vision condition	Nearsightedness; refractive error that does not allow the eye to focus on distant objects (see Fig. 13-6).
presbyopia	*presby-* old age *-opia* vision condition	Progressive loss of elasticity of the lens (usually accompanies aging), resulting in hyperopia.
strabismus		General term for a lack of coordination between the eyes, usually due to a muscle weakness or paralysis. Sometimes called a "squint," which refers to the patient's effort to correct the disorder.

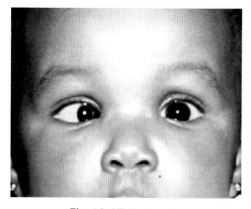

Fig. 13-17 Esotropia.

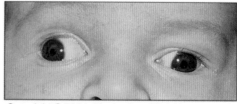

Fig. 13-18 Exotropia.

Terms Related to Visual Disturbances and Blindness (H53-H54)

Term	Word Origin	Definition
achromatopsia	*a-* no, not, without *chromat/o* color *-opsia* vision condition	Impairment of color vision. Inability to distinguish between certain colors because of abnormalities of the photopigments produced in the retina. Also called **color blindness**. Protanopia, deuteranopia, and tritanopia are types of achromatopsia due to respective defective L, M, and S cones.
amblyopia ex anopsia	*ambly/o* dull, dim *-opia* vision condition *ex* without *an-* no, not, without *-opsia* vision condition	Dull or dim vision due to disuse. Also called **lazy eye**.
diplopia	*dipl/o* double *-opia* vision condition	Double vision. Emmetropia (EM, Em) means normal vision.
hemianopsia	*hemi-* half *an-* no, not, without *-opsia* vision condition	Loss of half the visual field, often as the result of a cerebrovascular accident.
nyctalopia	*nyctal/o* night blindness *-opia* vision condition	Inability to see well in dim light. May be due to a vitamin A deficiency, retinitis pigmentosa, or choroidoretinitis.
photophobia	*phot/o* light *-phobia* condition of fear, sensitivity	Extreme sensitivity to light. The suffix *-phobia* here means "aversion," not "fear."
scotoma	*scot/o* darkness *-oma* mass, tumor	Area of decreased vision in the visual field. Commonly called a "blind spot."

Terms Related to Other Disorders of Eye and Adnexa (H55-H57)

Term	Word Origin	Definition
anisocoria	*an-* no, not, without *is/o* equal *cor/o* pupil *-ia* condition	Condition of unequally sized pupils, sometimes due to pressure on the optic nerve as a result of trauma or lesion (Fig. 13-19).
miosis	*mi/o* to close, constrict *-sis* state	Excessive and/or prolonged constriction of the pupil.

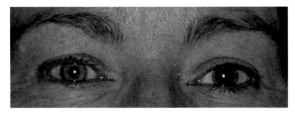

Fig. 13-19 Anisocoria. Note enlarged pupil in patient's left eye.

Term	Word Origin	Definition
mydriasis	*mydr/o* dilation *-iasis* state	Excessive and/or prolonged dilation of the pupil.
nystagmus		Involuntary back-and-forth eye movements due to a disorder of the labyrinth of the ear and/or parts of the nervous system associated with rhythmic eye movements.

⊗ Be Careful! *Do not confuse these similar terms:* esotropia, exotropia, entropion, *and* ectropion.

⊗ Be Careful! *Nyctalopia means* night blindness, *not* night vision.

Terms Related to Benign Neoplasms

Term	Word Origin	Definition
choroidal hemangioma	*choroid/o* choroid *-al* pertaining to *hemangi/o* blood vessel *-oma* tumor, mass	Tumor of the blood vessel layer under the retina (the choroid layer). May cause visual loss or retinal detachment.

Terms Related to Malignant Neoplasms

Term	Word Origin	Definition
intraocular melanoma	*intra-* within *ocul/o* eye *-ar* pertaining to *melan/o* dark, black *-oma* tumor, mass	Malignant tumor of the choroid, ciliary body, or iris that usually occurs in individuals in their 50s or 60s (Fig. 13-20).
retinoblastoma	*retin/o* retina *blast/o* embryonic, immature *-oma* tumor, mass	A rare form of cancer present at birth that arises from embryonic retinal cells (Fig. 13-21).

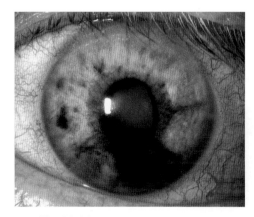

Fig. 13-20 Intraocular melanoma.

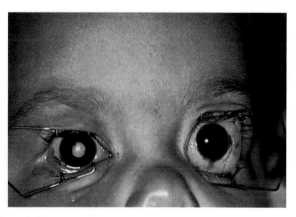

Fig. 13-21 Retinoblastoma. White pupil is a classic sign.

Exercise 5: Disorders of Ocular Muscles, Accommodation, Refraction, Visual Disturbances, Blindness, Neoplasms, and Other Disorders of the Eye and Adnexa

Match the terms to their definitions.

____	1. strabismus	A. turning inward of one or both eyes
____	2. esotropia	B. term for lack of coordination between the eyes
____	3. exotropia	C. nearsightedness
____	4. astigmatism	D. turning outward of one or both eyes
____	5. hypermetropia	E. malignant tumor of the choroid, ciliary body, or iris
____	6. myopia	F. extreme sensitivity to light
____	7. hemianopsia	G. tumor of the choroid layer
____	8. achromatopsia	H. excessive or prolonged constriction of the pupil
____	9. amblyopia ex anopsia	I. malcurvature of the cornea leading to blurred vision
____	10. photophobia	J. farsightedness
____	11. nystagmus	K. impairment of color vision
____	12. miosis	L. loss of half the visual field
____	13. choroidal hemangioma	M. involuntary back-and-forth eye movements
____	14. intraocular melanoma	N. dull or dim vision due to disuse

Build the terms.

15. visual condition of double_____

16. mass of darkness_____

17. condition of not equal pupil_____

18. state of dilation_____

19. tumor of embryonic retina_____

20. vision condition of old age_____

PROCEDURES

Terms Related to Diagnostic Procedures

Term	Word Origin	Definition
Amsler grid		Test to assess central vision and to help diagnose age-related macular degeneration (Fig. 13-22).
diopters		Level of measurement that quantifies refraction errors, including the amount of nearsightedness (negative numbers), farsightedness (positive numbers), and astigmatism.

Terms Related to Diagnostic Procedures—cont'd

Term	Word Origin	Definition
fluorescein staining		Use of a dye dropped into the eyes that allows differential staining of abnormalities of the cornea.
gonioscopy	*goni/o* angle *-scopy* viewing	Visualization of the angle of the anterior chamber of the eye; used to diagnose glaucoma and to inspect ocular movement.
ophthalmoscopy	*ophthalm/o* eye *-scopy* viewing	Any visual examination of the interior of the eye with an ophthalmoscope.
Schirmer tear test		Test to determine the amount of tear production; useful in diagnosing dry eye (xerophthalmia).
slit lamp examination		Part of a routine eye examination; used to examine the various layers of the eye. Medications may be used to dilate the pupils (mydriatics), numb the eye (anesthetics), or dye the eye (fluorescein staining).
tonometry	*ton/o* tone, tension *-metry* measuring	Measurement of intraocular pressure (IOP); used in the diagnosis of glaucoma. In Goldmann applanation tonometry, the eye is numbed and measurements are taken directly on the eye. In air-puff tonometry, a puff of air is blown onto the cornea (Fig. 13-23).
visual acuity (VA) assessment		Test of the clearness or sharpness of vision; also called the **Snellen test**. Normal vision is described as being 20/20. The top figure is the number of feet the examinee is standing from the Snellen chart; the bottom figure is the number of feet a normal person would be from the chart and still be able to read the smallest letters. Thus if the result is 20/40, the highest line that the individual can read is what a person with normal vision can read at 40 feet.
visual field (VF) test		Test to determine the area of physical space visible to an individual. A normal visual field is 65 degrees upward, 75 degrees downward, 60 degrees inward, and 90 degrees outward.

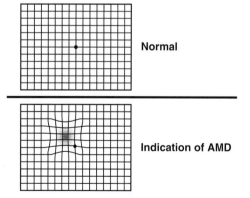

Fig. 13-22 Amsler grid. The patient looks at the central dot with one eye covered and notes the pattern of the lines. If any line in any direction is missing or wavy, the patient marks it in with a pencil or makes a note. The Amsler grid can be used to monitor macular degeneration to determine whether it is stable or progressing

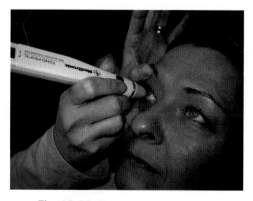

Fig. 13-23 Tono-pen tonometry.

Exercise 6: Diagnostic Procedures

Matching.

_____ 1. measure of the area of physical space visible to an individual   A. slit lamp exam
_____ 2. measurement of intraocular pressure   B. VA test
_____ 3. test of sharpness of vision   C. Schirmer test
_____ 4. visualization of angle of anterior chamber   D. fluorescein staining
_____ 5. test to measure central vision   E. VF test
_____ 6. test to determine amount of tear production   F. Amsler grid
_____ 7. exam of abnormalities of cornea   G. tonometry
_____ 8. part of routine eye exam of layers of the eye   H. gonioscopy
_____ 9. measurement units used to determine refraction errors   I. diopters

Terms Related to Procedures

Term	Word Origin	Definition
blepharoplasty	*blephar/o* eyelid *-plasty* surgically forming	Forming a new eyelid or restoring an eyelid. May be done to correct blepharoptosis or blepharochalasis (Fig. 13-24).
canthorrhaphy	*canth/o* corner (of eye) *-rrhaphy* suturing	Suturing the upper and lower eyelids to prevent them from opening. Also called **tarsorrhaphy** or **blepharorrhaphy**.
conjunctivoplasty	*conjunctiv/o* conjunctiva *-plasty* surgically forming	Forming a new or restored conjunctiva that may require the use of grafting procedures from the tissue of the cheek or other eye.
cyclodiathermy	*cycl/o* ciliary body *dia-* through *therm/o* temperature, heat *-y* process of, condition	Use of heat to destroy part of the ciliary body for the treatment of glaucoma. Destruction of the ciliary body reduces the amount of aqueous humor, reducing intraocular pressure. If light is used (instead of heat) the procedure is called **cyclophotocoagulation**.
enucleation of eyeball	*e-* out *nucle/o* nucleus *-ation* process of	Removal of the entire eyeball.
evisceration of eyeball	*e-* out *viscer/o* organ *-ation* process of	Removal of the contents of the eyeball, leaving the outer coat (the sclera) intact.

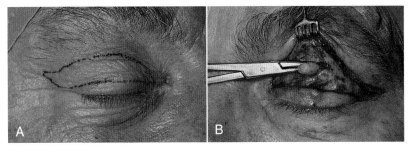

Fig. 13-24 Blepharorrhaphy.

Terms Related to Procedures—cont'd

Term	Word Origin	Definition
iridectomy	*irid/o* iris *-ectomy* cutting out	Cutting out all or part of the iris to allow aqueous humor to flow out of the anterior chamber. Used to treat closed-angle glaucoma.
iridoplasty	*irid/o* iris *-plasty* surgically forming	Forming a new or restored iris with laser treatment that allows the drainage of aqueous humor through an enhanced opening. Used to treat closed-angle glaucoma.
keratectomy	*kerat/o* cornea *-ectomy* cutting out	Cutting out part or all of the cornea to remove a lesion (Fig. 13-25).
keratoplasty	*kerat/o* cornea *-plasty* surgically forming	Forming a new or restored cornea. A transplantation of corneal tissue from a donor or the patient's own (autograft) cornea. May be either a full- or partial-thickness graft.
laser-assisted in-situ keratomileusis (LASIK)	*kerat/o* cornea *-mileusis* Greek word meaning "carving"	Flap procedure in which an excimer laser is used to remove material under the corneal flap. Corrects astigmatism, myopia, and hyperopia (Fig. 13-26).

Continued

 CPT Coding Alert!

Corneal hysteresis is a CPT code title that may cause some medical terminology students to blink! Hysteresis is an examination of the output of a structure based on former inputs. It does NOT relate to the uterus (hyster/o), but is derived from a different Greek word (hysteresis), meaning "a deficiency or to lag." In this case, the procedure is done to assist in the treatment of intraocular pressure and other corneal disorders.

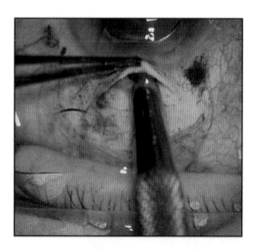

Fig. 13-25 Keratectomy performed using a punch.

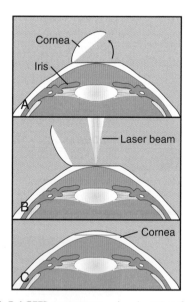

Fig. 13-26 LASIK surgery. A, A microkeratome is used to create a hinged cap of tissue, which is lifted off the cornea. **B,** An excimer laser is used to vaporize and reshape underlying tissue. **C,** Tissue cap is replaced.

To watch a demonstration of LASIK, click on **Animations.**

Terms Related to Procedures—cont'd

Term	Word Origin	Definition
phacoemulsification with/without intraocular lens (IOL)	*phac/o* lens *-emulsification* breaking down	Breaking down and removing the lens (with/without lens implant) to treat cataract. May be intracapsular **(ICCE),** in which the entire lens and capsule are removed, or extracapsular **(ECCE),** in which the lens capsule is left in place (Fig. 13-27).
radial keratotomy	*kerat/o* cornea *-tomy* cutting	Cutting the cornea in a spokelike fashion to flatten it and correct myopia.
tarsorrhaphy	*tars/o* tarsal plate *-rrhaphy* suturing	A partial suturing of the eyelids together (upper and lower lids) to protect the eye.
trabeculectomy	*trabecul/o* trabecula *-ectomy* cutting out	A cutting out of a piece of the trabecular meshwork to create an opening for drainage of the aqueous humor of the eye.
vitrectomy	*vitr/o* vitreous body, glassy *-ectomy* cutting out	Removal of part or all of the vitreous humor. Usually done as part of the procedure (scleral buckling) to treat a retinal detachment. In scleral buckling the vitreous is removed and a buckle is attached to the sclera to hold it away from the detached retinal layer. The sclera then is able to return to its normal proximity to the choroid layer and heal (Fig. 13-28).

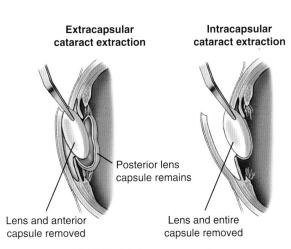

Fig. 13-27 Lens removal.

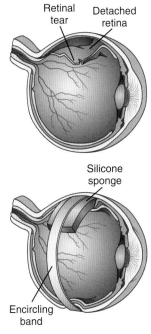

Fig. 13-28 Scleral buckling procedure.

Exercise 7: Procedures

Match the terms to their definitions

____ 1. phacoemulsification
____ 2. canthorrhaphy
____ 3. cyclodiathermy
____ 4. enucleation of eyeball
____ 5. evisceration of eyeball
____ 6. radial keratotomy
____ 7. iridoplasty
____ 8. keratectomy
____ 9. keratoplasty

A. breaking down and removing the lens to treat cataract
B. removal of the entire eyeball
C. cutting out part or all of the cornea to remove a lesion
D. removal of the contents of the eyeball
E. transplantation of corneal tissue from a donor or an autograft
F. suturing the upper and lower eyelids to prevent them from opening
G. forming a new or restored iris with laser treatment
H. use of heat to destroy part of the ciliary body to treat glaucoma
I. cutting the cornea in spokelike fashion to correct myopia

Translate the terms.

10. blepharoplasty_____

11. iridectomy_____

12. conjunctivoplasty_____

13. vitrectomy_____

PHARMACOLOGY

antibiotics: Medications used to treat bacterial infections. Examples include gentamicin (Garamycin) and ciprofloxacin (Ciloxan).

antiglaucoma drugs: Decrease the intraocular pressure by decreasing the amount of fluid in the eye or increasing the drainage. Examples include carbonic anhydrase inhibitors (dorzolamide), cholinergics (pilocarpine), prostaglandin agonists (latanoprost), beta blockers (levobunolol), and alpha-2 agonists (brimonidine).

antihistamines: Drugs used to treat allergic conditions such as itchy or watery eyes. Diphenhydramine (Benadryl) is a common oral OTC product used to treat allergies. Ketotifen (Zaditor) is an example of OTC eye drops.

cycloplegics: Induce paralysis of the ciliary body to allow examination of the eye. One example is atropine (Isopto Atropine) eye drops.

lubricants: Keep the eyes moist, mimicking natural tears.

miotics: Cause the pupils to constrict; often used to treat glaucoma. An example is echothiophate iodide (Phospholine Iodide).

mydriatics: Cause the pupils to dilate; used in diagnostic and refractive examination of the eye. An example is cyclopentolate (Cyclogyl).

ophthalmics: Drugs applied directly to the eye. These may be in the form of solutions or ointments.

topical anesthetics: Temporarily anesthetize the eye for the purpose of examination. An example includes tetracaine (Pliaglis).

Exercise 8: Pharmacology

Matching.

____ 1. used to treat allergic conditions
____ 2. used to constrict pupils
____ 3. used to allow examination of eye by paralyzing ciliary body
____ 4. used to dilate pupils
____ 5. used to keep eyes moist

A. mydriatics
B. cycloplegics
C. antihistamines
D. lubricants
E. miotics

RECOGNIZING SUFFIXES FOR PCS

Now that you've finished reading about the procedures for the eye and adnexa, take a look at this review of the *suffixes* used in their terminology. Each of these suffixes is associated with one or more root operations in the medical surgical section or one of the other categories in PCS.

Suffixes and Root Operations for the Eye and Adnexa

Suffix	Root Operation
-ectomy	Excision, resection
-plasty	Reposition, repair, replacement, supplement
-rrhaphy	Repair
-tomy	Drainage, repair

Abbreviations

Abbreviation	Meaning	Abbreviation	Meaning
ARMD, AMD	age-related macular degeneration	LASIK	laser-assisted in-situ keratomileusis
Astigm, As, Ast	astigmatism	MY	myopia
ECCE	extracapsular cataract extraction	OD	right eye
		OS	left eye
EM, Em	emmetropia	OU	each eye
ICCE	intracapsular cataract extraction	VA	visual acuity test
IOL	intraocular lens	VF	visual field test
IOP	intraocular pressure		

Note: The Institute for Safe Medication Practices has determined that the traditional abbreviations for the eye (OD, OS, OU) are to be considered as dangerous abbreviations because of the ease of confusing the letters used with those traditionally used to indicate the ears. Although these are mentioned, as they may be encountered in medical records, they should not be used. The preferred method of noting left, right, or each eye is to write out the words entirely.

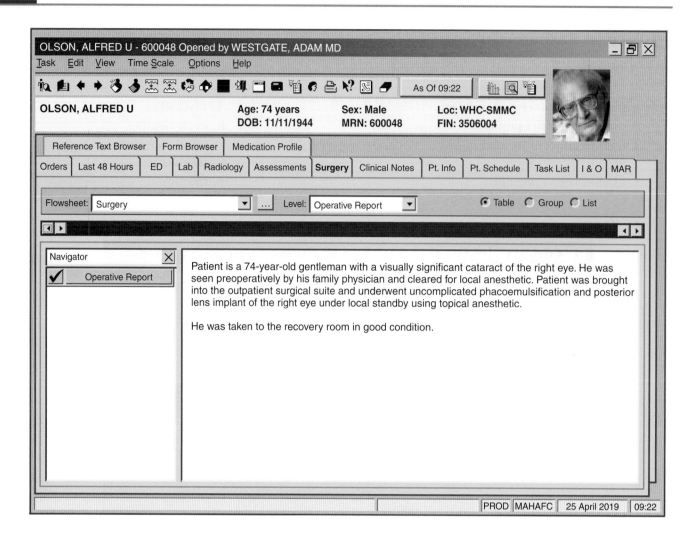

OLSON, ALFRED U - 600048 Opened by WESTGATE, ADAM MD

Task   Edit   View   Time Scale   Options   Help

As Of 09:22

OLSON, ALFRED U   Age: 74 years   Sex: Male   Loc: WHC-SMMC
                             DOB: 11/11/1944   MRN: 600048   FIN: 3506004

Reference Text Browser | Form Browser | Medication Profile

Orders | Last 48 Hours | ED | Lab | Radiology | Assessments | **Surgery** | Clinical Notes | Pt. Info | Pt. Schedule | Task List | I & O | MAR

Flowsheet: Surgery   ...   Level: Operative Report   ● Table   ○ Group   ○ List

Navigator

✓ Operative Report

Patient is a 74-year-old gentleman with a visually significant cataract of the right eye. He was seen preoperatively by his family physician and cleared for local anesthetic. Patient was brought into the outpatient surgical suite and underwent uncomplicated phacoemulsification and posterior lens implant of the right eye under local standby using topical anesthetic.

He was taken to the recovery room in good condition.

PROD MAHAFC 25 April 2019 09:22

Exercise 9: Operative Report

Using the operative report above, answer the following questions.

1. What is the condition that the procedure is intended to correct? _____

2. What does "preoperatively" mean? _____

3. Phacoemulsification means that the lens was _____

4. How do you know that he received a new lens? _____

5. What type of anesthetic was used during the surgery? _____

O'Connor Eye Associates
456 Humphrey St.
Philadelphia, PA 19117

Morgan Ophthalmology Associates
789 Henry Ave.
Philadelphia, PA 19118

August 12, 2021

Re: Mary Ellen Wright, DOB: 4/1/1980

Dear Dr. Morgan:

I have had the pleasure of treating Mary Ellen Wright for the past 11 years. She has asked me to summarize her treatment for you.

Ms. Wright had received comprehensive optometric care from her previous optometrist from 1995 to 2008. Her previous records reflected good binocular oculomotor function and good ocular health, including the absence of posterior vitreous detachment, retinal breaks, or peripheral retinal degeneration in either eye. She specifically denies any incidence of trauma, diplopia, or cephalgia. She also denies any personal or family history of glaucoma, strabismus, retinal disease, diabetes, hypertension, heart disease, or breathing problems. She is on no medications. Refractive correction for compound myopic astigmatism contained the following parameters:

Spectacle Correction: Right eye   7.50 - 1.00 × 165 20/20
                        Left eye   7.50 - 1.00 × 180 20/20
Contact Lenses: Right eye 20/15; Left eye 20/15

The contact lens fit showed a stable paralimbal soft lens fit with good centration, 360 degree corneal coverage, and 0.50 mm movement in each eye. Each lens surface contained a trace amount of scattered protein deposits.

She came for her last comprehensive examination without any visual or ocular complaints. She desired a new supply of disposable contact lenses. She reported clear and comfortable vision at distance, intermediate, and near with both her glasses and contact lenses.

Eye Health Assessment: Slit lamp examination revealed clean lids with good tonicity and apposition to the globe. The lashes and lid margins were clear of debris. There was no discharge from either eye. The corneas were clear with no fluorescein staining either eye. Pupils were equal, round, and reactive to light and accommodation without apparent defect. Intraocular pressures measured 10 mm Hg right eye, left eye at 1:30 pm with Goldmann applanation tonometry.

If any further information is needed, please feel free to contact me regarding this patient.

Sincerely,

Roland O'Connor, OD

Exercise 10: **Healthcare Report**

Using the healthcare report on the previous page, answer the following questions.

1. Mary Ellen denies diplopia and cephalgia. Explain these terms._____
   _____

2. Mary Ellen has been diagnosed with myopic astigmatism. In your own words, explain this visual disorder._____

3. What is the name of the test for glaucoma?_____

4. Explain the term *paralimbal.*_____

Go to Evolve to interactively build terms, label images, memorize word parts, and practice using terms that relate to the eye in context.

Match the word parts to their definitions.

WORD PART DEFINITIONS

Prefix/Suffix
-chalasia
ec-
eso-
extra-
-malacia
-metry
-opia
-opsia
pan-
-plasty
-ptosis
-scopy

Definition
1. _____ drooping, sagging, prolapse
2. _____ measuring
3. _____ viewing
4. _____ outside
5. _____ relaxation, slackening
6. _____ all
7. _____ softening
8. _____ vision condition
9. _____ surgically forming
10. _____ inward
11. _____ vision condition
12. _____ out

Combining Form
blephar/o
canth/o
core/o
cycl/o
dacry/o
dacryoaden/o
dacryocyst/o
goni/o
irid/o
kerat/o
lacrim/o
nyctal/o
ophthalm/o
opt/o
palpebr/o
papill/o
phac/o
phot/o
retin/o
scler/o
scot/o

Definition
13. _____ tears
14. _____ cornea
15. _____ tears
16. _____ eye
17. _____ lacrimal sac
18. _____ ciliary body
19. _____ vision
20. _____ darkness
21. _____ eyelid
22. _____ iris
23. _____ night blindness
24. _____ retina
25. _____ pupil
26. _____ light
27. _____ corner of eye
28. _____ optic disk
29. _____ eyelid
30. _____ angle
31. _____ lacrimal gland
32. _____ lens
33. _____ sclera

WORDSHOP

Prefixes	Combining Forms	Suffixes
a-	blephar/o	-ia
an-	canth/o	-iasis
dia-	chromat/o	-itis
eso-	cor/o	-opia
hemi-	cycl/o	-opsia
hyper-	dacryoaden/o	-phobia
pan-	is/o	-plasty
presby-	kerat/o	-ptosis
	metr/o	-rrhaphy
	mydr/o	-y
	ophthalm/o	
	phak/o	
	phot/o	
	therm/o	
	trop/o	

Build eye terms by combining the word parts above. Some word parts may be used more than once. Some may not be used at all. The number in parentheses indicates the number of word parts needed.

Definition	Term
1. condition of no lens (3)	
2. vision condition of no color (3)	
3. inflammation of the lacrimal gland (2)	
4. drooping of the eyelid (2)	
5. condition of fear of light (2)	
6. vision condition of old age (2)	
7. condition of turning inward (3)	
8. inflammation of all eye (3)	
9. vision condition of excessive measure (3)	
10. condition of not equal pupil (4)	
11. process of heat through the ciliary body (4)	
12. surgically forming the cornea (2)	
13. suturing the corner of the eye (2)	
14. state of dilation (2)	
15. vision condition of without half (3)	

Sort the terms into the correct categories.

TERM SORTING

Anatomy and Physiology	Pathology	Procedures

accommodation

Amsler grid

annulus of Zinn

aphakia

blepharitis

canthorrhaphy

canthus

chalazion

conjunctiva

conjunctivoplasty

cornea

cyclodiathermy

dacryocystitis

diopters

enucleation of eyeball

exophthalmos

fluorescein staining

glaucoma

gonioscopy

hyphema

iridoplasty

iris

keratomalacia

lacrimation

LASIK

limbus

macula lutea

nyctalopia

oculus sinistra

optic papillitis

palpebration

photophobia

pinguecula

pupil

radial keratotomy

retinoblastoma

Schlemm's canal

sclera

scotoma

slit lamp

strabismus

tonometry

uvea

VA

vitrectomy

Replace the highlighted words with the correct terms.

TRANSLATIONS

1. Maria was complaining of **extreme sensitivity to light** and **excessive lacrimation.**

2. Mr. M had **prolonged constriction of the pupil** and **adhesion of the lens to the cornea** and was subsequently diagnosed with **inflammation of the anterior uvea.**

3. The auto accident victim came to the ED with **a condition of unequally sized pupils** and **blood in the anterior chamber of the eye.**

4. During Michael's eye examination, it was discovered that he had red/green **impairment of color vision** and slight **nearsightedness.**

5. Patient R had **swelling of the optic disk.**

6. Rose's **disorder characterized by abnormal intraocular pressure** was tested with **measurement of intraocular pressure.**

7. Terrance had a **forming or restoring an eyelid** to correct his **drooping of the upper eyelid.**

8. The patient had **vitreous humor removed and a buckle attached to the sclera** to correct a **separation of the retina from the choroid layer.**

9. Mrs. Lawrence was worried about her daughter's "squint" and the ophthalmologist diagnosed **lack of coordination between the eyes.**

10. 75-year-old Anna Walker had a **test to assess central vision** and was diagnosed with **progressive destruction of the macula.**

11. A **test to determine the amount of tear production** was used to determine the degree of the patient's dry eye.

12. Mary Kate's **inability to see well in dim light** was a result of **a hereditary degenerative disease marked by a progressive loss of visual field.**

14 Ear and Mastoid Process

OBJECTIVES

☐ Recognize and use terms related to the anatomy and physiology of the ear.

☐ Recognize and use terms related to the pathology of the ear.

☐ Recognize and use terms related to procedures for the ear.

ICD-10-CM Example from Tabular
H92.0 Otalgia
    H92.01 Otalgia, right ear
    H92.02 Otalgia, left ear
    H92.03 Otalgia, bilateral
    H92.09 Otalgia, unspecified ear

ICD-10-PCS Example from Index
Myringectomy
    see Excision, Ear, Nose, Sinus **09B**
    see Resection, Ear, Nose, Sinus **09T**
Myringoplasty
    see Repair, Ear, Nose, Sinus **09Q**
    see Replacement, Ear, Nose, Sinus **09R**
    see Supplement, Ear, Nose, Sinus **09U**
Myringostomy
    see Drainage, Ear, Nose, Sinus **099**
Myringotomy
    see Drainage, Ear, Nose, Sinus **099**

hearing = acous/o,
   audi/o, aur/o, -acusis,
   -cusis

ear = ot/o

stone = petr/o

petrous bone = petros/o

mastoid process =
   mastoid/o

cartilage = chondr/o,
   cartilag/o

auricle, outer ear =
   auricul/o

helix, coil = helic/o

FUNCTIONS OF THE EAR

The ears provide an individual with the sense of **hearing** and balance, or equilibrium.

ANATOMY AND PHYSIOLOGY

The ear is regionally divided into the outer, middle, and inner ear (Fig. 14-1). Sound travels through air, bone, and fluid across these divisions.

The middle and inner ear are contained within the harder, protective petrous portion of the temporal bone. The **mastoid process** is a hard, small projection of the temporal bone full of air cells. Located behind the opening of the **external auditory canal**, the air cells of the mastoid are connected to the middle ear through a cavity termed the *mastoid antrum*. This connection is the conduit for infections from the middle ear to the mastoid process.

Outer (External) Ear

Sound waves are initially gathered by the flesh-covered elastic **cartilage** of the outer ear called the pinna, or **auricle** (Fig. 14-2). The auricular cartilage is folded into several distinct structures with separate names. The **helix** is the upper outer rim of the auricle, whereas the antihelix is the inner curve that is parallel to the helix. The antihelix has two "legs," or **crura** (*sing*, crus), that divide to form a

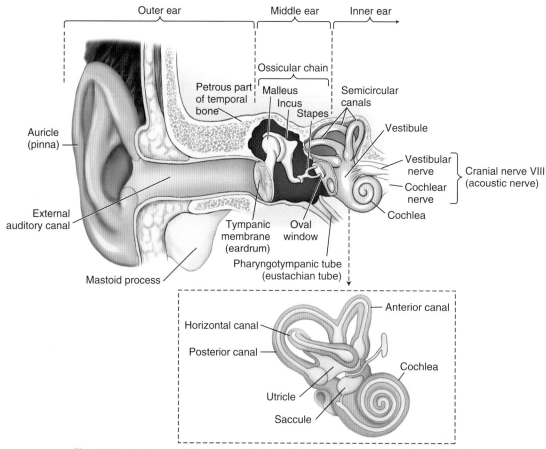

Fig. 14-1 Anatomy of the ear, with detail of the inner ear structures (*inset*).

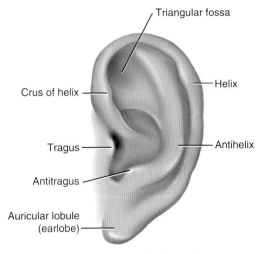

Triangular fossa

Crus of helix

Helix

Tragus

Antihelix

Antitragus

Auricular lobule
(earlobe)

Fig. 14-2 Auricle (pinna).

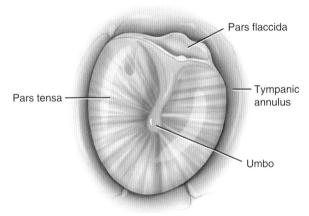

Pars flaccida

Pars tensa

Tympanic
annulus

Umbo

Fig. 14-3 The tympanic membrane.

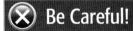

Be Careful!

A helix *is the upper outer rim of the auricle, while a* hallux *is the 1st (great) toe.*

shallow depression between them, referred to as the triangular fossa. The **tragus** is the fleshy tag of tissue with a tuft of hair on its underside that covers the opening of the external auditory canal. The antitragus is the small raised prominence that is opposite to the tragus. It is important to remember that elastic cartilage is covered by a layer of connective tissue called perichondrium. When this is separated from the cartilage by trauma, deformities of the pinna may occur. The **lobule**, usually referred to as the earlobe, is the only noncartilaginous part of the external ear. This fleshy protuberance is composed of adipose tissue.

The gathered sound is then funneled into the external auditory canal. The opening of the auditory canal is termed the **auditory** (acoustic) **meatus**. Earwax, or **cerumen**, is secreted by modified sweat glands within the external auditory canal and protects the ear with its antiseptic property and its stickiness, trapping foreign debris. It is moved out of the ear by the chewing movement of the jaw.

The **tympanic membrane (TM)**, or **eardrum**, marks the end of the external ear and the beginning of the middle ear (Fig. 14-3). This concave membrane of the eardrum is attached to an almost complete ring of bone called the tympanic annulus. The membrane is composed of a thick, taut part (the pars tensa) and a thin, flexible part (the pars flaccida). The center of the membrane is pulled inward, forming a shallow depression termed the *umbo*. Because the membrane is extremely delicate and vulnerable to perforation and infection, the additional terms naming structures of the eardrum are necessary to specify where an injury may occur.

perichondrium
  peri- = surrounding
  chondro/o = cartilage
  -ium = structure

cerumen = cerumin/o

**tympanic membrane,
  eardrum = tympan/o,
  myring/o**

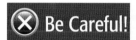

This chapter includes all the anatomy necessary to assign ICD-10 ear codes, including detail on the ossicular chain, the tympanic annulus, and the umbo. See Appendix H for a complete list of body parts and how they should be coded.

Middle Ear

The eardrum conducts sound to the air-filled tympanic cavity of the middle ear. The **eustachian tube**, also called the **auditory tube** or the **pharyngotympanic tube**, is a mucous membrane–lined connection between the middle ear and the throat. It functions to supply air for sound conduction and pressure equalization.

The three tiny bones in the middle ear are called the **ossicles**, or the **ossicular chain**, and are named for their shapes: the **malleus**, or hammer; the **incus** or anvil; and the **stapes** (*pl.* stapedes), or stirrup. The ossicles transmit the sound to the **oval window** through the stapes. The main cavity of the middle ear, opposite the tympanic membrane, is termed the *tympanic cavity proper*. Above the level of the eardrum is a separate space called the epitympanic recess, or attic. The attic contains the head of the malleus and the body of the incus. CPT uses the combining form attic/o in procedures related to the attic of the middle ear.

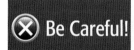

Be Careful! The combining form **salping/o** *can be used to name both the* fallopian tube and the eustachian tube.

Be Careful! **Malleus** *refers to one of the ossicles in the ear, whereas a* **malleolus** *may be one of the processes on the distal tibia and* fibula.

Inner Ear

Once sound is conducted to the oval window, it is transmitted to a structure called the **labyrinth**, or the inner ear. A membranous labyrinth is enclosed within a bony labyrinth. Between the two, and surrounding the inner labyrinth, is a fluid called **perilymph**. Within the membranous labyrinth is a fluid called **endolymph**. Hair cells within the inner ear fluids act as nerve endings that function as sensory receptors for hearing and equilibrium. Tiny calcium carbonate crystals called otoliths are attached to these hair cells and act as receptors to aid in balance. The outer, bony labyrinth is composed of three parts: the **vestibule**, the **semicircular canals**, and the **cochlea.** The vestibule and semicircular canals provide information about the body's sense of equilibrium, whereas the cochlea is an organ of hearing. Within the vestibule, two structures called the utricle and the saccule function to determine the body's static (nonmoving) equilibrium (Fig. 14-1, *inset*). A specialized patch of epithelium, called the **macula**, found in both the utricle and the saccule, provides information about the position of the head and a sense of acceleration and deceleration. The semicircular canals detect dynamic equilibrium or a sense of sudden rotation through the function of a structure called the **crista ampullaris**.

The cochlea receives the vibrations from the perilymph and transmits them to the cochlear duct, which is filled with endolymph. The transmission of sound continues through the endolymph to the **organ of Corti**, where the hearing receptor cells (hairs) stimulate a branch of the eighth cranial nerve, the **vestibulocochlear nerve**, to transmit the information to the temporal lobe of the brain.

Be Careful! *Do not confuse* **oral**, *meaning* pertaining to the mouth, *with* **aural**, *meaning* pertaining to the ear.

---

eustachian tube =
   salping/o

pharynotympanic
   pharyng/o = throat
   tympan/o = eardrum
   -ic = pertaining to

ossicle = ossicul/o

stapes = staped/o

epi- = above

labyrinth, inner ear =
   labyrinth/o

perilymph
   peri- = surrounding
   lymph/o = lymph

endolymph
   endo- = within
   lymph/o = lymph

otolith
   ot/o = ear
   lith/o = stone

vestibule = vestibul/o

cochlea = cochle/o

macula = macul/o

You can review the anatomy of the ear by clicking on **Body Spectrum**, then **Senses**.

 Exercise 1: **Anatomy of the Ear**

Match the combining forms with the correct parts of the ear. More than one answer may be correct.

_____ 1. eardrum
_____ 2. bone of the middle ear
_____ 3. stone
_____ 4. inner ear
_____ 5. hearing
_____ 6. eustachian tube
_____ 7. ear
_____ 8. stirrup-shaped ear bone
_____ 9. earwax
_____ 10. coil, helix
_____ 11. throat
_____ 12. cartilage

A. labyrinth/o
B. ossicul/o
C. cerumin/o
D. staped/o
E. myring/o
F. salping/o
G. chondr/o
H. audi/o
I. tympan/o
J. aur/o
K. petr/o
L. helic/o
M. pharyng/o
N. ot/o

Fill in the blanks.

13. The mucous membrane–lined structure that connects the ear to the throat is the _____.

14. The _____ is a hard, small projection of the temporal bone full of air cells.

15. The ear is regionally divided into the _____, _____, and _____ ears.

16. Another word for outer ear is _____ or _____.

17. The outer, bony labyrinth is composed of three parts: the _____, the_____,

and the _____.

18. The _____ and the _____ function within the vestibule to determine the

body's static (nonmoving) equilibrium.

To practice labeling the parts of the ear, click on **Label It**.

Combining Forms for Anatomy and Physiology of the Ear

Meaning	Combining Form	Meaning	Combining Form
antrum	antr/o	helix, coil	helic/o
auricle, pinna	auricul/o	labyrinth, inner ear	labyrinth/o
cartilage	chondr/o, cartilag/o	mastoid process	mastoid/o
cerumen, earwax	cerumin/o	ossicle, small bone	ossicul/o
cochlea	cochle/o	petrous bone	petros/o
ear	ot/o	spot, macula	macul/o
eardrum	tympan/o, myring/o	stapes	staped/o
eustachian tube	salping/o	stone	petr/o, lith/o
hearing	acous/o, audi/o, aur/o	vestibule	vestibul/o

Suffixes for Anatomy and Physiology of the Ear

Suffix	Meaning
-cusis, -acusis	hearing

PATHOLOGY

 CM Guideline Alert

B13. LATERALITY
Some ICD-10-CM codes indicate laterality, specifying whether the condition occurs on the left, right or is bilateral. If no bilateral code is provided and the condition is bilateral, assign separate codes for both the left and right side. If the side is not identified in the medical record, assign the code for the unspecified side.

Terms Related to Diseases of the External Ear (H60-H62)

Term	Word Origin	Definition
cholesteatoma, external ear	*chol/e* bile *steat/o* fat *-oma* mass, tumor	Cystic mass composed of epithelial cells and cholesterol. Can occur also in middle ear (Fig. 14-4).
exostosis of external ear	*ex-* out *oste/o* bone *-osis* abnormal condition	Bony growth usually due to chronic irritation.
otitis externa	*ot/o* ear *-itis* inflammation *extern/o* outer *-a* noun ending	Inflammation of the pinna/auricle (Fig. 14-5).
perichondritis, auricular	*peri-* around, surrounding *chondr/o* cartilage *-itis* inflammation	Inflammation of the perichondrium of the external ear. May result in a deformity referred to as "cauliflower ear."
stenosis of external ear canal, acquired	*stenosis* abnormal condition of narrowing	A narrowing of the auditory canal that develops after birth.

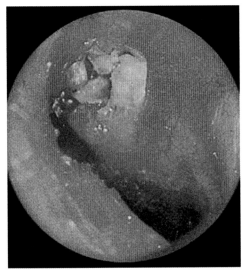

Fig. 14-4 Cholesteatoma.

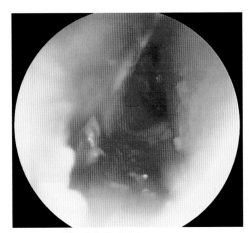

Fig. 14-5 Otitis externa.

Terms Related to Diseases of Middle Ear and Mastoid (H65-H75)

Term	Word Origin	Definition
ankylosis of ear ossicles	*ankyl/o* stiff *-osis* abnormal condition	Abnormal condition of stiffening of the tiny bones of the ear.
cholesteatoma of attic	*chol/e* bile *steat/o* fat *-oma* mass, tumor	Cystic mass of epithelial cells and cholesterol in the epitympanic recess.
eustachian salpingitis	*salping/o* eustachian tube *-itis* inflammation	Inflammation of the eustachian tube.
mastoiditis	*mastoid/o* mastoid process *-itis* inflammation	Inflammation of the mastoid process.

Terms Related to Diseases of Middle Ear and Mastoid (H65-H75)—cont'd

Term	Word Origin	Definition
myringitis	*myring/o* eardrum *-itis* inflammation	Inflammation of the eardrum. May be acute, chronic, or bullous (from the Latin meaning a bubble, but generally referring to a condition of blistering).
otitis media (OM)	*ot/o* ear *-itis* inflammation *medi/o* middle *-a* noun ending	Inflammation of the middle ear (Fig. 14-6). May be **suppurative** (as a result of an infection) or **nonsuppurative**, without infection. Nonsuppurative can be serous (with fluid) or sanguineous (with bloody discharge).
patulous eustachian tube	*patul/o* open *-ous* pertaining to	A continually open eustachian tube.
perforation of tympanic membrane	*tympan/o* eardrum *-ic* pertaining to	A puncture of the eardrum (Fig. 14-7).
petrositis	*petros/o* petrous bone *-itis* inflammation	Inflammation of the petrous portion of the temporal bone.
tympanosclerosis	*tympan/o* eardrum *-sclerosis* abnormal condition of hardening	Abnormal hardening of the eardrum. May be a result of scarring from use of polyethylene ventilating tubes to assist in drainage.

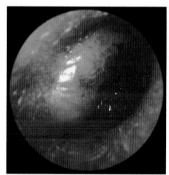

Fig. 14-6 Otitis media. Tympanic membrane is erythematous, opaque, and bulging.

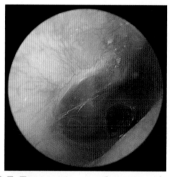

Fig. 14-7 Tympanic membrane perforation.

 Exercise 2: Diseases of the External and Middle Ear and Mastoid

Match the terms to their definitions.

_____ 1. stenosis of external ear canal
_____ 2. exostosis of external ear
_____ 3. perichondritis (auricular)
_____ 4. ankylosis of ear ossicles
_____ 5. eustachian salpingitis
_____ 6. petrositis
_____ 7. otitis externa
_____ 8. myringitis

A. narrowing of the auditory canal that develops after birth
B. abnormal condition of stiffening of the tiny bones of the ear
C. inflammation of the petrous portion of the temporal bone
D. inflammation of the pinna
E. "cauliflower ear"
F. inflammation of the eardrum
G. inflammation of the eustachian tube
H. bony growth usually due to chronic irritation

Translate the following terms.

9. tympanosclerosis_____

10. cholesteatoma_____

11. otitis media_____

Terms Related to Diseases of Inner Ear (H80-H83)

Term	Word Origin	Definition
aural vertigo	*aur/o* hearing *-al* pertaining to *vert/o* turn *-igo* condition	Dizziness associated with a disorder of the ear.
labyrinthitis	*labyrinth/o* inner ear, labyrinth *-itis* inflammation	Inflammation of the labyrinth, the inner ear.
Ménière's disease		Chronic condition of the inner ear characterized by vertigo, hearing loss, and tinnitus. Of unknown etiology.
otosclerosis	*ot/o* ear *-sclerosis* abnormal condition of hardening	Abnormal condition of hardening of the inner ear characterized by a development of spongy bone that can grow toward or away from the oval window. Usually results in progressive deafness. Also termed **vestibular neuritis**. Symptoms may be loss of balance and dizziness.
vestibular neuronitis	*vestibul/o* vestibule *-ar* pertaining to *neuron/o* nerve *-itis* inflammation	Inflammation of the vestibular nerve.

Terms Related to Other Disorders of the Ear (H90-H94)

Term	Word Origin	Definition
conductive hearing loss	*con-* with *duct/o* carry *-ive* pertaining to	Hearing loss resulting from damage to or malformation of the middle or outer ear.
diplacusis	*dipl/o* double *-acusis* hearing	Hearing disorder characterized by the perception of a single sound being two.
hyperacusis	*hyper-* above, excessive *-acusis* hearing	Hearing that is above normal. Patient is able to hear more acutely than normal.
otalgia	*ot/o* ear *-algia* pain	Pain in the ear. An earache.
otorrhagia	*ot/o* ear *-rrhagia* bursting forth	A rapid discharge of blood from one or both ears.
otorrhea	*ot/o* ear *-rrhea* discharge, flow	A discharge from the ears. If the discharge is purulent (pus filled), it is termed **otopyorrhea**.

Terms Related to Other Disorders of the Ear (H90-H94)—cont'd

Term	Word Origin	Definition
ototoxic hearing loss	*ot/o* ear *tox/o* poison *-ic* pertaining to	Hearing loss that is drug-induced.
presbycusis	*presby-* old age *-cusis* hearing	Loss of hearing due to the aging process.
sensorineural hearing loss	*sensor/i* sense *neur/o* nerve *-al* pertaining to	Hearing loss resulting from damage to the cochlea of the inner ear or auditory nerve.
tinnitus	*tinnit/o* jingling *-us* noun ending	Ringing in the ears.
transient ischemic deafness	*isch/o* hold back *-emic* blood condition	Intermittent hearing loss due to a lack of blood supply to the ear.

Terms Related to Benign Neoplasms

Term	Word Origin	Definition
acoustic neuroma	*acous/o* hearing *-tic* pertaining to *neur/o* nerve *-oma* mass, tumor	A benign tumor of the eighth cranial nerve (vestibulocochlear) that causes tinnitus, vertigo, and hearing loss. Also called **vestibular schwannoma**.
ceruminoma	*cerumin/o* cerumen, earwax *-oma* mass, tumor	A benign adenoma of the glands that produce earwax.

Exercise 3: Disorders of the Inner Ear, Other Disorders of the Ear, and Neoplasms

Fill in the blank.

_____ 1. otorrhagia
_____ 2. labyrinthitis
_____ 3. aural vertigo
_____ 4. ototoxic hearing loss
_____ 5. presbycusis
_____ 6. tinnitus
_____ 7. transient ischemic deafness
_____ 8. sensorineural hearing loss

A. dizziness caused by an ear disorder
B. hearing loss due to poisoning
C. ringing in the ears
D. hearing loss due to cochlea or auditory nerve damage
E. rapid discharge of blood from one or both ears
F. intermittent hearing loss due to lack of blood supply to the ear
G. hearing loss due to age
H. inflammation of the inner ear

Build the terms.

9. excessive hearing _____

10. inflammation of the inner ear _____

11. discharge from the ear _____

12. pain of the ear _____

13. mass of earwax _____

PROCEDURES

PCS Guideline Alert

BILATERAL BODY PART VALUES
B4.3 Bilateral body part values are available for a limited number of body parts. If the identical procedure is performed on contralateral body parts, and a bilateral body part value exists for that body part, a single procedure is coded using the bilateral body part value. If no bilateral body part value exists, each procedure is coded separately using the appropriate body part value.

CPT Coding Alert!

CPT details structures within the middle ear that ICD-10-PCS groups together. For example, an atticotomy is a cutting into the epitympanic recess to treat a cholesteatoma (a cystic mass of epithelial cells and cholesterol) of the middle ear.

Terms Related to Procedures of the Ear

Term	Word Origin	Definition
audiology, diagnostic	*audi/o* hearing *-logy* study of	A diagnostic study of an individual's ability to hear.
audiometry	*audi/o* hearing *-metry* measuring	The process of measuring hearing, usually with an instrument called an **audiometer**. The graphic representation of the results is called an **audiogram** (Fig. 14-8).
cochlear implant	*cochle/o* cochlea *-ar* pertaining to	Implanted device that assists those with hearing loss by electrically stimulating the cochlea (Fig. 14-9).
electrocochleography (ECOG)	*electr/o* electricity *cochle/o* cochlea *-graphy* recording	Recording the electrical activity of the cochlea to test hearing.

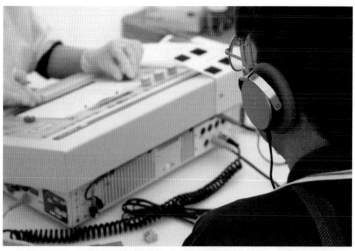

Fig. 14-8 Audiometry.

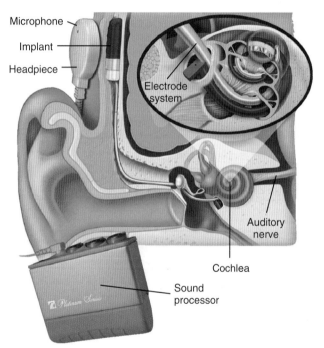

Microphone

Implant

Headpiece

Electrode system

Auditory nerve

Cochlea

Sound processor

Fig. 14-9 Cochlear implant.

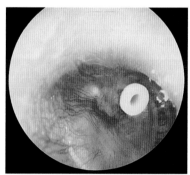

Fig. 14-10 Myringostomy tube in place.

Terms Related to to Procedures of the Ear—cont'd

Term	Word Origin	Definition
mastoidectomy	*mastoid/o* mastoid *-ectomy* cutting out	Cutting out part or all of the mastoid process to treat necrotic mastoiditis.
myringostomy	*myring/o* eardrum *-stomy* creating a new opening	Making a new opening in the eardrum. Done to promote drainage and/or allow the introduction of artificial tubes to maintain the opening (Fig. 14-10). Also called a **tympanostomy.**

Click on **Animations** to see a demonstration of a myringotomy.

Terms Related to to Procedures of the Ear—cont'd

Term	Word Origin	Definition
myringotomy	*myring/o* eardrum *-tomy* cutting	Cutting the eardrum to drain pus. Also called a **tympanotomy.**
ossiculectomy	*ossicul/o* small bone *-ectomy* cutting out	Cutting out part or all of the ossicles of the ear to treat ankylosis of ear ossicles.
otoplasty	*ot/o* ear *-plasty* surgically forming	Forming part or all of the ear. Done to correct malformations of the ear.
otoscopy	*ot/o* ear *-scopy* viewing	Process of viewing the ear using an **otoscope.**
paracentesis of tympanum	*para-* near, beside *-centesis* surgical puncture	Surgical puncture of the eardrum to drain fluids resulting from otitis media.
stapediolysis	*staped/o* stapes *-lysis* breaking down	Releasing the stapes to restore hearing in cases of otosclerosis.
stapedoplasty	*staped/o* stapes *-plasty* surgically forming	Forming part or all of the stapes. Reconstruction performed to restore hearing.
tympanometry	*tympan/o* eardrum, tympanum *-metry* measuring	Process of measuring the eardrum. A tympanogram is the resulting record. A **tympanometer** is the instrument that measures the function of the eardrum.
tympanoplasty	*tympan/o* eardrum, tympanum *-plasty* surgically forming	Forming part or all of the eardrum to reconstruct a perforated eardrum.
Universal Newborn Hearing Screening (UNHS) test		Test that uses otoacoustic emissions (OAEs), which are measured by the insertion of a probe into the baby's ear canal, and auditory brainstem response (ABR), which involves the placement of four electrodes on the baby's head to measure the change in electrical activity of the brain in response to sound while the baby is sleeping.

PCS Guideline Alert

B3.11a Inspection of a body part(s) performed in order to achieve the objective of a procedure is not coded separately.

Exercise 4: **Procedures**

Match the term to its definition.

___ 1. paracentesis of tympanum	A. surgical puncture of the eardrum
___ 2. ECOG	B. forming part or all of the stapes
___ 3. myringotomy	C. cutting the eardrum
___ 4. stapediolysis	D. cutting out part or all of the mastoid process
___ 5. mastoidectomy	E. forming part or all of the eardrum
___ 6. otoscopy	F. record of the eardrum
___ 7. ossiculectomy	G. recording the electrical activity of the cochlea to test hearing
___ 8. tympanogram	H. cutting out part or all of the ossicles
___ 9. stapedoplasty	I. process of viewing the ear
___ 10. tympanoplasty	J. releasing the stapes

Translate the following terms.

11. tympanometry_____

12. otoplasty_____

13. audiometry_____

PHARMACOLOGY

antibiotics: Treat bacterial infections. A commonly used oral agent to treat ear infections is amoxicillin (Amoxil). A topical example is ciprofloxacin with hydrocortisone (Cipro HC Otic).

ceruminolytics: Soften and break down earwax. An example is carbamide peroxide (Debrox).

decongestants: Relieve congestion associated with a cold, allergy, or sinus pressure. These drugs may be available as a nasal spray or an oral product. Examples include oxymetazoline (Kovanaze) and pseudoephedrine (Sudafed).

otics: Drugs applied directly to the external ear canal. These may be administered in the form of solutions, suspensions, or ointments.

 Exercise 5: **Pharmacology**

Matching.

___ 1. otics	A. drugs used to treat infection
___ 2. ceruminolytics	B. drugs used to relieve congestion
___ 3. antibiotics	C. drugs applied to the external ear canal
___ 4. decongestants	D. medications to soften and break down earwax

RECOGNIZING SUFFIXES FOR PCS

Now that you've finished reading about the procedures for the ear, take a look at this review of the *suffixes* used in their terminology. Each of these suffixes is associated with one or more root operations in the medical surgical section or one of the other categories in PCS.

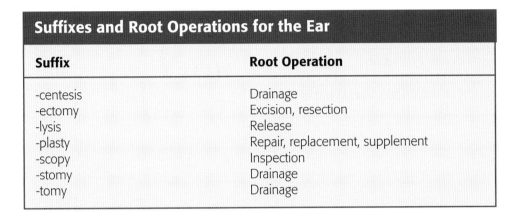

Suffixes and Root Operations for the Ear

Suffix	Root Operation
-centesis	Drainage
-ectomy	Excision, resection
-lysis	Release
-plasty	Repair, replacement, supplement
-scopy	Inspection
-stomy	Drainage
-tomy	Drainage

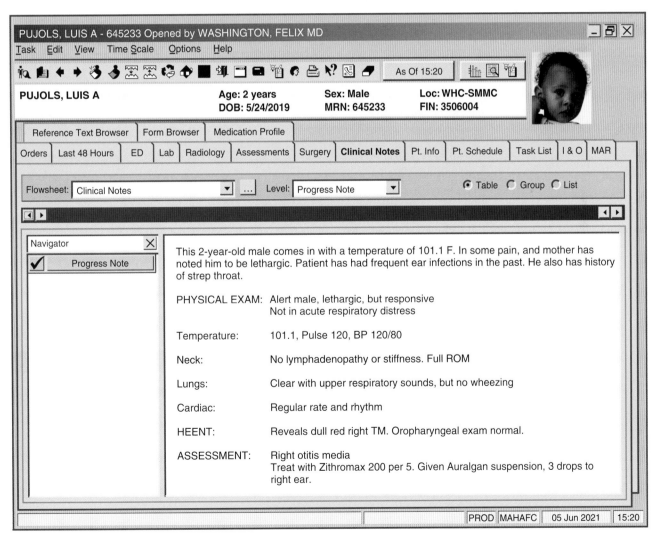

PUJOLS, LUIS A - 645233 Opened by WASHINGTON, FELIX MD

Task Edit View Time Scale Options Help

PUJOLS, LUIS A

| | Age: 2 years | Sex: Male | Loc: WHC-SMMC |
| | DOB: 5/24/2019 | MRN: 645233 | FIN: 3506004 |

Reference Text Browser | Form Browser | Medication Profile

Orders | Last 48 Hours | ED | Lab | Radiology | Assessments | Surgery | **Clinical Notes** | Pt. Info | Pt. Schedule | Task List | I & O | MAR

Flowsheet: Clinical Notes   Level: Progress Note   ⦿ Table ○ Group ○ List

Navigator

✓ Progress Note

This 2-year-old male comes in with a temperature of 101.1 F. In some pain, and mother has noted him to be lethargic. Patient has had frequent ear infections in the past. He also has history of strep throat.

PHYSICAL EXAM: Alert male, lethargic, but responsive
Not in acute respiratory distress

Temperature: 101.1, Pulse 120, BP 120/80

Neck: No lymphadenopathy or stiffness. Full ROM

Lungs: Clear with upper respiratory sounds, but no wheezing

Cardiac: Regular rate and rhythm

HEENT: Reveals dull red right TM. Oropharyngeal exam normal.

ASSESSMENT: Right otitis media
Treat with Zithromax 200 per 5. Given Auralgan suspension, 3 drops to right ear.

PROD | MAHAFC | 05 Jun 2021 | 15:20

Exercise 6: Progress Note

Using the progress note on the previous page, answer the following questions.

1. How do you know that the patient had no disease of his lymph glands? _____
_____

2. What term tells you that the patient did not exhibit a whistling sound made during breathing? _____
_____

3. The patient's right eardrum is examined and is found to be dull and red. What do you think TM stands
for? _____

4. What area of the throat appears normal on exam? _____
_____

5. The diagnosis is an inflammation of the middle ear. What is the term? _____
_____

Abbreviations

Abbreviation	Meaning	Abbreviation	Meaning
ABR	auditory brainstem response	UNHS	universal newborn hearing screening
ECOG	electrocochleography	AS	left ear
OAEs	otoacoustic emissions	AD	right ear
OM	otitis media	AU	each ear
TM	tympanic membrane		

Note: The Institute for Safe Medication Practices has determined that the traditional abbreviations for the ear (AS, AD, AU) are to be considered as Dangerous Abbreviations because of the ease of confusing the letters used with those traditionally used to indicate the eyes. Although these are mentioned, as they may be encountered in medical records, they should not be used. The preferred method of noting left, right, or each ear is to write out the words entirely.

Go to Evolve to interactively build terms, label images, memorize word parts, and practice using terms related to the ear in context.

Match the word parts to their definitions.

WORD PART DEFINITIONS

Prefix/Suffix
-acusis
endo-
-metry
-oma
peri-
-plasty
presby-
-sclerosis

Definition
1. _____old age
2. _____hearing
3. _____surgically forming
4. _____tumor, mass
5. _____surrounding
6. _____within
7. _____measuring
8. _____abnormal condition of hardening

Combining Form
acous/o
audi/o
auricul/o
cerumin/o
chondr/o
helic/o
labyrinth/o
myring/o
ot/o
salping/o
staped/o
tympan/o

Definition
9. _____stapes
10. _____helix, coil
11. _____earwax
12. _____eardrum
13. _____hearing
14. _____outer ear
15. _____cartilage
16. _____hearing
17. _____ear
18. _____inner ear
19. _____eardrum
20. _____eustachian tube

WORDSHOP

Prefixes	Combining Forms	Suffixes
hyper-	acous/o	-acusis
peri-	audi/o	-cusis
presby-	chol/e	-graphy
	chondr/o	-ia
	cochle/o	-ic
	dipl/o	-itis
	electr/o	-ium
	labyrinth/o	-lysis
	myring/o	-metry
	ot/o	-oma
	pharyng/o	-plasty
	staped/o	-rrhea
	steat/o	-sclerosis
	tympan/o	-tomy

Build ear terms by combining the word parts above. Some word parts may be used more than once. Some may not be used at all. The number in parentheses indicates the number of word parts needed.

Definition	Term
1. discharge, flow from the ear (2)	
2. old age hearing (2)	
3. surgically forming the eardrum (2)	
4. abnormal condition of hardening of the ear (2)	
5. inflammation of the inner ear (2)	
6. measuring hearing (2)	
7. structure surrounding cartilage (3)	
8. pertaining to the throat and eardrum (3)	
9. hearing double (2)	
10. excessive hearing (2)	
11. forming the stapes (2)	
12. cutting the eardrum (2)	
13. recording the electricity of the cochlea (3)	
14. tumor of bile fat (3)	

Sort the terms below into the correct categories.

TERM SORTING

Anatomy and Physiology	Pathology	Procedures

acoustic neuroma

audiometry

auricle

cerumen

ceruminoma

cochlea

cochlear implant

diplacusis

ECOG

endolymph

eustachian tube

helix

labyrinth

mastoidectomy

mastoiditis

Ménière's disease

myringitis

myringostomy

OM

organ of Corti

ossiculectomy

otalgia

otitis externa

otoplasty

otorrhea

otosclerosis

otoscopy

pinna

presbycusis

stapediolysis

stapes

tinnitus

tympanic membrane

tympanometry

tympanosclerosis

vestibule

UNHS

Replace the highlighted words with the correct terms.

TRANSLATIONS

1. The pediatrician used an **instrument to view the ear** to diagnose baby Grace's **inflammation of the middle ear.**

   _____
   _____

2. The 80-year-old patient was evaluated using **process of measuring hearing** and was found to have **loss of hearing due to the aging process.**

   _____
   _____
   _____

3. Mrs. M came to the ED complaining of **ringing in the ears** and vertigo and was eventually diagnosed with **benign tumor of the eighth cranial nerve.**

   _____
   _____
   _____

4. A bilateral **forming part of all of the ear** was performed to correct the patient's damaged earlobe.

   _____
   _____

5. Carl's hearing loss was caused by **development of bone around the oval window.**

   _____
   _____

6. Reginald's chronic **inflammation of the mastoid process** was treated with a **cutting out part or all of the mastoid process.**

   _____
   _____
   _____

7. Marcy Dielman had a **cutting out part or all of the ossicles of the ear** to treat her **abnormal condition of stiffening of the tiny bones of the ear.**

   _____
   _____
   _____

8. **Inflammation of the eustachian tube** and **inflammation of the eardrum** were making the child acutely uncomfortable.

   _____
   _____

9. Patient X was diagnosed with **abnormal hardening of the eardrum.**

   _____
   _____

10. Aurora Catalano was suffering from an unusual condition called **hearing disorder characterized by the perception of a single sound being two.**

    _____
    _____

Endocrine System and Nutritional and Metabolic Diseases

OBJECTIVES

☐ Recognize and use terms related to the anatomy and physiology of the endocrine system.

☐ Recognize and use terms related to the pathology of the endocrine system.

☐ Recognize and use terms related to the procedures for the endocrine system.

ICD-10-CM Example from Tabular

E20 Hypoparathyroidism

Excludes1 DiGeorge's syndrome (**D82.1**)

Postprocedural hypoparathyroidism (**E89.2**)

Tetany, NOS (**R29. 0**)

Transitory neonatal hypoparathyroidism (**P71.4**)

E20.0 Idiopathic hypoparathyroidism

E20.1 Pseudohypoparathyroidism

E20.8 Other hypoparathyroidism

E20.9 Hypoparathyroidism, unspecified

Parathyroid tetany

ICD-10-PCS Example from Index

Adrenalectomy

see Excision, Endocrine System **0GB**

see Resection, Endocrine System **0GT**

Adrenalorrhaphy

see Repair, Endocrine System **0GQ**

Adrenalotomy

see Drainage, Endocrine System **0G9**

FUNCTIONS OF THE ENDOCRINE SYSTEM

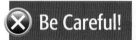

endocrine
endo- = within
-crine = to secrete

The **endocrine** and nervous systems work together and separately to achieve the delicate physiological balance necessary for survival, termed *homeostasis*. Whereas the nervous system uses electrical impulses and chemicals termed *neurotransmitters*, the endocrine system secretes chemical messengers called **hormones** into the bloodstream. Hormones play a major role in the regulation of **metabolism** (the conversion of energy), and nutritional disorders may be a cause or result of endocrine dysfunction. The term *neuroendocrine*, as in the term *neuroendocrine tumors*, is a recognition of the close relationship between the two systems. Nervous stimulation of the posterior lobe of the pituitary (neurohypophysis) causes secretion of hormones ADH and oxytocin.

> ⊗ **Be Careful!**   *Do not confuse* **aden/o,** *which means* gland, *with* **adren/o,** *which means the* adrenal gland.

ANATOMY AND PHYSIOLOGY

The endocrine system is composed of several single and paired ductless glands that secrete hormones into the bloodstream. The hormones regulate specific body functions by acting on target cells with receptor sites for those particular hormones only. See Fig. 15-1 for an illustration of the body with the locations of the endocrine glands.

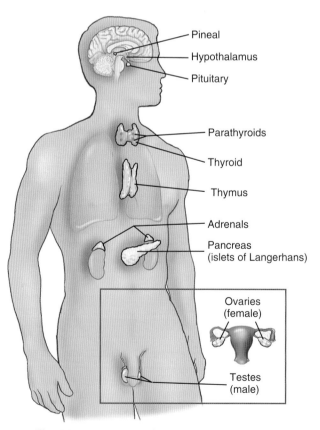

Fig. 15-1 Locations of the endocrine glands.

This chapter includes all the anatomy necessary to assign ICD-10 endocrine system codes, including detail on the mammillary body and the adenohypophysis. See Appendix H for a complete list of body parts and how they should be coded.

Pay attention to the General Guidelines for laterality for the endocrine system. Although some glands are singular, they may be coded for right and left segments.

Pituitary Gland

The **pituitary gland,** also known as the **hypophysis,** is a tiny gland located behind the optic nerve in the cranial cavity in a depression in the sphenoid bone called the **sella turcica.** The **hypothalamic infundibulum,** named for its funnel-like appearance, is the structure that attaches the pituitary to the hypothalamus directly superior to it in the brain. Sometimes called the *master gland* because of its role in controlling the functions of other endocrine glands, the hypophysis is composed of anterior and posterior lobes, each with their own function.

The **anterior lobe,** or **adenohypophysis,** is composed of glandular tissue and secretes hormones in response to stimulation by the hypothalamus. The **hypothalamus** sends hormones through blood vessels, which cause the adenohypophysis either to release or to inhibit the release of specific hormones. The adenohypophysis has a wide range of effects on the body, as Fig. 15-2 and the table below illustrate.

The **posterior lobe (neurohypophysis)** of the pituitary gland is composed of nervous tissue. The hormones that it secretes are produced in the hypothalamus, transported to the neurohypophysis directly through the tissue connecting the organs, and released from storage in the posterior lobe by neural stimulation from the hypothalamus. The two hormones released by this lobe are **antidiuretic hormone (ADH)** and **oxytocin (OT).** See the following table and Fig. 15-2 for the hormones secreted by the neurohypophysis and their effects.

pituitary gland =
   hypophys/o,
   pituitar/o, pituit/o

gland = **aden/o**

turning = **trop/o**

lobe = **lob/o**

hypothalamus
   hypo- = under, deficient
   thalam/o = thalamus
   -us = structure

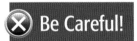 **Be Careful!**   *The combining form* **trop/o** *means* turning, *whereas* **troph/o** *means* development *or* nourishment.

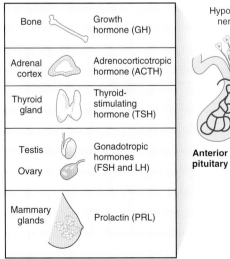

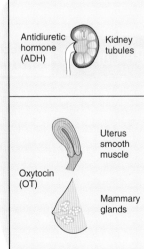

Fig. 15-2 Pituitary hormones. Principal anterior and posterior pituitary hormones and their target organs.

Adenohypophysis Hormones and Their Effects

Adenohypophysis Hormones	Effect
Adrenocorticotropic hormone (ACTH)	Stimulates the adrenal cortex to release steroids.
Gonadotropic hormones (includes **follicle-stimulating hormone [FSH]**, **luteinizing hormone [LH]**, and **interstitial cell-stimulating hormone [ICSH]**)	FSH stimulates the development of gametes in the respective sexes. LH stimulates ovulation in the female and the secretion of sex hormones in both the male and the female. ICSH stimulates production of reproductive cells in the male.
Growth hormone (GH) (also called **human growth hormone [hGH]** or **somatotropin hormone [STH]**)	Stimulates growth of long bones and skeletal muscle; converts proteins to glucose.
Prolactin (PRL) (also called **lactogenic hormone**)	Stimulates milk production in the breast.
Thyrotropin (also called **thyroid-stimulating hormone [TSH]**)	Stimulates thyroid to release two other thyroid hormones.

Neurohypophysis Hormones and Their Effects

Neurohypophysis Hormones	Effect
Antidiuretic hormone (ADH) (also called **vasopressin**)	Stimulates the kidneys to reabsorb water and return it to circulation; is also a vasoconstrictor, resulting in higher blood pressure.
Oxytocin (OT)	Stimulates the muscles of the uterus during the delivery of an infant and the muscles surrounding the mammary ducts to contract, releasing milk.

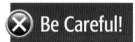 **Be Careful!** **Oxytocin,** a hormone, *should not be confused with* **oxytocia,** *which means* a rapid delivery.

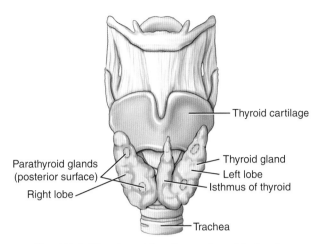

Fig. 15-3 The thyroid and parathyroid glands.

Thyroid Gland

The **thyroid gland** is a single organ, but is divided into right and left lobes that are joined by a thin structure termed the thyroid isthmus (Fig. 15-3). It is located in the anterior part of the neck and is bounded by the trachea behind it and the thyroid cartilage above it. It regulates the metabolism of the body and normal growth and development, and controls the amount of **calcium** (Ca) deposited into bone. The thyroid gland is composed of small sacs, called **follicles,** that absorb iodine. The sacs are surrounded by follicular cells that produce triiodothyronine (T_3) and thyroxine (T_4). Parafollicular cells in the thyroid produce and secrete calcitonin, which controls the amount of calcium in the blood. **Thyroid-stimulating hormone (TSH),** released by the anterior pituitary gland, causes the thyroid to release T_3 and T_4.

thyroid gland = thyr/o, thyroid/o

calcium = calc/o

Thyroid Gland Hormones and Their Effects

Thyroid Gland Hormone	Effect
Calcitonin	Regulates the amount of calcium in the bloodstream.
Tetraiodothyronine (also called **thyroxine** [T_4])	Increases cell metabolism.
Triiodothyronine (T_3)	Increases cell metabolism.

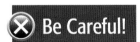 **Be Careful!**   *Don't confuse* **calc/o** *and* **calc/i,** *meaning* calcium, *with* **calic/o,** *meaning* calyx, *and* **kal/i,** *meaning* potassium.

Parathyroid Glands

The **parathyroids** are four small glands (right and left, superior and inferior) located on the posterior surface of the thyroid gland in the neck. They secrete **parathyroid hormone (PTH)** in response to a low level of calcium in the blood. When low calcium is detected, the PTH increases calcium by causing it to be released from the bone, which results in calcium reabsorption by the kidneys and the digestive system. PTH is inhibited by high levels of calcium.

parathyroid gland = parathyroid/o

Adrenal Glands (Suprarenals)

The **adrenal glands,** also called the **suprarenals,** are paired, one on top of each kidney. Different hormones are secreted by the two different parts of these

adrenal gland = adren/o

suprarenal
  supra- = above, upward
  ren/o = kidney
  -al = pertaining to

cortex = cortic/o
medulla = medull/o

glands: the external portion called the **adrenal cortex** and an internal portion called the **adrenal medulla.**

The adrenal cortex secretes three hormones that are called steroids.

The adrenal medulla is the inner portion of the adrenal gland. It produces sympathomimetic hormones that stimulate the fight-or-flight response to stress, similar to the action of the sympathetic nervous system.

Adrenal Cortex Hormones and Their Effects

Adrenal Cortex Hormones	Effect
Glucocorticoids (e.g., cortisol [hydrocortisone])	Respond to stress; have anti-inflammatory properties.
Mineralocorticoids (e.g., aldosterone)	Regulate blood volume, blood pressure, and electrolytes.
Gonadal steroids (sex hormones: estrogens, androgens and progestogens)	Responsible for secondary sex characteristics.

Adrenal Medulla Hormones and Their Effects

Adrenal Medulla Hormones (Catecholamines)	Effect
Dopamine	Dilates arteries and increases production of urine, blood pressure, and cardiac rate. Acts as a neurotransmitter in the nervous system.
Epinephrine (also called adrenaline)	Dilates bronchi, increases heart rate, raises blood pressure, dilates pupils, and elevates blood sugar levels.
Norepinephrine (also called noradrenaline)	Increases heart rate and blood pressure and elevates blood sugar levels for energy use.

pancreas = pancreat/o

exocrine
  exo- = outward
  -crine = to secrete

glucose, sugar = gluc/o, glyc/o, glycos/o

Pancreas

The pancreas, located inferior and posterior to the stomach, is a gland with both exocrine and endocrine functions (Fig. 15-4). The **exocrine function** is to release digestive enzymes through a duct into the small intestines. The **endocrine function,** accomplished through a variety of types of cells called **islets of Langerhans,** is to regulate the level of glucose in the blood by stimulating the liver. The two main types of islets of Langerhans are alpha and beta cells. **Alpha cells** produce the hormone glucagon, which increases the level of glucose in the blood when levels are low. **Beta cells** secrete **insulin,** which decreases the level of glucose in the blood when levels are high. Insulin is needed to transport glucose out of the bloodstream and into the cells. In the absence of glucose in the cells, proteins and fats are broken down, causing excessive fatty acids and **ketones** in the blood. Normally, these hormones regulate glucose levels through the metabolism of fats, carbohydrates, and proteins. See Fig. 15-5 for a diagram explaining the effects of insulin and glucagon.

To understand the role of insulin, click on **Animations.**

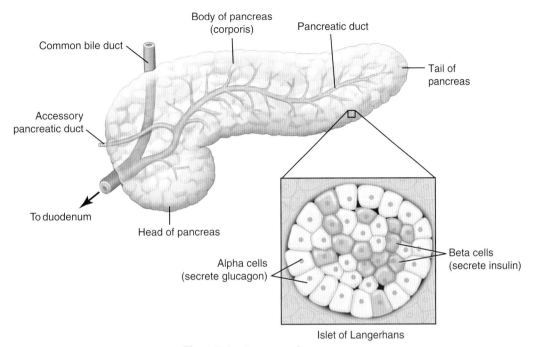

Fig. 15-4 The normal pancreas.

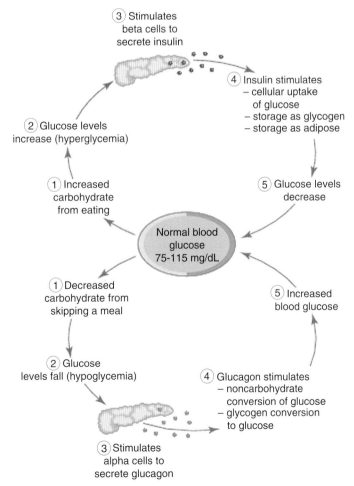

Fig. 15-5 Effects of insulin and glucagon.

thymus gland = thym/o

ketone = ket/o, keton/o

gonads, reproductive
organs = gonad/o

Thymus Gland

The **thymus** gland is located in the mediastinum above the heart. It releases a hormone called thymosin, which is responsible for stimulating key cells in the immune response. For more details, see Chapter 9 on the circulatory and lymphatic systems.

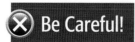 **Be Careful!**   *Do not confuse* **thyr/o,** *which means* thyroid, *and* **thym/o,** *which means* thymus.

Ovaries and Testes

The **ovaries** and **testes,** the female and male **gonads,** also act as endocrine glands, which influence reproductive functions.

Pineal Body

The **pineal** body (gland) is located in the center of the brain, functioning to secrete the hormone **melatonin,** thought to be responsible for inducing sleep.

 Note   Aside from the endocrine organs that have been discussed, there are a number of tiny arteriovenous structures that act as chemoreceptors throughout the body. These structures, called **glomera** *(sing.* glomus), "sense" changes in the blood and trigger needed adjustments by the endocrine and nervous systems. The glomera named are the aortic, carotid, coccygeal, and jugular bodies.

 Exercise 1: Endocrine Anatomy and Physiology

Match the endocrine word parts with their definitions.

____ 1. aden/o
____ 2. hypophys/o
____ 3. lob/o
____ 4. thalam/o
____ 5. thyr/o, thyroid/o
____ 6. calc/o, calc/i
____ 7. parathyroid/o
____ 8. adren/o
____ 9. ren/o
____ 10. cortic/o
____ 11. medull/o
____ 12. pancreat/o
____ 13. gluc/o, glyc/o, glycos/o
____ 14. thym/o
____ 15. ket/o, keton/o
____ 16. gonad/o
____ 17. endo-
____ 18. supra-
____ 19. exo-
____ 20. hypo-
____ 21. -crine

A. kidney
B. above
C. to secrete
D. calcium
E. outside
F. sugar, glucose
G. gland with exocrine and endocrine functions
H. reproductive organ
 I. gland
 J. medulla
K. within
L. ketone
M. gland in mediastinum
N. master gland
O. under
P. suprarenal gland
Q. cortex
R. gland regulating metabolism
 S. gland regulating calcium in the blood
T. lobe
U. thalamus

Exercise 2: Endocrine Anatomy and Physiology

Fill in the blanks.

1. The pituitary gland, the _____, is called the master gland because of its control over other endocrine glands.

2. The pituitary gland is stimulated by the _____.

3. The anterior lobe of the pituitary gland is also known as the _____.

4. The thyroid gland is responsible for regulation of the body's_____ and controls the amount of _____ deposited into bone.

5. Adrenal glands are named for their location above the _____.

6. The inner part of the adrenal gland is the adrenal _____, whereas the outer part of the adrenal gland is the adrenal_____.

7. The endocrine function of the pancreas regulates glucose in the blood through the hormones _____ _____ and _____.

8. Fatty acids and _____ are produced if glucose cannot pass out of the bloodstream into the cells to be metabolized.

9. The thymus gland is located in the _____ above the heart and is responsible for stimulating key cells in the _____response.

10. The _____ gland is located in the center of the brain, functioning to secrete the hormone _____, thought to be responsible for inducing _____.

To practice labeling the endocrine system, click on **Label It.**

Combining Forms for the Anatomy and Physiology of the Endocrine System

Meaning	Combining Form	Meaning	Combining Form
adrenal gland	adren/o, adrenal/o	medulla	medull/o
calcium	calc/o, calc/i	pancreas	pancreat/o
cortex	cortic/o	parathyroid gland	parathyroid/o
gland	aden/o	pituitary gland	hypophys/o, pituitar/o, pituit/o
glucose, sugar	gluc/o, glyc/o, glycos/o	thalamus	thalam/o
gonads	gonad/o	thymus gland	thym/o
ketone	ket/o, keton/o	thyroid gland	thyr/o, thyroid/o
kidney	ren/o, nephr/o	to secrete	crin/o
lobe	lob/o	turning	trop/o

Prefixes for the Anatomy of the Endocrine System

Prefix	Meaning
endo-	within
exo-	outward
hypo-	under, deficient
supra-	above

Suffixes for the Anatomy of the Endocrine System

Suffix	Meaning
-al	pertaining to
-crine	to secrete
-us, -is	structure

PATHOLOGY

Most of the pathology of the endocrine system is the result of either *hyper-* (too much) or *hypo-* (too little) hormonal secretion. Developmental issues also play a role in determining when the malfunction occurs and what the results will be.

Terms Related to Signs and Symptoms of Endocrine Disorders (R00-R99)

Term	Word Origin	Definition
anorexia	*an-* no, not, without *orex/o* appetite *-ia* condition	Lack of appetite. Anorexia nervosa is an eating disorder.
glycosuria	*glycos/o* sugar, glucose *-uria* urinary condition	Presence of glucose in the urine. May indicate diabetes mellitus. Also called **glucosuria.**
hyperalimentation	*hyper-* excessive, above *aliment/o* nutrition *-ation* process of	An excessive intake of food. May be used to describe overeating.
hyperglycemia	*hyper-* excessive, above *glyc/o* glucose, sugar *-emia* blood condition	Excessive glucose in the blood.
ketonuria	*keton/o* ketone *-uria* urinary condition	Presence of ketones in urine. May indicate diabetes mellitus or malnutrition.
paresthesia	*par-* abnormal *esthesi/o* feeling *-ia* condition	Abnormal sensation, such as prickling.
polydipsia	*poly-* many, much, excessive *dips/o* thirst *-ia* condition	Condition of excessive thirst.
polyphagia	*poly-* many, much, excessive *phag/o* to eat, swallow *-ia* condition	Condition of excessive appetite.
polyuria	*poly-* many, much, excessive *-uria* urinary condition	Condition of excessive urination.
prediabetes		A condition in which an individual's blood glucose level is higher than normal, but not high enough for a diagnosis of type 2 diabetes.
tetany		Continuous muscle spasms.

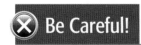 **Be Careful!**   **Anorexia** *is a simple lack of appetite.* **Anorexia nervosa** *is a serious eating disorder classified in the mental health chapter.*

Exercise 3: Signs and Symptoms

____ 1. hyperalimentation
____ 2. prediabetes
____ 3. tetany
____ 4. polydipsia
____ 5. anorexia
____ 6. polyphagia
____ 7. polyuria
____ 8. ketonuria

A. condition of excessive appetite
B. presence of ketones in urine
C. condition of excessive urination
D. excessive intake of food
E. condition in which blood glucose levels aren't high enough to be diagnosed as type 2 diabetes
F. condition of excessive thirst
G. lack of appetite
H. continuous muscle spasms

Translate the terms.

9. hyperglycemia _____

10. glycosuria _____

Terms Related to Thyroid Disorders (E00-E07)

Term	Word Origin	Definition
goiter		Enlargement of the thyroid gland, not due to a tumor (Fig. 15-6).
hyperthyroidism	*hyper-* excessive, above *thyroid/o* thyroid gland *-ism* condition	Excessive thyroid hormone production; also called **thyrotoxicosis,** the most common form of which is Graves' disease, which may be accompanied by exophthalmos, in which the eyeballs protrude from their orbits. The extreme form is called thyroid storm or thyroid crisis and is life threatening (Fig. 15-7).
hypothyroidism	*hypo-* deficient, under *thyroid/o* thyroid gland *-ism* condition	Deficient thyroid hormone production. If it occurs during childhood, it causes a condition called **cretinism,** which results in stunted mental and physical growth. The extreme adult form is called **myxedema,** which is characterized by facial and orbital edema.
thyroiditis	*thyroid/o* thyroid *-itis* inflammation	Inflammation of the thyroid. Hashimoto's thyroiditis is a chronic autoimmune form of thyroiditis.

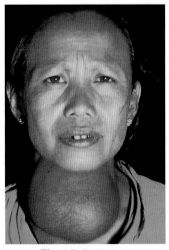

Fig. 15-6 Goiter.

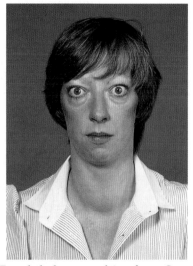

Fig. 15-7 Exophthalmos resulting from Graves' disease.

Terms Related to Diabetes Mellitus (E08-E13)

Term	Word Origin	Definition
diabetes mellitus (DM)		Diabetes mellitus is a group of metabolic disorders characterized by high glucose levels that result from inadequate amounts of insulin, resistance to insulin, or a combination of both. Secondary diabetes is a condition secondary to another condition or the result of a pancreatectomy. Complications include diabetic neuropathy, diabetic nephropathy, diabetic retinopathy (destruction of retina due to blockage of blood vessels), and ulcers of the foot and toes.
type 1 diabetes		Total lack of insulin production, resulting in glycosuria, polydipsia, polyphagia, polyuria, blurred vision, fatigue, and frequent infections. Thought to be an autoimmune disorder. Previously called **insulin-dependent diabetes mellitus (IDDM)** and **juvenile diabetes.**
type 2 diabetes		Deficient insulin production, with symptoms similar to type 1 diabetes. Cause unknown but associated with obesity and family history; previously called **non-insulin-dependent diabetes mellitus (NIDDM).**

 CM Guideline Alert

4a DIABETES MELLITUS
The diabetes mellitus codes are combination codes that include the type of diabetes mellitus, the body system affected, and the complications affecting that body system. As many codes within a particular category as are necessary to describe all of the complications of the disease may be used. They should be sequenced based on the reason for a particular encounter. Assign as many codes from categories E08-E13 as needed to identify all of the associated conditions that the patient has.

1) TYPE OF DIABETES
The age of a patient is not the sole determining factor, though most type 1 diabetics develop the condition before reaching puberty. For this reason, type 1 diabetes mellitus is also referred to as juvenile diabetes.

2) TYPE OF DIABETES MELLITUS NOT DOCUMENTED
If the type of diabetes mellitus is not documented in the medical record, the default is E11.-, Type 2 diabetes mellitus.

3) DIABETES MELLITUS AND THE USE OF INSULIN AND ORAL HYPOGLYCEMICS
If the documentation in a medical record does not indicate the type of diabetes but does indicate that the patient uses insulin, code E11, Type 2 diabetes mellitus, should be assigned. An additional code should be assigned from category Z79 to identify the long-term (current) use of insulin or oral hypoglycemic drugs. If the patient is treated with both oral medications and insulin, only the code for long-term (current) use of insulin should be assigned. Code Z79.4 should not be assigned if insulin is given temporarily to bring a type 2 patient's blood sugar under control during an encounter.

Note: This is a sample of some of the DM coding alerts. See the ICD-10-CM for the entire guidelines.

 Gestational diabetes mellitus is included in Chapter 7, Obstetric, Perinatal and Congenital Conditions.

Terms Related to Other Disorders of Glucose Regulation and Pancreatic Internal Secretion (E15-E16)		
Term	**Word Origin**	**Definition**
hypoglycemia	*hypo-* deficient, under *glyc/o* sugar, glucose *-emia* blood condition	Condition of deficient sugar in the blood. The opposite would be hyperglycemia—excessive sugar in the blood.
hyperinsulinism	*hyper-* excessive, above *insulin/o* insulin *-ism* condition	Oversecretion of insulin; seen in some newborns of diabetic mothers. Causes severe hypoglycemia.

Terms Related to Disorders of Other Endocrine Glands (E20-E35)		
Term	**Word Origin**	**Definition**
acromegaly and pituitary gigantism	*acro-* extremities *-megaly* enlargement	Acromegaly is the hypersecretion of somatotropin from adenohypophysis during adulthood; leads to an enlargement of the extremities (hands and feet), jaw, nose, and forehead (Fig. 15-8). Usually caused by an adenoma of the pituitary gland. Pituitary gigantism is hypersecretion that occurs during childhood.
Cushing's syndrome		Excessive secretion of cortisol by the adrenal cortex causes symptoms of obesity, leukocytosis, hirsutism (excessive hairiness), hypokalemia, hyperglycemia, and muscle wasting (Fig. 15-9).
diabetes insipidus (DI)		Deficiency of antidiuretic hormone (ADH), which causes the patient to excrete large quantities of urine (polyuria) and exhibit excessive thirst (polydipsia).
growth hormone deficiency (GHD)		Somatotropin deficiency due to dysfunction of the adenohypophysis during childhood results in dwarfism (Fig. 15-10). If during adulthood, patients may develop obesity and may experience weakness and cardiac difficulties.

Continued

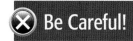 **Be Careful!**   *Do not confuse **diabetes mellitus** (a disorder of insulin) with **diabetes insipidus** (a disorder of antidiuretic hormone).*

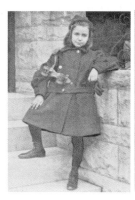 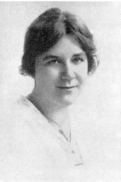 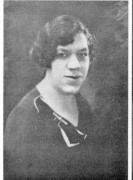 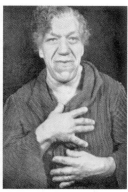

Fig. 15-8 The progression of acromegaly.

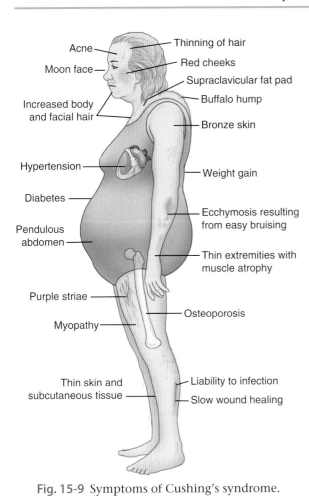

Acne
Moon face
Increased body and facial hair
Hypertension
Diabetes
Pendulous abdomen
Purple striae
Myopathy
Thin skin and subcutaneous tissue

Thinning of hair
Red cheeks
Supraclavicular fat pad
Buffalo hump
Bronze skin
Weight gain
Ecchymosis resulting from easy bruising
Thin extremities with muscle atrophy
Osteoporosis
Liability to infection
Slow wound healing

Fig. 15-9 Symptoms of Cushing's syndrome.

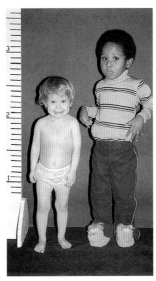

Fig. 15-10 The normal 3½-year-old boy is in the 50th percentile for height. The short 3-year-old girl exhibits the characteristic "Kewpie doll" appearance, suggesting a diagnosis of growth hormone (GH) deficiency.

Terms Related to Disorders of Other Endocrine Glands (E2Ø-E35)—cont'd

Term	Word Origin	Definition
hyperparathyroidism	*hyper-* excessive, above *parathyroid/o* parathyroid gland *-ism* condition	Overproduction of parathyroid hormone; symptoms include polyuria, hypercalcemia, hypertension, and kidney stones.
hypoparathyroidism	*hypo-* deficient *parathyroid/o* parathyroid gland *-ism* condition	Deficient parathyroid hormone production results in tetany, hypocalcemia, irritability, and muscle cramps.
hypopituitarism	*hypo-* deficient *pituitar/o* pituitary *-ism* condition	Deficiency or lack of all pituitary hormones, causing hypotension, weight loss, weakness; also includes Simmonds' disease and panhypopituitarism.
polycystic ovary syndrome (PCOS)	*poly-* many, much, excessive *cyst/o* sac *-ic* pertaining to	Bilateral presence of numerous cysts in the ovaries, caused by a hormonal abnormality leading to the secretion of androgens. Can cause acne, facial hair, and infertility (Fig. 15-11).
primary adrenocortical insufficiency		Insufficient secretion of adrenal cortisol from the adrenal cortex is manifested by gastric complaints, hypotension, dehydration, fatigue, and hyperpigmentation of skin and mucous membranes (Fig. 15-12). Also called **Addison's disease**.

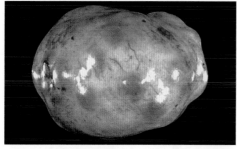

Fig. 15-11 Polycystic ovary syndrome. Multiple fluid-filled cysts in the ovary.

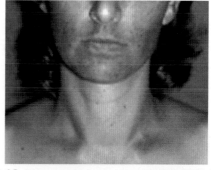

Fig. 15-12 Hyperpigmentation in Addison's disease.

Terms Related to Disorders of Other Endocrine Glands (E20-E35)—cont'd

Term	Word Origin	Definition
progeria	*pro-* forward, in front of *ger/o* old age *-ia* condition	Genetic condition of rapid aging. Also called **Hutchinson-Gilford progeria syndrome (HGPS).**
syndrome of inappropriate antidiuretic hormone (SIADH)		Oversecretion of ADH from the neurohypophysis, leading to severe hyponatremia and the inability to excrete diluted urine.

 Exercise 4: **Thyroid Disorders; Diabetes Mellitus; Glucose Regulation and Pancreatic Internal Secretion; and Disorders of Other Endocrine Glands**

Match the terms to their definitions.

_____ 1. goiter
_____ 2. myxedema
_____ 3. thyrotoxicosis
_____ 4. Hashimoto's thyroiditis
_____ 5. DM
_____ 6. type 1 diabetes
_____ 7. type 2 diabetes
_____ 8. hyperinsulinism
_____ 9. GHD
_____ 10. hyperparathyroidism
_____ 11. hypoparathyroidism
_____ 12. SIADH
_____ 13. panhypopituitarism
_____ 14. DI
_____ 15. Cushing's syndrome
_____ 16. Addison's disease
_____ 17. PCOS

A. disorder caused by excessive thyroid hormone production
B. extreme adult form of hypothyroidism
C. enlargement of the thyroid gland
D. deficient production of parathyroid hormone
E. deficiency of ADH, which causes polyuria and polydipsia
F. DM that results from total lack of insulin production
G. group of metabolic disorders characterized by high glucose levels as a result of inadequate amounts of insulin or resistance to insulin or both
H. chronic autoimmune form of thyroiditis
I. DM that results from deficient insulin production
J. bilateral presence of numerous cysts caused by hormonal abnormality leading to secretion of androgens
K. excessive secretion of cortisol by the adrenal cortex
L. oversecretion of ADH from the neurohypophysis, leading to severe hyponatremia and the inability to excrete diluted urine
M. insufficient secretion of adrenal cortisol from the adrenal cortex
N. deficiency or lack of all pituitary hormones
O. overproduction of parathyroid hormone
P. deficiency of somatotropin due to adenohypophysis dysfunction
Q. oversecretion of insulin

Build the terms.

18. condition of excessive thyroid gland_____

19. blood condition of deficient glucose_____

20. enlargement of the extremities_____

21. condition of before old age_____

Terms Related to Overweight, Obesity, and Other Hyperalimentation (E65-E68)

Term	Word Origin	Definition
adiposity	*adipos/o* full of fat *-ity* noun ending	Accumulation of adipose (fat) tissue in specific body areas.
morbid obesity	*morb/o* disease *-id* pertaining to	A condition of patients who are 50% to 100% over their ideal body weight. The body mass index (BMI) is used to measure the relationship between a person's height and weight to determine obesity.

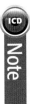

Note

BMI codes are divided into adult and pediatric codes. The adult codes record the BMI in categories from <19 to >70 using an individual's weight and height. The calculation is the division of the weight in kilograms divided by height in meters squared. A BMI of 19 to <25 is considered to be a normal BMI. In children, the BMI is calculated as a percentile of what is normal for a child's age and sex. Obesity is considered to be at or above the 95th percentile of children in that particular category.

Terms Related to Metabolic Disorders (E70-E88)

Term	Word Origin	Definition
cystic fibrosis (CF)	*cyst/o* sac *-ic* pertaining to *fibr/o* fiber *-osis* abnormal condition	Inherited disorder of the exocrine glands resulting in abnormal thick secretions of mucus that cause COPD. Caused by a defect in the gene that allows for the normal mucous secretions of the lungs to be diluted and excreted (Fig. 15-13).
dehydration	*de-* lack of *hydr/o* water *-ation* process of	Condition of deficient water in the body.
hemochromatosis	*hem/o* blood *chromat/o* color *-osis* abnormal condition	Abnormal condition of excessive iron deposits in body tissues. May lead to organ failure, arthritis and bronze coloration of skin.
hypercholesterolemia	*hyper-* excessive, above *cholesterol/o* cholesterol *-emia* blood condition	Excessive cholesterol, a waxy substance, in the blood.

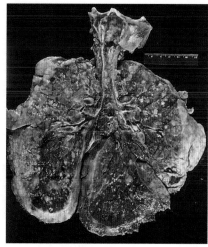

Fig. 15-13 Cystic fibrosis. Lungs of person with cystic fibrosis, showing extensive mucus plugging and dilation of the tracheobronchial tree.

Terms Related to Metabolic Disorders (E70-E88)—cont'd

Term	Word Origin	Definition
hyperlipidemia	*hyper-* excessive, above *lipid/o* fat *-emia* blood condition	Excessive fat in the blood. May be due to genetic causes.
hypocalcemia	*hypo-* deficient, under *calc/o* calcium *-emia* blood condition	Condition of deficient calcium (Ca) in the blood. The opposite would be hypercalcemia—excessive calcium in the blood.
hypokalemia	*hypo-* deficient, under *kal/i* potassium *-emia* blood condition	Condition of deficient potassium (K) in the blood. The opposite would be hyperkalemia—excessive potassium in the blood.
hyponatremia	*hypo-* deficient, under *natr/o* sodium *-emia* blood condition	Condition of deficient sodium (Na) in the blood. The opposite would be hypernatremia—excessive sodium in the blood.
hypovolemia	*hypo-* deficient, under *vol/o* volume *-emia* blood condition	Deficient volume of circulating blood.
ketoacidosis	*ket/o* ketone *acid/o* acid *-osis* abnormal condition	Excessive amount of ketone acids in the bloodstream.
phenylketonuria (PKU)		A deficiency of the enzyme phenylalanine hydroxylase, which is responsible for converting phenylalanine, found in certain foods, into tyrosine. Failure to treat this condition will lead to brain damage and developmental disabilities..
Tay-Sachs disease		A fatal genetic disorder in which lipids accumulate in the tissues and brain due to an enzyme deficiency.

Exercise 5: Overweight, Obesity, and Other Hyperalimentation and Metabolic Disorders

Match the terms to their definitions.

_____ 1. adiposity
_____ 2. morbid obesity
_____ 3. Tay-Sachs disease
_____ 4. dehydration
_____ 5. cystic fibrosis
_____ 6. phenylketonuria
_____ 7. hypovolemia
_____ 8. hypokalemia
_____ 9. ketoacidosis
_____ 10. hyponatremia
_____ 11. hemochromatosis

A. fatal genetic disorder in which lipids accumulate in the tissues and brain due to an enzyme deficiency
B. a condition of patients who are 50% to 100% over their ideal body weight
C. deficient volume of circulating blood
D. condition of deficient water in the body
E. excessive amount of ketone acids in the bloodstream
F. accumulation of fat tissue in specific body areas
G. inherited disorder of the exocrine glands resulting in thick secretions that cause COPD
H. condition of deficient sodium in the blood
I. condition of deficient potassium in the blood
J. deficiency of enzyme phenylalanine hydroxylase
K. excessive iron deposits in body tissues

Translate the terms.

11. hyperlipidemia_____.
12. hypocalcemia_____.
13. hypercholesterolemia_____.

Terms Related to Benign Neoplasms		
Term	**Word Origin**	**Definition**
pheochromocytoma	*phe/o* dark *chrom/o* color *cyt/o* cell *-oma* tumor, mass	Usually benign tumor of the adrenal medulla.
prolactinoma	*prolactin/o* prolactin *-oma* tumor, mass	Most common type of pituitary tumor (Fig. 15-14). Causes the pituitary to oversecrete prolactin.
thymoma	*thym/o* thymus *-oma* tumor, mass	Noncancerous tumor of epithelial origin that is often associated with myasthenia gravis.

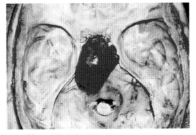

Fig. 15-14 Pituitary tumor.

Terms Related to Malignant Neoplasms

Term	Word Origin	Definition
islet cell carcinoma	*carcin/o* epithelial cancer *-oma* tumor, mass	Pancreatic cancer; fourth leading cause of cancer death in the United States. Treated surgically with a Whipple procedure (pancreatoduodenectomy).
malignant thymoma	*thym/o* thymus gland *-oma* tumor, mass	Rare cancer of the thymus gland.
thyroid carcinoma	*carcin/o* epithelial cancer *-oma* tumor, mass	The most common types of thyroid carcinoma are follicular and papillary. Both have high 5-year survival rates.

 Exercise 6: Neoplasms

Match the neoplasms with their definitions.

_____ 1. malignant thymoma
_____ 2. islet cell carcinoma
_____ 3. pheochromocytoma
_____ 4. thyroid carcinoma
_____ 5. thymoma
_____ 6. prolactinoma

A. most common type of pituitary tumor
B. rare cancer of the thymus gland
C. most common thyroid cancer
D. benign tumor of adrenal medulla
E. benign thymus tumor
F. pancreatic cancer

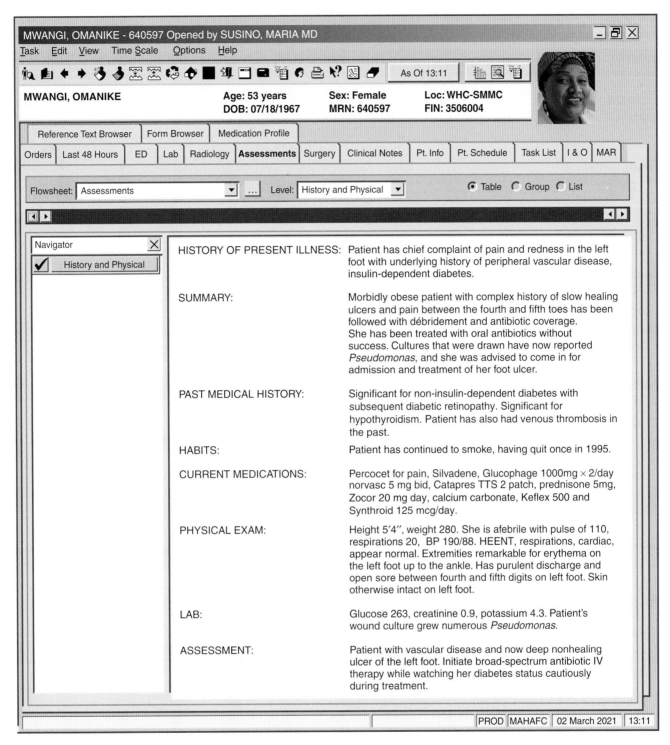

MWANGI, OMANIKE - 640597 Opened by SUSINO, MARIA MD

Task   Edit   View   Time Scale   Options   Help

MWANGI, OMANIKE | Age: 53 years DOB: 07/18/1967 | Sex: Female MRN: 640597 | Loc: WHC-SMMC FIN: 3506004

Reference Text Browser | Form Browser | Medication Profile

Orders | Last 48 Hours | ED | Lab | Radiology | **Assessments** | Surgery | Clinical Notes | Pt. Info | Pt. Schedule | Task List | I & O | MAR

Flowsheet: Assessments   Level: History and Physical   ● Table   ○ Group   ○ List

Navigator
✓ History and Physical

HISTORY OF PRESENT ILLNESS: Patient has chief complaint of pain and redness in the left foot with underlying history of peripheral vascular disease, insulin-dependent diabetes.

SUMMARY: Morbidly obese patient with complex history of slow healing ulcers and pain between the fourth and fifth toes has been followed with débridement and antibiotic coverage. She has been treated with oral antibiotics without success. Cultures that were drawn have now reported *Pseudomonas*, and she was advised to come in for admission and treatment of her foot ulcer.

PAST MEDICAL HISTORY: Significant for non-insulin-dependent diabetes with subsequent diabetic retinopathy. Significant for hypothyroidism. Patient has also had venous thrombosis in the past.

HABITS: Patient has continued to smoke, having quit once in 1995.

CURRENT MEDICATIONS: Percocet for pain, Silvadene, Glucophage 1000mg × 2/day norvasc 5 mg bid, Catapres TTS 2 patch, prednisone 5mg, Zocor 20 mg day, calcium carbonate, Keflex 500 and Synthroid 125 mcg/day.

PHYSICAL EXAM: Height 5'4", weight 280. She is afebrile with pulse of 110, respirations 20, BP 190/88. HEENT, respirations, cardiac, appear normal. Extremities remarkable for erythema on the left foot up to the ankle. Has purulent discharge and open sore between fourth and fifth digits on left foot. Skin otherwise intact on left foot.

LAB: Glucose 263, creatinine 0.9, potassium 4.3. Patient's wound culture grew numerous *Pseudomonas*.

ASSESSMENT: Patient with vascular disease and now deep nonhealing ulcer of the left foot. Initiate broad-spectrum antibiotic IV therapy while watching her diabetes status cautiously during treatment.

PROD | MAHAFC | 02 March 2021 | 13:11

Exercise 7: Admission History and Physical

Using the form above, answer the following questions.

1. Which type (number) of diabetes does this patient have? _____

2. What is the term for the eye disease that the patient has in her past history? _____

3. What index could Dr. Susino have used to determine whether the patient was morbidly obese? _____

4. What term tells you the patient has an underactive thyroid gland? _____

PROCEDURES

Terms Related to Diagnostic Tests

Term	Word Origin	Definition
A1c		Measure of average blood glucose during a 3-month time span. Used to monitor response to diabetes treatment. Also called **glycosylated hemoglobin** or **HbA1c.**
fasting plasma glucose (FPG)		After a period of fasting, blood is drawn. The amount of glucose present is used to measure the body's ability to break down and use glucose. 100-125 mg/dL = prediabetes; >126 = diabetes. Previously called fasting blood sugar (FBS).
hormone tests		Measure the amount of antidiuretic hormone (ADH), cortisol, growth hormone, or parathyroid hormone in the blood.
oral glucose tolerance test (OGTT)		Blood test to measure the body's response to a concentrated glucose solution. May be used to diagnose diabetes mellitus.
radioimmunoassay studies (RIA)		Nuclear medicine tests used to tag and detect hormones in the blood through the use of radionuclides.
sweat test		Method of evaluating sodium and chloride concentration in sweat as a means of diagnosing cystic fibrosis.
thyroid function tests (TFTs)		Blood tests done to assess T_3, T_4, and calcitonin. May be used to evaluate abnormalities of thyroid function.
total calcium		Measures the amount of calcium in the blood. Results may be used to assess parathyroid function, calcium metabolism, or cancerous conditions.
urine glucose		Used as a screen for or to monitor diabetes mellitus; a urine specimen is tested for the presence of glucose.
urine ketones		Test to detect presence of ketones in a urine specimen; may indicate diabetes mellitus or hyperthyroidism.

 ## Exercise 8: Diagnostic Procedures

Circle the correct answer.

1. Nuclear medicine tests used to tag and detect hormones in the blood are called *(magnetic resonance imaging, RIA).*

2. A test used to monitor a patient's response to diabetes treatment is *(urine ketone test, A1c).*

3. Parathyroid dysfunction may be detected through a blood test for parathyroid hormone or a test for *(urine glucose, total calcium).*

4. Which type of test can be used to screen for diabetes mellitus? *(urine glucose, total calcium).*

5. What tests are used to evaluate abnormalities of thyroid function? *(FPG, TFTs)*

Terms Related to Endocrine Procedures

Term	Word Origin	Definition
adrenalectomy	*adrenal/o* adrenal gland *-ectomy* cutting out	Bilateral removal of the adrenal glands to reduce excess hormone secretion.
adrenalorrhaphy	*adrenal/o* adrenal gland *-rrhaphy* suturing	Suturing the adrenal gland.
endoscopic retrograde pancreatography (ERP)	*endo-* within *-scopic* pertaining to viewing *pancreat/o* pancreas *-graphy* recording	The recording of the pancreas through the use of an endoscope (duodenoscope) and a contrast medium (Fig. 15-15).
pancreatectomy	*pancreat/o* pancreas *-ectomy* cutting out	Excision of all or part of the pancreas to remove a tumor or to treat an intractable inflammation of the pancreas.
pancreatoduodenectomy	*pancreat/o* pancreas *duoden/o* duodenum *-ectomy* cutting out	Excision of the head of the pancreas together with the duodenum. Used to treat pancreatic cancer. Also called **Whipple procedure.**
pancreatolithotomy	*pancreat/o* pancreas *-lithotomy* cutting out a stone	Cutting a stone from the pancreas.
parathyroidectomy	*parathyroid/o* parathyroid gland *-ectomy* cutting out	Removal of the parathyroid gland, usually to treat hyperparathyroidism.
pinealectomy	*pineal/o* pineal body *-ectomy* cutting out	Cutting out the pineal body.

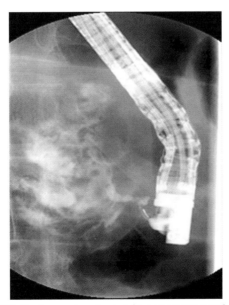

Fig. 15-15 Endoscopic retrograde pancreatography (ERP).

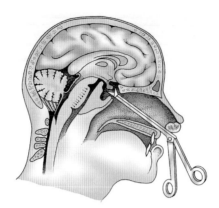

Fig. 15-16 Pituitectomy.

Terms Related to Endocrine Procedures—cont'd

Term	Word Origin	Definition
pituitectomy	*pituit/o* pituitary gland *-ectomy* cutting out	Excision of the pituitary gland; usually done to remove a pituitary tumor (Fig. 15-16). Also called **pituitarectomy.**
thyroidectomy	*thyroid/o* thyroid gland *-ectomy* cutting out	Removal of part or all of the thyroid gland to treat goiter, tumors, or hyperthyroidism that does not respond to medication. Removal of most, but not all, of this gland will result in a regrowth of the gland with normal function. If cancer is detected, a total thyroidectomy is performed.

CPT Coding Alert!

CPT requires a distinction between partial and total thyroidectomies to include details as to whether the isthmus is removed and whether the contralateral lobe is also removed.

 Exercise 9: **Procedures**

Build the terms.

1. cutting out the pancreas and duodenum_____

2. suturing an adrenal gland_____

3. cutting out a stone in the pancreas_____

4. viewing the thyroid gland_____

5. cutting out the pituitary gland_____

PHARMACOLOGY

Most of the pharmacological interventions for endocrine disorders are provided to correct imbalances, either inhibiting or replacing abnormal hormone levels.

antidiabetics: Manage glucose levels in the body when the pancreas or insulin receptors are no longer functioning properly. These drugs are also known as hypoglycemic agents and encompass various oral agents and replacement insulin. Type 1 diabetes mellitus typically requires insulin therapy, and management of type 2 diabetes mellitus begins with antidiabetic drugs such as metformin (Glucophage), glipizide (Glucotrol), or albiglutide (Tanzeum); insulin is typically used as a last resort. Fig. 15-17 shows an insulin pump in use by patient.

antithyroid agents: Treat hyperthyroidism. Examples include methimazole (Tapazole) and propylthiouracil (PTU).

corticosteroids: Mimic or replace the body's steroids normally produced by the adrenal glands. Underfunctioning adrenal cortices (Addison's disease) may be treated with prednisone (Deltasone). Corticosteroids are classified as glucosteroids and mineralocorticoids, depending on structure and function.

growth hormones: Treat various disease-causing growth inhibitions. Human growth hormone (hGH) is available as the prescription somatropin (Genotropin, Nutropin).

posterior pituitary hormones: Vasopressin (Vasostrict) and desmopressin acetate (DDAVP) are used to treat diabetes insipidus.

thyroid hormones: Treat hypothyroidism. Examples include natural thyroid hormones (Armour Thyroid) and levothyroxine (Levoxyl, Synthroid).

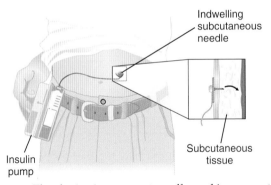

Fig. 15-17 Insulin pump. The device is worn externally and is connected to an indwelling subcutaneous needle, usually inserted into the abdomen.

 Exercise 10: **Pharmacology**

Match the pharmacological agent with the correct disease or disorder.

____ 1. insulin	A. Addison's disease
____ 2. prednisone	B. hypothyroidism
____ 3. vasopressin	C. diabetes mellitus
____ 4. Synthroid	D. diabetes insipidus

RECOGNIZING SUFFIXES FOR PCS

Now that you've finished reading about the procedures for the endocrine system, take a look at this review of the *suffixes* used in their terminology. Each of these suffixes is associated with one or more root operations in the medical surgical section or one of the other categories in PCS.

Suffixes and Root Operations for the Endocrine System

Suffix	Root Operation
-ectomy	Excision, resection
-lithotomy	Extirpation
-rrhaphy	Repair

Abbreviations

Abbreviation	Meaning
ACTH	adrenocorticotropic hormone
ADH	antidiuretic hormone
BMI	body mass index
Ca	calcium
CF	cystic fibrosis
DI	diabetes insipidus
DM	diabetes mellitus
ERP	endoscopic retrograde pancreatography
FBS	fasting blood sugar
FPG	fasting plasma glucose
FSH	follicle-stimulating hormone
GH	growth hormone
GHD	growth hormone deficiency
hGH	human growth hormone
HGPS	Hutchinson-Gilford progeria syndrome
ICSH	interstitial cell-stimulating hormone
IDDM	insulin-dependent diabetes mellitus

Abbreviation	Meaning
K	potassium
LH	luteinizing hormone
Na	sodium
NIDDM	non-insulin-dependent diabetes mellitus
OGTT	oral glucose tolerance test
OT	oxytocin
PCOS	polycystic ovary syndrome
PKU	phenylketonuria
PRL	prolactin
PTH	parathyroid hormone
RIA	radioimmunoassay studies
SIADH	syndrome of inappropriate antidiuretic hormone
STH	somatotropic hormone
T_3	triiodothyronine
T_4	thyroxine
TFTs	thyroid function tests
TSH	thyroid-stimulating hormone

Go to Evolve to interactively build terms, label images, memorize word parts, and practice using endocrine terms in context.

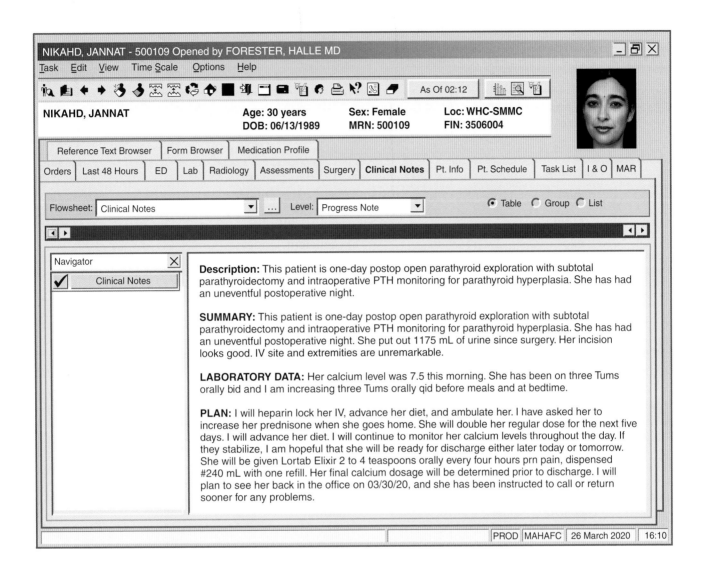

Description: This patient is one-day postop open parathyroid exploration with subtotal parathyroidectomy and intraoperative PTH monitoring for parathyroid hyperplasia. She has had an uneventful postoperative night.

SUMMARY: This patient is one-day postop open parathyroid exploration with subtotal parathyroidectomy and intraoperative PTH monitoring for parathyroid hyperplasia. She has had an uneventful postoperative night. She put out 1175 mL of urine since surgery. Her incision looks good. IV site and extremities are unremarkable.

LABORATORY DATA: Her calcium level was 7.5 this morning. She has been on three Tums orally bid and I am increasing three Tums orally qid before meals and at bedtime.

PLAN: I will heparin lock her IV, advance her diet, and ambulate her. I have asked her to increase her prednisone when she goes home. She will double her regular dose for the next five days. I will advance her diet. I will continue to monitor her calcium levels throughout the day. If they stabilize, I am hopeful that she will be ready for discharge either later today or tomorrow. She will be given Lortab Elixir 2 to 4 teaspoons orally every four hours prn pain, dispensed #240 mL with one refill. Her final calcium dosage will be determined prior to discharge. I will plan to see her back in the office on 03/30/20, and she has been instructed to call or return sooner for any problems.

Exercise 11: Progress Note

Using the progress note above, answer the following questions.

1. What does the abbreviation PTH stand for? _____

2. What term tells you that the patient did not have all of her parathyroid glands removed? _____

3. PTH regulates what mineral in the blood? _____

4. How do you know that the PTH monitoring was done while the surgery was taking place? _____

5. What term tells you that the surgery involved checking for an abnormal enlargement of the parathyroid? _____

Match the word parts to their definitions.

WORD PART DEFINITIONS

Prefix/Suffix	Definition
acro-	1. _____ recording
-crine	2. _____ urinary condition
-ectomy	3. _____ within
endo-	4. _____ excessive, above
-emia	5. _____ above, upward
exo-	6. _____ deficient, under
-graphy	7. _____ blood condition
hyper-	8. _____ outward
hypo-	9. _____ to secrete
poly-	10. _____ extremities
supra-	11. _____ many, much, excessive
-uria	12. _____ cutting out

Combining Form	Definition
aden/o	13. _____ potassium
adren/o	14. _____ pituitary
calc/o	15. _____ color
chrom/o	16. _____ sodium
crin/o	17. _____ glucose, sugar
cyt/o	18. _____ gonads
gluc/o	19. _____ parathyroid gland
glyc/o	20. _____ turning
gonad/o	21. _____ gland
hypophys/o	22. _____ thymus gland
kal/i	23. _____ sugar, glucose
natr/o	24. _____ dark
pancreat/o	25. _____ to secrete
parathyroid/o	26. _____ thyroid gland
phe/o	27. _____ thalamus
pituitar/o	28. _____ adrenal gland
thalam/o	29. _____ calcium
thym/o	30. _____ pancreas
thyr/o	31. _____ cell
trop/o	32. _____ pituitary gland

WORDSHOP

Prefixes	Combining Forms	Suffixes
acro-	acid/o	-al
hyper-	chrom/o	-ectomy
hypo-	cyt/o	-emia
poly-	dips/o	-ia
supra-	duoden/o	-ism
	glyc/o	-megaly
	kal/i	-oma
	ket/o	-osis
	natr/o	
	pancreat/o	
	phe/o	
	ren/o	
	thyroid/o	

Build endocrine terms by combining the word parts above. Some word parts may be used more than once. Some may not be used at all. The number in parentheses indicates the number of word parts needed.

Definition	Term
1. pertaining to above the kidney (3)	
2. blood condition of excessive glucose (3)	
3. condition of excessive thirst (3)	
4. condition of deficient thyroid gland (3)	
5. enlargement of the extremities (2)	
6. blood condition of deficient potassium (3)	
7. abnormal condition of ketone acid (3)	
8. tumor of dark color cell (4)	
9. cutting out the pancreas and duodenum (3)	
10. blood condition of deficient sodium (3)	

Sort the terms below into their correct categories.

TERM SORTING

Anatomy and Physiology	Pathology	Procedures

A1c

ADH

adiposity

adrenal cortex

adrenalectomy

calcitonin

Cushing's syndrome

cystic fibrosis

dehydration

DI

DM

ERP

FPC

GHD

glycosuria

hyperthyroidism

hypoglycemia

hypothalamus

insulin

islets of Langerhans

ketone

ketonuria

melatonin

metabolism

neurohypophysis

OGTT

oxytocin

pancreatoduodenectomy

parathyroid

pinealotomy

polydipsia

progeria

RIA

SIADH

suprarenals

TFTs

thymoma

thymosin

TSH

Replace the highlighted text with the correct terms.

TRANSLATIONS

1. After experiencing **condition of excessive thirst** and **condition of excessive urination**, Tilda was diagnosed with diabetes insipidus.

2. Victor's **protrusion of eyeballs from their orbits** was caused by **excessive thyroid hormone production**.

3. Moira went to the endocrinologist with symptoms of **condition of deficient calcium in the blood** and **continuous muscle spasms**. She was diagnosed with **deficient parathyroid hormone production**.

4. Soo Lin had hirsutism, easy bruising, **excessive sugar in the blood** and **condition of deficient potassium in the blood**, which led to a diagnosis of Cushing's disease.

5. The patient's **condition of oversecretion of insulin** caused a **condition of deficient sugar in the blood**.

6. Franco had **a pancreatic cancer**, which was treated with an **excision of the head of the pancreas and the duodenum**.

7. The patient with **total lack of insulin production** was diagnosed with **a blood test to measure the body's response to a concentrated glucose solution**.

8. A **removal of part or all of the thyroid gland** was performed to treat the patient's **enlargement of the thyroid gland not due to a tumor**.

9. Severe **condition of deficient sodium in the blood** and the inability to excrete diluted urine were two symptoms of **oversecretion of ADH from the neurohypophysis**.

10. After undergoing **a blood test done after fasting**, Mrs. Brown was diagnosed with **a deficient insulin production with symptoms similar to type 1 diabetes**.

11. When she was an adult, Martha developed **enlargement of the extremities** due to hypersecretion of somatotropin from the **anterior lobe of her pituitary gland**.

Illustration Credits

Beauchamp RD, et al: *Sabaston textbook of surgery: the biological basis of modern surgical practice*, ed 20, Elsevier, 2017 (Fig. 5-22)

Bird D, Robinson D: *Modern dental assisting*, ed 11, Philadelphia, 2015, Saunders (Fig. 5-12)

Black JM, Hawks JH, Keene A: *Medical-surgical nursing: clinical management for positive outcomes*, ed 8, Philadelphia, 2009, Saunders (Fig. 5-14, Fig. 6-11, Fig. 9-26 B, 9-35, 10-25A, Fig. 11-24B, 13-13)

Blumgart L: *Video Atlas: Liver, biliary & pancreatic surgery*, Philadelphia, 2011, Saunders (Fig. 5-32)

Bolognia JL: *Dermatology*, ed 3, St Louis, 2012, Mosby (Fig. 4-36, 5-11, 8-13)

Bonewit-West K: *Clinical procedures for medical assistants*, ed 9, Philadelphia, 2015, Saunders (Fig. 8-20)

Bork K, Brauninger W: *Skin diseases in clinical practice*, ed 2, Philadelphia, 1999, Saunders (Fig. 4-10)

Buck C: *Step-by-step medical coding*, ed 2015, St Louis, 2015, Saunders (Fig. 9-39)

Callen JP, Greer KE, Saller AS, et al: *Color atlas of dermatology*, ed 3, Philadelphia, 2003, Saunders (Fig. 4-5, 4-11, 4-12, 4-13, 4-17, 4-27, 11-10B)

Cameron M, Monroe L: *Physical rehabilitation*, St Louis, 2007, Saunders (Fig. 11-20)

Cooper K, Gosnell K: *Foundations and adult health nursing*, ed 7, St Louis, 2015, Mosby (Fig. 10-29D)

Copstead-Kirkhorn L, Banasik J: *Pathophysiology*, ed 5, St Louis, 2013, Saunders (Fig. 6-15)

Copyright iStock.com (Fig. A-2, A-3, 4-25A-C, 11-25AB).

Damjanov I: *Anderson's pathology*, ed 10, St Louis, 2000, Mosby (Fig. 3-26 A, 4-28, 5-30 A, 6-6 B, 6-19, 6-31, 8-17, 9-33, 13-21, 15-14)

Damjanov I: *Pathology: a color atlas*, St Louis, 2000, Mosby (Fig. 5-15, 5-16, Fig. 5-19, 5-21 B, 5-23, 9-21, 9-23, 10-9, 10-14, 11-13)

Damjanov I: *Pathology for the health professions*, 4e, St Louis, 2011, Saunders (Fig. 10-13)

Donatelli, Wooden: *Orthopedic physical therapy*, ed 4, St. Louis, 2009, Churchill Livingstone (Fig. 3-31)

Early PJ, Sodee DB: *Principles and practices of nuclear medicine*, ed 2, St Louis, 1994, Mosby (Fig. 10-23)

Eisen D, Lynch DP: *The mouth: diagnosis and treatment*, St Louis, 1998, Mosby (Fig. 5-13)

Eisenberg RL, Johnson N: *Comprehensive radiographic pathology*, ed 5, St Louis, 2012, Mosby (Fig. 3-26B, 10-25B)

Elkin MK, Perry AG, Potter PA: *Nursing intervention and clinical skills*, ed 4, St Louis, 2008, Mosby (Fig. 4-16)

Epstein E: *Common skin disorders*, ed 5, Philadelphia, 2001, Saunders (Fig. 4-9)

Fattahi T, Fernandes R: *Atlas of the oral and maxillofacial surgery clinics of North America*, vol 15-1, 2007, Saunders (Fig. 11-27)

Feldman M et al: *Sleisenger and Fordtran's gastrointestinal and liver disease*, ed 8, Philadelphia, 2006, Saunders (Fig. 1-1)

Fletcher CD: *Diagnostic histopathology of tumors*, ed 3, London, 2008, Churchill Livingstone (Fig. 9-32)

Fortinash KM: *Psychiatric mental health nursing*, ed 5, St Louis, 2012, Mosby (Fig. 12-4)

Frank ED, Long BW, Smith BJ: *Merrill's atlas of radiographic positions and radiologic procedures*, ed 12, St Louis, 2012, Mosby (Fig. 2-3 A, 2-4, 3-11, 3-16 B, 3-21 B, 3-8 B, 5-26, 5-31, 6-32, 6-35, 9-34, 9-38 A, 9-41)

Frazier MS, Drzymkowski JW: *Essentials of human diseases and conditions*, ed 4, Philadelphia, 2008, Saunders (Fig. 6-10 A)

Fuller JK: *Surgical technology*, ed 6, Philadelphia, 2013, Saunders (Fig. 1-10, 3-34 B, 4-37, 5-30 B, 13-24)

Goldman L, Ausiello DA: *Cecil Medicine*, ed 23, Philadelphia, 2008, Saunders (Fig. 8-15, 9-18, 10-5)

Habif TP: *Clinical dermatology*, ed 6, St Louis, 2015, Mosby (Fig. 4-18, 4-22, 4-26,4-31, 4-38)

Habif T et al: *Skin disease: diagnosis and treatment*, ed 3, St Louis, 2011, Mosby (Fig. 4-14, 4-15, 4-20)

Hagen-Ansert SL: *Textbook of diagnostic sonography*, ed 7, St Louis, 2012 (Fig. 6-38 B, 9-38 B)

Hallett J, Mills J, Earnshaw J, Reekers J, Rooke T: *Comprehensive vascular and endovascular surgery*, ed 2, Philadelphia, 2009, Mosby (Fig. 9-28)

Hansell D, et al: *Imaging of diseases of the chest*, ed 5, Edinburgh, 2009, Mosby (Fig. 10-21)

Harris P, et al: *Mosby's dictionary of medicine, nursing and health professions*, ed 9, St. Louis, 2013, Mosby (Fig. 13-19)

Henry M, Stapleton E: *EMT prehospital care*, ed 3, St Louis, 2007, Mosby (Fig. 9-27)

Herlihy B, Maebius NK: *The human body in health and illness*, ed 4, Philadelphia, 2011, Saunders (Fig. 8-5, 8-7, 11-25)

Hill MJ: *Skin disorders*, St Louis, 1994, Mosby (Fig. 4-19, 4-21)

Hore I, Bajaj Y, Denyer J, Martinez A.E., Mellerio J.E., Bibas T, Albert D. *The management of general and disease specific ENT problems in children with Epidermolysis Bullosa—A retrospective case note review*. International Journal of Pediatric Otorhinolaryngology. 2007; 71(3):385-391 (Fig. 14-5)

Huether S, McCance K: *Understanding pathophysiology*, 2012, ed 5, St Louis, 2008, Mosby (Fig. 9-25)

Hurst B, et al: *Uterine artery embolization for symptomatic uterine myomas*, Fertility and Sterility, 2000, vol 74, Issue 5, pages 855-869 (Fig. 6-41)

Ignatavicius DD, Workman ML: *Medical-surgical nursing: critical thinking for collaborative care*, ed 7, Philadelphia, 2013, Saunders (Fig. 4-35, 6-10 B, 6-28, 10-6, 10-28, 13-27, 13-28, 15-16)

Illyés A, Kiss R: *Shoulder muscle activity during pushing, pulling, elevation and overhead throw*, Journal of Electromyography and Kinesiology 15(3):282-289, 2005 (Fig. 3-35)

James S, Ashwill J: *Nursing care of children*, ed 4, St Louis, 2013, Saunders (Fig. 8-12)

Jarnagin WR: *Blumgart's Surgery of the Liver, Biliary Tract and Pancreas*, ed 5, Philadelphia, 2013, Saunders (Fig. 5-22)

Johns Hopkins Hospital, Engorn B, Flerlage J: *The Harriet Lane Handbook*, ed 20, Philadelphia, 2015, Saunders (Fig. 2-3B)

Kanski J, Bowling B: *Clinical ophthalmology*, ed 7, London, 2011, Saunders (Fig. 11-19)

Kanski J: *Clinical diagnosis in ophthalmology*, Edinburgh, 2006, Mosby (Fig. 13-15)

Kliegman R, Stanton B, St. Geme J, Schor N, Behrman R: *Nelson's textbook of pediatrics*, ed 20, St Louis, 2016, Saunders (Fig. 13-17)

Kostalnick C: *Mosby's textbook for long-term care nursing assistants*, ed 8, St Louis, 2019, Elsevier (Fig. 10-30)

Kozma R: *Artificial intelligence in the age of neural networks and brain computing*, ed 1, Cambridge, 2018, Elsevier (Fig. 12-3)

Kowalczyk N: *Radiographic pathology for technologists*, ed 6, St Louis, 2014, Mosby (Fig. 3-32 B, 3-33 B)

Kumar P, Clark ML: *Kumar and Clark's clinical medicine*, ed 7, Philadelphia, 2009, Saunders (Fig. 6-6 A, 6-18, 8-11)

Kumar V et al: *Robbins and Cotran pathologic basis of disease*, professional edition, ed 9, Philadelphia, 2015, Saunders (Fig. 11-22)

Kumar V et al: *Robbins basic pathology*, ed 9, Philadelphia, 2013, Saunders (Fig. 5-20, 11-23)

Kumar V et al: *Robbins basic pathology*, ed 8, Philadelphia, 2007, Saunders (Fig. 10-20)

LaTrenta G: *Atlas of aesthetic face and neck surgery*, Philadelphia, 2004, Saunders (Fig. 4-39)

Lewis S, et al: *Medical-surgical nursing: assessment and management of clinical problems*, ed 8, St Louis, 2011, Mosby (Fig. 3-34 A, 9-17B&C, 11-28, 13-23, 14-9)

Liberman L, Menell J: *Breast imaging reporting and data system (BI-RADS)*, Radiologic Clinics of North America, 2002, Vol 40, Issue 3, pages 409-430 (Fig. 6-34)

Lowdermilk DL, Perry SE, Bobak IM: *Maternity and women's health care*, ed 10, St Louis, 2012, Mosby (Fig. 4-30, 6-33, 6-39)

Mahan LK, Escott-Stump S: *Krause's food and nutrition therapy*, ed 13, Philadelphia, 2012, Saunders (Fig. 5-21 A)

Manster BJ, May D, Disler D: *Musculoskeletal imaging: the requisites*, ed 4, Philadelphia, 2013, Mosby (Fig. 3-30)

Marks JG Jr, Miller JJ: *Lookingbill & Marks' principles of dermatology*, ed 4, London, 2006, Saunders (Fig. 4-8)

McCance KL, Huether SE: *Pathophysiology: the biologic basis for disease in adults and children*, ed 6, St Louis, 2010, Mosby (Fig. 4-29, 4-34)

Mendelhoff A, Smith DE: *Acromegaly, diabetes, hypermetabolism, proteinuria, and heart failure*, Clinical Pathologic Conference, AMJM, 20:133, 1956 (Fig. 15-8)

Moran CA, Suster S: *Tumors and Tumor-like Conditions of the Lung and Pleura*, Philadelphia, 2010, Saunders (Fig. 10-19)

Mosby's medical nursing and allied health dictionary, ed 8, St Louis, 2009, Mosby (Fig. 6-16, 6-17)

Murray SS: *Foundations of maternal newborn & women's health nursing*, ed 5, Philadelphia, 2010, Saunders (Fig. 7-16)

Muscolino J: *Kinesiology*, ed 3, St Louis, 2017, Mosby (Fig. 3-10)

Nguyen Q, et al, *Retinal pharmacotherapy*, London, 2010, Saunders (Fig. 13-20)

Palay DA, Krachmer J: *Primary Care Ophthalmology*, ed 2, Philadelphia, 2005, Elsevier Mosby (Fig. 13-7)

Parrillo JE, Dellinger RP: *Critical Care Medicine*, ed 4, Philadelphia, 2014, Mosby (Fig. 9-29)

Perry AG, Hockenberry SE: *Maternal child nursing care*, ed 6, Elsevier, 2018 (Fig. 7-22)

Potter PA, Perry AG: *Fundamentals of nursing*, ed 8, St Louis, 2013, Mosby (Fig. 10-29 A-C)

Rakel D: *Integrative medicine*, ed 3, Philadelphia, 2012, Saunders (Fig. 13-22)

Rosai: *Rosai and Ackerman's surgical pathology*, ed 10, Edinburgh, 2011, Mosby (Fig. 10-10)

Sahani D, Samir A: *Abdominal imaging*, Philadelphia, 2011, Saunders (Fig. 6-20)

Schachner L, Hansen R: *Pediatric dermatology*, ed 4, London, 2011, Mosby (Fig. 7-8)

Seidel HM, et al: *Mosby's guide to physical examination*, ed 8, St Louis, 2015, Mosby. Courtesy Richard A. Buckingham, MD. Clinical Professor, Otolaryngology, Abraham Lincoln School of Medicine, University of Illinois, Chicago (Fig. 14-4)

Seidel HM, et al: *Mosby's guide to physical examination*, ed 7, St Louis, 2011, Mosby (Fig. 1-7, 3-15, 4-7, 4-33, 6-7, 13-8, 13-10, 13-11, 13-12)

Shapiro S: *Encyclopedia of Respiratory Medicine*, 2007, Saunders (Fig. 10-7)

Shiland BJ: *Shiland's Mastering Healthcare Terminology*, 5e, Philadelphia, 2015, Mosby (Fig. Appendix B B-10)

Slipman C, Derby R, Simeone F, Mayer T: *Interventional Spine: an algorithmic approach*, ed 1, Edinburgh, 2008, Saunders (Fig. 3-28)

Slovis: *Caffey's pediatric diagnostic imaging*, ed 11, Philadelphia, 2008, Mosby (Fig. 6-5 A)

Sorrentino S, Remmert L, Gorek B: *Mosby's essentials for nursing assistants*, ed 5, St Louis, 2014, Mosby (Fig. 11-12)

Sorrentino SA: *Assisting with patient care*, ed 2, St Louis, 2004, Mosby (Fig. 13-9)

Sorrentino SA: *Textbook for long-term care nursing assistants*, ed 6, St Louis, 2011, Mosby (Fig. 10-27)

Strachan M, Sharma S, Hunter J: *Davidson's 100 Clinical Cases*, ed 2, London, 2012, Churchill Livingstone (15-12).

Stuart GW, Laraia MT: *Principles and practice of psychiatric nursing*, ed 9, St Louis, 2009, Mosby (Fig. 12-1)

Stuart GW, Laraia MT: *Principles and practice of psychiatric nursing*, ed 10, St Louis, 2013, Mosby (Fig. 12-2)

The Centers for Disease Control (Fig. 4-32, 8-19)

Thibodeau GA, Patton KT: *Anatomy and physiology*, ed 8, St Louis, 2013, Mosby (Fig. 3-2, 3-8A, 8-3, Table 9-1, Table 9-2, Table 9-3, 11-4, 11-9)

Thibodeau GA, Patton KT: *The human body in health and disease*, ed 5, St Louis, 2010, Mosby (Fig. 11-7)

Van Rhee J: *Physician assistant board review*, ed 2, Philadelphia, 2010, Saunders (Fig. 10-8)

Vardaxis N: *A textbook of pathology*, ed 2, Sydney, 2010, Mosby (Fig. 7-7)

White S, Pharoah M: *Oral radiology*, ed 7, St Louis, 2014, Mosby (Fig. 5-24)

Wilson SF, Giddons JF: *Health assessment for nursing practice*, ed 4, St Louis, 2012, Mosby (Fig. 3-16 A , 4-6)

Yanoff M, Duker J, Augsburger J: *Ophthalmology*, ed 2, St Louis, 2004, Mosby (Fig. 13-18, 13-25)

Young AP, Proctor DB: *Kinn's the medical assistant*, ed 11, Philadelphia, 2011, Saunders (Fig. 3-20, 10-24)

Young N: *Bone marrow failure syndromes*, Philadelphia, 2000, Saunders (Fig. 8-10)

Zitelli BJ, Davis HW: *Atlas of pediatric physical diagnosis*, ed 5, St Louis, 2007, Mosby (Fig. 5-18)

Zitelli BJ, Davis HW: *Atlas of pediatric physical diagnosis*, ed 6, St Louis, 2012, Mosby (Fig. 11-18, 15-10)

Appendix A   Infectious and Parasitic Disease Basics

pathogen
path/o = disease
-gen = producing, produced by

The very first chapter of ICD-10, "Certain Infectious and Parasitic Diseases," presents a variety of concerns and questions for coders. Unlike the majority of chapters, it is not organized by body systems, but instead, is loosely organized around the **pathogens** that carry and transmit the ailments listed. The medical terms for each of the diseases are often very different from the particular microbe that causes it, and each set of terms has its own naming conventions. Attempting to apply strict logic to neatly compartmentalize these diseases will be met with frustration, as the structure of the chapter has its roots in the 16th century with John Graunt's examination of the London Bills of Mortality (Fig. A-1). Over 400 years of medical science (including the use of naked eye and electron microscopy) has occurred in the interim, so some categories include only one type of pathogen, while others group together diseases by their mode of transmission.

Medical terminology is a constantly evolving discipline, with new terms being added and older terms being deleted from the International Classification of Diseases. The WHO has published best practices for naming new diseases (2015) that includes the avoidance of using the names of individuals, animals, geographic locations, ethnic, or cultural references. Preference is given to signs and symptoms, severity, or the name of the pathogen. Disease names such as "consumption, quinsy, and king's evil" have now passed out of common usage. Covid-19 (sometimes referred to as the novel (meaning new) coronavirus disease recognized in 2019 is a good example of a disease that has used the new naming system. Because of newly emerging diseases, an understanding of the terminology and guidelines for coding this chapter is essential for accurately and completely coding a patient's given diagnoses.

The next revision, ICD-11, is rumored to be a major restructuring of the system with an expected four-fold increase in codes (from 14,400 to 55,000). The United States is not expected to adopt its own clinically modified version of the classification until at least 2023. Of special interest is a list of infectious diseases by agent and a dramatic increase in the codes to record infections resistant to antibiotics. Cur-

ICD-10-CM Guideline Alert!

OGCR 1.C. INFECTIONS RESISTANT TO ANTIBIOTICS
Many bacterial infections are resistant to current antibiotics. It is necessary to identify all infections documented as antibiotic resistant. Assign a code from category Z16, Resistance to antimicrobial drugs, following the infection code only if the infection code does not identify drug resistance.

rently, the guidelines only address MRSA (methicillin-resistant *Staphylococcus aureus*) and MSSA (methicillin-susceptible *Staphylococcus aureus*) conditions specifically.

The majority of terms in this chapter relate to communicable diseases. **Communicable diseases** are those that are easily acquired through a variety of means. Transmission can occur through close personal contact with another infected person (Ex. hugging), by ingesting or inhaling pathogen laden droplets, or by touching an object that an infected person has touched. **Noncommunicable diseases** (NCDs) are those that are inherited, or are congenital, degenerative, or the result of injury. Communicable diseases are caused by **pathogenic** microorganisms, and these particular diseases (the ones in this first chapter) cannot be readily assigned to a body system chapter (hence, the

pathogenic
path/o = disease
-genic = pertaining to produced by

protozoa
proto- = first
-zoa = animal
micro- = tiny, small

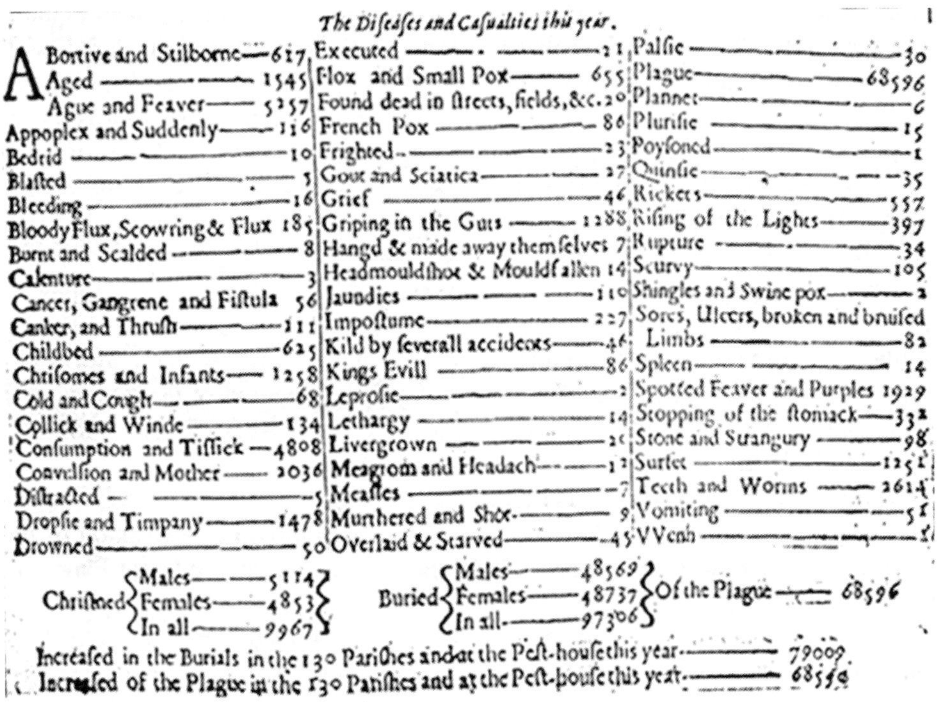

The Diseases and Casualties this year.

Abortive and Stilborne——617	Executed————————21	Palsie————————30
Aged————————1545	Flox and Small Pox————655	Plague————68596
Ague and Feaver————5257	Found dead in streets, fields, &c.—20	Planet————6
Appoplex and Suddenly——116	French Pox————86	Plurisie————15
Bedrid————10	Frighted————23	Poysoned————1
Blasted————5	Gout and Sciatica————27	Quinsie————35
Bleeding————16	Grief————46	Rickets————557
Bloody Flux, Scowring & Flux 185	Griping in the Guts————1288	Rising of the Lights——397
Burnt and Scalded————8	Hang'd & made away themselves 7	Rupture————34
Calenture————3	Headmouldshot & Mouldfallen 14	Scurvy————105
Cancer, Gangrene and Fistula 56	Jaundies————110	Shingles and Swine pox——2
Canker, and Thrush————111	Impostume————227	Sores, Ulcers, broken and bruised
Childbed————625	Kil'd by severall accidents——46	Limbs————82
Chrisomes and Infants——1258	Kings Evill————86	Spleen————14
Cold and Cough————68	Leprosie————2	Spotted Feaver and Purples 1929
Collick and Winde————134	Lethargy————14	Stopping of the stomack——332
Consumption and Tissick——4808	Livergrown————20	Stone and Strangury————98
Convulsion and Mother——2036	Meagrom and Headach————12	Surfet————1251
Distracted————5	Measles————7	Teeth and Worms————2614
Dropsie and Timpany————1478	Murthered and Shot————9	Vomiting————51
Drowned————50	Overlaid & Starved————45	Wenh————2

Christned { Males————5114	Buried { Males————48569	} Of the Plague——68596
Females————4853	Females————48737	
In all————9967	In all————97306	

Increased in the Burials in the 130 Parishes and at the Pest-house this year————79009.
Increased of the Plague in the 130 Parishes and at the Pest-house this year————68550

Fig. A-1 A summary page of causes of death from 1665.

"certain" infectious and parasitic disease title). Some of the diseases spread directly from one person to another, while others spread via a **vector**, a non-human carrier like a mosquito or tick (think malaria or Lyme disease). The internal structure of the chapter is organized largely by the infectious agents that cause the diseases. The infectious agents are termed microbes and include bacteria, viruses, helminths (worms), fungi, prions, **protozoa,** and parasites such as mites and lice. Note that the prefix "**micro-**" has a significant role in infectious disease terminology, as the majority of organisms are too tiny or small to be seen with the naked eye. The use of the microscope in identifying microorganisms is credited to the Dutch scientist Antonie Philips van Leeuwenhoek in the late 1600s. Leeuwenhoek is now known as the father of microbiology. The word "germ" comes to mind when thinking in the vernacular about pathogenic microbes. If germs are present in the body, one is at least a **host** (the organism/location where the pathogen multiplies) and is considered infected. If the germs have multiplied enough to cause signs and symptoms of disease, then one's body may fight the germs with its inflammatory process. If, instead of germs, one has parasites (think mites or lice), one may be infested.

To sort out a few similar, and possibly confusing terms, please note that **inflammation** is a protective response to irritation or injury, while **infection** is the presence of microorganisms where they do not normally reside. Many of the microorganisms in the digestive tract are normal and helpful, but if, for example, *E. coli* spreads to the urinary tract, it can result in a urinary tract infection. Note that an inflammation can result from an infection, with the signs and symptoms of redness, swelling, pain, and a fever, but an infection can also be asymptomatic (no symptoms) or subclinical (no signs or symptoms) and display no evidence of an immune response. The final term, **infestation**, is the presence of a large number of parasites, such that they cause disease or injury.

When you see the word **contagious**, it usually refers to a disease that is spread via physical contact between individuals. Some references consider the terms "contagious" and "infectious" to be synonymous, but "infectious" also has a definition that refers to spread of disease through air or water. All communicable diseases are infectious, but not all infectious diseases are communicable. For example, one can acquire a tetanus infection (commonly referred to as lockjaw), but that infection cannot be spread to another individual. The bacteria that causes tetanus would have to enter the body through a deep cut from infected soil, not from an infected person. Lyme disease is another example. It is acquired through the bite of a tick that introduces a bacterium into the body. An infected person cannot then transmit Lyme disease to another individual. So, both tetanus and Lyme disease are infectious, but not communicable.

PATHOGENS

The diseases in the chapter are largely grouped by the type of pathogens that cause them. In some instances, the mode of transmission is the grouping (sexually transmitted diseases), or an individual disease may be grouped by itself (tuberculosis). The following is a brief summary of what the pathogens are and how they are named. Keep in mind that the pathogen is not the disease, it is an individual microbe and in different locations/situations, it can cause different diseases. The naming of the pathogens generally consists of a two-word name that places the genus first, before the species. For the purpose of this appendix, only the type of pathogen, such as bacteria or virus, will be named in the tables, and the scientific names will not be included, as in many cases more than one species can cause different forms of a disease.

Bacteria

By far, the greatest number of pathogens that infect humans are bacteria (upward of 1 billion) (Fig. A-2). These one-celled creatures are so tiny that most are smaller than a period in a sentence (hence the need for a microscope to

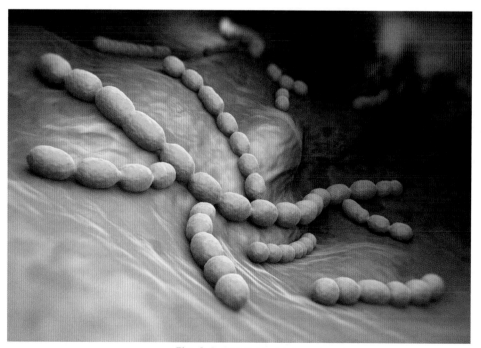

Fig. A-2 Streptococcus.

distinguish one from another, count them, and determine their stage of development). Yet, they are by far the largest of all of the microbes by a factor of 10 to 100 when compared to the next most numerous, viruses. Bacteria are named for their morphology and fall into three basic shapes: bacillus (rod shaped), coccus (spherical), and spirillum (spiral). The spirillum is divided into three subsets depending on the degree of curl in the spiral.

Aside from their shape, bacteria can be sorted into two main types depending on their type of cell wall. By using a dye to differentiate the two, they are classified as gram positive (staining with a purple color) and gram negative (staining with a pink color).

Viruses

Viruses are the second most common pathogen, although they do not qualify technically as microorganisms, because they do not reproduce and have no metabolism. They do, however, require a host to replicate themselves and are categorized by their shape, their size, and their type of genetic material. Those viruses that replicate themselves using DNA are the viruses that cause smallpox and the herpesviruses (chicken pox and cold sores). The RNA viruses are the cause of many common colds, influenza, measles, and mumps. Names of viruses may give a hint of the diseases that they cause, for example, respiratory syncytial virus (RSV), poliovirus (poliomyelitis), and human papillomavirus (HPV). Other viruses are named for their shape: coronavirus (crown-shaped), astrovirus (star-shaped), and rotavirus (wheel-shaped). Retroviruses are named for their use of an enzyme (reverse transcriptase) to use RNA instead of DNA to encode genetic information. The rotaviruses cause gastroenteritis, and the retroviruses cause AIDS and a variety of cancers. Fig. A-3 shows a microphotograph of the novel coronavirus.

Fungi

The fungi group includes yeasts and molds. Examples are histoplasmosis and ringworm (ascariasis). Yeast is a fungus that naturally occurs in the body. It plays a role in the healthy functioning of the digestive system. Too much yeast , however, can lead to infections. Candida yeast infections are commonly referred to as thrush (in the mouth) or diaper rash. Antibiotics often provide an opportunity for yeast to flourish when they kill off the normal bacterial population and provide the nonaffected yeast an opportunity to grow unchecked.

Protozoa

Protozoa are single-celled organisms that can be acquired through contaminated food or water. *Giardia lamblia* and *Cryptosporidium parvum* are two examples. Malaria, transmitted by the anopheles mosquito, is caused by the protozoan *Plasmodium*. Another example of a protozoan is the one that causes toxoplasmosis: *Toxoplasma gondii*. This protozoan is spread through contaminated food or through contact with cat feces.

Helminths

Helminths (common name *worms*) are multicellular organisms that may cause disease. Roundworms (ascariasis), hookworm, and whipworm are considered soil-transmitted helminths (STH), while trichinosis (*Trichinella spiralis*) is carried by pigs and is seen in improperly cooked pork.

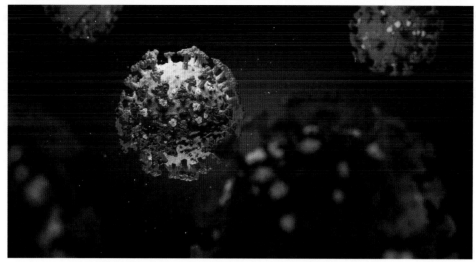

Fig. A-3 Microphotograph of the novel coronavirus.

Prions

Prions became the most recent addition to the classification when Stanley Prusiner named them as an infectious agent in transmissible spongiform encephalopathies (TSEs). Unlike other microbes, prions lack nucleic acid, a large biomolecule essential to life. The term *prion* is an interesting blend of "protein" and "infection." This type of etymology is referred to as a portmanteau, a blend of word parts that does not fit the normal rules of building medical terms. Other interesting examples of portmanteaus that may be familiar from English are *smog* ("smoke" and "fog") and *motel* (from "motor" and "hotel"). In healthcare, common portmanteaus are *botox* (from "botulism" and "toxin") and *caplet* (from "capsule" and "tablet") and of course, Covid-19 (from corona, virus, and disease).

Parasites

The last of the infectious diseases are the parasites lice and mites. A parasite is technically any organism that lives off of a host. Scabies is a parasitic infestation caused by mites and is characterized by a pruritic papular rash. Pediculosis is a parasitic infestation with lice and involves the head, body, or genital area. Pubic lice are termed phthiriasis pubis (*phthir/o* is from the Greek, meaning "wasting away").

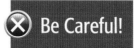 **Be Careful!** Acariasis *is a term for a rash caused by mites, while* ascariasis *is an infection of the small intestine by the roundworm* **Ascaris slumbricoide.**

Terms Related to Certain Infectious and Parasitic Diseases Tables

The following tables are arranged according to the classification's sequence of diseases and include the name of the disease, its word origins, the type of pathogen, and a short definition. The diseases that have been named centuries ago have names that do not fit neatly into medical terminology's word root and suffix schema. Diphtheria, cholera, and leprosy have names that are rooted in medical knowledge from the time they were initially documented. Locations (Lyme disease), discoverers (ehrlichiosis), and characteristics (whooping cough) are also used to name diseases in this chapter.

As always, English medical terminology is dependent on the same alphabet as mainstream English language. Terms for very different diseases can be spelled very similarly and be a source of confusion (see *ascariasis* and *acariasis*). Where this happens, a **Be Careful!** alert has been inserted.

Intestinal Infectious Diseases (A00-A09) and Tuberculosis (A15-A19)			
Term	**Word Origins**	**Pathogen Type/ Name**	**Definition**
cholera	Possibly from the Latin term meaning *a gutter*, referring to the body's role in expelling diarrhea.	bacteria	Bacterial (*Vibrio cholerae*) infection of the small intestine that is spread through contaminated food and water. Marked by acute diarrhea.
typhoid	*-oid* like, resembling Named for its similarity to another disease, typhus, which is spread by fleas and lice.	bacteria	Bacterial infection spread through contaminated food and water. Caused by *Salmonella typhi*.
enterocolitis due to *Clostridium difficile*	*enter/o* small intestines *col/o* large intestines *-itis* inflammation	bacteria	Common bacterial infection of the large intestine caused by the *Clostridium difficile* bacteria.
botulism food poisoning	*Botulism* is derived from the Latin term for sausage, as first cases were due to tainted sausage meat.	bacteria	Caused by food that is contaminated by the neurotoxin bacterium, *Clostridium botulinum*.
tuberculosis	Originally a "disease caused by swellings" (tubercules)	bacteria	Chronic infectious disorder caused by *Mycobacterium tuberculosis.* Multidrug-resistant tuberculosis (MDRTB) is fatal in 80% of cases.

Certain Zoonotic Bacterial Diseases and Other Bacterial Diseases (A20-A28 and A30-A49)

Term	Word Origins	Pathogen Type/Name	Definition
plague	From Latin meaning "epidemic that causes many deaths."	bacteria	A disease caused by the bacterium *Yersinia pestis*. Transmitted by fleas from rodents carrying the plague bacterium (*Yersinia pestis*) or by handling an animal infected with plague.
anthrax	*anthrac/o* black Named for the characteristic black skin lesions caused by the disease.	bacteria	A serious infectious disease caused by gram-positive, rod-shaped bacteria known as *Bacillus anthracis*.
leprosy	Named for the Latin term meaning "I peel," referring to the skin sores that develop.	bacteria	An infection caused by the bacterium *Mycobacterium leprae*. It can affect the nerves, skin, eyes, and lining of the nose. Also called **Hansen's disease**.
diphtheria	Named for a Greek term meaning "leathery," which refers to the covering that occurs on the back of the throat.	bacteria	An infection caused by the bacterium *Corynebacterium diphtheriae*. The thick covering in the back of the throat that develops can lead to difficulty breathing, heart failure, and paralysis.
pertussis	Tussis refers to a cough.	bacteria	A highly contagious respiratory disease caused by the bacterium *Bordetella pertussis*. Known for causing uncontrollable, violent coughing. After coughing, someone with pertussis often feels the need to take a deep breath, which results in a "whooping" sound. Also called **whooping cough**.
Legionnaires' disease	Named for outbreak at American Legion convention in Philadelphia, 1976	bacteria	Rare respiratory disease caused by *Legionella pneumophila*.

 ICD-10-CM Guideline Alert!

C.1.C INFECTIONS RESISTANT TO ANTIBIOTICS
Many bacterial infections are resistant to current antibiotics. It is necessary to identify all infections documented as antibiotic resistant. Assign a code from category Z16, Resistance to antimicrobial drugs, following the infection code only if the infection code does not identify drug resistance.

Infections with a Predominantly Sexual Mode of Transmission (A50-A64)

Term	Word Origins	Pathogen Type/Name	Definition
syphilis	unknown	bacteria	Multistage sexually transmitted infection (STI) caused by the spirochete *Treponema pallidum*. A highly infectious chancre appears in the first stage, usually on the genitals.
gonococcal infection	*gon/o* seed *-rrhea* discharge, flow	bacteria	Disease caused by the gram negative diploccous Neisseria gonorrhoeae bacterium. Manifests as inflammation of urethra, prostate, rectum, or pharynx. May be asymptomatic when in the cervix or fallopian tubes of women.
chlamydial infection	Named for the bacteria that causes it.	bacteria	Inflammation of the urethra caused by *chlamydia trachomatis*.
trichomoniasis	*trich/o* hair	protozoa	Common curable, pruritic vaginal infectious disease caused by the protozoan *Trichomonas*.

Other Spirochetal Disease, Rickettsioses and Viral and Prion Infections of the CNS (A65-A89)

Term	Word Origins	Pathogen Type/ Name	Definition
Lyme disease	Named for the location of first diagnosed cases: Lyme, Conn.	bacteria	Usually caused by the bacterium *Borrelia burgdorferi*. It is transmitted to humans through the bite of infected ticks. Typical symptoms include fever, headache, fatigue, and a characteristic skin rash called erythema migrans (bull's-eye rash). If left untreated, infection can spread to joints, the heart, and the nervous system.
typhus fever	From Ancient Greek meaning fever or stupor.	bacteria	**Typhus fevers** are a group of diseases caused by bacteria that are spread to humans by fleas and lice. The most common symptoms are fever, headaches, and sometimes rash.
ehrlichiosis	Named for the microbiologist Paul Ehrlich.	bacteria	Ehrlichiosis is the general name used to describe diseases caused by the bacteria *Ehrlichia chaffeensis*, *E. ewingii*, or *E. muris eauclairensis* in the United States.

Other Spirochetal Disease, Rickettsioses and Viral and Prion Infections of the CNS (A65-A89)—cont'd

Term	Word Origins	Pathogen Type/ Name	Definition
acute poliomyelitis	*poli/o* gray *myel/o* spinal cord *-itis* inflammation	virus	Inflammation of the gray matter of the spinal cord caused by a poliovirus. Severe formscause paralysis.
Creutzfeldt-Jakob disease (CJD)	Named for the doctors who reported the first cases.	prion	Creutzfeldt-Jakob disease (CJD) is a rare degenerative, fatal brain disorder. CJD usually appears in later life and runs a rapid course.
rabies	From Sanskrit meaning "to do violence"	virus	Rabies is a fatal but preventable viral disease that can spread to people and pets if they are bitten or scratched by a rabid animal infected with the rabies virus.

Arthropod-Borne Viral Fevers and Viral Hemorrhagic Fevers and Viral Infections Characterized By Skin and Mucous Membrane Lesions (A90-B09)

Term	Word Origins	Pathogen Type/Name	Definition
West Nile virus infection	Named for the Ugandan location where first seen.	virus	Viral infection spread by mosquitoes. Can vary in severity with symptoms of convulsions, fever, paralysis and coma.
Zika virus disease	Named for Ugandan forest where first seen.	virus	Viral infection spread by mosquitoes. Mild form is not serious, unless it affects a pregnant woman. Infants born to infected mothers may have microcephaly (smaller than normal heads).
varicella	unknown	virus	Highly contagious viral infection marked by skin eruptions. Also called **chicken pox**.
zoster [herpes zoster]	From herpes meaning "to creep" and zoster referring to a belt or girdle. No doubt a reference to the nature of the rash, which follows the peripheral nerves.	virus/herpes zoster	Acute, painful rash caused by reactivation of latent varicella-zoster virus. Also called **shingles**.
smallpox	Named for the characteristic skin eruptions.	virus	Easily communicable disease that appears to now be eradicated. Marked by skin eruptions. Also called **variola**.
rubeola	From the Latin *rubellus*, meaning *red*. No doubt a reference to the color of the rash.	virus	Highly contagious viral disease marked by red spots on skin, tongue and cheeks. Also called **measles**.
rubella	From Latin *rubellus*, meaning *red*.	virus	Mildly contagious disease with rash resembling rubeola. Also called **German measles**.

Continued

Arthropod-Borne Viral Fevers and Viral Hemorrhagic Fevers and Viral Infections Characterized By Skin and Mucous Membrane Lesions (A90-B09)—cont'd

Term	Word Origins	Pathogen Type/Name	Definition
verruca	From Latin, meaning "a wart".	virus	Common contagious epithelial growths, usually appearing on skin of hands, feet, legs, and face. Can be caused by one of 60 types of human papillomavirus (HPV). Also called **warts**.

 Be Careful!   *Do not confuse* varicella (chicken pox) *with* variola (smallpox).

 Be Careful!   *Do not confuse* rubeola (common measles) *with* rubella (German measles).

 ICD-10-CM Guideline Alert!

C.1.F. ZIKA VIRUS INFECTIONS
1) Code only confirmed cases
Code only a confirmed diagnosis of Zika virus (A92.5, Zika Virus diseases) as documented by the provider. This is an exception to the hospital inpatient guideline Section II, H.

In this context, "confirmation" does not require documentation of the type of test performed; the physician's diagnostic statement that the condition is confirmed is sufficient. This code should be assigned regardless of the stated mode of transmission.

Viral Hepatitis (B15-B19)

Term	Word Origins	Pathogen Type/Name	Definition
acute hepatitis A (HAV)	*hepat/o* liver *-itis* inflammation	virus	Inflammatory disease of liver transmitted through direct contact with fecally contaminated food or water.
acute hepatitis B (HBV)	*hepat/o* liver *-itis* inflammation	virus	Inflammatory disease of liver transmitted through contaminated blood or sexual contact.
other acute viral hepatitis	*hepat/o* liver *-itis* inflammation	virus	Inflammatory diseases of liver (usually hepatitis C) transmitted through blood transfusion, percutaneous inoculation, or sharing of needles.

Human Immunodeficiency Virus (HIV) Disease (B2Ø) and Other Viral Diseases (B25-B34)

Term	Word Origins	Pathogen Type/Name	Definition
human immunodeficiency virus (HIV) disease	*immun/o* immune	virus	Viral infection spread through bodily fluids that attacks the immune system. Includes acquired immunodeficiency syndrome (AIDS) and AIDS-related complex (ARC).
cytomegalovirus (CMV)	*cyt/o* cell *megal/o* large	virus	Common herpes-type viral infection that is usually mild, but may cause problems in individuals with weakened immune systems.
infectious parotitis	*parot/o* parotid gland *-itis* inflammation	virus	Viral disease of the salivary glands. May cause complications of testes and ovaries. Also called **mumps**.
infectious mononucleosis	*mono-* one *nucle/o* nucleus *-osis* abnormal condition	virus	Relatively benign infection caused by the Epstein-Barr virus. Symptoms include enlarged lymph glands, fever, and sore throat.

Note

HIV guidelines are noted in the Blood, Blood-Forming Organs, and the Immune Mechanism chapter.

Mycoses and Protozoal Diseases (B35-B64)

Term	Word Origins	Pathogen Type/ Name	Definition
tinea barbae	*Tinea* is from Latin, meaning a "gnawing worm." *Barbae* is from Latin, meaning a beard.	fungus	Fungal infection of the beard and facial hair.
tinea capitis	*capit/o* head	fungus	Fungal infection of the scalp. Also called **ringworm.**
tinea unguium	*ungu/o* nail	fungus	Fungal infection of the nails.
tinea manuum	*man/u* hand	fungus	Fungal infection of the hand.
tinea pedis	*ped/i* foot	fungus	Fungal infection of the foot.

Continued

Mycoses and Protozoal Diseases (B35-B64)—cont'd

Term	Word Origins	Pathogen Type/Name	Definition
tinea corporis	*corpor/o* body	fungus	Fungal infection of the body.
tinea cruris	*crur/o* leg	fungus	Fungal infection of the external genitalia and upper legs, particularly in warm weather. Also called "jock itch."
candidiasis	From the Latin meaning "white". *-iasis* abnormal condition Hence, an abnormal condition of whiteness, describing the appearance of the fungus on the body parts affected.	fungus	Candidiasis is a fungal infection caused by yeasts that belong to the genus *Candida* and become problematic when they are not kept in check. *Candida* normally lives in moist places such as the mouth, throat, gut, and vagina and on the skin and usually does not cause any problems.
histoplasmosis	unknown	fungus	Histoplasmosis is an infection caused by a fungus called *Histoplasma capsulatum* that lives in the environment, particularly in soil that contains large amounts of bird or bat droppings. It affects the lungs and is common among AIDS patients.
malaria	From the Italian word meaning "bad air," referring to the areas where mosquitoes tend to breed.	protozoa	Malaria is a mosquito-borne disease caused by a parasite. The most common parasite that is transmitted by the mosquito is of the species *Plasmodium*, although other species exist. People with malaria often experience fever, chills, and flu-like illness.
toxoplasmosis	*tox/o* poison *plasm/a* plasma *-osis* abnormal condition	protozoa	Toxoplasmosis is an infection caused by a parasite. This parasite is called *Toxoplasma gondii*. It can be found in cat feces and undercooked meat, especially venison, lamb, and pork.

Helminthiases, Pediculosis, Ascariasis and Other Infestations (B65-B89)

Term	Word Origins	Pathogen Type/Name	Definition
ascariasis	Named for the worm that causes the disease. *-iasis* abnormal condition	helminth	Ascaris, hookworm, and whipworm are parasitic worms. Ascaris parasites live in the intestine, and Ascaris eggs are passed in the feces of infected people.
pediculosis	From Latin meaning "infested with lice."	parasite	Parasitic infestation with lice, involving the head, body, or genital area.

Helminthiases, Pediculosis, Ascariasis and Other Infestations (B65-B89)—cont'd

Term	Word Origins	Pathogen Type/Name	Definition
acariasis	Named for Latin term for mite, "acarid." *-iasis* abnormal condition	parasite	Parasitic infestation caused by mites; characterized by pruritic papular rash. Scabies is an example of acarisasis.

 ### ICD-10-CM Guideline Alert!

As of the date that this text is being published, Covid-19 was assigned a code of B97.29 for confirmed cases. (Other coronavirus as the cause of diseases classified elsewhere). A separate code should also be assigned for the appropriate diagnosis code. An experimental code, U07.1, has been designated by WHO because of the diseases international public health emergency status.

AMA has also published a new code for antibody plasma testing: **86328** *Immunoassay for infectious agent antibody(ies), qualitative or semiquantitative, single step method (eg, reagent strip); severe acute respiratory syndrome coronavirus 2 (SARS-CoV-2) (Coronavirus disease [COVID-19])*

86769 *Antibody; severe acute respiratory syndrome coronavirus 2 (SARS-CoV-2) (Coronavirus disease [COVID-19])*

Coding charts with diagnoses from the **neoplasm** chapter of ICD-10-CM requires an understanding of the terminology describing the types of tumors, and the diagnostic and therapeutic procedures used to detect and treat each. Diagnostic coding guidelines determine how the tumor should be coded, depending on whether it is the original **cancer,** or one that has developed from it. Further detailed guidelines are given in regard to diagnoses that indicate admissions for treatments to either the original or subsequent formations. Coding the procedures used to diagnose and treat these various neoplasms necessitates an understanding of the terminology that is often used with cancer diagnosis and treatment, but is used less often with other pathologies.

Where there is life, there is cancer. Although the types of cancer and their incidence (the number of new cases diagnosed each year) may vary by geography, sex, race, age, and ethnicity, cancer exists in every population and has since ancient times. Archeologists have found evidence of cancer in dinosaur bones and human mummies. Written descriptions of cancer treatment have been discovered dating back to 1600 BC. The word *cancer* comes from the Greek word for *crab*. It was used by Hippocrates to describe the appearance of the most common type of cancer, carcinoma, as it invaded the tissue it inhabited.

neo- = new
-plasm = formation

cancer = carcin/o

NAMING MALIGNANT TUMORS

All cancers are **neoplasms** (new formations), but not all neoplasms are cancerous. Cancerous **tumors** are termed *malignant,* whereas noncancerous tumors are termed *benign.* Malignant tumors tend to grow rapidly and spread, and their cells do not resemble the cells of the tissue that they are invading. If they are removed, they often tend to recur. While still tumors, benign neoplasms grow slowly, do not spread, and their cells resemble the cells of the tissue that they inhabit. If a tumor is described as being "in situ," it means that the tumor cells have not invaded the tissue and are still in a very early stage. Naming tumors by their "type" is referred to as their **behavior,** or how they act in the body. Determining the behavior of a neoplasm is one of the first steps in determining how it should be treated.

In ICD-10-CM, C codes denote malignant tumors, while D codes indicate *in situ,* benign, uncertain, and unspecified behaviors.

The following tables summarize characteristics of benign and malignant tumors by body system. Note that a particular system does not always have all one type of cancer because organs are composed of a variety of tissues with different embryonic origins. The integumentary system has both carcinomas and sarcomas, because it is composed of epithelial and connective tissue.

Comparison of Benign and Malignant Neoplasms

Characteristics	Benign	Malignant
Mode of growth	Relatively slow growth by expansion; encapsulated; cells adhere to each other	Rapid growth; invades surrounding tissue by infiltration
Cells under microscopic examination	Resemble tissue of origin; well differentiated; appear normal	Do not resemble tissue of origin; vary in size and shape; abnormal appearance and function
Spread	Remains isolated	Metastasis; cancer cells carried by blood and lymphatics to one or more other locations; secondary tumors occur
Other properties	No tissue destruction; not prone to hemorrhage; may be smooth and freely movable	Ulceration and/or necrosis; prone to hemorrhage; irregular and less movable
Recurrence	Rare after excision	A common characteristic
Pathogenesis	Symptoms related to location with obstruction and/or compression of surrounding tissue or organs; usually not life threatening unless inaccessible	Cachexia; pain; fatal if not controlled

From Frazier MS, Drzymkowski JW: *Essentials of human diseases and conditions,* ed 6, Philadelphia, 2016, Saunders.

Coding Guidelines I.C.2

GENERAL GUIDELINES
To properly code a neoplasm it is necessary to determine from the record if the neoplasm is benign, in situ, malignant, or of uncertain histologic behavior. If malignant, any secondary (metastatic) sites should also be determined.

CARCINOGENESIS

Cancer is not *one* disease but a group of hundreds of diseases with similar characteristics. The shared characteristics are uncontrolled cell growth and a spread of altered cells. Different types of cancers have different occurrence rates and different causes.

Current research suggests that there is no single cause of cancer. Radiation, bacteria, viruses, genetics, diet, smoking (or exposure to tobacco smoke), alcohol, and other factors all contribute to the development of cancer termed **carcinogenesis.** Each of these factors is instrumental in disrupting the normal balance of cell growth and destruction within the body by causing a mutation in the deoxyribonucleic acid (DNA) of cells (Fig. B-l) Once this **mutation** takes place, a process of uncontrolled cell growth may begin. It is important to note that the cancer cells that replace normal cells no longer function to keep the body working. The only mission of cancer cells is to reproduce. Fig. B-2 illustrates the process of **apoptosis,** the body's normal restraining function to keep cell growth in check. Fig. B-3 shows the progression from normally

carcinogenesis
 carcin/o = cancer
 -genesis = production, origin

mutation
 mut/a = change
 -tion = process of

apoptosis
 apo- = away from
 -ptosis = falling

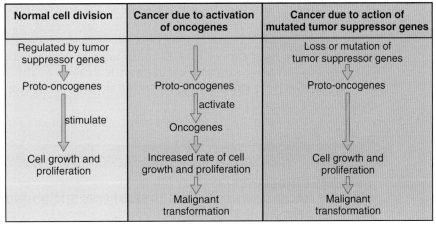

Fig. B-1 Normal cell growth vs. oncogenesis.

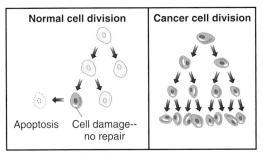

Fig. B-2 Apoptosis.

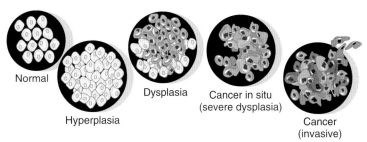

Fig. B-3 Progression of skin cancer from hyperplasia to cancer.

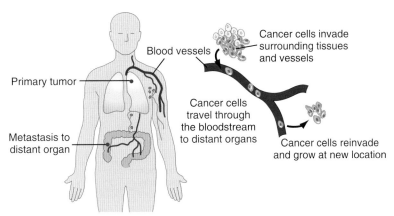

Fig. B-4 Metastasis.

functioning skin tissue to **hyperplasia,** to **dysplasia,** and finally to carcinoma in situ (CIS). The **histology** (literally, study of tissue) of the tumor will yield its tissue type and behavior. Cancer is a continuum—from tissue made up of normally functioning cells fulfilling their role to keep the body healthy, to tissue replaced by cancerous cells that no longer perform the work of the tissue and now perform only the function of reproducing themselves. Cancers are capable of destroying not only the tissue in which they originate (the primary site), but also other tissues through the process of **metastasis,** the spread of cancer. Metastasis can occur by direct extension to contiguous organs and tissues or to distant sites through blood (Fig. B-4) or lymphatic involvement. It

hyperplasia
   hyper- = excessive
   -plasia = condition of
      formation

dysplasia
   dys- = abnormal
   -plasia = condition of
      formation

metastasis
   meta- = beyond, change
   -stasis = controlling,
      stopping

histology
   hist/o = tissue
   -logy = study of

tumor = onc/o, -oma

neoplasm
   neo- = new
   -plasm = formation

embryonic = blast/o,
   -blast

carcinoma
   carcin/o = cancer
   -oma = tumor, mass

ectodermal
   ecto- = outer
   derm/o = skin
   -al = pertaining to

endodermal
   endo- = within
   derm/o = skin
   -al = pertaining to

mesodermal
   meso- = middle
   derm/o = skin
   -al = pertaining to

connective tissue cancer
   = sarc/o, -sarcoma

is important to note that the primary site is the site of origin, while the metastatic site, is a secondary site.

For example, a lung cancer may be a primary site (the site where the cancer began), while a liver cancer may develop later as a metastatic (secondary) site. That patient has lung cancer with metastatic growth to the liver. The abbreviation **mets** stands for **metatases,** the resultant secondary tumors that have traveled from the original site.

> ### Coding Guideline I.C.2
>
> **GENERAL GUIDELINES**
> **PRIMARY MALIGNANT NEOPLASMS OVERLAPPING SITE BOUNDARIES**
> A primary malignant neoplasm that overlaps two or more contiguous (next to each other) sites should be classified to the subcategory/code .8 ('overlapping lesion'), unless the combination is specifically indexed elsewhere. For multiple neoplasms of the same site that are not contiguous such as tumors in different quadrants of the same breast, codes for each site should be assigned.

Although the hundreds of known types of malignant tumors commonly share the characteristics listed previously, the names that they are given reflect their differences. All tissues (and hence organs) are derived from the progression of three embryonic germ layers that differentiate into specific tissues and organs. Tumors are generally divided into two broad categories and a varying number of other categories, based on their **embryonic** origin. Fig. B-5 illustrates the different types of cancers and where they occur.

- **Carcinomas:** Approximately 80% to 90% of malignant tumors are derived from the outer **(ectodermal)** and inner **(endodermal)** layers of the embryo that develop into epithelial tissue that either covers or lines the surfaces of the body. This category of cancer is divided into two main types. If derived from an organ or gland, it is an adenocarcinoma; if derived from squamous epithelium, it is a squamous cell carcinoma. Examples include gastric adenocarcinoma and squamous cell carcinoma of the lung.
- **Sarcomas** are derived from the middle **(mesodermal)** layer, which becomes connective tissue (bones, muscle, cartilage, blood vessels, and fat). Most end

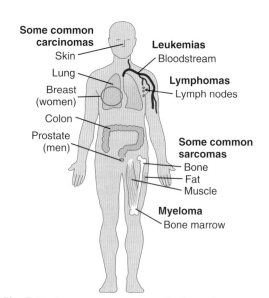

Fig. B-5 Common cancers and where they occur.

in the suffix **-*sarcoma***. Examples include osteosarcoma, chondrosarcoma, hemangiosarcoma, mesothelioma, and glioma.

- **Lymphomas** develop in lymphatic tissue (vessels, nodes, and organs, including the spleen, tonsils, and thymus gland). Lymphomas are solid cancers and may also appear outside of the sites of lymphatic organs in the stomach, breast, or brain; these are called **extranodal lymphomas.** All lymphomas may be divided into two categories: Hodgkin lymphoma and non-Hodgkin lymphoma.
- **Leukemia** is cancer of the bone marrow. An example is acute myelocytic leukemia.
- **Myelomas** arise from the plasma cells in the bone marrow. An example is multiple myeloma.
- **Mixed tumors** are a combination of cells from within one category or between two cancer categories. Examples are **teratocarcinoma** and **carcinosarcoma.**

STAGING AND GRADING

To treat cancer, the treating physician must determine the severity of the cancer, the grade, and its stage, or size and spread. Cancers at different grades and stages react differently to various treatments. Although one does not need to use staging and grading in coding tumors, it is helpful to understand the terminology used for assigning grades and stages and the roles they play in determining treatment protocols.

Grading (G) is the first means of affixing a value to a clinical opinion of the degree of **dedifferentiation (anaplasia)** of cancer cells, or how much the cells appear different from their original form. Healthy cells are well differentiated; cancer cells are poorly differentiated. The pathologist determines this difference and assigns a grade ranging from 1 to 4. The higher the grade, the more cancerous, or dedifferentiated, is the tissue sample. Grading is a measure of the cancer's *severity.*

The other means of determining the *size and spread* of the cancer from its original site is called **staging.** A number of systems are used to describe staging. Some are specific to the type of cancer; others are general systems. If staging is determined by various diagnostic techniques, it is referred to as **clinical staging.** If it is determined by the pathologist's report, it is called **pathologic staging.** An example is TNM staging. In this system, **T** stands for the size of the **tumor, N** stands for the number of lymph **nodes** positive for cancer, and **M** stands for the presence of distant **metastasis.** Summary staging puts together the TNM to give one number as a stage. Again, this helps the clinician to determine the type of treatment that is most effective. Fig. B-6 illustrates a staging system. Remember, if the cancer cells appear only at the original site and have not invaded the organ of origin, it is called **carcinoma in situ (CIS).**

extranodal
  extra- = outside
  nod/o = node
  -al = pertaining to

myeloma
  myel/o = bone marrow, spinal cord
  -oma = tumor, mass

teratocarcinoma
  terat/o = deformity
  -carcinoma = cancer of epithelial origin

carcinosarcoma
  carcin/o = cancer
  -sarcoma = connective tissue cancer

anaplasia
  ana- = up, apart
  -plasia = condition of formation

pathologic
  path/o = disease
  -logic = pertaining to studying

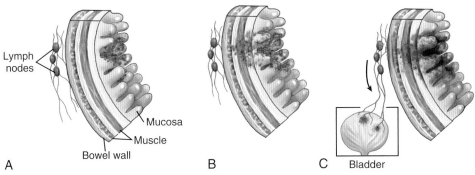

Fig. B-6 Staging of colon cancer. **A,** Stage I; **B,** stage II; **C,** stage III.

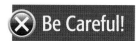 **Be Careful!** *Don't confuse* **sarc/o***, meaning* flesh, *with* **sacr/o,** *meaning* sacrum.

Combining and Adjective Forms for Oncology

Meaning	Combining Form	Adjective Form
change	mut/a	
disease	path/o	
embryo	blast/o	embryonic
node	nod/o	nodal
tumor	onc/o	

Prefixes for Oncology

Prefix	Meaning
ana-	up, apart
apo-	away from
dys-	abnormal
ecto-	outer
endo-	within
extra-	outside
hyper-	excessive
meso-	middle
meta-	beyond, change
neo-	new

Suffixes for Oncology

Suffix	Meaning
-carcinoma	cancer of epithelial origin
-genesis	production, origin
-oma	tumor, mass
-plasia	condition of formation
-plasm	formation
-ptosis	falling
-sarcoma	connective tissue cancer
-stasis	controlling, stopping

PATHOLOGY

Signs and Symptoms

The signs and symptoms of cancer are manifestations of how cancer cells replace the functions of healthy tissue. Some examples include anorexia (lack of appetite), bruising, leukocytosis (slight increase of white blood cells), fatigue, cachexia (wasting), and thrombocytopenia (deficiency of clotting cells).

 Coding Guideline I.C.g

SYMPTOMS, SIGNS, AND ABNORMAL FINDINGS LISTED IN CHAPTER 18 ASSOCIATED WITH NEOPLASMS
Symptoms, signs, and ill-defined conditions listed in Chapter 18 characteristic of, or associated with, an existing primary or secondary site malignancy cannot be used to replace the malignancy as principal or first-listed diagnosis, regardless of the number of admissions or encounters for treatment and care of the neoplasm.

Neoplasia by Body System

Body System	Organ	Benign Neoplasms	Malignant Neoplasms
Musculoskeletal (MS)	bone cartilage muscle	osteoma chondroma rhabdomyoma leiomyoma	Ewing sarcoma, osteosarcoma chondrosarcoma, rhabdomyosarcoma, leiomyosarcoma
Integumentary	skin	dermatofibroma	basal cell carcinoma, squamous cell carcinoma, malignant melanoma, Kaposi sarcoma
Gastrointestinal (GI)	esophagus stomach pancreas colon/rectum	leiomyoma polyp gastric adenoma	adenocarcinoma of the esophagus, stomach, pancreas, colon, and/or rectum
Urinary	kidney bladder	nephroma	hypernephroma/renal cell carcinoma, Wilms tumor/, nephroblastoma transitional cell carcinoma (bladder cancer)
Male reproductive	testis prostate	benign prostatic hyperplasia	seminoma, teratoma, adenocarcinoma of the prostate
Female reproductive	breast uterus ovaries cervix	fibrocystic changes in the breast fibroids ovarian cyst cervical dysplasia	infiltrating ductal adenocarcinoma of the breast, stromal endometrial carcinoma epithelial ovarian carcinoma, squamous cell carcinoma of the cervix

Neoplasia by Body System—cont'd

Blood/lymphatic/ immune	blood lymph vessels thymus gland	thymoma	leukemia non-Hodgkin lymphoma, Hodgkin-lymphoma malignant thymoma
Cardiovascular	blood vessels heart	hemangioma myxoma	hemangiosarcoma myxosarcoma
Respiratory	epithelial tissue of respiratory tract, lung, bronchus	papilloma of lung	adenocarcinoma of the lung, small cell carcinoma, mesothelioma, bronchogenic carcinoma
Nervous	Central nervous system (CNS; brain, spinal cord, meninges) Peripheral nervous system (PNS)	neuroma neurofibroma meningioma	glioblastoma multiforme
Endocrine	pituitary thyroid adrenal medulla	benign pituitary tumor pheochromocytoma	thyroid carcinoma
Eyes and ears	retina choroid acoustic nerve	choroidal hemangioma acoustic neuroma	retinoblastoma

See also neoplasm tables in Chapters 3 to 15.

DIAGNOSTIC PROCEDURES

Patient History

Along with the various clinical techniques described, the patient's history is especially important, including information regarding family history (for genetic information) and social history, such as tobacco and alcohol use, diet, and sexual history. A patient's smoking history is described in terms of "pack years." The number of pack years equals the average number of packs smoked per day multiplied by the number of years of smoking. For example: 1 pack/day × 25 years of smoking represents 25 pack years. A patient's current or former occupation may also shed light on the type of cancer. For example, exposure to asbestos, through an occupation of ship building or working with brake repair, may lead to a rare type of lung cancer—mesothelioma. Z codes may be used to specify personal history details.

Tumor Markers

Tumor marker tests measure the levels of a variety of biochemical substances detected in the blood, urine, or body tissues that often appear in higher than normal amounts in individuals with certain neoplasms. Because other factors may influence the amount of the tumor marker present, they are not intended to be used as a sole means of diagnosis. Examples include the following:

alpha fetoprotein (AFP) test: Increased levels may indicate liver or testicular cancer.

beta-2 microglobulin (B2M): Levels are elevated in multiple myeloma and chronic lymphocytic leukemia.

bladder tumor antigen (BTA): Present in the urine of patients with bladder cancer.

CA125: Used for ovarian cancer detection and management.

CA15-3: Levels are measured to determine the stage of breast cancer.

CA19-9: Levels are elevated in stomach, colorectal, and pancreatic cancers.

CA27-29: Used to monitor breast cancer; especially useful in testing for recurrences.

carcinoembryonic antigen (CEA): Monitors colorectal cancer when the disease has spread or after treatment to measure the patient's response.

human chorionic gonadotropin (hCG): Used as a screen for choriocarcinoma and testicular and ovarian cancers.

neuron-specific enolase (NSE): Used to measure the stage and/or patient's response to treatment of small cell cancer and neuroblastoma.

prostate-specific antigen (PSA): Increased levels may be due to benign prostatic hyperplasia/hypertrophy (BPH) or prostate cancer.

TA-90: Used to detect the spread of malignant melanoma.

Other lab tests include **fecal occult blood test (FOBT)** to test for colon cancer and **Papanicolaou test (Pap)** to test for cervical and vaginal cancer.

Biopsy (Bx)

See Chapter 4 for additional information on types of biopsies.

Imaging

computed tomography (CT) scans: CT scans provide information about a tumor's shape, size, and location, along with the source of its blood supply. They are useful in detecting, evaluating, and monitoring cancer, especially liver, pancreatic, bone, lung, and adrenal gland cancers. CT scans are also useful in staging cancer and guiding needles for aspiration biopsy (bx) (Fig. B-7).

magnetic resonance imaging (MRI): Areas of the body that are often difficult to image are possible to see with MRI because of its three-dimensional (3D) capabilities. MRI is useful in detecting cancer in the CNS and the MS system. It is also used to stage breast and endometrial cancer before surgery and to detect metastatic spread of cancer to the liver.

nuclear scans: Nuclear scans are useful in locating and staging cancer of the thyroid and the bone. A **positron emission tomography (PET) scan** provides information about the metabolism of an internal structure, along with its size and shape. It is primarily used for images of the brain, neck, colon, rectum, ovary, and lung. It may also help to identify more aggressive tumors (Fig. B-8). **Single-photon emission computed tomography (SPECT)** uses a rotating camera to create 3D images with the use of radioactive substances. It is useful in identifying metastases to the bone. *Monoclonal antibodies* are used to evaluate cancer of the prostate, colon, breast, and ovaries and melanoma.

radiography: Because tumors are usually denser than the tissue surrounding them, they may appear as a lighter shade of gray (blocking more radiation). Abdominal x-rays may reveal tumors of the stomach, liver, kidneys, and so on, whereas chest x-rays are useful in detecting lung cancer. If a contrast medium is used, as in an upper or lower GI series or intravenous urogram (IVU), tumors of the esophagus, rectum, colon, or kidneys may be detected. Another special type of x-ray is a **mammogram,** which is useful in the early detection of breast cancer. **Stereotactic (3D) mammography** may be used for an image-guided biopsy.

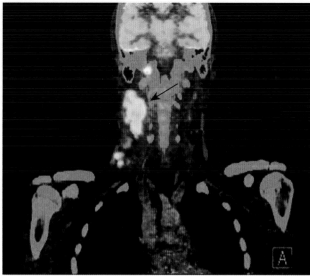

Fig. B-7 Computed tomography (CT) scan of needle biopsy of the liver clearly shows the needle in the liver on the left. (Courtesy Riverside Methodist Hospitals, Columbus, Ohio.)

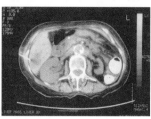

Fig. B-8 High-resolution positron emission tomography (PET) scan showing neck cancer *(arrow)*.

THERAPEUTIC INTERVENTIONS

Surgery

 Coding Guideline I.C.2.a

TREATMENT DIRECTED AT THE MALIGNANCY
If the treatment is directed at the malignancy, designate the malignancy as the principal diagnosis.

The only exception to this guideline is if a patient admission/encounter is solely for the administration of chemotherapy, immunotherapy or radiation therapy, assign the appropriate Z51.- code as the first-listed or principal diagnosis, and the diagnosis or problem for which the service is being performed as a secondary diagnosis.

 Coding Guideline I.C.2.b

TREATMENT OF SECONDARY SITE
When a patient is admitted because of a primary neoplasm with metastasis and treatment is directed toward the second site only, the secondary neoplasm is designated as the principal diagnosis even though the primary malignancy is still present.

The primary treatment for cancer has always been, and remains, removal of the tumor. When the tumor is relatively small and is present only in the organ that is removed, surgery is most effective.

The amount of tissue removed varies with the stage and grade of the cancer. In breast cancer surgery, for example, the types of surgery are as follows: **en bloc resection:** Removal of the cancerous tumor and the lymph nodes, **lumpectomy:** Removal of the tumor only.

lymph node dissection: The removal of clinically involved lymph nodes. **Lymph node mapping** determines a pattern of spread from the primary tumor site through the lymph nodes. The **sentinel node** is the first node in which lymphatic drainage occurs in a particular area. If this node is negative for cancer upon dissection, then the lymph system is free of cancer, and no other nodes need to be excised.

radical mastectomy: Removal of the breast containing the cancer, along with the lymph nodes and the muscle under the breast. When the surgical report discusses **margins,** it refers to the borders of normal tissue surrounding the cancer. A **wide margin resection** means that the cancer is removed with a significant amount of tissue around the tumor to ensure that all cancer cells are removed. If the margins are reported as negative, no cancer cells are seen. If the margins are reported as positive, cancer cells have been detected by the pathologist.

simple mastectomy: Removal of the breast containing the cancer.

 Coding Guideline I. C. e.2

PATIENT ADMISSION/ENCOUNTER SOLELY FOR ADMINISTRATION OF CHEMOTHERAPY, IMMUNOTHERAPY AND RADIATION THERAPY

If a patient admission/encounter is solely for the administration of chemotherapy, immunotherapy, or radiation therapy assign code Z51.0, Encounter for antineoplastic radiation therapy, or Z51.11, Encounter for antineoplastic immunotherapy as the first-listed or principal diagnosis. If a patient receives more than one of these therapies during the same admission more than one of these codes may be assigned, in any sequence.

The malignancy for which the therapy is being administered should be assigned as a secondary diagnosis.

RADIATION THERAPY

Approximately half of all cancer patients receive radiation. The goal of radiation therapy is to destroy the nucleus of the cancer cells, thereby destroying their ability to reproduce and spread.

Although radiation is usually started after removal of the tumor, sometimes it is done before removal to shrink the tumor. Some cancers may be treated solely with radiation.

three-dimensional conformal radiation therapy (3DCRT): Targeted radiation therapy that uses digital diagnostic imaging and specialized software to treat tumors without damaging surrounding tissue (Fig. B-9).

brachytherapy: The use of radiation placed directly on or within the cancer through the use of needles or beads containing radioactive gold, cobalt, or radium (Fig. B-10).

gamma knife surgery: A noninvasive type of surgery that uses gamma radiation to destroy a brain tumor.

intensity-modulated radiation therapy (IMRT): High-dosage radiation delivered via a beam that changes its dosage and shape.

brachytherapy
brachy- = short
-therapy = treatment

Systemic Therapy

bone marrow transplant (BMT): Patients who are incapable of producing healthy blood cells are given bone marrow from a matching donor to stimulate normal blood cell growth. Patients with specific types of leukemia may receive BMTs after chemotherapy has effectively destroyed the functioning of their own bone marrow.

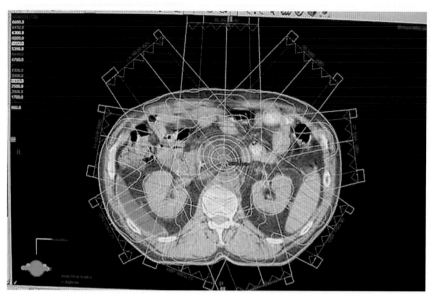

Fig. B-9 Dosimetry plan showing nine different radiation fields used to treat a pancreatic tumor.

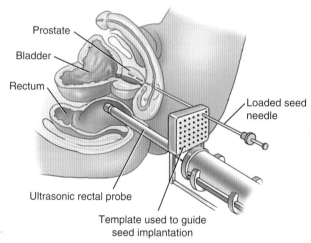

Prostate

Bladder

Rectum

Loaded seed needle

Ultrasonic rectal probe

Template used to guide seed implantation

Fig. B-10 Prostate brachytherapy. Radioactive seeds are implanted with a needle guided by sonography and a template grid.

chemotherapy: Chemotherapy is the circulation of cancer-destroying medicine throughout the body. Chemotherapy may also be used as an adjuvant (aid) to other forms of treatment to relieve symptoms or slow down the spread of cancer. Combination chemotherapy is the use of two or more anticancer drugs at one time.

complementary and alternative medicine (CAM) techniques: Prayer, massage, diet, exercise, and mind-body techniques constitute the majority of CAM methods used in cancer treatment. The US government has established the National Center for Complementary and Integrative Health, which reports on results of research studies on the use of CAM techniques for various disorders (http://www.nccam.nih.gov).

immunotherapy: Immunotherapy is the use of the body's own defense system to attack cancer cells.

Preventive Measures

vaccines: Two vaccines are currently in use to prevent specific cancers. The hepatitis B vaccine prevents hepatitis B with its sequelae of liver cancer and cirrhosis. The cervical cancer vaccine protects a woman against strains 16 and 18 of the human papillomavirus (HPV).

PHARMACOLOGY

Chemotherapy works by disrupting the cycle of cell replication. All cells go through a cycle of reproducing themselves, but, unlike cancer cells, they have a built-in mechanism that limits their growth. The side effects of cancer therapy (such as hair loss or nausea) are due to the inability of chemotherapeutic agents to differentiate between normal and cancerous cells. Thus cells that reproduce rapidly (such as hair cells or those that line the stomach) are also affected. It should also be noted that two or more chemotherapeutic agents usually are used together to effectively attack the cancer at various stages. This is referred to as a *drug protocol* or *plan*.

Most of the pharmaceuticals prescribed to treat cancer are referred to as *antineoplastic agents*. They accomplish the goal of slowing or stopping the progression of cancer in different ways:

alkylating agents: Interfere with DNA replication to lead to cancer cell death or dysfunction. Examples include cisplatin (Platinol AQ), nitrosoureas like carmustine (Gliadel), and nitrogen mustards like cyclophosphamide (Cytoxan).

antimetabolites: Replace compounds that cancer cells need to grow and/or replicate. Examples are methotrexate and fluorouracil (5-FU).

antineoplastic antibiotics: Prevent or delay cell replication. Examples include doxorubicin (Rubex, Adriamycin) and dactinomycin (Cosmegen).

antineoplastic hormones: Interfere with receptors for growth-stimulating proteins. Examples include flutamide (Eulexin) and tamoxifen (Nolvadex).

interleukins: Stimulate cells of the immune system to boost attacks on cancer cells. An example is aldesleukin (Proleukin).

mitotic inhibitors: Prevent cell division. An example is paclitaxel (Taxol).

vinca alkaloids: Prevent formation of chromosome spindles necessary for cell duplication. Examples include vincristine (Oncovin) and vinblastine (Velban).

chemotherapy
chem/o = drug, chemical
-therapy = treatment

Abbreviations

Abbreviations	Meaning
3DCRT	three-dimensional conformal radiation therapy
ACS	American Cancer Society
AFP	alpha fetoprotein (test)
B2M	beta-2 microglobulin
BMT	bone marrow transplant
BTA	bladder tumor antigen
Bx	biopsy
CA	cancer
CA125	tumor marker primarily for ovarian cancer
CA15-3	tumor marker to monitor breast cancer
CA19-9	tumor marker for pancreatic, stomach, and bile duct cancer
CA27-29	tumor marker to check for recurrence of breast cancer
CAM	complementary and alternative medicine
CEA	carcinoembryonic antigen
CIS	carcinoma in situ
CTR	certified tumor registrar
FOBT	fecal occult blood test
G	grade
GI	gastrointestinal
hCG	human chorionic gonadotropin
IMRT	intensity-modulated radiation therapy
IVU	intravenous urogram
mets	metastases
MS	musculoskeletal
NSE	neuron-specific enolase
Pap	Papanicolaou test for cervical/vaginal cancer
PET	positron emission tomography
PSA	prostate-specific antigen
SPECT	single-photon emission computed tomography
TA-90	tumor marker for spread of malignant melanoma
TNM	tumor-nodes-metastases (staging)

Appendix C   Pharmacology Basics

Simply stated, **pharmacology** is the study of drugs (also called *pharmaceuticals*). What is not so simple is the number of details that are involved with this field of study. Fortunately, many of the concepts and terms necessary to understand pharmacology are built from Greek and Latin word parts that will help you remember their definitions.

Pharmacists specialize in the preparation and dispensing of medications. Usually, these individuals work in a pharmacy—that is to say, a drugstore. They spend years studying the disciplines that make up pharmacology, such as **pharmacodynamics,** the action and effects of drugs on the tissues of the body; **pharmacokinetics,** the study of the movement of drugs through the body over time, and **pharmacotherapeutics,** the use of drugs in treating disease. See the table below for a breakdown of the word origins of these terms.

DRUG NAMES

Unlike diseases or procedures, each drug has at least three names. The **chemical name** is the scientific name that specifies the chemical composition of the drug. The **generic name** is its common name, often abbreviated from the chemical name. The copyrighted name that is given to the drug by its manufacturer is the **brand, trade, or proprietary name** and is accompanied by a symbol (an R with a circle around it, meaning "registered," or TM, meaning "trademark") next to it. The TM abbreviation is used until the U.S. Patent and Trademark Office has registered the name, after which the symbol ® is used. Federal law protects the patent (an exclusive right to make and sell the drug) on a new drug. The manufacturer has several years to sell its uniquely formulated and named medication before another company may use the "recipe."

Acetylsalicylic acid, aspirin, and Ecotrin are the chemical, generic, and brand names of a common over-the-counter (OTC) medication used to treat pain and inflammation.

DRUG SOURCES

Medications are manufactured from a variety of sources. Animal, botanical, and mineral sources are common, along with synthetic and recombinant DNA technology. Willow bark, for example, is the source of aspirin, while the foxglove plant is used to extract digitalis to control heart arrhythmias. Fish are the source of oil to supplement diets with vitamins A, D, and omega-3 fatty acids. Calcium is the essential component in Tums and Rolaids, which soothe an upset stomach. Penicillin is an example of an organic synthetic drug, and Humulin is a form of insulin that has been developed through the use of recombinant DNA technology.

Terms Related to Pharmacology Basics

Term	Word Origins	Definition
pharmacist	*pharmac/o* drugs *-ist* one who specializes	One who specializes in the preparation and dispensing of drugs.
pharmacodynamics	*pharmac/o* drugs *-dynamics* pertaining to power	The power of drugs (action and effects) on the body.
pharmacokinetics	*pharmac/o* drugs *-kinetics* pertaining to movement	The study of the movement of drugs through the body over time.
pharmacology	*pharmac/o* drugs *-logy* study of	The study of drugs.
pharmacotherapeutics	*pharmac/o* drugs *-therapeutics* pertaining to treatment	The use of drugs in treating disease

DRUG RESOURCES AND REGULATION

The **United States Pharmacopeia (USP)** is a guide to the approved formulas along with information for the preparation and dispensing of medications in the United States. The **National Formulary (NF)** is an official listing of the drugs that may be prescribed and/or dispensed over the counter. The *Physicians' Desk Reference (PDR)* is an annual commercial listing of pharmaceuticals in the United States. It is arranged by brand, generic, manufacturer, and product categories. Product information includes the drug's indications, contraindications, adverse reactions, warnings, and instructions. The **Food and Drug Administration (FDA)** enforces safety standards in the manufacture of drugs, foods, and cosmetics.

The **Drug Enforcement Agency (DEA),** under the Department of Justice, regulates distribution of drugs that have the potential for abuse and dependency.

Drugs that have the potential for abuse or dependency are designated "controlled substances" and are grouped into **drug schedules** (Table 1). They are denoted by the letter C along with a Roman numeral (I-V) indicating the number of the schedule. Schedule I (C-I) drugs are considered to have no medicinal use and have the highest potential for abuse and physical or mental dependency. As the schedule number increases, the level of potential abuse or dependency decreases. Schedule II drugs are those that have high potential for abuse or dependency but have valid medicinal uses and are available via prescription. Examples from Schedule II are meperidine (Demerol) and oxycodone (Percodan). Schedule V drugs have the lowest potential for abuse and include drugs that are available over the counter (given certain restrictions), such as cough syrups with codeine.

PHARMACODYNAMICS

Pharmacodynamics is the study of the action and effects of the drugs in the body. The action of a drug describes where and how it acts in the body. "Where" could be described as being **local** or **topical** (limited to the site of administration) or **systemic** (throughout the body). The "how" is the drug effect, or change in the body as the result of its use. This can be positive (the desired effect) or negative, a **side effect.** Side effects can include drowsiness, as in the case of some antihistamines. Side effects are considered to be mild, as opposed to the **toxic** (*toxic/o* = "poison") effect a drug may have when it is taken to excess. All drugs have a toxic level. **Adverse reactions** are unintended and undesirable effects that are more serious than side effects. Common side effects and adverse reactions are listed with information about the specific drug. **Teratogenic** drugs are those that are capable of causing birth defects.

Once a drug is introduced into the body, it can behave in a number of ways. A drug's desired effect is referred to as its **agonism.** *Agon/o* is a combining form meaning "struggle." In this term, it helps you to remember that the medication has been prescribed to overcome the disease—that is, to defeat it in the struggle for health.

If two drugs have their effects weakened by being given together, the effect is termed **antagonism.** Here the prefix *anti-*, meaning "against," has been added to show that the effect is *against* helping in the fight against the disease. Note that the "i" has been dropped from the prefix *anti-* in order to make the pronunciation of the term smoother.

If, however, the two drugs work together and have a stronger effect than they would individually, the effect is referred to as **synergism,** a condition of working together.

Using the prefix *syn-* again, we can decode the term for another effect, **idiosyncrasy.** Idiosyncrasy is an effect that occurs unexpectedly, a reaction to a drug that is unique to an individual.

With the exception of an idiosyncratic effect, physicians can monitor a patient's drug usage and make adjustments for the interaction of the various medications that he or she is prescribed. A potentially dangerous situation is that of **polypharmacy,** in which an individual will take medications that are not known to his or her doctor.

PHARMACOKINETICS

Most drugs have a predictable process in the body. Remember that the suffix *-kinetics* means "movement." The movement of a drug through the body is termed *pharmacokinetics.* The steps in this process begin with the drug's **absorption** (uptake) into the body (regardless of whether the drug was swallowed, injected, inhaled, or applied topically), and then its **distribution** (spreading) throughout the body. The drug is then usually **metabolized** (broken down, usually by the liver) and finally **excreted** (removed from the body). These steps can be abbreviated **ADME,** which stands for absorption, distribution, metabolism, excretion.

PHARMACOTHERAPEUTICS

Using medications to treat disease is the province of pharmacotherapeutics, but there are other reasons.

Table 1 Drug Classifications According to the Controlled Substances Act of 1970

Drug Schedule	Characteristics	Prescription Regulations	Examples
Schedule I	High potential for abuse, severe physical or psychological dependence No accepted medicinal use in United States For research use only	No accepted use in United States Marijuana may be used for cancer and glaucoma in states that have legalized medical marijuana or for some patients in research situations.	Narcotics—heroin (diacetylmorphine) Hallucinogens—mescaline (peyote), psilocybin (psychedelic mushrooms), lysergic acid diethylamide (LSD) Depressants—marijuana (cannabis), gamma-hydroxybutyric acid (GHB) Stimulants—MDMA (ecstasy), methylamphetamine (crystal meth)
Schedule II	High potential for abuse, severe physical or psychological dependence Accepted medicinal use with specific restrictions	Dispensed by prescription only Oral emergency orders for Schedule II drugs may be given, but physician must supply written prescription within 72 hr No refills without a new written prescription from the physician	**Narcotics**—opium, codeine, morphine (MS Contin), methadone (Dolophine), hydromorphone (Dilaudid), meperidine (Demerol), oxycodone (Oxycontin), fentanyl (Duragesic), hydrocodone with acetaminophen (Vicodin) **Stimulants**—methylphenidate (Ritalin), amphetamine salts (Adderall), cocaine **Depressants**—pentobarbital (Nembutal), secobarbital (Seconal)
Schedule III	Moderate potential for abuse, moderate to low psychological or physical dependence Accepted medicinal uses	Dispensed by prescription only May be refilled 5 times in 6 mo with prescription authorization by physician Prescription may be phoned to pharmacy	**Narcotics**—buprenorphine (Buprenex), paregoric (opium derivative), codeine combinations such as codeine with acetaminophen (Tylenol with Codeine #3) **Depressants**—butalbital (Fiorinal), ketamine (Ketalar), dronabinol (Marinol) **Stimulants**—benzphetamine (Didrex), phendimetrazine (Bontril) **Others**—testosterone (Aveed)
Schedule IV	Lower potential for abuse than Schedule III drugs Limited psychological and physical dependence Accepted medicinal uses	Dispensed by prescription only May be refilled 5 times in 6 mo with physician authorization Prescription may be phoned to pharmacy	**Narcotics**—pentazocine (Talwin), tramadol (Ultram) **Depressants**—phenobarbital (Donnatal), diazepam (Valium), chlordiazepoxide (Librium), alprazolam (Xanax), lorazepam (Ativan), triazolam (Halcion), meprobamate (Equanil), zolpidem (Ambien), eszopiclone (Lunesta), carisoprodol (Soma) **Stimulants**—phentermine (Adipex-P), diethylpropion (Tenuate), modafinil (Provigil)
Schedule V	Low potential for abuse Abuse may lead to limited physical or psychological dependence Accepted medicinal uses	OTC narcotic drugs in limited quantities sold by registered pharmacist Buyer must be 18 years of age, show ID, and sign for medications unless obtained with a prescription	**Narcotics**—preparations containing limited quantities of narcotics, such as cough syrups with codeine, diphenoxylate with atropine (Lomotil) **Depressants**—pregabalin (Lyrica)

From the Drug Enforcement Administration, U.S. Department of Justice, Washington, DC. Local DEA offices can provide current lists of medications on these schedules. State regulations can mandate different scheduling from the Federal Controlled Substance Act's designations.

Terms Related to Pharmacodynamics

Term	Word Origins	Definition
agonism	*agon/o* struggle *-ism* condition, state of	Condition of "struggle." The intended effect of a drug.
antagonism	*anti-* against *agon/o* struggle *-ism* condition, state of	Condition of "struggling against." The lessened effect that occurs when two drugs are given together.
idiosyncrasy	*idi/o* unique *syn-* together *cras/o* mixture *-y* process of, condition	Condition of a unique mixing together. An unusual reaction that occurs that is unique to the individual.
polypharmacy	*poly-* many *pharmac/o* drug *-y* process of, condition	Condition of many drugs.
synergism	*syn-* together *erg/o* work *-ism* condition, state of	Condition of working together.
teratogenic	*terat/o* deformity *-genic* pertaining to producing	Pertaining to producing a deformity
topical	*top/o* place, location *-ical* pertaining to	Pertaining to place (as in on the skin).
toxic	*tox/o* poison *-ic* pertaining to	Pertaining to poison.

The word *treat* can actually be broken into five different areas.

Drugs are prescribed for several reasons. Their purpose may be **curative** (killing a fungal infection), **diagnostic** (identifying a disorder or disease), **prophylactic** (preventive, as in a vaccine), **replacement** (such as hormone replacement), or **therapeutic** (to restore the body to its presymptom state, such as lowering a fever).

Pharmacotherapeutics is also concerned with **indications** (reasons for treatment; e.g., certain signs and symptoms) and **contraindications** (reasons *against* the use of a drug for treatment). An example of the latter would be the use of aspirin to treat pain in patients who have a clotting disorder. This would be contraindicated because aspirin has an anticoagulant (keeping the blood from clotting) effect along with its anti-inflammatory properties.

DRUG FORMS

Pills, elixirs and powders are all different forms of drugs that sound like compounds from a class that Harry Potter might take at Hogwarts Academy. Medications come in a variety of forms, the most familiar being liquid and solid.

The liquid medications can be divided into the aqueous, for those that are dissolved in water, and alcoholic, for those that are composed primarily of an alcoholic base. The aqueous solutions include emulsions, solutions, suspensions, lotions, liniments, syrups, and aerosols (drugs that are suspended in a mist). The alcoholic forms are drugs that are mixed with an alcohol base, such as tinctures and elixirs (alcohol along with water and sugar).

Examples of solid (and semisolid) medications can be divided into powders, tablets, capsules, ointments, troches (lozenges), creams, and transdermal products. Although you will study each of these individually and most are not composed of Greek or Latin word parts, consult the table below to give you some help with the terminology used for these forms.

ROUTES OF ADMINISTRATION

The means by which drugs are introduced into the body are called the *routes of administration*. In general, these are referred to as *enteral*, meaning "through the digestive system"; *parenteral*, meaning "by way of injection"; *inhaled*, meaning "through

Terms Related to Drug Forms

Term	Word Origins	Definition
aerosol	*aer/o* air *-sol* solution	Medication suspended within a mist
transdermal	*trans-* across, through *derm/o* skin *-al* pertaining to	Pertaining to through the skin. Medications that employ "patches" as a delivery system.

Terms Related to Routes of Administration

Term	Word Origin	Definition
buccal	*bucc/o* cheek *-al* pertaining to	Pertaining to the cheek
enteral	*enter/o* intestine *-al* pertaining to	Pertaining to the digestive system. A general category including the oral and rectal routes at either end of the digestive tract.
hypodermic	*hypo-* below *derm/o* skin *-ic* pertaining to	Pertaining to below the skin.
inhalation	*in-* in *hal/o* breathe *-ation* process of	The process of breathing in.
intradermal	*intra-* within *derm/o* skin *-al* pertaining to	Pertaining to within the skin.
intramuscular	*intra-* within *muscul/o* muscle *-ar* -pertaining to	Pertaining to within a muscle.

Continued

Terms Related to Routes of Administration–cont'd

Term	Word Origin	Definition
intravenous	*intra-* within *ven/o* vein *-ous* pertaining to	Pertaining to within a vein.
oral	*or/o* mouth *-al* pertaining to	Pertaining to the mouth.
parenteral	*par-* near, beside *enter/o* intestine *-al* pertaining to	Pertaining to "near the intestines." A general category for a route of administration that includes all injections, because they are given near, but not through, the digestive tract.
percutaneous	*per-* through *cutane/o* skin *-ous* pertaining to	Pertaining to through the skin.
rectal	*rect/o* rectum *-al* pertaining to	Pertaining to the rectum.
subcutaneous	*sub-* under, below *cutane/o* skin *-ous* pertaining to	Pertaining to under the skin.
sublingual	*sub-* under, below *lingu/o* tongue *-al* pertaining to	Pertaining to under the tongue.
topical	*top/o* place *-ical* pertaining to	Pertaining to place. A route of administration that applies a medication to the "place" of the surface of the skin.
transdermal	*trans-* through, across *derm/o* skin *-al* pertaining to	Pertaining to within the skin.

the lungs"; and *percutaneous,* meaning "through the skin." The table above gives a number of different routes with the derivations of the terms.

DRUG CLASSIFICATIONS

Drugs can be categorized into a variety of groupings, termed *drug classifications.* They can be grouped by their chemical similarity, their therapeutic effect, the body system that they affect, their action, and the area where the drug works (local or systemic). See the table for common classifications, their word origins, and their meanings.

PRESCRIPTIONS

The written directive for the preparation and administration of a specific drug is called a **prescription.** Literally, the origins of this term are the "process of writing before" the drug can be prepared. These are directions that are given by the prescriber as to the medication, the route of administration, the dosage, and the amount. Although you may hear the term "script" for a prescription, there are three other terms that share this word root.

Electronic prescribing (eprescribing) is an electronic transfer of your prescription to a pharmacy with the goal of a fast, accurate, and efficient means of transmission. While the content of what is needed

Terms Related to Drug Classifications

Term	Word Origin	Definition
analgesic	*an-* no, not, without *alges/o* pain *-ic* pertaining to	Drug to reduce pain.
anesthetic	*an-* no, not, without *esthesi/o* feeling, sensation *-ic* pertaining to	Drug to cause a loss of feeling or sensation.
antipyretic	*anti-* against *pyr/o* fever *-etic* pertaining to	Drug to reduce a fever.
diuretic	*di-* through, complete *ur/o* urine *-etic* pertaining to	Drug to increase the formation of urine.
hematinic	*hemat/o* blood *-inic* pertaining to a substance	Drug to increase the number of red blood cells (erythrocytes).
hypnotic	**hypn/o* sleep *-tic* pertaining to	Drug to promote sleep.
narcotic	*narc/o* stupor, dull the senses *-tic* pertaining to	Drug to relieve pain, dull senses, or induce sleep.
thrombolytic	*thromb/o* clot, clotting *-lytic* pertaining to destroying, dissolving	Drug to aid in the destruction of blood clots.

*Be careful! Don't confuse the prefix *hypo-*, meaning below or deficient, with the combining form *hypn/o,* meaning sleep.

in a prescription is the same, the eprescribing process helps eliminate errors due to handwriting and transcription problems.

The four parts of a prescription are the superscription, the inscription, the subscription, and the signature. The heading, which includes the date, patient name, address, and date of birth, is followed by the **superscription** (*super-* here means "above"), which contains the symbol R$_x$, meaning "to take." The next "script" term is the **inscription,** which is the part of the prescription where the physician has written in the names and amounts of the ingredients (HCTZ, 30mg). The **signature,** or **signa (sig.),** is the part of the prescription that tells the patient how the medication should be taken and for how long (e.g., two tablets, every morning, for 3 days). The final "script" term is the **subscription,** because it is written under the signature. It is the part of a prescription that gives directions for the number of doses, the quantity, and form of the drug.

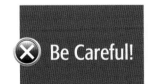
Be Careful!

Note that every prescription has a line for the prescriber writing the prescription to sign his or her name. This is not the same as the signature part of the prescription. There are also spaces for the prescriber to fill in his or her DEA# (if the prescription is for a controlled substance) and to specify the number (if any) of refills.

Terms Related to Prescription Terminology

Term	Word Origin	Definition
inscription	*in-* in *script/o* to write, writing *-ion* process of	The written direction of the names and amounts of a pharmaceutical.
prescription	*pre-* before *script/o* to write, writing *-ion* process of	The written directions for preparation and administration of a drug.
superscription	*super-* above *script/o* to write, writing *-ion* process of	The part of the prescription that is above the inscription. It contains the symbol Rx, meaning "to take" or "recipe."
subscription	*sub-* under *script/o* to write, writing *-ion* process of	The part of the prescription that is below the inscription. It contains the directions for number of doses, the quantity, and the form.

50 Commonly Prescribed Medications

Generic Name	Brand Name	Common Indication(s)
albuterol	Ventolin HFA, ProAir HFA	asthma, COPD
alendronate	Fosamax	osteoporosis
alprazolam	Xanax	anxiety, panic disorder
amlodipine	Norvasc	hypertension, coronary artery disease, angina
amoxicillin	Amoxil	bacterial infection
aripiprazole	Abilify	bipolar disorder, schizophrenia, major depressive disorder
atenolol	Tenormin	hypertension, angina, acute myocardial infarction
atorvastatin	Lipitor	hyperlipidemia
azithromycin	Zithromax	bacterial infection
budesonide	Pulmicort	asthma
carisoprodol	Soma	muscle spasm
carvedilol	Coreg	hypertension, heart failure, post-myocardial infarction
cephalexin	Keflex	bacterial infection
clopidogrel	Plavix	acute coronary syndrome, peripheral arterial disease
cyclobenzaprine	Flexeril	muscle spasm
digoxin	Lanoxin	atrial fibrillation, heart failure
escitalopram	Lexapro	major depressive disorder, generalized anxiety disorder
esomeprazole	Nexium	GERD
fluoxetine	Prozac	major depressive disorder, obsessive-compulsive disorder, panic disorder
fluticasone & salmeterol	Advair	COPD, asthma
furosemide	Lasix	hypertension, edema, congestive heart failure
gabapentin	Neurontin	epilepsy, postherpetic neuralgia
hydrochlorothiazide/triamterene	Maxzide	hypertension, edema
hydrocodone/acetaminophen	Vicodin	moderate to severe pain
ibuprofen	Motrin	inflammation

50 Commonly Prescribed Medications—cont'd

Generic Name	Brand Name	Common Indication(s)
insulin glargine	Lantus	diabetes mellitus
levothyroxine	Synthroid	hypothyroidism
liraglutide	Victoza	type 2 diabetes
lisinopril	Prinivil, Zestril	hypertension, heart failure, diabetic nephropathy, acute myocardial infarction
losartan	Cozaar	hypertension
memantine	Namenda	Alzheimer's disease
metformin	Glucophage	type 2 diabetes
methylphenidate	Concerta	attention-deficit hyperactivity disorder
methylprednisolone	Medrol	severe allergic conditions, Addison's disease, rheumatoid arthritis, SLE, severe psoriasis, severe seborrheic dermatitis, ulcerative colitis
metoprolol	Lopressor, Toprol XL	hypertension, angina pectoris, myocardial infarction
montelukast	Singulair	asthma, allergic rhinitis
isosorbide mononitrate	Imdur	angina pectoris
norgestimate/ethinyl estradiol	Ortho-Tri-Cyclen	oral contraception
prednisone	Deltasone	severe allergic conditions, Addison's disease, rheumatoid arthritis, SLE, severe psoriasis, severe seborrheic dermatitis, ulcerative colitis
rivaroxaban	Xarelto	nonvalvular atrial fibrillation, deep vein thrombosis, pulmonary embolism
sertraline	Zoloft	major depressive disorder, panic disorder, PTSD
sildenafil	Viagra	erectile dysfunction
simvastatin	Zocor	hyperlipidemia
sitagliptin	Januvia	type 2 diabetes
tamsulosin	Flomax	benign prostatic hyperplasia
tiotropium	Spiriva	COPD
tramadol	Ultram	moderate to severe pain
trazodone	Desyrel	major depressive disorder, insomnia
warfarin	Coumadin	venous thrombosis, pulmonary embolism, post-myocardial infarction, post-cerebrovascular accident
zolpidem	Ambien	insomnia

CODING INJURIES THAT RESULT FROM DRUGS

ICD-10-CM has guidelines for coding diagnoses for injuries that are the result of medical interventions related to drugs. These include adverse reactions (unexpected effects that includes allergic reactions), medication errors, overdoses (accidental or intentional), and underdoses. Table C-1 shows examples from the Table of Drugs and Chemicals that have codes for each of these circumstances. The category of underdosing is a relatively new one and is useful to capture events where patients are correctly prescribed a medication, but are either not taking it, or taking only part of the dosage. Additional Z codes, Factors influencing health status and contact with health services, are codes that may be used to indicate the intent and cause of the underdosing (intentional/unintentional, reasons that could be financial, age-related debility, or not otherwise specified).

Substance	Poisoning, Accidental (Unintentional)	Poisoning, Intentional Self-Harm	Poisoning, Assault	Poisoning, Undetermined	Adverse Effect	Underdosing
Furnace (coal burning) (domestic), gas from industrial	T58.2X1	T58.2X2	T58.2X3	T58.2X4	—	—
industrial	T58.8X1	T58.8X2	T58.8X3	T58.8X4	—	—
Furniture polish	T65.891	T65.892	T65.893	T65.894	—	—
Furosemide	T5Ø.1X1	T5Ø.1X2	T5Ø.1X3	T5Ø.1X4	T5Ø.1X5	T5Ø.1X6
Furoxone	T37.91	T37.92	T37.93	T37.94	T37.95	T37.96
Fursultiamine	T45.2X1	T45.2X2	T45.2X3	T45.2X4	T45.2X5	T45.2X6
Fusafungine	T36.8X1	T36.8X2	T36.8X3	T36.8X4	T36.8X5	T36.8X6
Fusel oil (any) (amyl) (butyl) (propyl), vapor	T51.3X1	T51.3X2	T51.3X3	T51.3X4	—	—
Fusidate (ethanolamine) (sodium)	T36.8X1	T36.8X2	T36.8X3	T36.8X4	T36.8X5	T36.8X6
Fusidic acid	T36.8X1	T36.8X2	T36.8X3	T36.8X4	T36.8X5	T36.8X6
Fytic acid, nonasodium	T5Ø.6X1	T5Ø.6X2	T5Ø.6X3	T5Ø.6X4	T5Ø.6X5	T5Ø.6X6

External Cause (T-Code)

Fig. C-1

 Guideline Alert!

19.E ADVERSE EFFECTS, POISONING, UNDERDOSING AND TOXIC EFFECTS

Codes in categories T36-T65 are combination codes that include the substance that was taken as well as the intent. No additional external cause code is required for poisonings, toxic effects, adverse effects and underdosing codes.

19.E.5 THE OCCURRENCE OF DRUG TOXICITY IS CLASSIFIED IN ICD-10-CM AS FOLLOWS:
(A) ADVERSE EFFECT
When coding an adverse effect of a drug that has been correctly prescribed and properly administered, assign the appropriate code for the nature of the adverse effect followed by the appropriate code for the adverse effect of the drug (T36-T5Ø). The code for the drug should have a 5th or 6th character "5" (for example, T36.ØX5-). Examples of the nature of an adverse effect are tachycardia, delirium, gastrointestinal hemorrhaging, vomiting, hypokalemia, hepatitis, renal failure, or respiratory failure.

(B) POISONING
When coding a poisoning or reaction to the improper use of a medication (e.g., overdose, wrong substance given or taken in error, wrong route of administration), first assign the appropriate code from categories (T36-T5Ø. The poisoning codes have an associated intent as their 5th or 6th character (accidental, intentional self-harm, assault and undetermined). If the intent of the poisoning is unknown or unspecified, code the intent as accidental intent. The undetermined

intent is only for use if the documentation in the record specifies that the intent cannot be determined. Use additional code(s) for all manifestations of poisonings.

If there is also a diagnosis of abuse or dependence of the substance, the abuse of dependence is assigned as an additional code.

(C) UNDERDOSING
Underdosing refers to taking less of a medication than is prescribed by a provider or a manufacturer's instruction. Discontinuing the use of a prescribed medication on the patient's own initiative (not directed by the patient's provider) is also classified as an underdosing. For underdosing, assign the code from categories T36-T5Ø (fifth or sixth character "6").

Codes for underdosing should never be assigned as principal or first-listed codes. If a patient has a relapse or exacerbation of the medical condition for which the drug is prescribed because of the reduction in dose, then the medical condition itself should be coded.

Noncompliance (Z91.12-, Z91.13- and Z91.14-) or complication of care (Y63.6-Y63.9) codes are to be used with an underdosing code to indicate intent, if known.

(D) TOXIC EFFECTS
When a harmful substance is ingested or comes in contact with a person, this is classified as a toxic effect. The toxic effect does are in categories T51-T65.

Toxic effect codes have an associated intent: accidental, intentional self-harm, assault and undetermined.

Appendix D

Word Parts and Definitions

Word Part	Meaning
-a	noun ending
a-	no, not, without, lack of
ab-	away from
abdomin/o	abdomen
-abrasion	scraping of
-ac	pertaining to
ac-	toward
acetabul/o	acetabulum (hip socket)
achill/o	Achilles tendon
acid/o	acid
acous/o	hearing
acro-	heights, extremes, extremities
acromi/o	acromion process
act/o, act/i	rays
acu-	sharp
-acusis	hearing
-ad	toward
ad-	toward
aden/o	gland
adenoid/o	adenoid (pharyngeal tonsil)
adip/o	fat
adipos/o	fat
adnex/o	accessory
adren/o	adrenal gland
adrenal/o	adrenal gland
aer/o	air
af-	toward
agglutin/o	clumping
agora-	marketplace
-al	pertaining to
-algia	pain
al/i, al/o	wing
aliment/o	nutrition
allo-	other, different
alveol/o	small cavity, alveolus
-alysis	breaking down
ambly/o	dull, dim
ambul/o	walking
amel/o	enamel

Word Part	Meaning
amni/o, amnion/o	amnion, inner fetal sac
-amnios	amnion, inner fetal sac
amphi-	both
amyl/o	starch
-an	pertaining to
an-	no, not, without
an/o	anus
ana-	up, apart, away
andr/o	male
angi/o	vessel
ankyl/o	stiffening
annul/o	annulus, ring
-ant	pertaining to
ante-	forward, in front of, before
anter/o	front
anthrop/o	man
anti-	against
antr/o	antrum, cavity
aort/o	aorta (largest artery)
-apheresis	removal
aphth/o	ulceration
apic/o	pointed extremity, apex
apo-	separate, away from
append/o, appendic/o	vermiform appendix, that which is added
appendicul/o	appendicular
-ar	pertaining to
-arche	beginning
arteri/o	artery
arteriol/o	arteriole (small artery)
arthr/o	articulation (joint)
articul/o	articulation (joint)
-ary	pertaining to
-ase	enzyme
astr/o	star
ather/o	fat, plaque
-atic	pertaining to
-ation	process of

Continued

Word Parts and Definitions—cont'd

Word Part	Meaning	Word Part	Meaning
atlant/o	1st cervical vertebra (atlas) (C1)	capn/o	carbon dioxide
-atory	pertaining to	carcin/o	epithelial cancer
atri/o	atrium	-carcinoma	cancer of epithelial origin
audi/o	hearing	cardi/o	heart
aur/o	hearing	cardiomy/o	heart muscle
auricul/o	auricle, pinna	-cardia	condition of the heart
auto-	self	carp/o	carpus (wrist)
axill/o	axilla (armpit)	cartilag/o	cartilage
axi/o	axial, axis bone (2nd cervical vertebra) (C2)	cata-	down
		caud/o	tail
azyg/o	without a yoke	caus/o	burning
bacteri/o	bacteria	cauter/i	burning
balan/o	glans penis	cec/o	cecum (first part of large intestine)
band/o	bands		
bartholin/o	Bartholin's gland	-cele	herniation, protrusion
bas/o	base, bottom	celi/o	abdomen
bi-	two	cellul/o	cell
bi/o	life, living	-centesis	surgical puncture
bil/i	bile	cephal/o	head
bin-	two	-cephalus	head
-blast	embryonic, immature	-ceps	heads
blast/o	embryonic, immature	cerebell/o	cerebellum
blephar/o	eyelid	cerebr/o	cerebrum
bol/o	to throw, throwing	cerumin/o	cerumen (earwax)
brachi/o	arm	cervic/o	neck, cervix
brady-	slow	-chalasia	condition of relaxation, slackening
brom/o	odor, stench	-chalasis	relaxation, slackening
bronch/o	bronchus	cheil/o	lips
bronchi/o	bronchus	chem/o	drug, chemical
bronchiol/o	bronchiole	chol/e	bile, gall
bucc/o	cheek	cholangi/o	bile vessel
bulb/o	globe	cholecyst/o	gallbladder
bunion/o	bunion	choledoch/o	common bile duct
burs/o	bursa	cholesterol/o	cholesterol
calc/o, calc/i	calcium	chondr/o	cartilage
calcane/o	calcaneus (heel bone)	chord/o	cord, spinal cord
calcul/o	stone, calculus	chori/o	chorion (outer fetal sac)
cali/o	calyx, calix	chorion/o	chorion (outer fetal sac)
calic/o	calyx, calix	choroid/o	choroid
calyc/o	calyx, calix	chrom/o	color
canalicul/o	canaliculus, little canal	chromat/o	color
canth/o	canthus (corner of eye)	chron/o	time
capit/o	head	chyl/o	lymph

Word Parts and Definitions—cont'd

Word Part	Meaning	Word Part	Meaning
chym/o	juice	crin/o	to secrete, secreting
cili/o	tiny hairs	-crine	to secrete, secreting
circum-	around	-crit	to separate, separating
cirrh/o	orange-yellow	crur/o	leg
-cision	cutting	cry/o	extreme cold
cistern/o	box, cistern	crypt-	hidden
-clasis	intentional breaking	cuboid/o	cuboid bone, box-shaped
-clast	breaking down	cubit/o	elbow, forearm
claustr/o	closing	culd/o	cul-de-sac (rectouterine pouch)
clav/i	clavicle (collarbone)	cune/o	cuneiform bone
clavicul/o	clavicle (collarbone)	-cusis	hearing
cleid/o	clavicle (collarbone)	cusp/o	point, cusp
clitorid/o	clitoris	cut/o	skin
-clysis	washing	cutane/o	skin
coagul/o	clotting	cyan/o	blue
-coagulation	process of clotting	cycl/o	ciliary body, recurring, round
coccyg/o	coccyx (tailbone)	-cyesis	pregnancy, gestation
cochle/o	cochlea	-cyst	sac
columell/o	columella	cyst/o	bladder, sac
coll/o	neck	cyt/o	cell
col/o	colon (large intestine)	-cyte	cell
colon/o	colon (large intestine)	-cytosis	condition of abnormal increase in cells
colp/o	vagina	dacry/o	tear
con-	together	dacryoaden/o	lacrimal gland
condyl/o	condyle, knob	dacryocyst/o	lacrimal sac
coni/o	dust	dactyl/o	digitus (finger or toe)
conjunctiv/o	conjunctiva	de-	down, lack of
contra-	opposite, against	delt/o	triangle, deltoid muscle
cor/o	pupil	dendr/o	dendrite, tree
corac/o	coracoid process of the scapula	densit/o	density
cord/o	cord, spinal cord	dent/i	teeth
cordi/o	heart	-derma	skin condition
core/o	pupil	derm/o	skin
corne/o	cornea	dermat/o	skin
coron/o	crown, heart	-desis	binding
corpor/o	body	dextr/o	right
corrug/o	wrinkled	di-	two, both
cortic/o	cortex (outer portion)	dia-	through, complete
cost/o	costa (rib)	diaphragm/o	diaphragm
cox/o	coxa (hip)	diaphragmat/o	diaphragm
crani/o	skull	digit/o	finger or toe
crepit/o	crackling	dipl/o	double
cret/o	to grow		

Continued

Word Parts and Definitions—cont'd

Word Part	Meaning
dips/o	thirst
dis-	bad, abnormal, apart
disc/o	disc
dist/o	far
diverticul/o	diverticulum, pouch
dors/o, dors/i	back
-drome	to run, running
duct/o	to carry, carrying
duoden/o	duodenum
dur/o	dura mater, hard
dynam/o	power
-dynia	pain
dys-	bad, difficult, painful, abnormal
-e	noun ending
e-	outward, out
-eal	pertaining to
ec-	out, outward
echo-	sound, reverberation
-ectasia	condition of expansion, dilation
-ectasis	expansion, dilation
-ectomy	cutting out
-edema	swelling
ef-	away from
electr/o	electricity
-emesis	vomiting, vomit
-emia	blood condition
-emphraxis	obstructing, crushing
-emulsification	breaking down
en-	in
encephal/o	brain
end-	within
endo-	within
endocardi/o	inner lining of the heart
endometri/o	endometrium, inner lining of cervix
-ent	pertaining to
enter/o	small intestines, intestines
eosin/o	rosy-colored
epi-	above, upon
epicardi/o	epicardium
epicondyl/o	epicondyle
epididym/o	epididymis
epiglott/o	epiglottis

Word Part	Meaning
epiplo/o	omentum
episi/o	vulva (external female genitalia)
epitheli/o	epithelium
erythemat/o	red
erythr/o	red
eschar/o	scab
-esis	state of
eso-	inward
esophag/o	esophagus
esthesi/o	feeling, sensation
-esthetica	feeling, sensation
ethmoid/o	ethmoid bone, sieve
eu-	healthy, normal
ex-	out
exanthemat/o	rash
-exeresis	tearing out
-exia	condition
exo-	outside
extra-	outside
extern/o	outer
faci/o	face
fasci/o	fascia
fec/a	feces, stool
femor/o	femur (thigh bone)
fer/o	to bear, carry
-ferous	pertaining to carrying
fetish/o	charm
fet/o	fetus
fibr/o	fiber
fibrin/o	fibrous substance
fibul/o	fibula (lower lateral leg bone)
-fida	to split, splitting
fimbri/o	fimbria
fissur/o	deep cleft or groove
flex/o	to bend, bending
fluor/o	to flow, flowing
-flux	to flow, flowing
follicul/o	follicle
foramin/o	hole, foramen
-form	shape
fornic/o	arched structure, fornix
foss/o	hollow, depression
fren/o	frenulum (of tongue and lip)

Word Parts and Definitions—cont'd

Word Part	Meaning
frenul/o	frenulum (of tongue and lip)
front/o	front, forehead
fund/o	fundus (base, bottom)
-fusion	process of pouring
galact/o	milk
gangli/o	ganglion
ganglion/o	ganglion
gastr/o	stomach
-gen	producing
-geneic	pertaining to produced by
-genesis	production, origin
-genic	pertaining to produced by
geni/o	chin
-genous	pertaining to originating from
gen/u	knee
ger/o	old age
germ/i	sprout
gingiv/o	gums
glauc/o	gray, bluish green
glen/o	glenoid cavity (arm socket)
-glia	glia cell, glue
-globin	protein substance
-globulin	protein substance
globulin/o, globin/o	protein
glomerul/o	glomerulus
gloss/o	tongue
gluc/o	sugar, glucose
glucos/o	sugar, glucose
glute/o	gluteus (buttocks)
glyc/o	sugar, glucose
glycos/o	sugar, glucose
gnath/o	jaw, entire
-gnosis	state of knowledge
gon/o	seed
gonad/o	gonad, sex organ
goni/o	angle
-grade	flow
-gram	record, recording
granul/o	little grain
-graph	instrument to record
-graphy	recording
gravid/o	pregnancy, gestation

Word Part	Meaning
-gravida	pregnancy, gestation
gryph/o	curved
gyn/e	female, woman
gynec/o	female, woman
halit/o	breath
hal/o	to breathe, breathing
halluc/o	hallux (great toe)
hedon/o	pleasure
helic/o	helix, coil
hem/o	blood
hemangi/o	blood vessel
hemat/o	blood
hemi-	half
hepat/o	liver
herni/o	hernia
hiat/o	an opening
hidr/o	sweat
hidraden/o	sudoriferous gland (sweat gland)
hil/o	hilum
hist/o	tissue
home/o	same
homo-	same
humer/o	humerus (upper arm bone)
humor/o	liquid
hydatid/i	water drop
hydr/o	water, fluid
hymen/o	hymen
hyoid/o	hyoid bone
hyper-	excessive, above
hypn/o	sleep
hypo-	deficient, below, under, decreased
hypophys/o	hypophysis, pituitary
hyster/o	uterus
-ia	condition, state of
-iac	pertaining to
-iacal	pertaining to abnormal condition
-iasis	condition, presence of
-ic	pertaining to
ichthy/o	fishlike
-icle	small, tiny
-id	pertaining to
-igo	condition

Continued

Word Parts and Definitions—cont'd

Word Part	Meaning
ile/o	ileum (third part small intestines)
ili/o	ilium (superior, widest pelvic bone)
immun/o	safety, protection
-in	substance
in-	in, not
indur/o	to make hard
-ine	pertaining to
infer/o	downward
infra-	down, under
inguin/o	groin
insulin/o	insulin
inter-	between
intestin/o	intestine
intra-	within
-ion	process of
-ior	pertaining to
ipsi-	same
ir/o	iris
irid/o	iris
-is	structure, thing, noun ending
is/o	equal
isch/o	hold back, suppress
ischem/o	hold back
ischi/o	ischium (lower part of pelvic bone)
-ism	condition, state of
-ismus	spasm
-itis	inflammation
-itic	pertaining to
-ity	noun ending
-ium	structure, membrane
-ive	pertaining to
-ization	process
jejun/o	second part of small intestine, jejunum
jugul/o	throat, neck
kal/i	potassium
kary/o	nucleus
kerat/o	hard, horny, cornea
ket/o	ketone
keton/o	ketone
-kine	movement

Word Part	Meaning
-kinesis	movement
-kinin	movement substance
klept/o	to steal, stealing
kyph/o	roundback
labi/o	lips, labia
labyrinth/o	labyrinth (inner ear)
lacrim/o	tear
lact/o	milk
-lalia	condition of babbling
lamin/o	lamina, thin plate
lapar/o	abdomen
-lapse	fall
laryng/o	larynx (voice box)
later/o	side
leiomy/o	smooth muscle
-lepsy	seizure
-leukin	white substance
leuk/o	white
levo-	left
lex/o	word, speech
ligament/o	ligament
ligat/o	to tie, tying
-ligation	tying
limb/o	limbus
lingu/o	tongue
lip/o	fat
lipid/o	lipid, fat
-listhesis	slipping
lith/o	stone, calculus
-lithotomy	cutting out a stone
lob/o	lobe, section
lobul/o	small lobe
log/o	study
-logist	one who specializes in the study of
-logous	pertaining to origin
-logy	study of
long/o	long
lord/o	swayback
lumb/o	lower back
lumin/o	lumen (space within vessel)
lun/o	moon

Word Parts and Definitions—cont'd

Word Part	Meaning
lymph/o	lymph
lymphaden/o	lymph gland (lymph node)
lymphangi/o	lymph vessel
lymphat/o	lymph
lys/o	breakdown, dissolve
-lysis	breaking down, dissolving, loosening, freeing from adhesions
-lytic	pertaining to breaking down
macro-	large
macul/o	macula, macule, macula lutea, spot
mal-	bad, poor
-malacia	softening
malleol/o	distal process of lower leg, little malleolus
mamm/o	breast
mandibul/o	lower jaw
-mania	condition of madness
man/o	pressure, scanty
man/u, man/i	hand
manubri/o	manubrium of the breastbone, handle
mast/o	breast
mastoid/o	mastoid process
maxill/o	maxilla (upper jaw bone)
maxim/o	large
meat/o	meatus (opening)
medi/o	middle
mediastin/o	mediastinum (space between lungs)
medull/o	medulla, inner portion
-megaly	enlargement
melan/o	black, dark
-mileusis	carving
men/o	menstruation, menses
mening/o	meninges
meningi/o	meninges
menisc/o	meniscus, crescent
menstru/o	menstruation
ment/o	mind, chin
mer/o	thigh
mesenter/o	mesentery, midgut
meta-	beyond, change

Word Part	Meaning
metacarp/o	metacarpus (hand bone)
metatars/o	metatarsus (foot bone)
-meter	instrument to measure
metr/o	uterus, measure
metri/o	uterus
-metry	measuring
micro-	small
mid-	middle
mi/o	to close, constrict
-mileusis	carving
mitochondri/o	mitochondria
mol/o	molar
mono-	one
morb/o	disease
morph/o	shape, form
muc/o	mucus
mucos/o	mucus
multi-	many
mur/o	wall
muscul/o	muscle
my/o	muscle, to shut
myc/o	fungus
mydr/o	dilation
myel/o	bone marrow, spinal cord
myocardi/o	myocardium (heart muscle)
myometri/o	muscle layer of the uterus
myos/o	muscle
myring/o	eardrum
myx/o	mucus
narc/o	sleep, stupor
nas/o	nose
nat/i	birth
nat/o	birth, born
natr/o	sodium
navicul/o	navicular bone
necr/o	death, dead
neo-	new
nephr/o	kidney
nervos/o	nervous
neur/o	nerve
neuron/o	nerve
neutr/o	neutral

Continued

Word Parts and Definitions—cont'd

Word Part	Meaning
nev/o	nevus, birthmark
nid/o	nest
noct/i	night
nod/o	node, knot
-noia	condition of mind
non-	not
nos/o	disease
nuch/o	neck
nucle/o	nucleus
nulli-	none
nyctal/o	night
nymph/o	woman, female
o/o	ovum, egg, female sex cell
occipit/o	occiput
occlus/o	to close, closing, a blockage
ocul/o	eye
odont/o	teeth
-oid	resembling, like
-ole	small, tiny
olecran/o	elbow
olig/o	scanty, few
-oma	tumor, mass
-omatous	pertaining to a tumor
oment/o	omentum
omphal/o	umbilicus (navel)
onc/o	tumor
-on	structure
-one	hormone, substance that forms
oneir/o	dream
onych/o	nail
oophor/o	ovary (female gonad)
ophthalm/o	eye
-opia	vision condition
-opsia	vision condition
-opsy	viewing
opt/o	vision
optic/o	vision
or/o	mouth, oral cavity
orbit/o	orbit
orch/o	testis, testicle (male gonad)
orchi/o	testis, testicle (male gonad)
orchid/o	testis, testicle (male gonad)
orex/o	appetite

Word Part	Meaning
organ/o	organ, viscus
orth/o	straight, upright
-os	condition
-ose	pertaining to, full of
-osis	abnormal condition
oss/i	bone
osse/o	bone
ossicul/o	ossicle (tiny bone)
oste/o	bone
-osus	noun ending
ot/o	ear
-ous	pertaining to
ov/i	ovum (egg) (female sex cell)
ov/o	ovum (egg) (female sex cell)
ovari/o	ovary (female gonad)
ovul/o	ovum (female sex cell)
ox/i, ox/o	oxygen
oxy-	oxygen
palat/o	palate, roof of mouth, palatine bone
pallid/o	globus pallidum
palm/o	palm
palpebr/o	eyelid
pan-	all
pancreat/o	pancreas
papill/o	papilla, nipple, optic disk
papul/o	papule, pimple
par-	beside, near
-para	delivery, parturition
para-	near, beside, abnormal
parathyroid/o	parathyroid
parenchym/o	parenchyma
-paresis	slight paralysis
-pareunia	intercourse
pariet/o	wall, partition
part/o	parturition (delivery)
-partum	parturition (delivery)
patell/o, patell/a	patella (kneecap)
path/o	disease
-pathy	disease process
patul/o	open
-pause	stop, cease
pector/o	chest

Word Parts and Definitions—cont'd

Word Part	Meaning
ped/o	foot, child
pedicul/i	lice
pelv/i, pelv/o	pelvis
pen/i	penis
-penia	condition of deficiency
-pepsia	digestion
per-	through
peri-	surrounding, around
pericardi/o	sac surrounding the heart, pericardium
perimetri/o	perimetrium, outer layer of uterus
perine/o	perineum
peritone/o	peritoneum
perone/o	fibula, lower lateral leg bone
petros/o	petrous bone
petr/o	stone
-pexy	fixation, suspension
phac/o	lens
phag/o	to eat, swallow
-phagia	condition of eating, swallowing
phak/o	lens
phalang/o	phalanx (finger/toe bones)
phall/o	penis
pharmac/o	drug
pharyng/o	pharynx (throat)
phas/o	speech
phe/o	dark
-phil	attraction
phil/o	attraction
-philia	condition of attraction
phleb/o	vein
-phobia	condition of fear, extreme sensitivity
phon/o	sound, voice
phor/o	to carry, to bear
phot/o	light
phren/o	diaphragm, mind, phrenic nerve
-phthisis	wasting
physi/o	growth
-physis	growth
phyt/o	growth
pil/o	hair
pineal/o	pineal body (gland)

Word Part	Meaning
pituit/o	pituitary gland
pituitar/o	pituitary
placent/o	placenta
-plakia	condition of patches
plant/o	sole of foot
plas/o	formation
-plasia	condition of formation, development
-plasm	condition of formation
plasm/a	plasma
plasm/o	plasma
plast/o	formation
-plastic	pertaining to formation
-plastin	forming substance
-plasty	surgically forming
-plegia	paralysis
pleur/o	pleura, membrane surrounding lungs
-plication	fold, plica
-pnea	breathing
pne/o	to breathe, breathing
pneum/o	lung, air
pneumat/o	lung, air
pneumon/o	lung
-poiesis	formation, production
-poietin	forming substance
pol/o	pole
pollic/o	pollex (thumb)
poli/o	gray, grey
poly-	many, much, excessive, frequent
polyp/o	polyp
poplite/o	back of knee
por/o	passage
port/o	gate
post-	behind, after
poster/o	back
posth/o	foreskin
prax/o	purposeful movement
pre-	before, in front of
precordi/o	precordium
preputi/o	prepuce (foreskin)
presby-	old age
primi-	first

Continued

Word Parts and Definitions—cont'd

Word Part	Meaning
pro-	forward, in front of, in favor of
proct/o	rectum and anus
prolactin/o	prolactin
prostat/o	prostate
proxim/o	near
prurit/o	itching
pseud/o	false
psych/o	mind
pteryg/o	wing
-ptosis	drooping, prolapse, falling
ptyal/o	saliva
-ptysis	spitting
pub/o	pubis, anterior pelvic bone
puerper/o	puerperium
pulmon/o	lung
pupill/o	pupil
purpur/o	purple
pustul/o	pustule
py/o	pus
pyel/o	renal pelvis
pylor/o	pylorus
pyr/o	fever, fire
quadra-	four
quadri-	four
rach/i, rachi/o	spinal column, backbone
radi/o	radius (lower lateral arm bone), rays
radicul/o	nerve root, spinal nerve root
re-	back, backward, again
rect/o	rectum, straight
ren/o	kidney
retin/o	retina
retro-	backward
rhabdomy/o	striated (skeletal) muscle
rheumat/o	watery flow
rhin/o	nose
rhiz/o	spinal nerve root, nerve root
rhythm/o	rhythm
rhytid/o	wrinkle
rib/o	ribose
rot/o	wheel
-rrhagia, -rrhage	bursting forth

Word Part	Meaning
-rrhagic	pertaining to bursting forth
-rrhaphy	suturing
-rrhea	discharge, flow
-rrheic	pertaining to discharge
-rrhexis	rupture
rug/o	rugae, ridge
sacr/o	sacrum
sagitt/o	arrow, separating the sides
salping/o	fallopian or eustachian tube
-salpinx	fallopian or eustachian tube
sarc/o	flesh
-sarcoma	connective tissue cancer
scaphoid/o	scaphoid bone
scapul/o	scapula (shoulder blade)
-schisis	split
schiz/o	split
scler/o	sclera, hard
-sclerosis	abnormal condition of hardening
scoli/o	curvature
-scope	instrument to view
-scopic	pertaining to viewing
-scopy	viewing
scot/o	dark
scrot/o	scrotum (sac holding testes)
sebac/o	sebum, oil
seb/o	sebum, oil
semi-	half
semin/i	semen
sensor/i	sense
sept/o	septum, wall, partition
septic/o	infection
sequestr/o	sequestrum (bone fragment)
ser/o	serum
serrat/o	notched
sial/o	saliva
sialaden/o	salivary gland
sialodoch/o	salivary duct
sider/o	iron
-siderin	iron substance
sigmoid/o	sigmoid colon
sin/o	sinus, cavity
sinistr/o	left

Word Parts and Definitions—cont'd

Word Part	Meaning
sinus/o	sinus, cavity
-sis	state of, condition
skelet/o	skeleton
somat/o	body
-some	body
som/o	body
somn/o	sleep
-spadias	a rent or tear
-spasm	spasm; sudden, involuntary contraction
sperm/o	spermatozoon (male sex cell)
spermat/o	spermatozoon (male sex cell)
sphenoid/o, sphen/o	sphenoid
spher/o	sphere
spin/o	spine
spir/o	to breathe, breathing
splen/o	spleen
spondyl/o	vertebra, backbone, spine
squam/o	scaly
-stalsis	contraction
staped/o	stapes (third ossicle in ear)
-stasis	controlling, stopping
steat/o	fat
-stenosis	abnormal condition of narrowing
ster/o	steroid
stern/o	sternum (breastbone)
steth/o	chest
-sthenia	condition of strength
stiti/o	space
stom/o	an opening, a mouth
stomat/o	mouth, oral cavity
-stomy	making a new opening
strom/o	stroma (supportive tissue)
styl/o	styloid process (temporal bone)
sub-	under, below
sudor/i	sweat
sulc/o	sulcus, groove
super/o	upward
supra-	upward, above
sur/o	calf
sympath/o	to feel with

Word Part	Meaning
syn-	together, joined
syndesm/o	ligament (structure connecting bone)
synovi/o	synovium
synov/o	synovial membrane
-synthesis	bring together
system/o	system
-tabes	wasting
tachy-	fast, rapid
tal/o	talus bone
tars/o	tarsus (anklebone), flat surface
tax/o	order, coordination
tel/e	end, far, complete
tempor/o	temporal bone
ten/o	tendon (structure connecting bones)
tend/o	tendon (structure connecting bones)
tendin/o	tendon (structure connecting bones)
tendon/o	tendon (structure connecting bones)
tens/o	stretching, pressure
-tension	process of stretching, pressure
terat/o	deformity
test/o	testis, testicle (male gonad)
testicul/o	testis, testicle (male gonad)
tetra-	four
thalam/o	thalamus
thalass/o	sea
thel/e	nipple
-therapy	treatment
therm/o	heat, temperature
thorac/o	thorax (chest)
-thorax	chest (pleural cavity)
thromb/o	clotting, clot
-thrombin	clotting substance
thym/o	thymus gland, mind
-thymia	condition/state of mind
thyr/o	thyroid gland, shield
thyroid/o	thyroid gland
tibi/o	tibia (shinbone)
-tic	pertaining to
till/o	to pull

Continued

Word Parts and Definitions—cont'd

Word Part	Meaning	Word Part	Meaning
tinnit/o	jingling	uter/o	uterus
-tion	process of	uve/o	uvea
-tocia	parturition, delivery	uvul/o	uvula
-tome	instrument to cut	vag/o	vagus nerve
-tomy	cutting	vagin/o	vagina
ton/o	tension, tone	valv/o	valve
tonsill/o	tonsil	valvul/o	valve
top/o	place, location	varic/o	varices
tox/o	poison	vas/o	vessel, ductus deferens, vas deferens
toxic/o	poison		
trabecul/o	little beam	vascul/o	vessel
trache/o	trachea (windpipe)	ven/o	vein
trachel/o	uterine cervix	ventr/o	belly side
tract/o	to pull, pulling, tract, pathway	ventricul/o	ventricle
trans-	through, across	venul/o	venule, small vein
-tresia	condition of an opening	verm/o	worm
tri-	three	vers/o	to turn
trich/o	hair	-verse	to turn
trigon/o	trigone	-version	process of turning
-tripsy	crushing	vert/o	turn
-tripter	machine to crush	vertebr/o	vertebra, spine, backbone
-trite	instrument to crush	vesic/o	bladder
trochanter/o	trochanter	vesicul/o	small sac, seminal vesicle, blister
trop/o	to turn, turning	vestibul/o	vestibule (small space at entrance to canal)
troph/o	development, nourishment		
-trophy	process of nourishment	vill/o	villus
tub/o	tube, pipe	viscer/o	viscera, organ
tubercul/o	tubercle, a swelling	vitre/o, vitr/o	vitreous humor, glassy
turbin/o	turbinate bone	vol/o	volume
tympan/o	eardrum, drum	vomer/o	vomer
-ule	small	vulgar/o	common
uln/o	ulna (lower medial arm bone)	vuls/o	to pull
-um	structure, thing, membrane	vulv/o	vulva (external female genitalia)
umbilic/o	umbilicus (navel)	xen/o	foreign
ungu/o	nail	xer/o	dry
uni-	one	xiph/i, xiph/o	xiphoid process, sword
-ure	condition	-y	condition, process of
ur/o	urine, urinary system	-zation	process of
ureter/o	ureter	zo/o	animal
urethr/o	urethra	zygom/o	zygoma (cheekbone)
-uria	urinary condition	zygomat/o	zygoma (cheekbone)
urin/o	urine, urinary system	zygomatic/o	zygomaticus (cheek muscle)
-us	structure, thing		

Definitions and Word Parts

Meaning	Word Part
abdomen	abdomin/o, celi/o, lapar/o
abnormal	para-, dys-
abnormal condition	-osis
abnormal condition of hardening	-sclerosis
abnormal condition of narrowing	-stenosis
above	hyper-, supra-
above, upon	epi-
accessory	adnex/o
acetabulum	acetabul/o
Achilles tendon	achill/o
acid	acid/o
acromion	acromi/o, acromion/o
adenoid (pharyngeal tonsil)	adenoid/o
adrenal gland	adren/o, adrenal/o
again	re-
against	anti-, contra-
air	aer/o, pneum/o, pneumat/o
all	pan-
alveolus, small cavity	alveol/o
amnion	amni/o
amnion (inner fetal sac)	-amnios
angle	goni/o
animal	zo/o
anklebone (tarsal bone)	tars/o
annulus, ring	annul/o
antrum, cavity	antr/o
anus	an/o
aorta (largest artery)	aort/o
apart, away	ana-
apex, pointed extremity	apic/o
appendicular	appendicul/o
appendix, vermiform	append/o, appendic/o
appetite	orex/o
arched structure, fornix	fornic/o
arm	brachi/o

Meaning	Word Part
armpit (axilla)	axill/o
around	circum-, peri-
arrow, separating the sides	sagitt/o
arteriole (small artery)	arteriol/o
artery	arteri/o
articulation	articul/o, arthr/o
atlas bone (1st cervical vertebra) (C1)	atlant/o
atrium	atri/o
attraction	phil/o, -phil
away from	ab-, ef-, apo-
axilla	axill/o
axis bone (2nd cervical vertebra), axial	axi/o
back	dors/o, dors/i, poster/o
backbone	rachi/o, rach/i, vertebr/o, spondyl/o
back of knee	poplite/o
back, again	re-
backward	retro-, re-
bacteria	bacteri/o
bad, abnormal, apart	dis-
bad, difficult, painful, abnormal	dys-
bad, poor	mal-
bands	band/o
Bartholin's gland	bartholin/o
base, bottom	bas/o
bear, carry	fer/o, phor/o, duct/o
before, in front of	pre-
beginning	-arche
behind, after	post-
belly side	ventr/o
below	hypo-, sub-
bend, bending	flex/o
beside, near	par-, para-
between	inter-
beyond, change	meta-
bile, gall	bil/i, chol/e

Continued

Definitions and Word Parts

Meaning	Word Part
bile duct, common	choledoch/o
bile vessel	cholangi/o
binding	-desis
birth, born	nat/i, nat/o
black, dark	melan/o
bladder	vesic/o
bladder, sac	cyst/o
blister, small sac	vesicul/o
blood	hem/o, hemat/o
blood condition	-emia
blood vessel	hemangi/o
blue	cyan/o
bluish green	glauc/o
body	corpor/o, somat/o, som/o, -some
bone	oss/i, osse/o, oste/o
bone fragment, sequestrum	sequestr/o
bone marrow, spinal cord	myel/o
both	amphi-, di-
bottom	bas/o
box, cistern	cistern/o
brain	encephal/o
breakdown, dissolve	lys/o
breaking down	-lysis, -clast, -emulsification
breast	mamm/o, mast/o
breastbone (sternum)	stern/o
breath	halit/o
breathe, breathing	pne/o
breathing, to breathe	-pnea, spir/o, hal/o
bring together	-synthesis
bronchiole	bronchiol/o
bronchus	bronch/o, bronchi/o
bunion	bunion/o
burning	cauter/i, caus/o
bursa	burs/o
bursting forth	-rrhagia, -rrhage
buttocks	glute/o
calcaneus	calcane/o
calcium	calc/o
calculus, stone	calcul/o
calf	sur/o

Meaning	Word Part
calyx, calix	cali/o, calic/o, calyc/o
canaliculus, little canal	canalicul/o
cancer	carcin/o
cancer of epithelial origin	-carcinoma
canthus (corner of eye)	canth/o
carbon dioxide	capn/o
carpus, wrist	carp/o
carry, carrying	duct/o
carry, to bear	phor/o, fer/o
cartilage	cartilag/o, chondr/o
carving	-mileusis
cecum (first part of large intestine)	cec/o
cell	cellul/o, cyt/o, -cyte
cerebellum	cerebell/o
cerebrum	cerebr/o
cerumen, earwax	cerumin/o
cervix	cervic/o, trachel/o
change, beyond	meta-
charm	fetish/o
cheek	bucc/o
cheekbone (zygoma)	zygom/o, zygomat/o
cheek muscle, zygomaticus	zygomatic/o
chest (thorax)	pector/o, steth/o, thorac/o
chest (pleural cavity)	-thorax
childbirth, labor, delivery	-tocia
child, foot	ped/o
chin	ment/o, geni/o
cholesterol	cholesterol/o
choroid	choroid/o
chorion (outer fetal sac)	chori/o, chorion/o
ciliary body	cycl/o
cistern, box	cistern/o
clavicle	clav/i, clavicul/o, cleid/o
clitoris	clitorid/o
close, closing, a blockage	occlus/o
close, constrict	mi/o
closing	claustr/o
clotting, clotting process	coagul/o
clotting, clot	-thrombin, thromb/o
clumping	agglutin/o

Definitions and Word Parts

Meaning	Word Part
cochlea	cochle/o
collarbone (clavicle)	cleid/o, clavicul/o, clav/i
colon	col/o, colon/o
color	chrom/o, chromat/o
columella	columell/o
common	vulgar/o
common bile duct	choledoch/o
complete	dia-
condition	-igo
condition of abnormal increase in cells	-cytosis
condition of an opening	-tresia
condition of attraction	-philia
condition of babbling	-lalia
condition of deficiency	-penia
condition of eating, swallowing	-phagia
condition of expansion, dilation	-ectasia
condition of fear, extreme sensitivity	-phobia
condition of formation, development	-plasia, -plasm
condition of madness	-mania
condition of mind	-noia
condition of patches	-plakia
condition of relaxation, slackening	-chalasia
condition of strength	-sthenia
condition of the heart	-cardia
condition, presence of	-iasis
condition, state of	-exia, -ia, -ism
condition, state of mind	-thymia, -noia
condyle, knob	condyl/o
conjunctiva	conjunctiv/o
connective tissue cancer	-sarcoma
contraction	-stalsis
controlling, stopping	-stasis
coordination, order	tax/o
coracoid process	corac/o
cord, spinal cord	chord/o, cord/o
cornea	corne/o, kerat/o
cortex (outer portion)	cortic/o
costa, rib	cost/o

Meaning	Word Part
crackling	crepit/o
crown	coron/o
crushing	-tripsy
crushing, obstructing	-emphraxis
cul-de-sac, rectouterine pouch	culd/o
cuneiform bone	cune/o
curvature	scoli/o
curved	gryph/o
cusp, point	cusp/o
cutting	-cision, -tomy
cutting out	-ectomy
cutting out a stone	-lithotomy
dark	phe/o, scot/o
death, dead	necr/o
deficient, below, under	hypo-
deformity	terat/o
delivery, parturition	-para, part/o, -partum
deltoid muscle, triangle	delt/o
dendrite, tree	dendr/o
density	densit/o
depression, hollow	foss/o
development	troph/o
diaphragm	diaphragm/o, diaphragmat/o
diaphragm, mind	phren/o
digestion	-pepsia
digit, digitus	digit/o
dilation	mydr/o
disc	disc/o
discharge, flow	-rrhea
disease	path/o, morb/o, nos/o
disease process	-pathy
dissolve, dissolving	lys/o, -lysis
distal process of lower leg, malleolus	malleol/o
diverticulum, pouch	diverticul/o
double	dipl/o
down	cata-, infra-
down, lack of	de-
downward	infer/o
dream	oneir/o
drooping, prolapse	-ptosis

Continued

Definitions and Word Parts

Meaning	Word Part
drug, chemical	chem/o, pharmac/o
dry	xer/o
ductus deferens, vas deferens	vas/o
dull, dim	ambly/o
duodenum	duoden/o
dura mater	dur/o
dust	coni/o
ear	ot/o
earwax, cerumen	cerumin/o
eardrum, drum	myring/o, tympan/o
eat, swallow	phag/o
egg	o/o, ovul/o, ov/o, ov/i
elbow	olecran/o
elbow (forearm)	cubit/o
electricity	electr/o
embryonic, immature	-blast, blast/o
enamel	amel/o
end, far, complete	tel/e
endocardium (inner lining of the heart)	endocardi/o
endometrium	endometri/o
enlargement	-megaly
enzyme	-ase
epicardium	epicardi/o
epicondyle	epicondyl/o
epididymis	epididym/o
epiglottis	epiglott/o
epithelium	epitheli/o
equal	is/o
esophagus	esophag/o
ethmoid bone	ethmoid/o
excessive, above	hyper-, poly-
expansion, dilation	-ectasis, -ectasia
extreme cold	cry/o
extremities, heights	acro-
eye	ocul/o, ophthalm/o
eyelid	blephar/o, palpebr/o
face	faci/o
falling, drooping, prolapse	-lapse, -ptosis
fallopian tube	salping/o, -salpinx
far	tel/e, dist/o
fascia	fasci/o

Meaning	Word Part
fast, rapid	tachy-
fat	adip/o, adipos/o, steat/o
fat	lip/o, lipid/o
fatty plaque	ather/o
feces, stool	fec/a
feel with	sympath/o
feeling, sensation	esthesi/o, -esthetica
female, woman	gynec/o, gyn/e, nymph/o
female gonad, ovary	ovari/o, oophor/o
femur (thighbone)	femor/o
fetus	fet/o
fever, fire	pyr/o
few, scanty	olig/o
fiber	fibr/o
fibrous substance	fibrin/o
fibula	fibul/o, perone/o
fimbria	fimbri/o
finger or toe (digitus)	dactyl/o, digit/o
finger/toe bones (phalanx)	phalang/o
first	primi-
fishlike	ichthy/o
fissure, deep cleft	fissur/o
fixation, suspension	-pexy
flesh	sarc/o
flow	-grade
flow, flowing	fluor/o, -flux
fold, plica	plic/o
follicle	follicul/o
foot, child	ped/o
foramen	foramin/o
foreign	xen/o
foreskin (prepuce)	preputi/o, posth/o
formation, production	plas/o, plast/o, -poiesis
forming substance	-plastin, -poietin
fornix	fornic/o
forward, in front of	ante-, pro-
four	quadri-, quadra-, tetra-
frenulum (of tongue and lip)	fren/o, frenul/o
frequent	poly-

Definitions and Word Parts

Meaning	Word Part	Meaning	Word Part
front	anter/o, front/o	hernia	herni/o
fungus	myc/o	herniation, protrusion	-cele
fundus (base, bottom)	fund/o	hidden	crypt-
gallbladder	cholecyst/o	hilum	hil/o
ganglion	gangli/o, ganglion/o	hip (coxa)	cox/o
gate	port/o	hip socket, acetabulum	acetabul/o
gestation	-cyesis, -gravida, gravid/o	hold back, suppress	isch/o
		hold back blood flow	ischem/o
gland	aden/o	hole, foramen	foramin/o
glans penis	balan/o	hollow, depression	foss/o
glenoid cavity (arm socket)	glen/o	hormone, substance that forms	-one
globus pallidum	pallid/o	humerus (upper arm bone)	humer/o
glomerulus	glomerul/o		
glucose, sugar	gluc/o, glucos/o, glyc/o, glycos/o	hymen	hymen/o
		hyoid bone	hyoid/o
glue, glia cell	-glia	ileum	ile/o
gonad, sex organ	gonad/o	ilium (superior, widest pelvic bone)	ili/o
gray	poli/o		
great toe, hallux	halluc/o	immature, embryonic	-blast, blast/o
groin	inguin/o	in	en-, in-
grow	cret/o	in favor of	pro-
growth	physi/o, -physis, phyt/o	in front of, before	ante-, pre-, pro-
gums	gingiv/o	incision, cutting	-tomy
hair	pil/o, trich/o	infection	septic/o
hairs, tiny	cili/o	inflammation	-itis
half	hemi-, semi-	inner ear (labyrinth)	labyrinth/o
hallux, great toe	halluc/o	inner fetal sac, amnion	amni/o, amnion/o, -amnios
hand	man/u, man/i		
hard (dura mater)	dur/o	inner lining of heart	endocardi/o
hard, horny, cornea	kerat/o	inner lining of uterus	endometri/o
hard, sclera	scler/o	instrument to crush	-trite
head	capit/o, cephal/o, -cephalus	instrument to cut	-tome
		instrument to measure	-meter
healthy, normal	eu-	instrument to record	-graph
hearing	acous/o, audi/o, aur/o, -acusis, -cusis	instrument to view	-scope
		insulin	insulin/o
heart	cardi/o, cordi/o, coron/o	intentional breaking	-clasis
heat, temperature	therm/o	intestine	intestin/o, enter/o
heelbone (calcaneus)	calcane/o	inward	eso-
heights, extremes, extremities	acro-	iris	ir/o, irid/o
		iron	sider/o
helix, coil	helic/o	iron substance	-siderin
hemorrhoid	hemorrhoid/o	ischium	ischi/o

Continued

Definitions and Word Parts

Meaning	Word Part	Meaning	Word Part
itching	prurit/o	lymph gland (lymph node)	lymphaden/o
jaw, entire	gnath/o	lymph vessel	lymphangi/o
jejunum	jejun/o	machine to crush	-tripter
jingling	tinnit/o	macula, macula lutea	macul/o
joined	syn-	macule	macul/o
joint (articulation)	arthr/o, articul/o	making a new opening	-stomy
juice	chym/o	male	andr/o
ketone	ket/o, keton/o	male gonad	test/o, testicul/o, orch/o, orchi/o, orchid/o
kidney	nephr/o, ren/o	male sex cell, spermatozoon	spermat/o, sperm/o
kneecap (patella)	patell/o, patell/a	man	anthrop/o
knowledge (state of)	-gnosis	manubrium of breastbone	manubri/o
labyrinth	labyrinth/o	many	multi-
lacrimal gland	dacryoaden/o	many, much, excessive	poly-
lacrimal sac	dacryocyst/o	marketplace	agora-
lamina, thin plate	lamin/o	mass	-oma
large	macro-	mastoid process	mastoid/o
large intestine (colon)	col/o, colon/o	measuring	-metry
larynx, voice box	laryng/o	meatus (opening)	meat/o
left	levo-, sinistr/o	mediastinum	mediastin/o
leg	crur/o	medulla	medull/o
lens	phac/o, phak/o	meninges	mening/o, meningi/o
lice	pedicul/i	meniscus	menisc/o
life, living	bi/o	menstruation, menses	menstru/o, men/o
ligament	ligament/o, syndesm/o	mesentery, midgut	mesenter/o
light	phot/o	metacarpus (hand bone)	metacarp/o
limbus	limb/o	metatarsus (foot bone)	metatars/o
lipid, fat	lipid/o, lip/o	middle	medi/o, meso-, mid-
lips	cheil/o	midgut, mesentery	mesenter/o
lips (labia)	labi/o	milk	galact/o, lact/o
liquid	humor/o	mind	ment/o, phren/o, psych/o
little beam	trabecul/o	mitochrondria	mitochondri/a
little grain	granul/o	molar	mol/o
liver	hepat/o	moon	lun/o
lobe, section	lob/o	mouth, oral cavity	or/o, stomat/o, stom/o
long	long/o	movement	-kine, -kinesis
lower back	lumb/o	movement substance	-kinin
lower jaw	mandibul/o	mucus	muc/o, mucos/o, myx/o
lumen (space within vessel)	lumin/o	muscle	muscul/o, my/o, myos/o
lung, air	pneum/o, pneumat/o	myocardium (heart muscle)	myocardi/o, cardiomy/o
lung	pneumon/o, pulmon/o		
lymph	lymph/o, lymphat/o, chyl/o		

Definitions and Word Parts

Meaning	Word Part
myometrium	myometri/o
nail	onych/o, ungu/o
navel	omphal/o, umbilic/o
navicular bone	navicul/o
near	proxim/o
near, beside, abnormal	para-, par-
neck	nuch/o, coll/o
neck, cervix	cervic/o
neck, throat	jugul/o
nerve	neur/o, neuron/o
nerve root	radicul/o, rhiz/o
nervous	nervos/o
nest	nid/o
neutral	neutr/o
nevus, birthmark	nev/o
new	neo-
night	noct/i, nyctal/o
nipple	thel/e
nipple	papill/o
no, not, without	a-, an-, in-, non-
node, knot	nod/o
none	nulli-
nose	nas/o, rhin/o
notched	serrat/o
nourishment	troph/o, -trophy
noun ending	-a, -e, -is, -ity, -um, -osus
nucleus	kary/o, nucle/o
nutrition	aliment/o
obstructing, crushing	-emphraxis
occiput	-occipit/o
odor, stench	brom/o
old age	ger/o, presby-
omentum	oment/o, epiplo/o
one	mono-, uni-
open	patul/o
opening	hiat/o, meat/o
opening, a mouth	stom/o
opposite, against	contra-
optic disk	papill/o
orange-yellow	cirrh/o
orbit	orbit/o
order, coordination	tax/o

Meaning	Word Part
organ, viscera	organ/o, viscer/o
origin, production	-genesis
ossicle	ossicul/o
other, different	allo-
out, outward	ec-, ex-
outer fetal sac, chorion	chorion/o, chori/o
outside	exo-, extra-
outward	e-
ovary	oophor/o, ovari/o
ovum, egg	o/o, ovul/o, ov/o, ov/i
oxygen	ox/i, ox/o, oxy-
pain	-algia, -dynia
palate, roof of mouth, palatine bone	palat/o
palm	palm/o
pancreas	pancreat/o
papilla	papill/o
papule	papul/o
paralysis	-plegia
paralysis, slight	-paresis
parathyroid	parathyroid/o
parenchyma	parenchym/o
parturition, delivery	part/o, -partum, -para
passage	por/o
patella	patell/a, patell/o
pelvis	pelv/i, pelv/o
penis	pen/i, phall/o
pericardium (sac surrounding heart)	pericardi/o
perimetrium (outer layer of uterus)	perimetri/o
perineum	perine/o
peritoneum	peritone/o
pertaining to	-ac, -al, -an, -ant, -ar, -ary, -atic, -eal, -ent, -iac, -ic, -id, -ine, -ior, -itic, -ive, -ous, -tic
pertaining to abnormal condition	-iacal
pertaining to breaking down	-lytic
pertaining to bursting forth	-rrhagic
pertaining to carrying	-ferous
pertaining to discharge	-rrheic
pertaining to formation	-plastic

Continued

Definitions and Word Parts

Meaning	Word Part
pertaining to origin	-logous
pertaining to originating from	-genous
pertaining to produced by	-genic, -geneic
pertaining to viewing	-scopic
pertaining to, full of	-ose
petrous bone	petros/o
phalanx	phalang/o
pharyngeal tonsil, adenoid	adenoid/o
pharynx, throat	pharyng/o
phrenic nerve	phren/o
pimple	papul/o
pituitary, hypophysis	hypophys/o, pituitar/o, pituit/o
place, location	top/o
placenta	placent/o
plasma	plasm/a, plasm/o
pleasure	hedon/o
pleura (membrane surrounding lungs)	pleur/o
plica	plic/o
point, cusp	cusp/o
pointed extremity, apex	apic/o
poison	tox/o, toxic/o
pole	pol/o
pollex, thumb	pollic/o
polyp	polyp/o
potassium	kal/i
pouch, diverticulum	diverticul/o
power	dynam/o
precordium	precordi/o
pregnancy, gestation	-cyesis, gravid/o, -gravida
prepuce (foreskin)	preputi/o, posth/o
presence of	-iasis
pressure	man/o
pressure, stretching	-tension
process of	-ation, -ion, -zation, -tion, -y, -ization
process of clotting	-coagulation
process of pouring	-fusion
process of stretching, pressure	-tension

Meaning	Word Part
process of turning	-version
producing	-gen
production	-genesis, -poiesis
prolactin	prolactin/o
prolapse	-ptosis
prostate	prostat/o
protection, safety	immun/o
protein	globin/o, globulin/o
protein substance	-globin, -globulin
pubis, anterior pelvic bone	pub/o
puerperium	puerper/o
pull, pulling	tract/o, till/o, vuls/o
pupil	cor/o, core/o, pupill/o
purple	purpur/o
purposeful movement	prax/o
pus	py/o
pustule	pustul/o
pylorus	pylor/o
radius	radi/o
rapid, fast	tachy-
rash	exanthemat/o
rays	radi/o, act/o
record, recording	-gram
recording	-graphy
rectouterine pouch (cul-de-sac)	culd/o
rectum and anus	proct/o
rectum, straight	rect/o
recurring, round	cycl/o
red	erythr/o, erythemat/o
relaxation, slackening	-chalasis
removal	-apheresis
renal pelvis	pyel/o
rent or tear	-spadias
resembling, like	-oid
retina	retin/o
reverberation, sound	echo-
rhythm	rhythm/o
rib (costa)	cost/o
ribose	rib/o
right	dextr/o

Definitions and Word Parts

Meaning	Word Part
ring, annulus	annul/o
rosy, dawn colored	eosin/o
roundback	kyph/o
rugae, ridge	rug/o
run, running	-drome
rupture	-rrhexis
sac surrounding the heart	pericardi/o
sacrum	sacr/o
safety, protection	immun/o
saliva	sial/o, ptyal/o
salivary duct	sialodoch/o
salivary gland	sialaden/o
same	home/o, homo-, ipsi-
scab	eschar/o
scaly	squam/o
scanty, few	olig/o
scanty, thin	man/o
scaphoid bone	scaphoid/o
scapula (shoulder blade)	scapul/o
sclera, hard	scler/o
scraping of	-abrasion
scrotum	scrot/o
sea	thalass/o
sebum, oil	seb/o, sebac/o
secrete, secreting	crin/o, -crine
seed	gon/o
seizure	-lepsy
self	auto-
semen	semin/i
sensation	esthesi/o, -esthetica
sense	sensor/i
sensitivity, fear	-phobia
separate, separating	-crit
separate, away	apo-
septum	sept/o
sequestrum (bone fragment)	sequestr/o
serum	ser/o
shape, form	morph/o, -form
sharp	acu-
shinbone (tibia)	tibi/o
shoulder blade (scapula)	scapul/o
shut	my/o

Meaning	Word Part
side	later/o
sigmoid colon	sigmoid/o
sinus, cavity	sin/o, sinus/o
skeleton	skelet/o
skin	cut/o, cutane/o, derm/o, dermat/o
skin condition	-derma
skull	crani/o
slackening	-chalasia, -chalasis
sleep, stupor	narc/o, somn/o, hypn/o
slight paralysis	-paresis
slipping	-listhesis
slow	brady-
small	micro-, -ole, -ule, -icle
small cavity, alveolus	alveol/o
small intestines, intestines	enter/o
small lobe	lobul/o
small sac, seminal vesicle	vesicul/o
smooth muscle	leiomy/o
sodium	natr/o
softening	-malacia
sole of foot	plant/o
sound	echo-
sound, voice	phon/o
space	stiti/o
spasm	-spasm, -ismus
speech	phas/o
spermatozoon	sperm/o, spermat/o
sphenoid	sphenoid/o, sphen/o
sphere	spher/o
spinal column	rachi/o, rach/i
spinal cord	cord/o, myel/o, chord/o
spinal nerve root	rhiz/o, radicul/o
spine	spin/o, vertebr/o, spondyl/o
spitting	-ptysis
spleen	splen/o
split	schiz/o, -schisis, -fida
split, splitting	-fida
spot, macula lutea, macule	macul/o
sprout	germ/i

Continued

Definitions and Word Parts

Meaning	Word Part
stapes	staped/o
star	astr/o
starch	amyl/o
state of	-esis, -sis, -ia, -ism
state of relaxation	-chalasis
steal, stealing	klept/o
steroid	ster/o
stiffening	ankyl/o
stomach	gastr/o
stone (calculus)	calcul/o, lith/o
stone	petr/o
stop, cease	-pause
stopping, controlling	-stasis
straight, upright	orth/o
straight	rect/o
stretching	tens/o
striated (skeletal) muscle	rhabdomy/o
stroma (supportive tissue)	strom/o
structure, membrane, thing	-um, -ium
structure, thing, noun ending	-us, -on, -is
study	log/o
study of	-logy
styloid process	styl/o
substance	-in, -one
sudoriferous gland	hidraden/o
sugar, glucose	glycos/o, glucos/o, gluc/o, glyc/o
sulcus, groove	sulc/o
surgical puncture	-centesis
surgically forming	-plasty
surrounding, around	peri-
suspension, fixation	-pexy
suturing	-rrhaphy
swallow, eat	phag/o
swayback	lord/o
sweat	hidr/o, sudor/i
sweat gland (sudoriferous gland)	hidraden/o
swelling	-edema, tubercul/o
synovium	synovi/o, synov/o

Meaning	Word Part
system	system/o
tail	caud/o
tailbone (coccyx)	coccyg/o
talus bone	tal/o
tarsus (anklebone), flat surface	tars/o
tear	dacry/o, lacrim/o
tearing out	-exeresis
teeth	dent/i, odont/o
temporal bone	tempor/o
tendon	ten/o, tend/o, tendin/o, tendon/o
tension, tone	ton/o
testis, testicle	orch/o, orchi/o, orchid/o, test/o, testicul/o
thalamus	thalam/o
thigh	mer/o
thirst	dips/o
thorax, chest	thorac/o
three	tri-
throat (pharynx)	pharyng/o
throat, neck	jugul/o
through	per-
through, across	trans-
through, complete	dia-
throw, throwing	bol/o
thumb, pollex	pollic/o
thymus gland, mind	thym/o
thyroid gland	thyroid/o
thyroid gland, shield	thyr/o
tie, tying	ligat/o, -ligation
time	chron/o
tiny hairs	cili/o
tissue	hist/o
to flow, flowing	fluor/o
toe/finger bone, phalanx	phalang/o
together	con-
together, joined	syn-
tongue	gloss/o, lingu/o
tonsil	tonsill/o
tonsil (pharyngeal), adenoid	adenoid/o
toward	ac-, ad-, -ad, af-

Definitions and Word Parts

Meaning	Word Part
trabecula	trabecul/o
treatment	-therapy
tree	dendr/o
triangle, deltoid	delt/o
trigone	trigon/o
trochanter	trochanter/o
tube, fallopian	-salpinx
tube, fallopian or eustachian	salping/o
tube, pipe	tub/o
tumor	onc/o
tumor, mass	-oma
tubercle, a swelling	tubercul/o
turbinate bone	turbin/o
turn, turning	trop/o, vers/o, vert/o, -verse
two	bi-, bin-
two (both)	di-
tying	-ligation
ulceration	aphth/o
ulna	uln/o
umbilicus (navel)	omphal/o, umbilic/o
under, below	sub-, hypo-
up, apart, away	ana-
upper jaw bone (maxilla)	maxill/o
upward	super/o, supra-
ureter	ureter/o
urethra	urethr/o
urinary condition	-uria
urine, urinary system	ur/o, urin/o
uterus	hyster/o, metr/o, metri/o, uter/o
uvea	uve/o
uvula	uvul/o
vagina	colp/o, vagin/o
vagus nerve	vag/o
valve	valv/o, valvul/o
varices	varic/o
vas deferens	vas/o
vein	phleb/o, ven/o
ventricle	ventricul/o

Meaning	Word Part
venule (small vein)	venul/o
vertebra, backbone	spondyl/o, rach/i, rachi/o
vessel	angi/o, vascul/o, vas/o
vessel, ductus deferens, vas deferens	vas/o
vestibule	vestibul/o
viewing	-opsy, -scopy
villus	vill/o
vision	opt/o, optic/o
vision condition	-opia, -opsia
vitreous humor, glassy	vitre/o, vitr/o
voice	phon/o
voice box (larynx)	laryng/o
volume	vol/o
vomer	vomer/o
vomiting	-emesis
vulva	episi/o, vulv/o
walking	ambul/o
wall, partition, septum	pariet/o, sept/o
washing	-clysis
wasting	-phthisis, -tabes
water, fluid	hydr/o
water drop	hydatid/i
watery flow	rheumat/o
wheel	rot/o
white	leuk/o
white substance	-leukin
windpipe (trachea)	trache/o
wing	pteryg/o, al/o, al/i
within	end, endo-, intra-
woman, female	nymph/o, gyn/e, gynec/o
word, speech	lex/o
worm	verm/o
wrinkle	rhytid/o
wrinkled	corrug/o
wrist (carpus)	carp/o
xiphoid process	xiph/i, xiph/o
zygoma (cheek bone)	zygom/o, zygomat/o
zygomaticus (cheek muscle)	zygomatic/o

Abbreviations

Abbreviation	Meaning	Abbreviation	Meaning
#	fracture	Astigm, As, Ast	astigmatism
A	action	AU	each ear
AAMT	American Association of Medical Transcriptionists	AV	atrioventricular
		basos	basophils
A, B, AB, O	blood types	BBB	blood-brain barrier; bundle branch block
ABR	auditory brainstem response		
ACL	anterior cruciate ligament	BCC	basal cell carcinoma
ACTH	adrenocorticotropic hormone	BD, BP	bipolar disorder
AD	Alzheimer's disease	BE	barium enema
AD	right ear	BM	bowel movement
ADH	antidiuretic hormone	BMI	body mass index
ADHD	attention-deficit/hyperactivity disorder	BMP	basic metabolic panel
		BMT	bone marrow transplant
AEB	atrial ectopic beats	BP	blood pressure
AF	atrial fibrillation	BPD	borderline personality disorder
AFP	alpha fetoprotein test		
ABG	arterial blood gases	BPH	benign prostatic hyperplasia/ hypertrophy
AIDS	acquired immunodeficiency syndrome		
		BPM	beats per minute
ALL	acute lymphocytic leukemia	BS	barium swallow
ALP	alkaline phosphatase	BUN	blood urea nitrogen
ALPS	autoimmune lymphoproliferative syndrome	bx, Bx	biopsy
		C1-C7	first through seventh cervical vertebrae
ALS	amyotrophic lateral sclerosis		
ALT	alanine transaminase	C1-C8	cervical nerves
AMA	American Medical Association	C2	second cervical vertebra
AMI	acute myocardial infarction	Ca	calcium
AML	acute myelogenous leukemia	CABG	coronary artery bypass graft
ANS	autonomic nervous system	CAD	coronary artery disease
ant	anterior	CAPD	continuous ambulatory peritoneal dialysis
AP	anteroposterior		
APA	American Psychiatric Association	CBC	complete blood cell (count)
ARDS	acute respiratory distress syndrome	CF	cystic fibrosis
		CHF	congestive heart failure
ARF	acute renal failure; acute respiratory failure	CIN	cervical intraepithelial neoplasia
		CIN III	cervical intraepithelial neoplasia; cervical dysplasia
ARMD, AMD	age-related macular degeneration		
AS	aortic stenosis	CK, CPK	creatine phosphokinase
AS	left ear	CKD	chronic kidney disease
ASD	atrial septal defect	Cl	chloride

Abbreviations—cont'd

Abbreviation	Meaning
CLL	chronic lymphocytic leukemia
CLO test	campylobacter-like organism test
CML	chronic myelogenous leukemia
CMP	comprehensive metabolic panel
CNS	central nervous system
CO_2	carbon dioxide
COPD	chronic obstructive pulmonary disease
CP	cerebral palsy
CPAP	continuous positive airway pressure
CR	closed reduction
CREF	closed reduction external fixation
CRP	C-reactive protein
CS	cesarean section
CSF	cerebrospinal fluid
CST	contraction stress test
CT scan	computed tomography scan
CTS	carpal tunnel syndrome
CV	cardiovascular
CVA	cerebrovascular accident
CVS	chorionic villus sampling
CWP	coal workers' pneumoconiosis
cx	cervix
CXR	chest x-ray
D&C	dilation and curettage
D1-D12	first through twelfth dorsal vertebrae
DAP	Draw-a-Person Test
DEXA, DXA	dual-energy x-ray absorptiometry
DI	diabetes insipidus
DIC	disseminated intravascular coagulopathy
diff	differential WBC count
DIP	distal interphalangeal joint
DJD	degenerative joint disease
DLE	disseminated lupus erythematosus
DM	diabetes mellitus
DOE	dyspnea on exertion
DSM	*Diagnostic and Statistical Manual of Mental Disorders*

Abbreviation	Meaning
DTs	delirium tremens
DUB	dysfunctional uterine bleeding
DVT	deep vein thrombosis
EBV	Epstein-Barr virus
ECCE	extracapsular cataract extraction
ECG, EKG	electrocardiogram
ECHO	echocardiography
ECOG	electrocochleography
ECT	electroconvulsive therapy
ED	erectile dysfunction
EDD	estimated delivery date
EEG	electroencephalogram
EF	external fixation
EGD	esophagogastroduodenoscopy
EM, em	emmetropia
EMG	electromyography
EOC	epithelial ovarian cancer
eosins	eosinophils
ERCP	endoscopic retrograde cholangiopancreatography
ERP	endoscopic retrograde pancreatography
ESR	erythrocyte sedimentation rate
ESRD	end-stage renal disease
ESWL	extracorporeal shock wave lithotripsy
FB	foreign body
FBS	fasting blood sugar
FOBT	fecal occult blood test
FPG	fasting plasma glucose
FSH	follicle-stimulating hormone
FTA-ABS	fluorescent treponemal antibody absorption test
Fx	fracture
G6PD	glucose-6-phosphate dehydrogenase
GAD	generalized anxiety disorder
GAF	global assessment of functioning
GB	gallbladder
Gc	gonococcus, gonococcal
GCT	germ cell tumor
GERD	gastroesophageal reflux disease
GFR	glomerular filtration rate

Continued

Abbreviations—cont'd

Abbreviation	Meaning
GGT	gamma-glutamyl transferase
GH	growth hormone
GHD	growth hormone deficiency
GI	gastrointestinal
GVHD	graft-versus-host disease
HAA	hepatitis-associated antigen
HAV	hepatitis A virus
Hb	hemoglobin
HBV	hepatitis B virus
hCG	human chorionic gonadotropin
Hct	hematocrit; packed-cell volume
HCV	hepatitis C virus
HD	hemodialysis
HDL	high-density lipoproteins
HDN	hemolytic disease of the newborn
HELLP	hemolytic elevated liver enzymes low platelet count
HF	heart failure
Hgb	hemoglobin
hGH	human growth hormone
HGPS	Hutchinson-Gilford progeria syndrome
HHN	handheld nebulizer
HIV	human immunodeficiency virus
HPV	human papillomavirus
HSC	hematopoietic stem cell
HSG	hysterosalpingography
HSV	herpes simplex virus
HSV-1	herpes simplex virus-1
HSV-2	herpes simplex virus-2; herpes genitalis
I	insertion
I&D	incision and drainage
IBD	inflammatory bowel disease
IBS	irritable bowel syndrome
IC	interstitial cystitis
ICCE	intracapsular cataract extraction
ICD	International Classification of Diseases
ICSH	interstitial cell-stimulating hormone
IDC	infiltrating ductal carcinoma

Abbreviation	Meaning
IDDM	insulin-dependent diabetes mellitus
IF	internal fixation
Ig	immunoglobulin
IM	intramuscular
inf	inferior
IOL	intraocular lens
IOP	intraocular pressure
ITA	internal thoracic artery
IQ	intelligence quotient
K	potassium
KS	Kaposi's sarcoma
L1-L5	first through fifth lumbar vertebrae; lumbar nerves
LA	left atrium
LASIK	laser-assisted in situ keratomileusis
lat	lateral
LCA	left circumflex artery; left coronary artery
LCL	lateral collateral ligament
LDH	lactate dehydrogenase
LDL	low-density lipoproteins
LEEP	loop electrocautery excision procedure
LES	lower esophageal sphincter
LFTs	liver function tests
LGA	light for gestational age
LH	luteinizing hormone
LLL	left lower lobe
LLQ	lower left quadrant
LMP	last menstrual period
LP	lumbar puncture
LUL	left upper lobe
LUQ	left upper quadrant
LV	left ventricle
LVAD	left ventricular assist device
lymphs	lymphocytes
MCH	mean corpuscular hemoglobin
MCHC	mean corpuscular hemoglobin concentration
MCI	mild cognitive impairment
MCL	medial collateral ligament

Abbreviations—cont'd

Abbreviation	Meaning
MD	muscular dystrophy; medical doctor
MDI	metered-dose inhaler
MDR TB	multidrug-resistant tuberculosis
MHA-TP	microhemagglutination assay for *Treponema pallidum*
MIDCAB	minimally invasive direct coronary artery bypass
MMPI	Minnesota Multiphasic Personality Inventory
MR	mental retardation; mitral regurgitation
MRI	magnetic resonance imaging
MS	multiple sclerosis; mitral stenosis; musculoskeletal
MSE	mental status examination
MV	mitral valve
MVP	mitral valve prolapse
MY	myopia
Na	sodium
NCSE	Neurobehavioral Cognitive Status Examination
neuts	neutrophils
NGU	nongonococcal urethritis
NIDDM	non-insulin-dependent diabetes mellitus (type 2 diabetes)
NK	natural killer cell
NSCLC	non–small cell lung cancer
NSR	normal sinus rhythm
NST	nonstress test
NSTEMI	non–ST elevation myocardial infarction
O	origin
O_2	oxygen
OA	osteoarthritis
OAEs	otoacoustic emissions
OCD	obsessive-compulsive disorder
OCPD	obsessive-compulsive personality disorder
OD	right eye
ODD	oppositional defiant disorder
OGTT	oral glucose tolerance test
OM	otitis media

Abbreviation	Meaning
OR	open reduction
ORIF	open reduction internal fixation
OS	left eye
OT	oxytocin
OU	each eye
PA	posteroanterior; pulmonary artery
PAC	premature atrial contractions
PCL	posterior cruciate ligament
PCOS	polycystic ovary syndrome
PCV	packed-cell volume; hematocrit
PD	Parkinson's disease; panic disorder
PDA	patent ductus arteriosus
PDD	pervasive developmental disorder
PE	pulmonary embolism
PEEP	positive end-expiratory pressure
PEG	percutaneous endoscopic gastrostomy
PET scan	positron emission tomography scan
PFT	pulmonary function test
PID	pelvic inflammatory disease
PIP	proximal interphalangeal joint
PKU	phenylketonuria
plats	platelets; thrombocytes
PMB	postmenopausal bleeding
PMNs, polys	polymorphonucleocytes
PMS	premenstrual syndrome
PNS	peripheral nervous system
pos	posterior
PPB	positive pressure breathing
PPD	purified protein derivative
PPS	postpolio syndrome
PRL	prolactin
PSA	prostate-specific antigen
PSG	polysomnography
PSV	pressure support ventilation
PT	prothrombin time
PTCA	percutaneous transluminal coronary angioplasty
PTH	parathyroid hormone
PTSD	post-traumatic stress disorder

Continued

Abbreviations—cont'd

Abbreviation	Meaning
PTT	partial thromboplastin time
PUD	peptic ulcer disease
PUPP	pruritic urticarial papules and plaques
PUVA	psoralen plus ultraviolet A
PV	pulmonary vein
PVC	premature ventricular contraction
PVD	peripheral vascular disease
QFT	quantiferon-TB gold test
RA	rheumatoid arthritis; right atrium
RBC	red blood cell (count)
RCA	right coronary artery
RHD	rheumatic heart disease
RIA	radioimmunoassay studies
RLL	right lower lobe
RLQ	right lower quadrant
RML	right middle lobe
ROM	range of motion
RPR	rapid plasma reagin
RSV	respiratory syncytial virus
RUL	right upper lobe
RUQ	right upper quadrant
RV	right ventricle
S1-S5	first sacral through fifth sacral vertebrae; sacral nerves
SA	sinoatrial
SAD	seasonal affective disorder
SAH	subarachnoid hemorrhage
SARS	severe acute respiratory syndrome
SCLC	small cell lung cancer
SCC	squamous cell carcinoma
SDD	specific developmental disorders
segs	segmented neutrophils
SG	skin graft
SGA	small for gestational age
SGPT	serum glutamic-pyruvic transaminase
SIADH	syndrome of inappropriate antidiuretic hormone
SIRS	systemic inflammatory response syndrome
SLE	systemic lupus erythematosus

Abbreviation	Meaning
SNS	somatic nervous system
SOB	shortness of breath
SSS	sick sinus syndrome
ST	aspartate transaminase
stabs	band cells
STD	sexually transmitted disease
STEMI	ST elevation myocardial infarction
STH	somatotropic hormone
STSG	split-thickness skin graft
sup	superior
SVT	superficial vein thrombosis
T1-T12	first through twelfth thoracic vertebrae; thoracic nerves
T_3	triiodothyronine
T_4	thyroxine
TAH-BSO	total abdominal hysterectomy with bilateral salpingo-oophorectomy
TAT	Thematic Apperception Test
TB	tuberculosis
TBI	traumatic brain injury
TCC	transitional cell carcinoma
TEE	transesophageal echocardiogram
TEF	tracheoesophageal fistulization
TENS	transcutaneous electrical nerve stimulation
TFTs	thyroid function tests
THR	total hip replacement
TIA	transient ischemic attack
TKR	total knee replacement
TM	tympanic membrane
TMJ	temporomandibular joint
TMR	transmyocardial revascularization
TPN	total parenteral nutrition
TS	tricuspid stenosis
TSH	thyroid-stimulating hormone
TTTS	twin-to-twin transfusion syndrome
TUIP	transurethral incision of the prostate
TUMT	transurethral microwave thermotherapy

Abbreviations—cont'd

Abbreviation	Meaning
TUR	transurethral resection
TURP	transurethral resection of the prostate
TV	tricuspid valve
UA	urinalysis
UAE	uterine artery embolization
UCL	ulnar collateral ligament
uE3	unconjugated estriol
UNHS	universal newborn hearing screening
UPJ	ureteropelvic junction
UTI	urinary tract infection
VA	visual acuity
VAP	ventilator-associated pneumonia

Abbreviation	Meaning
VBAC	vaginal birth after cesarean section
VD	venereal disease
VDRL	Venereal Disease Research Laboratory
VEB	ventricular ectopic beats
VF	visual field
VSD	ventricular septal defect
VT	ventricular tachycardia
WAIS	Wechsler Adult Intelligence Scale
WBC	white blood cell (count)
WISC	Wechsler Intelligence Scale for Children

Institute for Safe Medication Practices

ISMP's List of *Error-Prone Abbreviations, Symbols,* and *Dose Designations*

The abbreviations, symbols, and dose designations found in this table have been reported to ISMP through the ISMP National Medication Errors Reporting Program (ISMP MERP) as being frequently misinterpreted and involved in harmful medication errors. They should **NEVER** be used when communicating medical information. This includes internal communications, telephone/verbal prescriptions, computer-generated labels, labels for drug storage bins, medication administration records, as well as pharmacy and prescriber computer order entry screens.

Abbreviations	Intended Meaning	Misinterpretation	Correction
µg	Microgram	Mistaken as "mg"	Use "mcg"
AD, AS, AU	Right ear, left ear, each ear	Mistaken as OD, OS, OU (right eye, left eye, each eye)	Use "right ear," "left ear," or "each ear"
OD, OS, OU	Right eye, left eye, each eye	Mistaken as AD, AS, AU (right ear, left ear, each ear)	Use "right eye," "left eye," or "each eye"
BT	Bedtime	Mistaken as "BID" (twice daily)	Use "bedtime"
cc	Cubic centimeters	Mistaken as "u" (units)	Use "mL"
D/C	Discharge or discontinue	Premature discontinuation of medications if D/C (intended to mean "discharge") has been misinterpreted as "discontinued" when followed by a list of discharge medications	Use "discharge" and "discontinue"
IJ	Injection	Mistaken as "IV" or "intrajugular"	Use "injection"
IN	Intranasal	Mistaken as "IM" or "IV"	Use "intranasal" or "NAS"
HS	Half-strength	Mistaken as bedtime	Use "half-strength" or "bedtime"
hs	At bedtime, hours of sleep	Mistaken as half-strength	
IU**	International unit	Mistaken as IV (intravenous) or 10 (ten)	Use "units"
o.d. or OD	Once daily	Mistaken as "right eye" (OD-oculus dexter), leading to oral liquid medications administered in the eye	Use "daily"
OJ	Orange juice	Mistaken as OD or OS (right or left eye); drugs meant to be diluted in orange juice may be given in the eye	Use "orange juice"
Per os	By mouth, orally	The "os" can be mistaken as "left eye" (OS-oculus sinister)	Use "PO," "by mouth," or "orally"
q.d. or QD**	Every day	Mistaken as q.i.d., especially if the period after the "q" or the tail of the "q" is misunderstood as an "i"	Use "daily"
qhs	Nightly at bedtime	Mistaken as "qhr" or every hour	Use "nightly"
qn	Nightly or at bedtime	Mistaken as "qh" (every hour)	Use "nightly" or "at bedtime"
q.o.d. or QOD**	Every other day	Mistaken as "q.d." (daily) or "q.i.d. (four times daily) if the "o" is poorly written	Use "every other day"
q1d	Daily	Mistaken as q.i.d. (four times daily)	Use "daily"
q6PM, etc.	Every evening at 6 PM	Mistaken as every 6 hours	Use "daily at 6 PM" or "6 PM daily"
SC, SQ, sub q	Subcutaneous	SC mistaken as SL (sublingual); SQ mistaken as "5 every;" the "q" in "sub q" has been mistaken as "every" (e.g., a heparin dose ordered "sub q 2 hours before surgery" misunderstood as every 2 hours before surgery)	Use "subcut" or "subcutaneously"
ss	Sliding scale (insulin) or ½ (apothecary)	Mistaken as "55"	Spell out "sliding scale;" use "one-half" or "½"
SSRI	Sliding scale regular insulin	Mistaken as selective-serotonin reuptake inhibitor	Spell out "sliding scale (insulin)"
SSI	Sliding scale insulin	Mistaken as Strong Solution of Iodine (Lugol's)	
i/d	One daily	Mistaken as "tid"	Use "1 daily"
TIW or tiw	3 times a week	Mistaken as "3 times a day" or "twice in a week"	Use "3 times weekly"
U or u**	Unit	Mistaken as the number 0 or 4, causing a 10-fold overdose or greater (e.g., 4U seen as "40" or 4u seen as "44"); mistaken as "cc" so dose given in volume instead of units (e.g., 4u seen as 4cc)	Use "unit"
UD	As directed ("ut dictum")	Mistaken as unit dose (e.g., diltiazem 125 mg IV infusion "UD" misinterpreted as meaning to give the entire infusion as a unit [bolus] dose)	Use "as directed"

Dose Designations and Other Information	Intended Meaning	Misinterpretation	Correction
Trailing zero after decimal point (e.g., 1.0 mg)**	1 mg	Mistaken as 10 mg if the decimal point is not seen	Do not use trailing zeros for doses expressed in whole numbers
"Naked" decimal point (e.g., .5 mg)**	0.5 mg	Mistaken as 5 mg if the decimal point is not seen	Use zero before a decimal point when the dose is less than a whole unit
Abbreviations such as mg. or mL. with a period following the abbreviation	mg mL	The period is unnecessary and could be mistaken as the number 1 if written poorly	Use mg, mL, etc. without a terminal period

Institute for Safe Medication Practices

ISMP's List of *Error-Prone Abbreviations, Symbols,* and *Dose Designations* (continued)

Dose Designations and Other Information	Intended Meaning	Misinterpretation	Correction
Drug name and dose run together (especially problematic for drug names that end in "l" such as Inderal40 mg; Tegretol300 mg)	Inderal 40 mg Tegretol 300 mg	Mistaken as Inderal 140 mg Mistaken as Tegretol 1300 mg	Place adequate space between the drug name, dose, and unit of measure
Numerical dose and unit of measure run together (e.g., 10mg, 100mL)	10 mg 100 mL	The "m" is sometimes mistaken as a zero or two zeros, risking a 10- to 100-fold overdose	Place adequate space between the dose and unit of measure
Large doses without properly placed commas (e.g., 100000 units; 1000000 units)	100,000 units 1,000,000 units	100000 has been mistaken as 10,000 or 1,000,000; 1000000 has been mistaken as 100,000	Use commas for dosing units at or above 1,000, or use words such as 100 "thousand" or 1 "million" to improve readability

Drug Name Abbreviations	Intended Meaning	Misinterpretation	Correction
To avoid confusion, do not abbreviate drug names when communicating medical information. Examples of drug name abbreviations involved in medication errors include:			
APAP	acetaminophen	Not recognized as acetaminophen	Use complete drug name
ARA A	vidarabine	Mistaken as cytarabine (ARA C)	Use complete drug name
AZT	zidovudine (Retrovir)	Mistaken as azathioprine or aztreonam	Use complete drug name
CPZ	Compazine (prochlorperazine)	Mistaken as chlorpromazine	Use complete drug name
DPT	Demerol-Phenergan-Thorazine	Mistaken as diphtheria-pertussis-tetanus (vaccine)	Use complete drug name
DTO	Diluted tincture of opium, or deodorized tincture of opium (Paregoric)	Mistaken as tincture of opium	Use complete drug name
HCl	hydrochloric acid or hydrochloride	Mistaken as potassium chloride (The "H" is misinterpreted as "K")	Use complete drug name unless expressed as a salt of a drug
HCT	hydrocortisone	Mistaken as hydrochlorothiazide	Use complete drug name
HCTZ	hydrochlorothiazide	Mistaken as hydrocortisone (seen as HCT250 mg)	Use complete drug name
MgSO4**	magnesium sulfate	Mistaken as morphine sulfate	Use complete drug name
MS, MSO4**	morphine sulfate	Mistaken as magnesium sulfate	Use complete drug name
MTX	methotrexate	Mistaken as mitoxantrone	Use complete drug name
PCA	procainamide	Mistaken as patient controlled analgesia	Use complete drug name
PTU	propylthiouracil	Mistaken as mercaptopurine	Use complete drug name
T3	Tylenol with codeine No. 3	Mistaken as liothyronine	Use complete drug name
TAC	triamcinolone	Mistaken as tetracaine, Adrenalin, cocaine	Use complete drug name
TNK	TNKase	Mistaken as "TPA"	Use complete drug name
ZnSO4	zinc sulfate	Mistaken as morphine sulfate	Use complete drug name

Stemmed Drug Names	Intended Meaning	Misinterpretation	Correction
"Nitro" drip	nitroglycerin infusion	Mistaken as sodium nitroprusside infusion	Use complete drug name
"Norflox"	norfloxacin	Mistaken as Norflex	Use complete drug name
"IV Vanc"	intravenous vancomycin	Mistaken as Invanz	Use complete drug name

Symbols	Intended Meaning	Misinterpretation	Correction
ʒ ♏	Dram Minim	Symbol for dram mistaken as "3" Symbol for minim mistaken as "mL"	Use the metric system
x3d	For three days	Mistaken as "3 doses"	Use "for three days"
> and <	Greater than and less than	Mistaken as opposite of intended; mistakenly use incorrect symbol; "< 10" mistaken as "40"	Use "greater than" or "less than"
/ (slash mark)	Separates two doses or indicates "per"	Mistaken as the number 1 (e.g., "25 units/10 units" misread as "25 units and 110" units)	Use "per" rather than a slash mark to separate doses
@	At	Mistaken as "2"	Use "at"
&	And	Mistaken as "2"	Use "and"
+	Plus or and	Mistaken as "4"	Use "and"
°	Hour	Mistaken as a zero (e.g., q2° seen as q 20)	Use "hr," "h," or "hour"
Φ or ⊘	zero, null sign	Mistaken as numerals 4, 6, 8, and 9	Use 0 or zero, or describe intent using whole words

**These abbreviations are included on The Joint Commission's "minimum list" of dangerous abbreviations, acronyms, and symbols that must be included on an organization's "Do Not Use" list, effective January 1, 2004. Visit www.jointcommission.org for more information about this Joint Commission requirement.

© ISMP 2013. Permission is granted to reproduce material with proper attribution for internal use within healthcare organizations. Other reproduction is prohibited without written permission from ISMP. Report actual and potential medication errors to the ISMP National Medication Errors Reporting Program (ISMP MERP) via the Web at www.ismp.org or by calling 1-800-FAIL-SAF(E).

INSTITUTE FOR SAFE MEDICATION PRACTICES

www.ismp.org

Urine Reference Values*

Analyte	Conventional Units	SI Units
Acetone and acetoacetate, qualitative	Negative	Negative
Albumin		
Qualitative	Negative	Negative
Quantitative	10-100 mg/24 h	0.15-1.5 µmol/d
Amylase/creatinine clearance ratio	0.01-0.04	0.01-0.04
Bilirubin, qualitative	Negative	Negative
Creatinine	15-25 mg/kg/24 h	0.13-0.22 mmol/kg/d
Glucose (as reducing substance)	<250 mg/24 h	<250 mg/d
Hemoglobin and myoglobin, qualitative	Negative	Negative
pH	4.6-8.0	4.6-8.0
Protein, total		
Qualitative	Negative	Negative
Quantitative	10-150 mg/24 h	10-150 mg/d
Protein/creatinine ratio	<0.2	<0.2
Specific gravity		
Random specimen	1.003-1.030	1.003-1.030
24-hour collection	1.015-1.025	1.015-1.025
Urobilinogen	0.5-4.0 mg/24 h	0.6-6.9 µmol/d

*Values may vary depending on the method used.

Hematology Reference Values

Test	Conventional Units	SI Units
Cell Counts		
Erythrocytes		
Males	4.6-6.2 million/mm^3	4.6-6.2 × 10^{12}/L
Females	4.2-5.4 million/mm^3	4.2-5.4 × 10^{12}/L
Children (varies with age)	4.5-5.1 million/mm^3	4.5-5.1 × 10^{12}/L
Leukocytes, total	4500-11,000/mm^3	
Leukocytes, Differential Counts		
Myelocytes	0%	0/L
Band neutrophils	3%-5%	150-400 × 10^6/L
Segmented neutrophils	54%-62%	3000-5800 × 10^6/L
Lymphocytes	25%-33%	1500-3000 × 10^6/L
Monocytes	3%-7%	300-500 × 10^6/L
Eosinophils	1%-3%	50-250 × 10^6/L
Basophils	0%-1%	15-50 × 10^6/L
Platelets	150,000-400,000/mm^3	150-400 × 10^9/L
Reticulocytes	25,000-75,000/mm^3	25-75 × 10^9/L
Coagulation Tests		
Bleeding time (template)	2.75-8.0 min	2.75-8.0 min
Coagulation time (glass tube)	5-15 min	5-15 min
D-Dimer	<0.5 μg/mL	<0.5 mg/L
Factor VIII and other coagulation factors	50%-150% of normal	0.5-1.5 of normal
Fibrin split products (Thrombo-Wellco test)	<10 μg/mL	<10 mg/L
Fibrinogen	200-400 mg/dL	2.0-4.0 g/L
Partial thromboplastin time, activated (aPTT)	20-35 s	20-35 s
Prothrombin time (PT)	12.0-14.0 s	12.0-14.0 s
Corpuscular Values of Erythrocytes		
Mean corpuscular hemoglobin (MCH)	26-34 pg/cell	26-34 pg/cell
Mean corpuscular volume (MCV)	80-96 μm^3	80-96 fL
Mean corpuscular hemoglobin concentration (MCHC)	32-36 g/dL	320-360 g/L
Hematocrit		
Males	40-54 mL/dL	0.40-0.54
Females	37-47 mL/dL	0.37-0.47
Newborns	49-54 mL/dL	0.49-0.54
Children (varies with age)	35-49 mL/dL	0.35-0.49
Hemoglobin		
Males	13.0-18.0 g/dL	8.1-11.2 mmol/L
Females	12.0-16.0 g/dL	7.4-9.9 mmol/L
Newborns	16.5-19.5 g/dL	10.2-12.1 mmol/L
Children (varies with age)	11.2-16.5 g/dL	7.0-10.2 mmol/L
Hemoglobin A$_{1c}$	3%-5% of total	0.03-0.05 of total
Sedimentation Rate (ESR)		
Westergren: Males	0-15 mm/h	0-15 mm/h
Females	0-20 mm/h	0-20 mm/h

Blood Chemistry Reference Values

Analyte	Conventional Units	SI Units
Acid phosphatase, serum (thymolphthalein monophosphate substrate)	0.1-0.6 U/L	0.1-0.6 U/L
Alanine aminotransferase (ALT) serum (SGPT)	1-45 U/L	1-45 U/L
Albumin, serum	3.3-5.2 g/dL	33-52 g/L
Alkaline phosphatase (ALP), serum		
Adult	35-150 U/L	35-150 U/L
Adolescent	100-500 U/L	100-500 U/L
Child	100-350 U/L	100-350 U/L
Anion gap, serum, calculated	8-16 mEq/L	8-16 mmol/L
Aspartate aminotransferase (AST) serum (SGOT)	1-36 U/L	1-36 U/L
Bilirubin, serum		
Conjugated	0.1-0.4 mg/dL	1.7-6.8 μmol/L
Total	0.3-101 mg/dL	5.1-19.0 μmol/L
Calcium, serum	8.4-10.6 mg/dL	2.10-2.65 mmol/L
Chloride, serum or plasma	96-106 mEq/L	96-106 mmol/L
Cholesterol, serum or ethylenediaminetetraacetic acid (EDTA) plasma		
Desirable range	<200 mg/dL	<5.20 mmol/L
Low-density lipoprotein (LDL) cholesterol	60-180 mg/dL	1.55-4.65 mmol/L
High-density lipoprotein (HDL) cholesterol	30-80 mg/dL	0.80-2.05 mmol/L
Creatine kinase (CK), serum		
Males	55-170 U/L	55-170 U/L
Females	30-135 U/L	30-135 U/L
Creatinine, serum	0.6-1.2 mg/dL	50-110 μmol/L
Gamma-glutamyltransferase (GGT), serum	5-40 U/L	5-40 U/L
Glucose, fasting, plasma or serum	70-115 mg/dL	3.9-6.4 nmol/L
Iron, serum	74-175 μg/dL	13-31 μmol/L
Lactate dehydrogenase (LD), serum	110-220 U/L	110-220 U/L
Phosphate, inorganic, serum		
Adult	3.0-4.5 mg/dL	1.0-1.5 mmol/L
Child	4.0-7.0 mg/dL	1.3-2.3 mmol/L
Potassium		
Serum	3.5-5.0 mEq/L	3.5-5.0 mmol/L
Plasma	3.5-4.5 mEq/L	3.5-4.5 mmol/L
Protein, serum, electrophoresis		
Total	6.0-8.0 g/dL	60-80 g/L
Albumin	3.5-5.5 g/dL	35-55 g/L
Globulins		
Alpha$_1$	0.2-0.4 g/dL	2.0-4.0 g/L
Alpha$_2$	0.5-0.9 g/dL	5.0-9.0 g/L

Blood Chemistry Reference Values—cont'd

Analyte	Conventional Units	SI Units
Beta	0.6-1.1 g/dL	6.0-11.0 g/L
Gamma	0.7-1.7 g/dL	7.0-17.0 g/L
Sodium, serum or plasma	135-145 mEq/L	135-145 mmol/L
Thyroxine (T_4), serum	4.5-12.0 µg/dL	58-154 nmol/L
Triglycerides, serum, 12-h fast	40-150 mg/dL	0.4-1.5 g/L
Triiodothyronine (T_3), serum	70-190 ng/dL	1.1-2.9 nmol/L
Triiodothyronine uptake, resin (T_3RU)	25%-38%	0.25-0.38
Urea, serum or plasma	24-49 mg/dL	4.0-8.2 nmol/L
Urea nitrogen, serum or plasma	11-23 mg/dL	8.0-16.4 nmol/L

From *Mosby's dictionary of medical, nursing, and health professions,* ed 10, St Louis, 2016, Mosby.

Tests of Immunological Function Reference Values

Test	Conventional Units	SI Units
Complement, serum		
C3	85-175 mg/dL	0.85-1.75 g/L
C4	15-45 mg/dL	150-450 mg/L
Total hemolytic (CH_{50})	150-250 U/mL	150-250 U/mL
Immunoglobulins, serum, adult		
IgG	640-1350 mg/dL	6.4-13.5 g/L
IgA	70-310 mg/dL	0.70-3.1 g/L
IgM	90-350 mg/dL	0.90-3.5 g/L
IgD	0.0-6.0 mg/dL	0.0-60 mg/L
IgE	0.0-430 ng/dL	0.0-430 µg/L

Urine reference values, chemistry reference values, and tests of immunological function reference values blood from *Mosby's dictionary of medical, nursing, and health professions,* ed 10, St Louis, 2016, Mosby.
Hematology reference values from Bope ET: *Conn's current therapy 2020,* Philadelphia, 2020, Saunders.

Appendix H

Body Part Key

If You See This Body Part	Code to This Body Part
Abdominal aortic plexus	Abdominal Sympathetic Nerve
Abdominal esophagus	Esophagus, Lower
Abductor hallucis muscle	Foot Muscle, Right Foot Muscle, Left
Accessory cephalic vein	Cephalic Vein, Right Cephalic Vein, Left
Accessory obturator nerve	Lumbar Plexus
Accessory phrenic nerve	Phrenic Nerve
Accessory spleen	Spleen
Acetabulofemoral joint	Hip Joint, Right Hip Joint, Left
Achilles tendon	Lower Leg Tendon, Right Lower Leg Tendon, Left
Acromioclavicular ligament	Shoulder Bursa and Ligament, Right Shoulder Bursa and Ligament, Left
Acromion (process)	Scapula, Right Scapula, Left
Adductor brevis muscle	Upper Leg Muscle, Right Upper Leg Muscle, Left
Adductor hallucis muscle	Foot Muscle, Right Foot Muscle, Left
Adductor longus muscle Adductor magnus muscle	Upper Leg Muscle, Right Upper Leg Muscle, Left
Adenohypophysis	Pituitary Gland
Alar ligament of axis	Head and Neck Bursa and Ligament
Alveolar process of mandible	Mandible, Right Mandible, Left
Alveolar process of maxilla	Maxilla, Right Maxilla, Left
Anal orifice	Anus
Anatomical snuffbox	Lower Arm and Wrist Muscle, Right Lower Arm and Wrist Muscle, Left
Angular artery	Face Artery
Angular vein	Face Vein, Right Face Vein, Left
Annular ligament	Elbow Bursa and Ligament, Right Elbow Bursa and Ligament, Left
Anorectal junction	Rectum

Body Part Key — cont'd

If You See This Body Part	Code to This Body Part
Ansa cervicalis	Cervical Plexus
Antebrachial fascia	Subcutaneous Tissue and Fascia, Right Lower Arm Subcutaneous Tissue and Fascia, Left Lower Arm
Anterior (pectoral) lymph node	Lymphatic, Right Axillary Lymphatic, Left Axillary
Anterior cerebral artery	Intracranial Artery
Anterior cerebral vein	Intracranial Vein
Anterior choroidal artery	Intracranial Artery
Anterior circumflex humeral artery	Axillary Artery, Right Axillary Artery, Left
Anterior communicating artery	Intracranial Artery
Anterior cruciate ligament (ACL)	Knee Bursa and Ligament, Right Knee Bursa and Ligament, Left
Anterior crural nerve	Femoral Nerve
Anterior facial vein	Face Vein, Right Face Vein, Left
Anterior intercostal artery	Internal Mammary Artery, Right Internal Mammary Artery, Left
Anterior interosseous nerve	Median Nerve
Anterior lateral malleolar artery	Anterior Tibial Artery, Right Anterior Tibial Artery, Left
Anterior lingual gland	Minor Salivary Gland
Anterior medial malleolar artery	Anterior Tibial Artery, Right Anterior Tibial Artery, Left
Anterior spinal artery	Vertebral Artery, Right Vertebral Artery, Left
Anterior tibial recurrent artery	Anterior Tibial Artery, Right Anterior Tibial Artery, Left
Anterior ulnar recurrent artery	Ulnar Artery, Right Ulnar Artery, Left
Anterior vagal trunk	Vagus Nerve
Anterior vertebral muscle	Neck Muscle, Right Neck Muscle, Left
Antihelix Antitragus	External Ear, Right External Ear, Left External Ear, Bilateral
Antrum of Highmore	Maxillary Sinus, Right Maxillary Sinus, Left
Aortic annulus	Aortic Valve
Aortic arch Aortic intercostal artery	Thoracic Aorta
Apical (subclavicular) lymph node	Lymphatic, Right Axillary Lymphatic, Left Axillary
Apneustic center	Pons

Continued

Body Part Key — cont'd

If You See This Body Part	Code to This Body Part
Aqueduct of Sylvius	Cerebral Ventricle
Aqueous humor	Anterior Chamber, Right Anterior Chamber, Left
Arachnoid mater	Cerebral Meninges Spinal Meninges
Arcuate artery	Foot Artery, Right Foot Artery, Left
Areola	Nipple, Right Nipple, Left
Arterial canal (duct)	Pulmonary Artery, Left
Aryepiglottic fold Arytenoid cartilage	Larynx
Arytenoid muscle	Neck Muscle, Right Neck Muscle, Left
Ascending aorta	Thoracic Aorta
Ascending palatine artery	Face Artery
Ascending pharyngeal artery	External Carotid Artery, Right External Carotid Artery, Left
Atlantoaxial joint	Cervical Vertebral Joint
Atrioventricular node	Conduction Mechanism
Atrium dextrum cordis	Atrium, Right
Atrium pulmonale	Atrium, Left
Auditory tube	Eustachian Tube, Right Eustachian Tube, Left
Auerbach's (myenteric) plexus	Abdominal Sympathetic Nerve
Auricle	External Ear, Right External Ear, Left External Ear, Bilateral
Auricularis muscle	Head Muscle
Axillary fascia	Subcutaneous Tissue and Fascia, Right Upper Arm Subcutaneous Tissue and Fascia, Left Upper Arm
Axillary nerve	Brachial Plexus
Bartholin's (greater vestibular) gland	Vestibular Gland
Basal (internal) cerebral vein	Intracranial Vein
Basal nuclei	Basal Ganglia
Basilar artery	Intracranial Artery
Basis pontis	Pons
Biceps brachii muscle	Upper Arm Muscle, Right Upper Arm Muscle, Left
Biceps femoris muscle	Upper Leg Muscle, Right Upper Leg Muscle, Left
Bicipital aponeurosis	Subcutaneous Tissue and Fascia, Right Lower Arm Subcutaneous Tissue and Fascia, Left Lower Arm

Body Part Key — cont'd

If You See This Body Part	Code to This Body Part
Bicuspid valve	Mitral Valve
Body of femur	Femoral Shaft, Right Femoral Shaft, Left
Body of fibula	Fibula, Right Fibula, Left
Bony labyrinth	Inner Ear, Right Inner Ear, Left
Bony orbit	Orbit, Right Orbit, Left
Bony vestibule	Inner Ear, Right Inner Ear, Left
Botallo's duct	Pulmonary Artery, Left
Brachial (lateral) lymph node	Lymphatic, Right Axillary Lymphatic, Left Axillary
Brachialis muscle	Upper Arm Muscle, Right Upper Arm Muscle, Left
Brachiocephalic artery Brachiocephalic trunk	Innominate Artery
Brachiocephalic vein	Innominate Vein, Right Innominate Vein, Left
Brachioradialis muscle	Lower Arm and Wrist Muscle, Right Lower Arm and Wrist Muscle, Left
Broad ligament	Uterine Supporting Structure
Bronchial artery	Thoracic Aorta
Buccal gland	Buccal Mucosa
Buccinator lymph node	Lymphatic, Head
Buccinator muscle	Facial Muscle
Bulbospongiosus muscle	Perineum Muscle
Bulbourethral (Cowper's) gland	Urethra
Bundle of His Bundle of Kent	Conduction Mechanism
Calcaneocuboid joint	Tarsal Joint, Right Tarsal Joint, Left
Calcaneocuboid ligament	Foot Bursa and Ligament, Right Foot Bursa and Ligament, Left
Calcaneofibular ligament	Ankle Bursa and Ligament, Right Ankle Bursa and Ligament, Left
Calcaneus	Tarsal, Right Tarsal, Left
Capitate bone	Carpal, Right Carpal, Left
Cardia	Esophagogastric Junction
Cardiac plexus	Thoracic Sympathetic Nerve
Cardioesophageal junction	Esophagogastric Junction

Continued

Body Part Key — cont'd

If You See This Body Part	Code to This Body Part
Caroticotympanic artery	Internal Carotid Artery, Right Internal Carotid Artery, Left
Carotid glomus	Carotid Body, Left Carotid Body, Right Carotid Bodies, Bilateral
Carotid sinus	Internal Carotid Artery, Right Internal Carotid Artery, Left
Carotid sinus nerve	Glossopharyngeal Nerve
Carpometacarpal (CMC) joint	Metacarpocarpal Joint, Right Metacarpocarpal Joint, Left
Carpometacarpal ligament	Hand Bursa and Ligament, Right Hand Bursa and Ligament, Left
Cauda equina	Lumbar Spinal Cord
Cavernous plexus	Head and Neck Sympathetic Nerve
Celiac (solar) plexus Celiac ganglion	Abdominal Sympathetic Nerve
Celiac lymph node	Lymphatic, Aortic
Celiac trunk	Celiac Artery
Central axillary lymph node	Lymphatic, Right Axillary Lymphatic, Left Axillary
Cerebral aqueduct (Sylvius)	Cerebral Ventricle
Cerebrum	Brain
Cervical esophagus	Esophagus, Upper
Cervical facet joint	Cervical Vertebral Joint Cervical Vertebral Joints, 2 or more
Cervical ganglion	Head and Neck Sympathetic Nerve
Cervical interspinous ligament Cervical intertransverse ligament Cervical ligamentum flavum	Head and Neck Bursa and Ligament
Cervical lymph node	Lymphatic, Right Neck Lymphatic, Left Neck
Cervicothoracic facet joint	Cervicothoracic Vertebral Joint
Choana	Nasopharynx
Chondroglossus muscle	Tongue, Palate, Pharynx Muscle
Chorda tympani	Facial Nerve
Choroid plexus	Cerebral Ventricle
Ciliary body	Eye, Right Eye, Left
Ciliary ganglion	Head and Neck Sympathetic Nerve
Circle of Willis	Intracranial Artery
Circumflex iliac artery	Femoral Artery, Right Femoral Artery, Left

Body Part Key — cont'd

If You See This Body Part	Code to This Body Part
Claustrum	Basal Ganglia
Coccygeal body	Coccygeal Glomus
Coccygeus muscle	Trunk Muscle, Right Trunk Muscle, Left
Cochlea	Inner Ear, Right Inner Ear, Left
Cochlear nerve	Acoustic Nerve
Columella	Nose
Common digital vein	Foot Vein, Right Foot Vein, Left
Common facial vein	Face Vein, Right Face Vein, Left
Common fibular nerve	Peroneal Nerve
Common hepatic artery	Hepatic Artery
Common iliac (subaortic) lymph node	Lymphatic, Pelvis
Common interosseous artery	Ulnar Artery, Right Ulnar Artery, Left
Common peroneal nerve	Peroneal Nerve
Condyloid process	Mandible, Right Mandible, Left
Conus arteriosus	Ventricle, Right
Conus medullaris	Lumbar Spinal Cord
Coracoacromial ligament	Shoulder Bursa and Ligament, Right Shoulder Bursa and Ligament, Left
Coracobrachialis muscle	Upper Arm Muscle, Right Upper Arm Muscle, Left
Coracoclavicular ligament Coracohumeral ligament	Shoulder Bursa and Ligament, Right Shoulder Bursa and Ligament, Left
Coracoid process	Scapula, Right Scapula, Left
Corniculate cartilage	Larynx
Corpus callosum	Brain
Corpus cavernosum Corpus spongiosum	Penis
Corpus striatum	Basal Ganglia
Corrugator supercilii muscle	Facial Muscle
Costocervical trunk	Subclavian Artery, Right Subclavian Artery, Left
Costoclavicular ligament	Shoulder Bursa and Ligament, Right Shoulder Bursa and Ligament, Left
Costotransverse joint	Thoracic Vertebral Joint Thoracic Vertebral Joints, 2 to 7 Thoracic Vertebral Joints, 8 or more

Continued

Body Part Key — cont'd

If You See This Body Part	Code to This Body Part
Costotransverse ligament	Thorax Bursa and Ligament, Right Thorax Bursa and Ligament, Left
Costovertebral joint	Thoracic Vertebral Joint Thoracic Vertebral Joints, 2 to 7 Thoracic Vertebral Joints, 8 or more
Costoxiphoid ligament	Thorax Bursa and Ligament, Right Thorax Bursa and Ligament, Left
Cowper's (bulbourethral) gland	Urethra
Cranial dura mater	Dura Mater
Cranial epidural space	Epidural Space
Cranial subarachnoid space	Subarachnoid Space
Cranial subdural space	Subdural Space
Cremaster muscle	Perineum Muscle
Cribriform plate	Ethmoid Bone, Right Ethmoid Bone, Left
Cricoid cartilage	Larynx
Cricothyroid artery	Thyroid Artery, Right Thyroid Artery, Left
Cricothyroid muscle	Neck Muscle, Right Neck Muscle, Left
Crural fascia	Subcutaneous Tissue and Fascia, Right Upper Leg Subcutaneous Tissue and Fascia, Left Upper Leg
Cubital lymph node	Lymphatic, Right Upper Extremity Lymphatic, Left Upper Extremity
Cubital nerve	Ulnar Nerve
Cuboid bone	Tarsal, Right Tarsal, Left
Cuboideonavicular joint	Tarsal Joint, Right Tarsal Joint, Left
Culmen	Cerebellum
Cuneiform cartilage	Larynx
Cuneonavicular joint	Tarsal Joint, Right Tarsal Joint, Left
Cuneonavicular ligament	Foot Bursa and Ligament, Right Foot Bursa and Ligament, Left
Cutaneous (transverse) cervical nerve	Cervical Plexus
Deep cervical fascia	Subcutaneous Tissue and Fascia, Anterior Neck
Deep cervical vein	Vertebral Vein, Right Vertebral Vein, Left
Deep circumflex iliac artery	External Iliac Artery, Right External Iliac Artery, Left
Deep facial vein	Face Vein, Right Face Vein, Left

Body Part Key — cont'd

If You See This Body Part	Code to This Body Part
Deep femoral (profunda femoris) vein	Femoral Vein, Right Femoral Vein, Left
Deep femoral artery	Femoral Artery, Right Femoral Artery, Left
Deep palmar arch	Hand Artery, Right Hand Artery, Left
Deep transverse perineal muscle	Perineum Muscle
Deferential artery	Internal Iliac Artery, Right Internal Iliac Artery, Left
Deltoid fascia	Subcutaneous Tissue and Fascia, Right Upper Arm Subcutaneous Tissue and Fascia, Left Upper Arm
Deltoid ligament	Ankle Bursa and Ligament, Right Ankle Bursa and Ligament, Left
Deltoid muscle	Shoulder Muscle, Right Shoulder Muscle, Left
Deltopectoral (infraclavicular) lymph node	Lymphatic, Right Upper Extremity Lymphatic, Left Upper Extremity
Dentate ligament	Dura Mater
Denticulate ligament	Spinal Cord
Depressor anguli oris muscle Depressor labii inferioris muscle Depressor septi nasi muscle Depressor supercilii muscle	Facial Muscle
Dermis	Skin
Descending genicular artery	Femoral Artery, Right Femoral Artery, Left
Diaphragma sellae	Dura Mater
Distal radioulnar joint	Wrist Joint, Right Wrist Joint, Left
Dorsal digital nerve	Radial Nerve
Dorsal metacarpal vein	Hand Vein, Right Hand Vein, Left
Dorsal metatarsal artery	Foot Artery, Right Foot Artery, Left
Dorsal metatarsal vein	Foot Vein, Right Foot Vein, Left
Dorsal scapular artery	Subclavian Artery, Right Subclavian Artery, Left
Dorsal scapular nerve	Brachial Plexus
Dorsal venous arch	Foot Vein, Right Foot Vein, Left
Dorsalis pedis artery	Anterior Tibial Artery, Right Anterior Tibial Artery, Left
Duct of Santorini	Pancreatic Duct, Accessory

Continued

Body Part Key — cont'd

If You See This Body Part	Code to This Body Part
Duct of Wirsung	Pancreatic Duct
Ductus deferens	Vas Deferens, Right Vas Deferens, Left Vas Deferens, Bilateral Vas Deferens
Duodenal ampulla	Ampulla of Vater
Duodenojejunal flexure	Jejunum
Dural venous sinus	Intracranial Vein
Earlobe	External Ear, Right External Ear, Left External Ear, Bilateral
Eighth cranial nerve	Acoustic Nerve
Ejaculatory duct	Vas Deferens, Right Vas Deferens, Left Vas Deferens, Bilateral Vas Deferens
Eleventh cranial nerve	Accessory Nerve
Encephalon	Brain
Ependyma	Cerebral Ventricle
Epidermis	Skin
Epiploic foramen	Peritoneum
Epithalamus	Thalamus
Epitrochlear lymph node	Lymphatic, Right Upper Extremity Lymphatic, Left Upper Extremity
Erector spinae muscle	Trunk Muscle, Right Trunk Muscle, Left
Esophageal artery	Thoracic Aorta
Esophageal plexus	Thoracic Sympathetic Nerve
Ethmoidal air cell	Ethmoid Sinus, Right Ethmoid Sinus, Left
Extensor carpi radialis muscle Extensor carpi ulnaris muscle	Lower Arm and Wrist Muscle, Right Lower Arm and Wrist Muscle, Left
Extensor digitorum brevis muscle	Foot Muscle, Right Foot Muscle, Left
Extensor digitorum longus muscle	Lower Leg Muscle, Right Lower Leg Muscle, Left
Extensor hallucis brevis muscle	Foot Muscle, Right Foot Muscle, Left
Extensor hallucis longus muscle	Lower Leg Muscle, Right Lower Leg Muscle, Left
External anal sphincter	Anal Sphincter
External auditory meatus	External Auditory Canal, Right External Auditory Canal, Left

Body Part Key — cont'd

If You See This Body Part	Code to This Body Part
External maxillary artery	Face Artery
External naris	Nose
External oblique aponeurosis	Subcutaneous Tissue and Fascia, Trunk
External oblique muscle	Abdomen Muscle, Right Abdomen Muscle, Left
External popliteal nerve	Peroneal Nerve
External pudendal artery	Femoral Artery, Right Femoral Artery, Left
External pudendal vein	Greater Saphenous Vein, Right Greater Saphenous Vein, Left
External urethral sphincter	Urethra
Extradural space	Epidural Space
Facial artery	Face Artery
False vocal cord	Larynx
Falx cerebri	Dura Mater
Fascia lata	Subcutaneous Tissue and Fascia, Right Upper Leg Subcutaneous Tissue and Fascia, Left Upper Leg
Femoral head	Upper Femur, Right Upper Femur, Left
Femoral lymph node	Lymphatic, Right Lower Extremity Lymphatic, Left Lower Extremity
Femoropatellar joint Femorotibial joint	Knee Joint, Right Knee Joint, Left
Fibular artery	Peroneal Artery, Right Peroneal Artery, Left
Fibularis brevis muscle Fibularis longus muscle	Lower Leg Muscle, Right Lower Leg Muscle, Left
Fifth cranial nerve	Trigeminal Nerve
First cranial nerve	Olfactory Nerve
First intercostal nerve	Brachial Plexus
Flexor carpi radialis muscle Flexor carpi ulnaris muscle	Lower Arm and Wrist Muscle, Right Lower Arm and Wrist Muscle, Left
Flexor digitorum brevis muscle	Foot Muscle, Right Foot Muscle, Left
Flexor digitorum longus muscle	Lower Leg Muscle, Right Lower Leg Muscle, Left
Flexor hallucis brevis muscle	Foot Muscle, Right Foot Muscle, Left
Flexor hallucis longus muscle	Lower Leg Muscle, Right Lower Leg Muscle, Left
Flexor pollicis longus muscle	Lower Arm and Wrist Muscle, Right Lower Arm and Wrist Muscle, Left
Foramen magnum	Occipital Bone, Right Occipital Bone, Left

Continued

Body Part Key — cont'd

If You See This Body Part	Code to This Body Part
Foramen of Monro (intraventricular)	Cerebral Ventricle
Foreskin	Prepuce
Fossa of Rosenmuller	Nasopharynx
Fourth cranial nerve	Trochlear Nerve
Fourth ventricle	Cerebral Ventricle
Fovea	Retina, Right Retina, Left
Frenulum labii inferioris	Lower Lip
Frenulum labii superioris	Upper Lip
Frenulum linguae	Tongue
Frontal lobe	Cerebral Hemisphere
Frontal vein	Face Vein, Right Face Vein, Left
Fundus uteri	Uterus
Galea aponeurotica	Subcutaneous Tissue and Fascia, Scalp
Ganglion impar (ganglion of Walther)	Sacral Sympathetic Nerve
Gasserian ganglion	Trigeminal Nerve
Gastric lymph node	Lymphatic, Aortic
Gastric plexus	Abdominal Sympathetic Nerve
Gastrocnemius muscle	Lower Leg Muscle, Right Lower Leg Muscle, Left
Gastrocolic ligament Gastrocolic omentum	Greater Omentum
Gastroduodenal artery	Hepatic Artery
Gastroesophageal (GE) junction	Esophagogastric Junction
Gastrohepatic omentum	Lesser Omentum
Gastrophrenic ligament Gastrosplenic ligament	Greater Omentum
Gemellus muscle	Hip Muscle, Right Hip Muscle, Left
Geniculate ganglion	Facial Nerve
Geniculate nucleus	Thalamus
Genioglossus muscle	Tongue, Palate, Pharynx Muscle
Genitofemoral nerve	Lumbar Plexus
Glans penis	Prepuce
Glenohumeral joint	Shoulder Joint, Right Shoulder Joint, Left
Glenohumeral ligament	Shoulder Bursa and Ligament, Right Shoulder Bursa and Ligament, Left
Glenoid fossa (of scapula)	Glenoid Cavity, Right Glenoid Cavity, Left

Body Part Key — cont'd

If You See This Body Part	Code to This Body Part
Glenoid ligament (labrum)	Shoulder Bursa and Ligament, Right Shoulder Bursa and Ligament, Left
Globus pallidus	Basal Ganglia
Glossoepiglottic fold	Epiglottis
Glottis	Larynx
Gluteal lymph node	Lymphatic, Pelvis
Gluteal vein	Hypogastric Vein, Right Hypogastric Vein, Left
Gluteus maximus muscle Gluteus medius muscle Gluteus minimus muscle	Hip Muscle, Right Hip Muscle, Left
Gracilis muscle	Upper Leg Muscle, Right Upper Leg Muscle, Left
Great auricular nerve	Cervical Plexus
Great cerebral vein	Intracranial Vein
Great saphenous vein	Greater Saphenous Vein, Right Greater Saphenous Vein, Left
Greater alar cartilage	Nose
Greater occipital nerve	Cervical Nerve
Greater splanchnic nerve	Thoracic Sympathetic Nerve
Greater superficial petrosal nerve	Facial Nerve
Greater trochanter	Upper Femur, Right Upper Femur, Left
Greater tuberosity	Humeral Head, Right Humeral Head, Left
Greater vestibular (Bartholin's) gland	Vestibular Gland
Greater wing	Sphenoid Bone, Right Sphenoid Bone, Left
Hallux	1st Toe, Right 1st Toe, Left
Hamate bone	Carpal, Right Carpal, Left
Head of fibula	Fibula, Right Fibula, Left
Helix	External Ear, Right External Ear, Left External Ear, Bilateral
Hepatic artery proper	Hepatic Artery
Hepatic flexure	Ascending Colon
Hepatic lymph node	Lymphatic, Aortic
Hepatic plexus	Abdominal Sympathetic Nerve
Hepatic portal vein	Portal Vein

Continued

Body Part Key — cont'd

If You See This Body Part	Code to This Body Part
Hepatogastric ligament	Lesser Omentum
Hepatopancreatic ampulla	Ampulla of Vater
Humeroradial joint Humeroulnar joint	Elbow Joint, Right Elbow Joint, Left
Hyoglossus muscle	Tongue, Palate, Pharynx Muscle
Hyoid artery	Thyroid Artery, Right Thyroid Artery, Left
Hypogastric artery	Internal Iliac Artery, Right Internal Iliac Artery, Left
Hypopharynx	Pharynx
Hypophysis	Pituitary Gland
Hypothenar muscle	Hand Muscle, Right Hand Muscle, Left
Ileal artery Ileocolic artery	Superior Mesenteric Artery
Ileocolic vein	Colic Vein
Iliac crest	Pelvic Bone, Right Pelvic Bone, Left
Iliac fascia	Subcutaneous Tissue and Fascia, Right Upper Leg Subcutaneous Tissue and Fascia, Left Upper Leg
Iliac lymph node	Lymphatic, Pelvis
Iliacus muscle	Hip Muscle, Right Hip Muscle, Left
Iliofemoral ligament	Hip Bursa and Ligament, Right Hip Bursa and Ligament, Left
Iliohypogastric nerve Ilioinguinal nerve	Lumbar Plexus
Iliolumbar artery	Internal Iliac Artery, Right Internal Iliac Artery, Left
Iliolumbar ligament	Trunk Bursa and Ligament, Right Trunk Bursa and Ligament, Left
Iliotibial tract (band)	Subcutaneous Tissue and Fascia, Right Upper Leg Subcutaneous Tissue and Fascia, Left Upper Leg
Ilium	Pelvic Bone, Right Pelvic Bone, Left
Incus	Auditory Ossicle, Right Auditory Ossicle, Left
Inferior cardiac nerve	Thoracic Sympathetic Nerve
Inferior cerebellar vein Inferior cerebral vein	Intracranial Vein
Inferior epigastric artery	External Iliac Artery, Right External Iliac Artery, Left
Inferior epigastric lymph node	Lymphatic, Pelvis

Body Part Key — cont'd

If You See This Body Part	Code to This Body Part
Inferior genicular artery	Popliteal Artery, Right Popliteal Artery, Left
Inferior gluteal artery	Internal Iliac Artery, Right Internal Iliac Artery, Left
Inferior gluteal nerve	Sacral Plexus
Inferior hypogastric plexus	Abdominal Sympathetic Nerve
Inferior labial artery	Face Artery
Inferior longitudinal muscle	Tongue, Palate, Pharynx Muscle
Inferior mesenteric ganglion	Abdominal Sympathetic Nerve
Inferior mesenteric lymph node	Lymphatic, Mesenteric
Inferior mesenteric plexus	Abdominal Sympathetic Nerve
Inferior oblique muscle	Extraocular Muscle, Right Extraocular Muscle, Left
Inferior pancreaticoduodenal artery	Superior Mesenteric Artery
Inferior phrenic artery	Abdominal Aorta
Inferior rectus muscle	Extraocular Muscle, Right Extraocular Muscle, Left
Inferior suprarenal artery	Renal Artery, Right Renal Artery, Left
Inferior tarsal plate	Lower Eyelid, Right Lower Eyelid, Left
Inferior thyroid vein	Innominate Vein, Right Innominate Vein, Left
Inferior tibiofibular joint	Ankle Joint, Right Ankle Joint, Left
Inferior turbinate	Nasal Turbinate
Inferior ulnar collateral artery	Brachial Artery, Right Brachial Artery, Left
Inferior vesical artery	Internal Iliac Artery, Right Internal Iliac Artery, Left
Infraauricular lymph node	Lymphatic, Head
Infraclavicular (deltopectoral) lymph node	Lymphatic, Right Upper Extremity Lymphatic, Left Upper Extremity
Infrahyoid muscle	Neck Muscle, Right Neck Muscle, Left
Infraparotid lymph node	Lymphatic, Head
Infraspinatus fascia	Subcutaneous Tissue and Fascia, Right Upper Arm Subcutaneous Tissue and Fascia, Left Upper Arm
Infraspinatus muscle	Shoulder Muscle, Right Shoulder Muscle, Left
Infundibulopelvic ligament	Uterine Supporting Structure
Inguinal canal Inguinal triangle	Inguinal Region, Right Inguinal Region, Left Inguinal Region, Bilateral

Body Part Key — cont'd

If You See This Body Part	Code to This Body Part
Interatrial septum	Atrial Septum
Intercarpal joint	Carpal Joint, Right Carpal Joint, Left
Intercarpal ligament	Hand Bursa and Ligament, Right Hand Bursa and Ligament, Left
Interclavicular ligament	Shoulder Bursa and Ligament, Right Shoulder Bursa and Ligament, Left
Intercostal lymph node	Lymphatic, Thorax
Intercostal muscle	Thorax Muscle, Right Thorax Muscle, Left
Intercostal nerve Intercostobrachial nerve	Thoracic Nerve
Intercuneiform joint	Tarsal Joint, Right Tarsal Joint, Left
Intercuneiform ligament	Foot Bursa and Ligament, Right Foot Bursa and Ligament, Left
Intermediate cuneiform bone	Tarsal, Right Tarsal, Left
Internal (basal) cerebral vein	Intracranial Vein
Internal anal sphincter	Anal Sphincter
Internal carotid plexus	Head and Neck Sympathetic Nerve
Internal iliac vein	Hypogastric Vein, Right Hypogastric Vein, Left
Internal maxillary artery	External Carotid Artery, Right External Carotid Artery, Left
Internal naris	Nose
Internal oblique muscle	Abdomen Muscle, Right Abdomen Muscle, Left
Internal pudendal artery	Internal Iliac Artery, Right Internal Iliac Artery, Left
Internal pudendal vein	Hypogastric Vein, Right Hypogastric Vein, Left
Internal thoracic artery	Internal Mammary Artery, Right Internal Mammary Artery, Left Subclavian Artery, Right Subclavian Artery, Left
Internal urethral sphincter	Urethra
Interphalangeal (IP) joint	Finger Phalangeal Joint, Right Finger Phalangeal Joint, Left Toe Phalangeal Joint, Right Toe Phalangeal Joint, Left
Interphalangeal ligament	Hand Bursa and Ligament, Right Hand Bursa and Ligament, Left Foot Bursa and Ligament, Right Foot Bursa and Ligament, Left

Body Part Key — cont'd

If You See This Body Part	Code to This Body Part
Interspinalis muscle	Trunk Muscle, Right Trunk Muscle, Left
Interspinous ligament	Trunk Bursa and Ligament, Right Trunk Bursa and Ligament, Left
Intertransversarius muscle	Trunk Muscle, Right Trunk Muscle, Left
Intertransverse ligament	Trunk Bursa and Ligament, Right Trunk Bursa and Ligament, Left
Interventricular foramen (Monro)	Cerebral Ventricle
Interventricular septum	Ventricular Septum
Intestinal lymphatic trunk	Cisterna Chyli
Ischiatic nerve	Sciatic Nerve
Ischiocavernosus muscle	Perineum Muscle
Ischiofemoral ligament	Hip Bursa and Ligament, Right Hip Bursa and Ligament, Left
Ischium	Pelvic Bone, Right Pelvic Bone, Left
Jejunal artery	Superior Mesenteric Artery
Jugular body	Glomus Jugulare
Jugular lymph node	Lymphatic, Right Neck Lymphatic, Left Neck
Labia majora Labia minora	Vulva
Labial gland	Upper Lip Lower Lip
Lacrimal canaliculus Lacrimal punctum Lacrimal sac	Lacrimal Duct, Right Lacrimal Duct, Left
Laryngopharynx	Pharynx
Lateral (brachial) lymph node	Lymphatic, Right Axillary Lymphatic, Left Axillary
Lateral canthus	Upper Eyelid, Right Upper Eyelid, Left
Lateral collateral ligament (LCL)	Knee Bursa and Ligament, Right Knee Bursa and Ligament, Left
Lateral condyle of femur	Lower Femur, Right Lower Femur, Left
Lateral condyle of tibia	Tibia, Right Tibia, Left
Lateral cuneiform bone	Tarsal, Right Tarsal, Left
Lateral epicondyle of femur	Lower Femur, Right Lower Femur, Left
Lateral epicondyle of humerus	Humeral Shaft, Right Humeral Shaft, Left

Continued

Body Part Key — cont'd

If You See This Body Part	Code to This Body Part
Lateral femoral cutaneous nerve	Lumbar Plexus
Lateral malleolus	Fibula, Right Fibula, Left
Lateral meniscus	Knee Joint, Right Knee Joint, Left
Lateral nasal cartilage	Nose
Lateral plantar artery	Foot Artery, Right Foot Artery, Left
Lateral plantar nerve	Tibial Nerve
Lateral rectus muscle	Extraocular Muscle, Right Extraocular Muscle, Left
Lateral sacral artery	Internal Iliac Artery, Right Internal Iliac Artery, Left
Lateral sacral vein	Hypogastric Vein, Right Hypogastric Vein, Left
Lateral sural cutaneous nerve	Peroneal Nerve
Lateral tarsal artery	Foot Artery, Right Foot Artery, Left
Lateral temporomandibular ligament	Head and Neck Bursa and Ligament
Lateral thoracic artery	Axillary Artery, Right Axillary Artery, Left
Latissimus dorsi muscle	Trunk Muscle, Right Trunk Muscle, Left
Least splanchnic nerve	Thoracic Sympathetic Nerve
Left ascending lumbar vein	Hemiazygos Vein
Left atrioventricular valve	Mitral Valve
Left auricular appendix	Atrium, Left
Left colic vein	Colic Vein
Left coronary sulcus	Heart, Left
Left gastric artery	Gastric Artery
Left gastroepiploic artery	Splenic Artery
Left gastroepiploic vein	Splenic Vein
Left inferior phrenic vein	Renal Vein, Left
Left inferior pulmonary vein	Pulmonary Vein, Left
Left jugular trunk	Thoracic Duct
Left lateral ventricle	Cerebral Ventricle
Left ovarian vein Left second lumbar vein	Renal Vein, Left
Left subclavian trunk	Thoracic Duct
Left subcostal vein	Hemiazygos Vein
Left superior pulmonary vein	Pulmonary Vein, Left
Left suprarenal vein Left testicular vein	Renal Vein, Left

Body Part Key — cont'd

If You See This Body Part	Code to This Body Part
Leptomeninges	Cerebral Meninges Spinal Meninges
Lesser alar cartilage	Nose
Lesser occipital nerve	Cervical Plexus
Lesser splanchnic nerve	Thoracic Sympathetic Nerve
Lesser trochanter	Upper Femur, Right Upper Femur, Left
Lesser tuberosity	Humeral Head, Right Humeral Head, Left
Lesser wing	Sphenoid Bone, Right Sphenoid Bone, Left
Levator anguli oris muscle	Facial Muscle
Levator ani muscle	Trunk Muscle, Right Trunk Muscle, Left
Levator labii superioris alaeque nasi muscle Levator labii superioris muscle	Facial Muscle
Levator palpebrae superioris muscle	Upper Eyelid, Right Upper Eyelid, Left
Levator scapulae muscle	Neck Muscle, Right Neck Muscle, Left
Levator veli palatini muscle	Tongue, Palate, Pharynx Muscle
Levatores costarum muscle	Thorax Muscle, Right Thorax Muscle, Left
Ligament of head of fibula	Knee Bursa and Ligament, Right Knee Bursa and Ligament, Left
Ligament of the lateral malleolus	Ankle Bursa and Ligament, Right Ankle Bursa and Ligament, Left
Ligamentum flavum	Trunk Bursa and Ligament, Right Trunk Bursa and Ligament, Left
Lingual artery	External Carotid Artery, Right External Carotid Artery, Left
Lingual tonsil	Tongue
Locus ceruleus	Pons
Long thoracic nerve	Brachial Plexus
Lumbar artery	Abdominal Aorta
Lumbar facet joint	Lumbar Vertebral Joint Lumbar Vertebral Joints, 2 or more
Lumbar ganglion	Lumbar Sympathetic Nerve
Lumbar lymph node	Lymphatic, Aortic
Lumbar lymphatic trunk	Cisterna Chyli
Lumbar splanchnic nerve	Lumbar Sympathetic Nerve
Lumbosacral facet joint	Lumbosacral Joint

Continued

Body Part Key — cont'd

If You See This Body Part	Code to This Body Part
Lumbosacral trunk	Lumbar Nerve
Lunate bone	Carpal, Right Carpal, Left
Lunotriquetral ligament	Hand Bursa and Ligament, Right Hand Bursa and Ligament, Left
Macula	Retina, Right Retina, Left
Malleus	Auditory Ossicle, Right Auditory Ossicle, Left
Mammary duct Mammary gland	Breast, Right Breast, Left Breast, Bilateral
Mammillary body	Hypothalamus
Mandibular nerve	Trigeminal Nerve
Mandibular notch	Mandible, Right Mandible, Left
Manubrium	Sternum
Masseter muscle	Head Muscle
Masseteric fascia	Subcutaneous Tissue and Fascia, Face
Mastoid (postauricular) lymph node	Lymphatic, Right Neck Lymphatic, Left Neck
Mastoid air cells	Mastoid Sinus, Right Mastoid Sinus, Left
Mastoid process	Temporal Bone, Right Temporal Bone, Left
Maxillary artery	External Carotid Artery, Right External Carotid Artery, Left
Maxillary nerve	Trigeminal Nerve
Medial canthus	Lower Eyelid, Right Lower Eyelid, Left
Medial collateral ligament (MCL)	Knee Bursa and Ligament, Right Knee Bursa and Ligament, Left
Medial condyle of femur	Lower Femur, Right Lower Femur, Left
Medial condyle of tibia	Tibia, Right Tibia, Left
Medial cuneiform bone	Tarsal, Right Tarsal, Left
Medial epicondyle of femur	Lower Femur, Right Lower Femur, Left
Medial epicondyle of humerus	Humeral Shaft, Right Humeral Shaft, Left
Medial malleolus	Tibia, Right Tibia, Left

Body Part Key — cont'd

If You See This Body Part	Code to This Body Part
Medial meniscus	Knee Joint, Right Knee Joint, Left
Medial plantar artery	Foot Artery, Right Foot Artery, Left
Medial plantar nerve Medial popliteal nerve	Tibial Nerve
Medial rectus muscle	Extraocular Muscle, Right Extraocular Muscle, Left
Medial sural cutaneous nerve	Tibial Nerve
Median antebrachial vein Median cubital vein	Basilic Vein, Right Basilic Vein, Left
Median sacral artery	Abdominal Aorta
Mediastinal lymph node	Lymphatic, Thorax
Meissner's (submucous) plexus	Abdominal Sympathetic Nerve
Membranous urethra	Urethra
Mental foramen	Mandible, Right Mandible, Left
Mentalis muscle	Facial Muscle
Mesoappendix Mesocolon	Metacarpal ligament
Metacarpophalangeal ligament Mesentery	Hand Bursa and Ligament, Right Hand Bursa and Ligament, Left
Metatarsal ligament	Foot Bursa and Ligament, Right Foot Bursa and Ligament, Left
Metatarsophalangeal (MTP) joint	Metatarsal-Phalangeal Joint, Right Metatarsal-Phalangeal Joint, Left
Metatarsophalangeal ligament	Foot Bursa and Ligament, Right Foot Bursa and Ligament, Left
Metathalamus	Thalamus
Midcarpal joint	Carpal Joint, Right Carpal Joint, Left
Middle cardiac nerve	Thoracic Sympathetic Nerve
Middle cerebral artery	Intracranial Artery
Middle cerebral vein	Intracranial Vein
Middle colic vein	Colic Vein
Middle genicular artery	Popliteal Artery, Right Popliteal Artery, Left
Middle hemorrhoidal vein	Hypogastric Vein, Right Hypogastric Vein, Left
Middle rectal artery	Internal Iliac Artery, Right Internal Iliac Artery, Left
Middle suprarenal artery	Abdominal Aorta
Middle temporal artery	Temporal Artery, Right Temporal Artery, Left

Continued

Body Part Key — cont'd

If You See This Body Part	Code to This Body Part
Middle turbinate	Nasal Turbinate
Mitral annulus	Mitral Valve
Molar gland	Buccal Mucosa
Musculocutaneous nerve	Brachial Plexus
Musculophrenic artery	Internal Mammary Artery, Right Internal Mammary Artery, Left
Musculospiral nerve	Radial Nerve
Myelencephalon	Medulla Oblongata
Myenteric (Auerbach's) plexus	Abdominal Sympathetic Nerve
Myometrium	Uterus
Nail bed Nail plate	Fingernail Toenail
Nasal cavity	Nose
Nasal concha	Nasal Turbinate
Nasalis muscle	Facial Muscle
Nasolacrimal duct	Lacrimal Duct, Right Lacrimal Duct, Left
Navicular bone	Tarsal, Right Tarsal, Left
Neck of femur	Upper Femur, Right Upper Femur, Left
Neck of humerus (anatomical)(surgical)	Humeral Head, Right Humeral Head, Left
Nerve to the stapedius	Facial Nerve
Neurohypophysis	Pituitary Gland
Ninth cranial nerve	Glossopharyngeal Nerve
Nostril	Nose
Obturator artery	Internal Iliac Artery, Right Internal Iliac Artery, Left
Obturator lymph node	Lymphatic, Pelvis
Obturator muscle	Hip Muscle, Right Hip Muscle, Left
Obturator nerve	Lumbar Plexus
Obturator vein	Hypogastric Vein, Right Hypogastric Vein, Left
Obtuse margin	Heart, Left
Occipital artery	External Carotid Artery, Right External Carotid Artery, Left
Occipital lobe	Cerebral Hemisphere
Occipital lymph node	Lymphatic, Right Neck Lymphatic, Left Neck

Body Part Key — cont'd

If You See This Body Part	Code to This Body Part
Occipitofrontalis muscle	Facial Muscle
Olecranon bursa	Elbow Bursa and Ligament, Right Elbow Bursa and Ligament, Left
Olecranon process	Ulna, Right Ulna, Left
Olfactory bulb	Olfactory Nerve
Ophthalmic artery	Internal Carotid Artery, Right Internal Carotid Artery, Left
Ophthalmic nerve	Trigeminal Nerve
Ophthalmic vein	Intracranial Vein
Optic chiasma	Optic Nerve
Optic disc	Retina, Right Retina, Left
Optic foramen	Sphenoid Bone, Right Sphenoid Bone, Left
Orbicularis oculi muscle	Upper Eyelid, Right Upper Eyelid, Left
Orbicularis oris muscle	Facial Muscle
Orbital fascia	Subcutaneous Tissue and Fascia, Face
Orbital portion of ethmoid bone Orbital portion of frontal bone Orbital portion of lacrimal bone Orbital portion of maxilla Orbital portion of palatine bone Orbital portion of sphenoid bone Orbital portion of zygomatic bone	Orbit, Right Orbit, Left
Oropharynx	Pharynx
Ossicular chain	Auditory Ossicle, Right Auditory Ossicle, Left
Otic ganglion	Head and Neck Sympathetic Nerve
Oval window	Middle Ear, Right Middle Ear, Left
Ovarian artery	Abdominal Aorta
Ovarian ligament	Uterine Supporting Structure
Oviduct	Fallopian Tube, Right Fallopian Tube, Left
Palatine gland	Buccal Mucosa
Palatine tonsil	Tonsils
Palatine uvula	Uvula
Palatoglossal muscle Palatopharyngeal muscle	Tongue, Palate, Pharynx Muscle
Palmar (volar) digital vein Palmar (volar) metacarpal vein	Hand Vein, Right Hand Vein, Left

Continued

Body Part Key — cont'd

If You See This Body Part	Code to This Body Part
Palmar cutaneous nerve	Median Nerve Radial Nerve
Palmar fascia (aponeurosis)	Subcutaneous Tissue and Fascia, Right Hand Subcutaneous Tissue and Fascia, Left Hand
Palmar interosseous muscle	Hand Muscle, Right Hand Muscle, Left
Palmar ulnocarpal ligament	Wrist Bursa and Ligament, Right Wrist Bursa and Ligament, Left
Palmaris longus muscle	Lower Arm and Wrist Muscle, Right Lower Arm and Wrist Muscle, Left
Pancreatic artery	Splenic Artery
Pancreatic plexus	Abdominal Sympathetic Nerve
Pancreatic vein	Splenic Vein
Pancreaticosplenic lymph node Paraaortic lymph node	Lymphatic, Aortic
Pararectal lymph node	Lymphatic, Mesenteric
Parasternal lymph node Paratracheal lymph node	Lymphatic, Thorax
Paraurethral (Skene's) gland	Vestibular Gland
Parietal lobe	Cerebral Hemisphere
Parotid lymph node	Lymphatic, Head
Parotid plexus	Facial Nerve
Pars flaccida	Tympanic Membrane, Right Tympanic Membrane, Left
Patellar ligament	Knee Bursa and Ligament, Right Knee Bursa and Ligament, Left
Patellar tendon	Knee Tendon, Right Knee Tendon, Left
Pectineus muscle	Upper Leg Muscle, Right Upper Leg Muscle, Left
Pectoral (anterior) lymph node	Lymphatic, Right Axillary Lymphatic, Left Axillary
Pectoral fascia	Subcutaneous Tissue and Fascia, Chest
Pectoralis major muscle Pectoralis minor muscle	Thorax Muscle, Right Thorax Muscle, Left
Pelvic splanchnic nerve	Abdominal Sympathetic Nerve Sacral Sympathetic Nerve
Penile urethra	Urethra
Pericardiophrenic artery	Internal Mammary Artery, Right Internal Mammary Artery, Left
Perimetrium	Uterus
Peroneus brevis muscle Peroneus longus muscle	Lower Leg Muscle, Right Lower Leg Muscle, Left

Body Part Key — cont'd

If You See This Body Part	Code to This Body Part
Petrous part of temporal bone	Temporal Bone, Right Temporal Bone, Left
Pharyngeal constrictor muscle	Tongue, Palate, Pharynx Muscle
Pharyngeal plexus	Vagus Nerve
Pharyngeal recess	Nasopharynx
Pharyngeal tonsil	Adenoids
Pharyngotympanic tube	Eustachian Tube, Right Eustachian Tube, Left
Pia mater	Cerebral Meninges Spinal Meninges
Pinna	External Ear, Right External Ear, Left External Ear, Bilateral
Piriform recess (sinus)	Pharynx
Piriformis muscle	Hip Muscle, Right Hip Muscle, Left
Pisiform bone	Carpal, Right Carpal, Left
Pisohamate ligament Pisometacarpal ligament	Hand Bursa and Ligament, Right Hand Bursa and Ligament, Left
Plantar digital vein	Foot Vein, Right Foot Vein, Left
Plantar fascia (aponeurosis)	Subcutaneous Tissue and Fascia, Right Foot Subcutaneous Tissue and Fascia, Left Foot
Plantar metatarsal vein Plantar venous arch	Foot Vein, Right Foot Vein, Left
Platysma muscle	Neck Muscle, Right Neck Muscle, Left
Plica semilunaris	Conjunctiva, Right Conjunctiva, Left
Pneumogastric nerve	Vagus Nerve
Pneumotaxic center Pontine tegmentum	Pons
Popliteal ligament	Knee Bursa and Ligament, Right Knee Bursa and Ligament, Left
Popliteal lymph node	Lymphatic, Right Lower Extremity Lymphatic, Left Lower Extremity
Popliteal vein	Femoral Vein, Right Femoral Vein, Left
Popliteus muscle	Lower Leg Muscle, Right Lower Leg Muscle, Left
Postauricular (mastoid) lymph node	Lymphatic, Right Neck Lymphatic, Left Neck
Postcava	Inferior Vena Cava

Continued

Body Part Key — cont'd

If You See This Body Part	Code to This Body Part
Posterior (subscapular) lymph node	Lymphatic, Right Axillary Lymphatic, Left Axillary
Posterior auricular artery	External Carotid Artery, Right External Carotid Artery, Left
Posterior auricular nerve	Facial Nerve
Posterior auricular vein	External Jugular Vein, Right External Jugular Vein, Left
Posterior cerebral artery	Intracranial Artery
Posterior chamber	Eye, Right Eye, Left
Posterior circumflex humeral artery	Axillary Artery, Right Axillary Artery, Left
Posterior communicating artery	Intracranial Artery
Posterior cruciate ligament (PCL)	Knee Bursa and Ligament, Right Knee Bursa and Ligament, Left
Posterior facial (retromandibular) vein	Face Vein, Right Face Vein, Left
Posterior femoral cutaneous nerve	Sacral Plexus
Posterior inferior cerebellar artery (PICA)	Intracranial Artery
Posterior interosseous nerve	Radial Nerve
Posterior labial nerve Posterior scrotal nerve	Pudendal Nerve
Posterior spinal artery	Vertebral Artery, Right Vertebral Artery, Left
Posterior tibial recurrent artery	Anterior Tibial Artery, Right Anterior Tibial Artery, Left
Posterior ulnar recurrent artery	Ulnar Artery, Right Ulnar Artery, Left
Posterior vagal trunk	Vagus Nerve
Preauricular lymph node	Lymphatic, Head
Precava	Superior Vena Cava
Prepatellar bursa	Knee Bursa and Ligament, Right Knee Bursa and Ligament, Left
Pretracheal fascia	Subcutaneous Tissue and Fascia, Anterior Neck
Prevertebral fascia	Subcutaneous Tissue and Fascia, Posterior Neck
Princeps pollicis artery	Hand Artery, Right Hand Artery, Left
Procerus muscle	Facial Muscle
Profunda brachii	Brachial Artery, Right Brachial Artery, Left
Profunda femoris (deep femoral) vein	Femoral Vein, Right Femoral Vein, Left

Body Part Key — cont'd

If You See This Body Part	Code to This Body Part
Pronator quadratus muscle Pronator teres muscle	Lower Arm and Wrist Muscle, Right Lower Arm and Wrist Muscle, Left
Prostatic urethra	Urethra
Proximal radioulnar joint	Elbow Joint, Right Elbow Joint, Left
Psoas muscle	Hip Muscle, Right Hip Muscle, Left
Pterygoid muscle	Head Muscle
Pterygoid process	Sphenoid Bone, Right Sphenoid Bone, Left
Pterygopalatine (sphenopalatine) ganglion	Head and Neck Sympathetic Nerve
Pubic ligament	Trunk Bursa and Ligament, Right Trunk Bursa and Ligament, Left
Pubis	Pelvic Bone, Right Pelvic Bone, Left
Pubofemoral ligament	Hip Bursa and Ligament, Right Hip Bursa and Ligament, Left
Pudendal nerve	Sacral Plexus
Pulmoaortic canal	Pulmonary Artery, Left
Pulmonary annulus	Pulmonary Valve
Pulmonary plexus	Vagus Nerve Thoracic Sympathetic Nerve
Pulmonic valve	Pulmonary Valve
Pulvinar	Thalamus
Pyloric antrum Pyloric canal Pyloric sphincter	Stomach, Pylorus
Pyramidalis muscle	Abdomen Muscle, Right Abdomen Muscle, Left
Quadrangular cartilage	Nasal Septum
Quadrate lobe	Liver
Quadratus femoris muscle	Hip Muscle, Right Hip Muscle, Left
Quadratus lumborum muscle	Trunk Muscle, Right Trunk Muscle, Left
Quadratus plantae muscle	Foot Muscle, Right Foot Muscle, Left
Quadriceps (femoris)	Upper Leg Muscle, Right Upper Leg Muscle, Left
Radial collateral carpal ligament	Wrist Bursa and Ligament, Right Wrist Bursa and Ligament, Left
Radial collateral ligament	Elbow Bursa and Ligament, Right Elbow Bursa and Ligament, Left

Continued

Body Part Key — cont'd

If You See This Body Part	Code to This Body Part
Radial notch	Ulna, Right Ulna, Left
Radial recurrent artery	Radial Artery, Right Radial Artery, Left
Radial vein	Brachial Vein, Right Brachial Vein, Left
Radialis indicis	Hand Artery, Right Hand Artery, Left
Radiocarpal joint	Wrist Joint, Right Wrist Joint, Left
Radiocarpal ligament Radioulnar ligament	Wrist Bursa and Ligament, Right Wrist Bursa and Ligament, Left
Rectosigmoid junction	Sigmoid Colon
Rectus abdominis muscle	Abdomen Muscle, Right Abdomen Muscle, Left
Rectus femoris muscle	Upper Leg Muscle, Right Upper Leg Muscle, Left
Recurrent laryngeal nerve	Vagus Nerve
Renal calyx Renal capsule Renal cortex	Kidney, Right Kidney, Left Kidneys, Bilateral Kidney
Renal plexus	Abdominal Sympathetic Nerve
Renal segment	Kidney, Right Kidney, Left Kidneys, Bilateral Kidney
Renal segmental artery	Renal Artery, Right Renal Artery, Left
Retroperitoneal lymph node	Lymphatic, Aortic
Retroperitoneal space	Retroperitoneum
Retropharyngeal lymph node	Lymphatic, Right Neck Lymphatic, Left Neck
Retropubic space	Pelvic Cavity
Rhinopharynx	Nasopharynx
Rhomboid major muscle Rhomboid minor muscle	Trunk Muscle, Right Trunk Muscle, Left
Right ascending lumbar vein Right atrioventricular valve	Azygos Vein Tricuspid Valve
Right auricular appendix	Atrium, Right
Right colic vein	Colic Vein
Right coronary sulcus	Heart, Right
Right gastric artery	Gastric Artery

Body Part Key — cont'd

If You See This Body Part	Code to This Body Part
Right gastroepiploic vein	Superior Mesenteric Vein
Right inferior phrenic vein	Inferior Vena Cava
Right inferior pulmonary vein	Pulmonary Vein, Right
Right jugular trunk	Lymphatic, Right Neck
Right lateral ventricle	Cerebral Ventricle
Right lymphatic duct	Lymphatic, Right Neck
Right ovarian vein Right second lumbar vein	Inferior Vena Cava
Right subclavian trunk	Lymphatic, Right Neck
Right subcostal vein	Azygos Vein
Right superior pulmonary vein	Pulmonary Vein, Right
Right suprarenal vein Right testicular vein	Inferior Vena Cava
Rima glottidis	Larynx
Risorius muscle	Facial Muscle
Round ligament of uterus	Uterine Supporting Structure
Round window	Inner Ear, Right Inner Ear, Left
Sacral ganglion	Sacral Sympathetic Nerve
Sacral lymph node	Lymphatic, Pelvis
Sacral splanchnic nerve	Sacral Sympathetic Nerve
Sacrococcygeal ligament	Trunk Bursa and Ligament, Right Trunk Bursa and Ligament, Left
Sacrococcygeal symphysis	Sacrococcygeal Joint
Sacroiliac ligament Sacrospinous ligament Sacrotuberous ligament	Trunk Bursa and Ligament, Right Trunk Bursa and Ligament, Left
Salpingopharyngeus muscle	Tongue, Palate, Pharynx Muscle
Salpinx	Fallopian Tube, Right Fallopian Tube, Left
Saphenous nerve	Femoral Nerve
Sartorius muscle	Upper Leg Muscle, Right Upper Leg Muscle, Left
Scalene muscle	Neck Muscle, Right Neck Muscle, Left
Scaphoid bone	Carpal, Right Carpal, Left
Scapholunate ligament Scaphotrapezium ligament	Hand Bursa and Ligament, Right Hand Bursa and Ligament, Left
Scarpa's (vestibular) ganglion	Acoustic Nerve
Sebaceous gland	Skin
Second cranial nerve	Optic Nerve

Continued

Body Part Key — cont'd

If You See This Body Part	Code to This Body Part
Sella turcica	Sphenoid Bone, Right Sphenoid Bone, Left
Semicircular canal	Inner Ear, Right Inner Ear, Left
Semimembranosus muscle Semitendinosus muscle	Upper Leg Muscle, Right Upper Leg Muscle, Left
Septal cartilage	Nasal Septum
Serratus anterior muscle	Thorax Muscle, Right Thorax Muscle, Left
Serratus posterior muscle	Trunk Muscle, Right Trunk Muscle, Left
Seventh cranial nerve	Facial Nerve
Short gastric artery	Splenic Artery
Sigmoid artery	Inferior Mesenteric Artery
Sigmoid flexure	Sigmoid Colon
Sigmoid vein	Inferior Mesenteric Vein
Sinoatrial node	Conduction Mechanism
Sinus venosus	Atrium, Right
Sixth cranial nerve	Abducens Nerve
Skene's (paraurethral) gland	Vestibular Gland
Small saphenous vein	Lesser Saphenous Vein, Right Lesser Saphenous Vein, Left
Solar (celiac) plexus	Abdominal Sympathetic Nerve
Soleus muscle	Lower Leg Muscle, Right Lower Leg Muscle, Left
Sphenomandibular ligament	Head and Neck Bursa and Ligament
Sphenopalatine (pterygopalatine) ganglion	Head and Neck Sympathetic Nerve
Spinal dura mater	Dura Mater
Spinal epidural space	Epidural Space
Spinal subarachnoid space	Subarachnoid Space
Spinal subdural space	Subdural Space
Spinous process	Cervical Vertebra Thoracic Vertebra Lumbar Vertebra
Spiral ganglion	Acoustic Nerve
Splenic flexure	Transverse Colon
Splenic plexus	Abdominal Sympathetic Nerve
Splenius capitis muscle	Head Muscle
Splenius cervicis muscle	Neck Muscle, Right Neck Muscle, Left
Stapes	Auditory Ossicle, Right Auditory Ossicle, Left

Body Part Key — cont'd

If You See This Body Part	Code to This Body Part
Stellate ganglion	Head and Neck Sympathetic Nerve
Stensen's duct	Parotid Duct, Right Parotid Duct, Left
Sternoclavicular ligament	Shoulder Bursa and Ligament, Right Shoulder Bursa and Ligament, Left
Sternocleidomastoid artery	Thyroid Artery, Right Thyroid Artery, Left
Sternocleidomastoid muscle	Neck Muscle, Right Neck Muscle, Left
Sternocostal ligament	Thorax Bursa and Ligament, Right Thorax Bursa and Ligament, Left
Styloglossus muscle	Tongue, Palate, Pharynx Muscle
Stylomandibular ligament	Head and Neck Bursa and Ligament
Stylopharyngeus muscle	Tongue, Palate, Pharynx Muscle
Subacromial bursa	Shoulder Bursa and Ligament, Right Shoulder Bursa and Ligament, Left
Subaortic (common iliac) lymph node	Lymphatic, Pelvis
Subclavicular (apical) lymph node	Lymphatic, Right Axillary Lymphatic, Left Axillary
Subclavius muscle	Thorax Muscle, Right Thorax Muscle, Left
Subclavius nerve	Brachial Plexus
Subcostal artery	Thoracic Aorta
Subcostal muscle	Thorax Muscle, Right Thorax Muscle, Left
Subcostal nerve	Thoracic Nerve
Submandibular ganglion	Facial Nerve Head and Neck Sympathetic Nerve
Submandibular gland	Submaxillary Gland, Right Submaxillary Gland, Left
Submandibular lymph node	Lymphatic, Head
Submaxillary ganglion	Head and Neck Sympathetic Nerve
Submaxillary lymph node	Lymphatic, Head
Submental artery	Face Artery
Submental lymph node	Lymphatic, Head
Submucous (Meissner's) plexus	Abdominal Sympathetic Nerve
Suboccipital nerve	Cervical Nerve
Suboccipital venous plexus	Vertebral Vein, Right Vertebral Vein, Left
Subparotid lymph node	Lymphatic, Head
Subscapular (posterior) lymph node	Lymphatic, Right Axillary Lymphatic, Left Axillary

Continued

Body Part Key — cont'd

If You See This Body Part	Code to This Body Part
Subscapular aponeurosis	Subcutaneous Tissue and Fascia, Right Upper Arm Subcutaneous Tissue and Fascia, Left Upper Arm
Subscapular artery	Axillary Artery, Right Axillary Artery, Left
Subscapularis muscle	Shoulder Muscle, Right Shoulder Muscle, Left
Substantia nigra	Basal Ganglia
Subtalar (talocalcaneal) joint	Tarsal Joint, Right Tarsal Joint, Left
Subtalar ligament	Foot Bursa and Ligament, Right Foot Bursa and Ligament, Left
Subthalamic nucleus	Basal Ganglia
Superficial circumflex iliac vein	Greater Saphenous Vein, Right Greater Saphenous Vein, Left
Superficial epigastric artery	Femoral Artery, Right Femoral Artery, Left
Superficial epigastric vein	Greater Saphenous Vein, Right Greater Saphenous Vein, Left
Superficial palmar arch	Hand Artery, Right Hand Artery, Left
Superficial palmar venous arch	Hand Vein, Right Hand Vein, Left
Superficial temporal artery	Temporal Artery, Right Temporal Artery, Left
Superficial transverse perineal muscle	Perineum Muscle
Superior cardiac nerve	Thoracic Sympathetic Nerve
Superior cerebellar vein Superior cerebral vein	Intracranial Vein
Superior clunic (cluneal) nerve	Lumbar Nerve
Superior epigastric artery	Internal Mammary Artery, Right Internal Mammary Artery, Left
Superior genicular artery	Popliteal Artery, Right Popliteal Artery, Left
Superior gluteal artery	Internal Iliac Artery, Right Internal Iliac Artery, Left
Superior gluteal nerve	Lumbar Plexus
Superior hypogastric plexus	Abdominal Sympathetic Nerve
Superior labial artery	Face Artery
Superior laryngeal artery	Thyroid Artery, Right Thyroid Artery, Left
Superior laryngeal nerve	Vagus Nerve
Superior longitudinal muscle	Tongue, Palate, Pharynx Muscle
Superior mesenteric ganglion	Abdominal Sympathetic Nerve

Body Part Key — cont'd

If You See This Body Part	Code to This Body Part
Superior mesenteric lymph node	Lymphatic, Mesenteric
Superior mesenteric plexus	Abdominal Sympathetic Nerve
Superior oblique muscle	Extraocular Muscle, Right Extraocular Muscle, Left
Superior olivary nucleus	Pons
Superior rectal artery	Inferior Mesenteric Artery
Superior rectal vein	Inferior Mesenteric Vein
Superior rectus muscle	Extraocular Muscle, Right Extraocular Muscle, Left
Superior tarsal plate	Upper Eyelid, Right Upper Eyelid, Left
Superior thoracic artery	Axillary Artery, Right Axillary Artery, Left
Superior thyroid artery	External Carotid Artery, Right External Carotid Artery, Left Thyroid Artery, Right Thyroid Artery, Left
Superior turbinate	Nasal Turbinate
Superior ulnar collateral artery	Brachial Artery, Right Brachial Artery, Left
Supraclavicular (Virchow's) lymph node	Lymphatic, Right Neck Lymphatic, Left Neck
Supraclavicular nerve	Cervical Plexus
Suprahyoid lymph node	Lymphatic, Head
Suprahyoid muscle	Neck Muscle, Right Neck Muscle, Left
Suprainguinal lymph node	Lymphatic, Pelvis
Supraorbital vein	Face Vein, Right Face Vein, Left
Suprarenal gland	Adrenal Gland, Left Adrenal Gland, Right Adrenal Glands, Bilateral Adrenal Gland
Suprarenal plexus	Abdominal Sympathetic Nerve
Suprascapular nerve	Brachial Plexus
Supraspinatus fascia	Subcutaneous Tissue and Fascia, Right Upper Arm Subcutaneous Tissue and Fascia, Left Upper Arm
Supraspinatus muscle	Shoulder Muscle, Right Shoulder Muscle, Left
Supraspinous ligament	Trunk Bursa and Ligament, Right Trunk Bursa and Ligament, Left
Suprasternal notch	Sternum
Supratrochlear lymph node	Lymphatic, Right Upper Extremity Lymphatic, Left Upper Extremity

Continued

Body Part Key — cont'd

If You See This Body Part	Code to This Body Part
Sural artery	Popliteal Artery, Right Popliteal Artery, Left
Sweat gland	Skin
Talocalcaneal (subtalar) joint	Tarsal Joint, Right Tarsal Joint, Left
Talocalcaneal ligament	Foot Bursa and Ligament, Right Foot Bursa and Ligament, Left
Talocalcaneonavicular joint	Tarsal Joint, Right Tarsal Joint, Left
Talocalcaneonavicular ligament	Foot Bursa and Ligament, Right Foot Bursa and Ligament, Left
Talocrural joint	Ankle Joint, Right Ankle Joint, Left
Talofibular ligament	Ankle Bursa and Ligament, Right Ankle Bursa and Ligament, Left
Talus bone	Tarsal, Right Tarsal, Left
Tarsometatarsal joint	Metatarsal-Tarsal Joint, Right Metatarsal-Tarsal Joint, Left
Tarsometatarsal ligament	Foot Bursa and Ligament, Right Foot Bursa and Ligament, Left
Temporal lobe	Cerebral Hemisphere
Temporalis muscle Temporoparietalis muscle	Head Muscle
Tensor fasciae latae muscle	Hip Muscle, Right Hip Muscle, Left
Tensor veli palatini muscle	Tongue, Palate, Pharynx Muscle
Tenth cranial nerve	Vagus Nerve
Tentorium cerebelli	Dura Mater
Teres major muscle Teres minor muscle	Shoulder Muscle, Right Shoulder Muscle, Left
Testicular artery	Abdominal Aorta
Thenar muscle	Hand Muscle, Right Hand Muscle, Left
Third cranial nerve	Oculomotor Nerve
Third occipital nerve	Cervical Nerve
Third ventricle	Cerebral Ventricle
Thoracic aortic plexus	Thoracic Sympathetic Nerve
Thoracic esophagus	Esophagus, Middle
Thoracic facet joint	Thoracic Vertebral Joint Thoracic Vertebral Joints, 2 to 7 Thoracic Vertebral Joints, 8 or more
Thoracic ganglion	Thoracic Sympathetic Nerve

Body Part Key — cont'd

If You See This Body Part	Code to This Body Part
Thoracoacromial artery	Axillary Artery, Right Axillary Artery, Left
Thoracolumbar facet joint	Thoracolumbar Vertebral Joint
Thymus gland	Thymus
Thyroarytenoid muscle	Neck Muscle, Right Neck Muscle, Left
Thyrocervical trunk	Thyroid Artery, Right Thyroid Artery, Left
Thyroid cartilage	Larynx
Tibialis anterior muscle Tibialis posterior muscle	Lower Leg Muscle, Right Lower Leg Muscle, Left
Tracheobronchial lymph node	Lymphatic, Thorax
Tragus	External Ear, Right External Ear, Left External Ear, Bilateral
Transversalis fascia	Subcutaneous Tissue and Fascia, Trunk
Transverse (cutaneous) cervical nerve	Cervical Plexus
Transverse acetabular ligament	Hip Bursa and Ligament, Right Hip Bursa and Ligament, Left
Transverse facial artery	Temporal Artery, Right Temporal Artery, Left
Transverse humeral ligament	Shoulder Bursa and Ligament, Right Shoulder Bursa and Ligament, Left
Transverse ligament of atlas	Head and Neck Bursa and Ligament
Transverse scapular ligament	Shoulder Bursa and Ligament, Right Shoulder Bursa and Ligament, Left
Transverse thoracis muscle	Thorax Muscle, Right Thorax Muscle, Left
Transversospinalis muscle	Trunk Muscle, Right Trunk Muscle, Left
Transversus abdominis muscle	Abdomen Muscle, Right Abdomen Muscle, Left
Trapezium bone	Carpal, Right Carpal, Left
Trapezius muscle	Trunk Muscle, Right Trunk Muscle, Left
Trapezoid bone	Carpal, Right Carpal, Left
Triceps brachii muscle	Upper Arm Muscle, Right Upper Arm Muscle, Left
Tricuspid annulus	Tricuspid Valve
Trifacial nerve	Trigeminal Nerve
Trigone of bladder	Bladder

Continued

Body Part Key — cont'd

If You See This Body Part	Code to This Body Part
Triquetral bone	Carpal, Right Carpal, Left
Trochanteric bursa	Hip Bursa and Ligament, Right Hip Bursa and Ligament, Left
Twelfth cranial nerve	Hypoglossal Nerve
Tympanic cavity	Middle Ear, Right Middle Ear, Left
Tympanic nerve	Glossopharyngeal Nerve
Tympanic part of temporal bone	Temporal Bone, Right Temporal Bone, Left
Ulnar collateral carpal ligament	Wrist Bursa and Ligament, Right Wrist Bursa and Ligament, Left
Ulnar collateral ligament	Elbow Bursa and Ligament, Right Elbow Bursa and Ligament, Left
Ulnar notch	Radius, Right Radius, Left
Ulnar vein	Brachial Vein, Right Brachial Vein, Left
Umbilical artery	Internal Iliac Artery, Right Internal Iliac Artery, Left
Ureteral orifice	Ureter, Right Ureter, Left Ureters, Bilateral Ureter
Ureteropelvic junction (UPJ)	Kidney Pelvis, Right Kidney Pelvis, Left
Ureterovesical orifice	Ureter, Right Ureter, Left Ureters, Bilateral Ureter
Uterine artery	Internal Iliac Artery, Right Internal Iliac Artery, Left
Uterine cornu	Uterus
Uterine tube	Fallopian Tube, Right Fallopian Tube, Left
Uterine vein	Hypogastric Vein, Right Hypogastric Vein, Left
Vaginal artery	Internal Iliac Artery, Right Internal Iliac Artery, Left
Vaginal vein	Hypogastric Vein, Right Hypogastric Vein, Left
Vastus intermedius muscle Vastus lateralis muscle Vastus medialis muscle	Upper Leg Muscle, Right Upper Leg Muscle, Left
Ventricular fold	Larynx
Vermiform appendix	Appendix
Vermilion border	Upper Lip Lower Lip

Body Part Key — cont'd

If You See This Body Part	Code to This Body Part
Vertebral arch	Cervical Vertebra Thoracic Vertebra Lumbar Vertebra
Vertebral canal	Spinal Canal
Vertebral foramen Vertebral lamina Vertebral pedicle	Cervical Vertebra Thoracic Vertebra Lumbar Vertebra
Vesical vein	Hypogastric Vein, Right Hypogastric Vein, Left
Vestibular (Scarpa's) ganglion Vestibular nerve Vestibulocochlear nerve	Acoustic Nerve
Virchow's (supraclavicular) lymph node	Lymphatic, Right Neck Lymphatic, Left Neck
Vitreous body	Vitreous, Right Vitreous, Left
Vocal fold	Vocal Cord, Right Vocal Cord, Left
Volar (palmar) digital vein	Hand Vein, Right
Volar (palmar) metacarpal vein	Hand Vein, Left
Vomer bone	Nasal Septum
Vomer of nasal septum	Nasal Bone
Xiphoid process	Sternum
Zonule of Zinn	Lens, Right Lens, Left
Zygomatic process of frontal bone	Frontal Bone, Right Frontal Bone, Left
Zygomatic process of temporal bone	Temporal Bone, Right Temporal Bone, Left
Zygomaticus muscle	Facial Muscle

Answers to Exercises and Review Questions

Chapter 1

Exercise 1
1. C   2. D   3. E   4. B   5. F   6. A
7. I   8. H   9. G   10. E   11. F   12. C
13. B   14. D   15. A   16. J   17. K

Exercise 2
1. C   2. D   3. A   4. E   5. B   6. F

Exercise 3
1. B   2. D   3. E   4. A   5. C

Exercise 4
1. ophthalm/o (eye) + -logy (the study of)
   Def: the study of the eye
2. ot/o (ear) + -plasty (surgically forming)
   Def: surgically forming the ear
3. gastr/o (stomach) + -algia (pain)
   Def: stomach pain
4. arthr/o (joint) + -scope (instrument to view)
   Def: instrument to view a joint
5. rhin/o (nose) + -tomy (cutting)
   Def: cutting the nose

Exercise 5
1. E   2. G   3. J   4. I   5. H   6. A
7. C   8. D   9. F   10. B

11. cardi/o (heart) + -megaly (enlargement)
    Def: enlargement of the heart
12. oste/o (bone) + -malacia (softening)
    Def: softening of bone
13. valvul/o (valve) + -itis (inflammation)
    Def: inflammation of a valve
14. cephal/o (head) + -ic (pertaining to)
    Def: pertaining to the head
15. gastr/o (stomach) + -ptosis (prolapse)
    Def: prolapse of the stomach

Exercise 6
1. E   2. I   3. H   4. F   5. J   6. C
7. D   8. A   9. G   10. B

11. arthr/o (joint) + -centesis (surgical puncture)
    Def: surgical puncture of a joint
12. spir/o (breathing) + -meter (instrument to measure)
    Def: instrument to measure breathing
13. hyster/o (uterus) + -scopy (viewing)
    Def: viewing the uterus
14. cyst/o (bladder) + -scope (instrument to view)
    Def: instrument to view the bladder
15. splen/o (spleen) + -ectomy (cutting out)
    Def: cutting out the spleen

Exercise 7
1. C   2. H   3. F   4. I   5. B   6. D
7. E   8. J   9. A   10. G

11. sub- (under) + hepat/o (liver) + -ic (pertaining to)
    Def: pertaining to under the liver
12. peri- (surrounding) + cardi/o (heart) + -um (structure)
    Def: structure surrounding the heart
13. dys- (difficult) + pne/o (breathing) + -ic (pertaining to)
    Def: pertaining to difficult breathing
14. per- (through) + cutane/o (skin) + -ous (pertaining to)
    Def: pertaining to through the skin
15. hypo- (deficient) + glyc/o (sugar, glucose) + -emia (blood condition)
    Def: blood condition of deficient glucose

Exercise 8
1. esophagi
2. larynges
3. fornices
4. pleurae
5. diagnoses
6. myocardia
7. cardiomyopathies
8. hepatitides

Chapter 1 Review

Word Part Definitions:
1. inter-
2. per-
3. par-
4. intra-
5. anti-
6. a-
7. peri-
8. para-
9. pre-
10. poly-
11. sub-
12. dys-
13. -dynia
14. -rrhea
15. -stenosis
16. -oma
17. -tripter
18. -itis
19. -rrhage
20. -scopy
21. -sclerosis
22. -tomy
23. -plasty

24. -ectomy
25. -graphy
26. -metry
27. -rrhaphy
28. -stomy
29. -osis
30. -pathy
31. -ar
32. -ia

Wordshop:
1. anophthalmia
2. parotid
3. subhepatic
4. gastroenteritis
5. ophthalmoscope
6. pericardium
7. colostomy
8. mammography
9. endoscopy
10. tonsillectomy
11. cystocele
12. cervical
13. cephalgia
14. hypodermic
15. splenomegaly

Chapter 2

Exercise 1
1. D   2. E   3. A   4. C   5. B

Exercise 2
1. C   2. A   3. D   4. B

Exercise 3
1. D   2. F   3. A   4. B   5. H   6. C
7. E   8. G   9. I

Exercise 4
1. pertaining to within the lumen
2. pertaining to a hilum
3. pertaining to surrounding the apex
4. pertaining to the antrum
5. pertaining to a vestibule
6. pertaining to the fundus
7. pertaining to the surface of an organ
8. lumen
9. hilum
10. apex
11. body (corporis)
12. sinuses

Exercise 5
1. F   2. H   3. C   4. A   5. G   6. E
7. I   8. B   9. K   10. D   11. J

Exercise 6
1. J   2. G   3. A   4. I   5. D   6. E
7. H   8. B   9. C   10. F

Exercise 7
1. the study of cells
2. one who specializes in the study of disease
3. viewing dead (tissue)
4. one who specializes in the study of tissues
5. viewing living (tissue)

Exercise 8
1. G   2. M   3. J   4. K   5. R   6. A
7. P   8. D   9. T   10. B   11. F   12. I
13. Q   14. C   15. S   16. N   17. E   18. O
19. H   20. L

Exercise 9
1. I   2. P   3. N   4. L   5. M   6. J
7. R   8. B   9. K   10. F   11. D   12. O
13. G   14. A   15. Q   16. E   17. C   18. H

Exercise 10
1. C   2. A   3. F   4. K   5. I   6. J
7. L   8. E   9. D   10. H   11. G   12. B

Exercise 11
1. esophagus
2. esophagus and stomach
3. The closest to point of origin and middle parts of the esophagus were normal.
4. distal esophagus

Exercise 12
1. D   2. C   3. B   4. A   5. E

Exercise 13
1. epigastric
2. lumbar
3. hypogastric
4. iliac or inguinal
5. hypochondriac

Exercise 14
1. transverse plane
2. midsagittal plane
3. frontal or coronal plane

Exercise 15
1. toes
2. inner
3. during
4. front to back

Exercise 16
1. closest to the wrist
2. backward

3. pertaining to the back of the body
4. posteroanterior (back to front)

Chapter 2 Review

Word Part Definitions:
1. epi-
2. ante-
3. uni-
4. endo-
5. bi-
6. af-
7. ipsi-
8. contra-
9. ef-
10. meta-
11. viscer/o
12. infer/o
13. anter/o
14. dist/o
15. medi/o
16. axill/o
17. super/o
18. proxim/o
19. sinistr/o
20. brachi/o
21. caud/o
22. crur/o
23. later/o
24. dextr/o
25. poster/o
26. hist/o
27. corpor/o
28. cephal/o
29. crani/o
30. cyt/o
31. inguin/o
32. cervic/o
33. thorac/o
34. lapar/o

Wordshop:
1. midsagittal
2. bilateral
3. dextrad
4. posteroanterior
5. thoracic
6. abdominopelvic
7. lumbar
8. contralateral
9. cytoplasm
10. superior
11. inguinal
12. histology
13. hypogastric
14. ipsilateral
15. intracranial

Term Sorting:
Organization of the Body: apex, cytoplasm, hilum, lumen, nucleus, organ, sinus, stroma, system, vestibule
Positional and Directional: afferent, anterior, distal, efferent, lateral, posterior, prone, superior, supine
Body Cavities and Planes: coronal, cranial, midsagittal, pleural, sagittal, spinal, thoracic, transverse, pelvic
Abdominal Regions and Quadrants: epigastric, hypochondriac, hypogastric, iliac, inguinal, lumbar, umbilical

Translations:
1. plantar, palmar
2. antecubital
3. bilateral
4. buccal
5. biopsy
6. lumen
7. thoracic
8. distal
9. mediastinum
10. contralateral
11. supine
12. inguinal
13. thoracic, coxal
14. epigastric

Chapter 3

Exercise 1
1. E	2. J	3. F	4. L	5. H	6. N
7. B	8. O	9. G	10. C	11. K	12. M
13. A	14. D	15. I			

16. build, break down
17. diaphysis, epiphyses
18. periosteum, endosteum
19. depressions, processes
20. antrum
21. long, short, flat, irregular, sesamoid
22. skull, vertebrae, ribcage
23. shoulder and pelvic girdles, and upper and lower extremities
24. head and facial bones, upper bones, lower bones
25. cortical bone is denser and stronger, while cancellous bone is weaker and more open

Exercise 2
1. I	2. K	3. F	4. G	5. N	6. J
7. M	8. B	9. E	10. D	11. A	12. O
13. C	14. H	15. L	16. P		

17. sub- (below) + mandibul/o (mandible) + -ar (pertaining to)
    Def: pertaining to below the mandible
18. cost/o (ribs) + chondr/o (cartilage) + -al (pertaining to)
    Def: pertaining to ribs and cartilage
19. lumb/o (lower back) + sacr/o (sacrum) + -al (pertaining to)
    Def: pertaining to the lower back and sacrum
20. thorac/o (chest) + -ic (pertaining to)
    Def: pertaining to the chest
21. sub- (below) + stern/o (breastbone) + -al (pertaining to)
    Def: pertaining to below the breastbone

Exercise 3

1. F	2. I	3. G	4. H	5. A	6. J
7. C	8. D	9. E	10. B	11. P	12. N
13. K	14. O	15. Q	16. R	17. T	18. L
19. U	20. S	21. M	22. V	23. X	24. W

25. inter- (between) + phalang/o (finger/toe bones) + -eal (pertaining to)
    Def: pertaining to between the finger or toe bones
26. humer/o (humerus) + uln/o (ulna) + -ar (pertaining to)
    Def: pertaining to the humerus and ulna
27. infra- (below) + patell/a (patella) + -ar (pertaining to)
    Def: pertaining to below the patella
28. femor/o (femur) + -al (pertaining to)
    Def: pertaining to the femur
29. supra- (above) + clavicul/o (clavicle) + -ar (pertaining to)
    Def: pertaining to above the clavicle

Exercise 4

1. H	2. I	3. A	4. F	5. B	6. G
7. C	8. J	9. D	10. E		

Exercise 5

1. H	2. F	3. A	4. B	5. C	6. G
7. E	8. J	9. I	10. D		

Exercise 6

1. G	2. C	3. I	4. M	5. O	6. B
7. A	8. N	9. H	10. D	11. E	12. F
13. K	14. L	15. J			

Exercise 7

1. N	2. L	3. F	4. A	5. M	6. K
7. J	8. C	9. H	10. I	11. D	12. G
13. B	14. E				

Exercise 8

1. E	2. H	3. A	4. C	5. J	6. B
7. I	8. F	9. D	10. G	11. Q	12. K
13. N	14. T	15. S	16. O	17. P	18. M
19. L	20. R				

Exercise 9

1. DIP is the articulation between the two far bones while PIP is the articulation between the two near bones (in relation to the head).
2. bend
3. right thumb
4. thumb

Exercise 10

1. arthrosis
2. bunion
3. contracture
4. crepitus
5. gout
6. osteophytosis
7. rheumatoid arthritis
8. TMJ
9. ankylosing spondylitis
10. herniated intervertebral disk
11. lordosis
12. sciatica
13. spinal stenosis
14. SLE
15. scleroderma
16. inflammation (-itis) bone (oste/o) joint (arthr/o)
    Term: osteoarthritis
17. inflammation (-itis) many (poly-) muscle (myos/o)
    Term: polymyositis
18. condition of slipping (-listhesis) vertebrae (spondyl/o)
    Term: spondylolisthesis
19. abnormal condition (-osis) vertebrae (spondyl/o)
    Term: spondylosis
20. abnormal condition (-osis) curvature (scoli/o)
    Term: scoliosis
21. abnormal condition (-osis) round back (kyph/o)
    Term: kyphosis

Exercise 11

1. costochondritis
2. Baker's cyst
3. bursitis
4. osteitis deformans
5. plantar fasciitis
6. rhabdomyolysis
7. osteomalacia
8. lateral epicondylitis
9. osteomyelitis

10. chondr/o (cartilage) + -malacia (softening)
    Def: softening of the cartilage
11. oste/o (bone) + -por/o (passage) + -osis
    (abnormal condition)
    **Def: abnormal condition of passages
    (empty spaces) in the bone**
12. tendin/o (tendon) + -itis (inflammation)
    Def: inflammation of a tendon
13. fibr/o (fiber) + my/o (muscle) + -algia (pain)
    Def: pain of muscle fiber

Exercise 12
1. A   2. D   3. F   4. G   5. I   6. E
7. B   8. H   9. C

Exercise 13
1. subluxation, dislocation
2. sprain
3. strain
4. compartment syndrome

Exercise 14
1. C   2. A   3. D   4. B

5. rhabdomy/o (skeletal muscle) -oma (tumor)
    Term: rhabdomyoma
6. oste/o (bone) -oma (tumor)
    Term: osteoma
7. leiomy/o (smooth muscle) -oma (tumor)
    Term: leiomyoma
8. chondr/o (cartilage) -oma (tumor)
    Term: chondroma
9. -osis (abnormal condition) ex- (out) oste/o (bone)
    Term: exostosis

Exercise 15
1. humerus; upper arm bone
2. closest to her shoulder
3. comminuted—crushed or shattered into
    multiple pieces
4. fibromyalgia
5. it hurts to move her arm in toward her body

Exercise 16
1. E   2. A   3. D   4. C   5. F   6. B
7. I   8. H   9. G

10. cutting out (-ectomy) dead bone (sequestr/o)
    Term: sequestrectomy
11. fixation (-pexy) kneecap (patell/a)
    Term: patellapexy
12. measuring (-metry) density (densit/o)
    Term: densitometry
13. cutting out (-ectomy) cartilage (chondr/o)
    Term: chondrectomy
14. surgically forming (-plasty) chin (geni/o)
    Term: genioplasty

15. breaking (-clasis) bone (oste/o)
    Term: osteoclasis
16. recording (-graphy) disc (disc/o)
    Term: discography

Exercise 17
1. I   2. H   3. C   4. G   5. A   6. D
7. B   8. E   9. F

10. arthr/o (joint) + -centesis (surgical puncture)
    Def: surgical puncture of a joint
11. arthr/o (joint) + -desis (binding)
    Def: binding a joint
12. my/o (muscle) + -pexy (fixation)
    Def: fixation of a muscle
13. electr/o (electricity) + my/o (muscle) + -graphy
    (recording)
    **Def: recording the electricity of a
    muscle**
14. ten/o (tendon) + my/o (muscle) + -plasty
    (surgically forming)
    **Def: surgically forming a tendon and
    muscle**

Exercise 18
1. bisphosphonates
2. disease-modifying antirheumatic drugs
    (DMARDs)
3. inflammation and pain
4. muscle relaxants

Exercise 19
1. osteoarthritis
2. the front of the knee
3. the kneecap
4. near the patella
5. cutting of a joint
6. turned out to the side
7. instrument to cut bone
8. extension beyond the normal range of motion

Chapter 3 Review

Word Part Definitions:
1. -desis
2. -algia
3. -centesis
4. -sarcoma
5. -malacia
6. -listhesis
7. peri-
8. -clasis
9. -physis
10. -osis
11. cleid/o
12. oste/o
13. gnath/o

14. rhabdomy/o
15. humer/o
16. carp/o
17. zygomat/o
18. femor/o
19. cervic/o
20. spondyl/o
21. chondr/o
22. myel/o
23. dactyl/o
24. phalang/o
25. cost/o
26. my/o
27. olecran/o
28. coccyg/o
29. patell/a
30. arthr/o
31. mandibul/o
32. scapul/o

Wordshop:
1. periosteum
2. polymyositis
3. intervertebral
4. chondromalacia
5. osteosarcoma
6. rhabdomyolysis
7. osteophytosis
8. arthrodesis
9. myopexy
10. chondroectomy
11. discography
12. spondylosyndesis
13. bursocentesis
14. leiomyoma
15. genioplasty

Term Sorting:
Anatomy and Physiology: articulation, cartilage, costa, diaphysis, digitus, endosteum, humerus, lamellae, ligament, osteogenesis, perichondrium, radius, scapula, sternum, ulna
Pathology: arthrosis, bunion, bursitis, chondromalacia, contracture, fibromyalgia, osteomyelitis, osteoporosis, osteosarcoma, rhabdomyoma, sciatica, SLE, spondylolisthesis, tendinitis, TMJ
Procedures: amputation, arthrocentesis, arthrodesis, arthrography, arthrotomy, carpectomy, densitometry, EMG, genioplasty, laminectomy, meniscectomy, osteoclasis, patellapexy, sacrectomy, scapulopexy

Translations:
1. chondromalacia, Baker's cyst
2. arthrocentesis, hemarthrosis
3. reduction, clavicle

4. osteophytoses, interphalangeal joints
5. kyphosis, osteoporosis
6. osteomyelitis, radius
7. plantar fasciitis, tendinitis
8. electromyography, polymyositis
9. greenstick, humerus
10. Colles' fracture, hairline fracture
11. bunionectomy, bunion
12. discectomy, herniated intervertebral disc
13. achillorrhaphy, sprain

Chapter 4

Exercise 1
1. B   2. I   3. M   4. A   5. E   6. H
7. F   8. J   9. C   10. K   11. D   12. G
13. L   14. N   15. O   16. P   17. Q

Exercise 2
1. the nail bed is the tissue under the nail; the nail plate is the actual nail
2. palm
3. an instrument for compression of blood vessels to control blood flow to and from the fingertip
4. the nail root

Exercise 3
1. E   2. F   3. C   4. A   5. B   6. D
7. C   8. D   9. A   10. E   11. B   12. D
13. E   14. C   15. A   16. B

Exercise 4
1. pemphigus
2. contact dermatitis
3. cellulitis
4. seborrheic dermatitis
5. pruritus
6. psoriasis
7. pilonidal cyst
8. impetigo
9. actinic keratosis
10. urticaria
11. furuncle
12. atopic dermatitis
13. inflammation (-itis) navel (omphal/o)
    Term: omphalitis
14. pertaining to (-al) hair (pil/o) nest (nid/o)
    Term: pilonidal
15. condition (-ia) nail (onych/o)
    Term: onychia
16. condition (-ia) beside (par-) nail (onych/o)
    Term: paronychia

Exercise 5
1. abnormal condition (-osis) curved (gryph/o) nail (onych/o)
    Term: onychogryphosis

2. softening (-malacia) nail (onych/o)
   Term: onychomalacia
3. abnormal condition (-osis) hidden (crypt-) nail (onych/o)
   Term: onychocryptosis
4. abnormal condition (-osis) excessive (hyper-) hair (trich/o)
   Term: hypertrichosis
5. inflammation (-itis) hair follicle (follicul/o)
   Term: folliculitis
6. abnormal condition (-osis) gray (poli/o)
   Term: poliosis
7. abnormal condition (-osis) no (an-) sweat (hidr/o)
   Term: anhidrosis
8. abnormal condition (-osis) odor (brom/o) sweat (hidr/o)
   Term: bromhidrosis
9. inflammation (-itis) sweat gland (hidraden/o)
   Term: hidradenitis
10. development (-trophy) abnormal (dys-) nail (onych/o)
    Term: onychodystrophy

Exercise 6
1. F   2. H   3. G   4. I   5. J   6. C
7. E   8. A   9. D   10. B

Exercise 7
1. D   2. C   3. F   4. B   5. H   6. A
7. G   8. E

9. pediculosis
10. herpes simplex virus
11. scabies
12. dermatomycosis

Exercise 8
1. C   2. A   3. D   4. B

Exercise 9
1. C   2. D   3. A   4. B

5. dermat/o (skin) + fibr/o (fiber) + -oma (tumor)
   Def: fibrous tumor of the skin
6. angi/o (vessel) + -oma (tumor)
   Def: tumor of a vessel
7. lip/o (fat) + -oma (tumor, mass)
   Def: fatty tumor

Exercise 10
1. excisional
2. needle aspiration
3. incisional
4. exfoliation
5. punch

6. F   7. C   8. E   9. B   10. G   11. A
12. D

Exercise 11
1. pruritic means pertaining to itching
2. no previous history of dermatitis
3. elevated and containing fluid
4. rash

Exercise 12
1. A. skin graft from self
   B. skin graft from another human
   C. skin graft from another species
2. full-thickness graft
3. dermatome
4. laser therapy
5. débridement
6. cauterization
7. cryosurgery
8. curettage
9. incision and drainage
10. shaving
11. occlusive therapy
12. Mohs surgery
13. cutting out (-ectomy) wrinkle (rhytid/o)
    Term: rhytidectomy
14. cutting out (-ectomy) fat (lip/o)
    Term: lipectomy
15. surgically forming (-plasty) eyelid (blephar/o)
    Term: blepharoplasty
16. scraping of (-abrasion) skin (derm/o)
    Term: dermabrasion
17. surgically forming (-plasty) skin (dermat/o)
    Term: dermatoplasty
18. surgically forming (-plasty) nail (onych/o)
    Term: onychoplasty

Exercise 13
1. D   2. C   3. A   4. B   5. E   6. G
7. F

Exercise 14
1. superficial partial-thickness burns extend into the papillary layer of the dermis
2. bulla, blisters, epidermal loss, erythema
3. circumscribed, elevated lesion containing fluid and smaller than ½ cm

Chapter 4 Review

Word Part Definitions:
1. hyper-
2. -osis
3. -lysis
4. -oma
5. -ule
6. crypt-
7. -derma
8. -itis
9. par-

10. -trophy
11. hidr/o
12. melan/o
13. onych/o or ungu/o
14. chrom/o
15. rhytid/o
16. follicul/o
17. vascul/o
18. papul/o
19. macul/o
20. vesicul/o
21. xer/o
22. ungu/o or onych/o
23. kerat/o
24. hidraden/o
25. cutane/o
26. pedicul/i
27. seb/o
28. eschar/o
29. squam/o
30. pil/o
31. adip/o
32. myc/o

Wordshop:
1. hypertrichosis
2. atrophy
3. rhytidectomy
4. seborrheic
5. paronychia
6. anhidrosis
7. blepharoplasty
8. onychomalacia
9. folliculitis
10. dyschromia
11. subcutaneous
12. dermatomycosis
13. dermatofibroma
14. onycholysis
15. onychocryptosis

Term Sorting:
Anatomy and Physiology: corium, cuticle, dermis, epidermis, eponychium, follicle, keratin, lunula, melanocyte, papilla, paronychium, perspiration, sebaceous gland, sebum
Pathology: alopecia, angioma, atrophy, dermatomycosis, dyschromia, eczema, furuncle, hyperhidrosis, onychomycosis, paronychia, plaque, tinea pedis, urticaria, verruca, vesicle
Procedures: allograft, blepharoplasty, curettage, cryosurgery, debridement, dermatoplasty, escharotomy, excisional bx, liposuction, Mantoux test, onychectomy, rhytidectomy, Tzanck test, Wood's light, xenograft

Translations:
1. tinea pedis
2. pruritus
3. hyperhidrosis
4. onychocryptosis, paronychia
5. keloid
6. impetigo, papules, vesicles
7. pediculosis
8. acne vulgaris
9. Mohs surgery, basal cell carcinoma (BCC)
10. verruca, cryosurgery
11. escharotomy, allograft
12. rhytidectomy, blepharoplasty
13. pressure ulcer, decubitus ulcer or bedsore

Chapter 5

Exercise 1
1. K   2. H   3. D   4. E   5. L   6. G
7. I   8. B   9. J   10. C   11. M   12. F
13. A

Exercise 2
1. L   2. H   3. F   4. I   5. D   6. G
7. B   8. M   9. J   10. K   11. A   12. C
13. O   14. N   15. E

Exercise 3
1. H   2. C   3. L   4. A   5. K   6. Q
7. J   8. M   9. N   10. S   11. B   12. E
13. G   14. O   15. T   16. P   17. R   18. I
19. F   20. D

Exercise 4
A:
1. H   2. I   3. M   4. G   5. N   6. L
7. O   8. J   9. F   10. B   11. P   12. E
13. D   14. K   15. A   16. C
B:
1. J   2. A   3. F   4. B   5. G   6. K
7. I   8. E   9. H   10. C   11. D

Exercise 5
1. G   2. D   3. A   4. C   5. B   6. E
7. F   8. H   9. M   10. K   11. I   12. L
13. J

Exercise 6
1. pharynx, esophagus, stomach, pylorus, duodenum
2. close to
3. the fundus
4. cardiac sphincter, gastroesophageal sphincter

Exercise 7
1. C   2. D   3. H   4. F   5. E   6. A
7. G   8. B

9. pain (-algia) stomach (gastr/o)
Term: gastralgia
10. difficult (dys-) swallowing condition (-phagia)
Term: dysphagia
11. abnormal condition (-osis) breath (halit/o)
Term: halitosis

Exercise 8
1. D   2. B   3. F   4. G   5. E   6. C
7. A   8. H

9. gingiv/o (gums) + -itis (inflammation)
Def: inflammation of the gums
10. gloss/o (tongue) + -itis (inflammation)
Def: inflammation of the tongue
11. an- (without) + odont/o (teeth) + -ia (condition)
Def: condition of being without teeth
12. sialoaden/o (salivary gland) + -itis (inflammation)
Def: inflammation of a salivary gland
13. cheil/o (lips) + -itis (inflammation)
Def: inflammation of the lips

Exercise 9
1. B   2. D   3. C   4. A

5. gastr/o (stomach) + -itis (inflammation)
Def: inflammation of the stomach
6. a- (without) + -chalasia (condition of relaxation)
Def: condition of not relaxing (of the LES)
7. dys- (bad, abnormal, painful) + -pepsia (digestion condition)
Def: condition of bad or painful digestion
8. esophag/o (esophagus) + -itis (inflammation)
Def: inflammation of the esophagus

Exercise 10
1. G   2. B   3. F   4. H   5. C   6. D
7. E   8. A

Exercise 11
1. J   2. H   3. F   4. K   5. D   6. I
7. C   8. B   9. G   10. E   11. A

12. drooping (-ptosis) rectum and anus (proct/o)
Term: proctoptosis
13. inflammation (-itis) diverticulum (diverticul/o)
Term: diverticulitis
14. inflammation (-itis) rectum and anus (proct/o)
Term: proctitis
15. abnormal condition (-osis) diverticulum (diverticul/o)
Term: diverticulosis

Exercise 12
1. B   2. C   3. A   4. D   5. F   6. E
7. G   8. H

9. inflammation (-itis) gallbladder (cholecyst/o)
Term: cholecystitis
10. inflammation (-itis) liver (hepat/o)
Term: hepatitis
11. presence of (-iasis) stones (lith/o) common bile duct (choledoch/o)
Term: choledocholithiasis
12. inflammation (-itis) bile vessels (cholangi/o)
Term: cholangitis
13. inflammation (-itis) peritoneum (peritone/o)
Term: peritonitis
14. inflammation (-itis) pancreas (pancreat/o)
Term: pancreatitis
15. vomiting (-emesis) blood (hemat/o)
Term: hematemesis

Exercise 13
1. polyps
2. hepatocellular carcinoma/hepatoma
3. adenocarcinoma
4. odontogenic tumor

Exercise 14
1. F   2. E   3. A   4. G   5. H   6. C
7. I   8. B   9. D   10. J

Exercise 15
1. D   2. C   3. B   4. G   5. E   6. J
7. H   8. I   9. A   10. F

11. palat/o (palate) + -plasty (surgically forming)
Def: surgically forming the palate
12. esophag/o (esophagus) + gastr/o (stomach) + duoden/o (duodenum) + -scopy (viewing)
Def: viewing the esophagus, stomach, and duodenum
13. gastr/o (stomach) + -plasty (surgically forming)
Def: surgically forming the stomach
14. stomat/o (mouth) + -plasty (surgically forming)
Def: surgically forming the mouth

Exercise 16
1. E   2. A   3. G   4. C   5. B   6. D
7. F

8. append/o (appendix) + -ectomy (cutting out)
Def: cutting out the appendix
9. colon/o (large intestine) + -scopy (viewing)
Def: viewing the large intestine
10. col/o (large intestine) + -stomy (making a new opening)
Def: making a new opening in the large intestine

11. peritone/o (peritoneum) + -centesis (surgical puncture)
    Def: surgical puncture of the peritoneum
12. proct/o (rectum and anus) + -clysis (washing)
    Def: cleansing the rectum and anus
13. herni/o (hernia) + -rrhaphy (suturing)
    Def: suturing a hernia

Exercise 17
1. recording (-graphy) bile vessel (cholangi/o)
   Term: cholangiography
2. cutting out (-ectomy) common bile duct (choledoch/o)
   Term: choledochectomy
3. cutting out (-ectomy) liver (hepat/o)
   Term: hepatectomy
4. cutting out a stone (-lithotomy) common bile duct (choledoch/o)
   Term: choledocholithotomy
5. cutting out (-ectomy) gallbladder (cholecyst/o)
   Term: cholecystectomy

Exercise 18
1. E   2. C   3. D   4. F   5. A   6. B

Exercise 19
1. colonoscopy
2. colonoscope
3. diverticula
4. pertaining to surrounding the rectum

Exercise 20
1. cholelithiasis means the condition of stones in the gallbladder
2. cholecystitis
3. laparoscopic cholecystectomy
4. back

Chapter 5 Review

Word Part Definitions:
1. -rrhea
2. -scopy
3. -stomy
4. -chalasia
5. -rrhaphy
6. -emesis
7. -iasis
8. -phagia
9. -stalsis
10. -pepsia
11. gloss/o
12. gingiv/o
13. lip/o
14. bil/i

15. esophag/o
16. sial/o
17. cholangi/o
18. choledoch/o
19. stomat/o
20. epiplo/o
21. gastr/o
22. proct/o
23. cheil/o
24. hepat/o
25. bucc/o
26. odont/o
27. an/o
28. cholecyst/o
29. pharyng/o
30. lumin/o
31. col/o
32. enter/o

Wordshop:
1. gastroesophageal
2. gastroplasty
3. periodontal
4. gastritis
5. colostomy
6. proctoclysis
7. esophagogastroduodenoscopy
8. cholecystectomy
9. gastrostomy
10. dysphagia
11. hepatomegaly
12. sialodochoplasty
13. glossorrhaphy
14. choledocholithiasis
15. anodontia

Term Sorting:
Anatomy and Physiology: chyme, defecation, deglutition, duodenum, esophagus, frenulum, ileum, mastication, omentum, peristalsis, philtrum, plicae, retroperitoneum, rugae
Pathology: achalasia, anodontia, anorectal fistula, aphthous stomatitis, appendicitis, ascites, cheilitis, cholelithiasis, cirrhosis, dyspepsia, femoral hernia, halitosis, ileus, ptyalism
Procedures: appendectomy, BE, cecopexy, cholangiography, enteral nutrition, ERCP, gastroplasty, glossorrhaphy, herniorrhaphy, hyperalimentation, peritoneocentesis, sialoadenectomy, stomatoplasty, total bilirubin

Translations:
1. colonoscopy, polypectomy
2. hepatitis, jaundice
3. inguinal hernia, herniorrhaphy
4. stool guaiac test
5. cholelithiasis, cholecystectomy

6. colostomy, Crohn's disease
7. flatus, diarrhea
8. appendicitis, peritonitis
9. gingivitis, periodontal disease
10. dyspepsia, gastralgia, pyrosis
11. peritoneocentesis, ascites
12. anastomosis, gastroduodenostomy

Chapter 6

Exercise 1
1. C   2. F   3. D   4. A   5. E   6. G
7. B   8. L   9. J   10. H   11. M   12. I
13. K

14. trans- (through) + urethr/o (urethra) + -al (pertaining to)
    Def: pertaining to through the urethra
15. para- (near) + nephr/o (kidney) + -ic (pertaining to)
    Def: pertaining to near the kidney
16. retro- (backward) + peritone/o (peritoneum) + -al (pertaining to)
    Def: pertaining to backward (behind) of the peritoneum
17. supra- (above) + ren/o (kidney) + -al (pertaining to)
    Def: pertaining to above the kidney
18. peri- (around) + vesic/o (bladder) + -al (pertaining to)
    Def: pertaining to around the bladder

Exercise 2
1. K   2. O   3. G   4. B   5. M   6. A
7. F   8. N   9. C   10. L   11. I   12. D
13. J   14. E   15. H   16. P

17. painful (dys-) urinary condition (-uria)
    Term: dysuria
18. excessive, frequent (poly-) urinary condition (-uria)
    Term: polyuria
19. abnormal condition (-osis) water (hydr/o) kidney (nephr/o)
    Term: hydronephrosis

Exercise 3
1. H   2. B   3. E   4. L   5. A   6. I
7. C   8. G   9. K   10. D   11. F   12. J
13. M

14. nephr/o (kidney) + -ptosis (drooping, prolapse)
    Def: drooping or prolapse of the kidney
15. cyst/o (urinary bladder) + -itis (inflammation)
    Def: inflammation of the urinary bladder

16. nephr/o (kidney) + blast/o (embryonic) + -oma (tumor)
    Def: embryonic tumor of the kidney

Exercise 4
1. J   2. A   3. D   4. H   5. B   6. G
7. E   8. I   9. C   10. F

11. cutting out (-ectomy) bladder (cyst/o)
    Term: cystectomy
12. complete (dia-) breaking down (-lysis) blood (hem/o)
    Term: hemodialysis
13. removing a stone (-lithotomy) kidney (nephr/o)
    Term: nephrolithotomy
14. crushing (-tripsy) stone (lith/o)
    Term: lithotripsy

Exercise 5
1. D   2. E   3. A   4. F   5. C   6. B

Exercise 6
1. post lithotripsy
2. urinary incontinence
3. ureter
4. lithotripsy
5. voiding okay
6. no edema

Exercise 7
1. D   2. K   3. A   4. G   5. B   6. I
7. J   8. L   9. H   10. F   11. E   12. C

Exercise 8
1. D   2. F   3. H   4. J   5. L   6. E
7. I   8. A   9. K   10. G   11. M   12. B
13. C

14. inflammation (-itis) glans penis (balan/o)
    Term: balanitis
15. condition (-ia) no (a-) living, animal (zo/o) sperm (sperm/o)
    Term: azoospermia
16. inflammation (-itis) prostate (prostat/o)
    Term: prostatitis
17. herniation, protrusion (-cele) water, fluid (hydr/o)
    Term: hydrocele
18. inflammation (-itis) glans penis (balan/o), foreskin (posth/o)
    Term: balanoposthitis

Exercise 9
1. condylomata
2. syphilis
3. nongonococcal urethritis
4. gonorrhea
5. chancres

6. asymptomatic
7. human papillomavirus
8. herpes simplex virus-2 (HSV-2)

Exercise 10
1. C   2. E   3. D   4. B   5. A

6. tumor (-oma) semen (semin/i)
   Term: seminoma
7. gland (aden/o) cancer of epithelial origin
   (-carcinoma)
   Term: adenocarcinoma

Exercise 11
1. F   2. B   3. A   4. K   5. D   6. C
7. G   8. J   9. E   10. H   11. I

12. surgically forming (-plasty) glans penis (balan/o)
    Term: balanoplasty
13. suspending (-pexy) testis (orchi/o)
    Term: orchiopexy
14. recording (-graphy) epididymis (epididym/o)
    seminal vesicle (vesicul/o)
    Term: epididymovesiculography
15. tying (-ligation) vessel (vas/o)
    Term: vasoligation

Exercise 12
1. D   2. A   3. B   4. E   5. C

Exercise 13
1. BPH is abnormal enlargement of the prostate
   gland around the urethra, leading to difficulty
   in urination.
2. A. painful urination
   B. inability to hold urine
   C. need to urinate more frequently than usual
      or normal
   D. blood in the urine
3. two lobes
4. transurethral resection of the prostate
5. around or surrounding the prostate

Exercise 14
1. E   2. F   3. A   4. A   5. B   6. G
7. C   8. D   9. F   10. A   11. B   12. H
13. I

14. supra- (above) + cervic/o (cervix) + -al
    (pertaining to)
    Def: pertaining to above the cervix
15. intra- (within) + uter/o (uterus) + -ine
    (pertaining to)
    Def: pertaining to within the uterus
16. pre- (before) + menstru/o (menstruation) + -al
    (pertaining to)
    Def: pertaining to before menstruation

17. trans- (through) + vagin/o (vagina) + -al
    (pertaining to)
    Def: pertaining to through the vagina

Exercise 15
1. B, J   2. D, F   3. G   4. A, I   5. L   6. E, K
7. H   8. C   9. M

10. inter- (between) + labi/o (labia) + -al
    (pertaining to)
    Def: pertaining to between the labia
11. intra- (within) + mamm/o (breast) + -ary
    (pertaining to)
    Def: pertaining to within the breast

Exercise 16
1. galact/o (milk) + -rrhea (discharge, flow)
   Def: discharge of milk
2. gynec/o (female) + mast/o (breast) + -ia
   (condition)
   Def: female breast condition
3. mast/o (breast) + -dynia (pain)
   Def: pain of the breast
4. mast/o (breast) + -ptosis (sagging)
   Def: sagging of the breast
5. bartholin/o (Bartholin's gland) + -itis
   (inflammation)
   **Def: inflammation of a Bartholin's
   gland**
6. cervic/o (cervix) + -itis (inflammation)
   Def: inflammation of the cervix
7. oophor/o (ovary) + -itis (inflammation)
   Def: inflammation of the ovary
8. salping/o (fallopian tube) + -itis (inflammation)
   Def: inflammation of a fallopian tube
9. vulv/o (vulva) + -itis (inflammation)
   Def: inflammation of the vulva

Exercise 17
1. polymenorrhea
2. menometrorrhagia
3. amenorrhea
4. metrorrhagia
5. menorrhagia
6. oligomenorrhea
7. dysmenorrhea
8. dysfunctional uterine bleeding
9. premenstrual syndrome
10. postmenopausal bleeding
11. cervical intraepithelial neoplasia
12. herniation (-cele) urinary bladder (cyst/o)
    Term: cystocele
13. painful (dys-) intercourse (-pareunia)
    Term: dyspareunia
14. pertaining to (-al) endometrium (endometri/o)
    excessive (hyper-) development (-plasia)
    Term: endometrial hyperplasia

15. abnormal condition (-osis) endometrium (endometri/o)
    Term: endometriosis
16. blood (hemat/o) fallopian tube (-salpinx)
    Term: hematosalpinx
17. drooping (-ptosis) uterus (hyster/o)
    Term: hysteroptosis
18. herniation (-cele) rectum (rect/o)
    Term: rectocele
19. pain (-dynia) vulva (vulv/o)
    Term: vulvodynia

Exercise 18
1. D   2. C   3. B   4. A   5. E   6. G
7. K   8. J   9. I   10. H   11. F

Exercise 19
1. C   2. B   3. L   4. O   5. H   6. P
7. F   8. J   9. G   10. N   11. Q   12. I
13. K   14. M   15. A   16. E   17. D

18. hyster/o (uterus) + trachel/o (cervix) + -plasty (surgically forming)
    Def: surgically forming the uterine cervix
19. colp/o (vagina) + -pexy (suspending)
    Def: suspending of the vagina
20. hyster/o (uterus) + salping/o (fallopian tube) + -graphy (recording)
    Def: recording of the uterus and fallopian tubes
21. salping/o (fallopian tube) + -lysis (breaking down)
    Def: breaking down (adhesions) of the fallopian tubes
22. mamm/o (breast) + -plasty (surgically forming)
    Def: surgically forming the breast

Exercise 20
1. total abdominal hysterectomy
2. bilateral salpingo-oophorectomy (TAH-BSO)
3. dyspareunia
4. endometriosis
5. dysmenorrhea
6. menorrhagia
7. supine position
8. low transverse incision

Chapter 6 Review

Word Part Definitions–Urinary:
1. -lithotomy
2. -iasis
3. -lysis
4. -tripsy
5. -osis
6. -scopy
7. -pexy
8. -ptosis
9. -uria
10. -esis
11. hydr/o
12. cyst/o or vesic/o
13. ureter/o
14. py/o
15. noct/i
16. trigon/o
17. urethr/o
18. ur/o
19. lith/o
20. meat/o
21. nephr/o or ren/o
22. olig/o
23. glomerul/o
24. ren/o or nephr/o
25. calic/o
26. pyel/o
27. hil/o
28. vesic/o or cyst/o
29. cortic/o

Wordshop–Urinary:
1. perivesical
2. nephrolithotomy
3. cystoscope
4. trigonitis
5. dysuria
6. hematuria
7. nephropathy
8. ureterolithiasis
9. anuria
10. lithotripsy
11. uremia
12. hemodialysis
13. polyuria
14. urethrolysis
15. nephrostomy

Term Sorting–Urinary:
Anatomy and Physiology: calyx, cortex, glomeruli, hilum, loop of Henle, medulla, micturition, nephron, parenchymal tissue, renal corpuscle, renal pelvis, trigone, urethra, urinary meatus, urine
Pathology: ARF, CKD, cystitis, enuresis, hematuria, hydronephrosis, incontinence, nephroblastoma, nephroptosis, nocturia, pyonephrosis, renal adenoma, urethral stricture UTI, urolithiasis
Procedures: BUN, CAPD, cystectomy, cystoscopy, GFR, hemodialysis, lithotripsy, meatotomy, nephrolithotomy, nephropexy, nephrostomy, renal dialysis, urethrolysis, urinalysis, vesicotomy

Translations—Urinary:
1. urinary retention, vesical tenesmus
2. blood urea nitrogen (BUN), creatinine clearance test
3. hematuria, urolithiasis
4. nephrolithiasis, lithotripsy
5. urinary tract infection (UTI), enuresis
6. cystoscope, interstitial cystitis
7. oliguria, extrarenal uremia
8. nephroptosis, nephropexy
9. hydronephrosis
10. pyonephrosis
11. vesicoureteral reflux
12. renal dialysis, renal transplant

Word Part Definitions—Reproductive:
1. trans-
2. hyper-
3. -salpinx
4. -one
5. -rrhea
6. -rrhagia
7. -ptosis
8. -cele
9. a-
10. -ligation
11. -genesis
12. -plasia
13. semin/i
14. balan/o
15. orchid/o
16. preputi/o
17. vesicul/o
18. phall/o
19. vas/o
20. olig/o
21. trachel/o
22. galact/o
23. mamm/o
24. leiomy/o
25. o/o
26. men/o
27. colp/o
28. hyster/o
29. culd/o
30. salping/o
31. oophor/o
32. episi/o

Wordshop—Reproductive:
1. oligospermia
2. vesiculitis
3. hysterosalpingography
4. balanoplasty
5. dysmenorrhea
6. galactorrhea

7. mastoptosis
8. vasoligation
9. endometriosis
10. azoospermia
11. colpopexy
12. polymenorrhea
13. epididymotomy
14. hysterotracheloplasty

Term Sorting—Reproductive:
Anatomy and Physiology: areola, corpora cavernosa, corpus luteum, epididymis, gametes, menarche, menopause, menstruation, mons pubis, ovulation, prepuce, puberty, rectouterine pouch, spermatogenesis, tunica vaginalis
Pathology: amenorrhea, BPH, endometriosis, epididymitis, hematosalpinx, HPV, hysteroptosis, leiomyosarcoma, menorrhagia, mittelschmerz, oligospermia, PID, seminoma, vulvodynia
Procedures: colposcopy, D&C, epididymotomy, epididymo-vesiculography, hysteropexy, mammoplasty, oophorectomy, orchiopexy, phalloplasty, prostatectomy, salpingolysis, tubal ligation, TUIP, vasoligation, vasovasostomy

Translations—Reproductive:
1. oligospermia
2. dysmenorrhea, dyspareunia
3. benign prostatic hyperplasia (BPH), transurethral incision of the prostate (TUIP)
4. mastectomy, infiltrating ductal carcinoma (IDC)
5. circumcision, phimosis
6. hysterosalpingography, salpingitis
7. vasectomy, vasovasostomy
8. hysterectomy, leiomyosarcoma
9. orchidectomy, nonseminoma
10. mastoptosis, mastodynia
11. epididymo-vesiculography, spermatocele of epididymis

Chapter 7

Exercise 1
1. E 2. L 3. H 4. K 5. A 6. G
7. D 8. I 9. J 10. C 11. B 12. F
13. M

14. multigravida
15. blastocyst
16. dizygotic, monozygotic
17. zygote, embryo, fetus
18. amnion, chorion
19. umbilical cord
20. parturition
21. none

Exercise 2

1. G   2. C   3. N   4. K   5. D   6. I
7. A   8. L   9. E   10. M   11. B   12. J
13. F   14. H

15. chori/o (chorion) + -carcinoma (cancer of epithelial origin)
Def: cancer of the chorionic membrane
16. hypo- (deficient) galact/o (milk) + -ia (condition)
Def: condition of deficient milk production
17. poly- (excessive) + hydr/o (water, fluid) + -amnios (amnion)
Def: excessive amniotic fluid
18. placent/o (placenta) + -itis (inflammation)
Def: inflammation of the placenta

Exercise 3

1. D   2. A   3. C   4. E   5. B

6. amni/o (amnion) + -centesis (surgical puncture)
Def: surgical puncture of the amnion
7. episi/o (vulva) + -tomy (cutting)
Def: cutting of the vulva
8. pelv/i (pelvis) + -metry (measuring)
Def: measuring the pelvis

Exercise 4

1. OCP
2. barrier method
3. condoms
4. IUDs
5. abortifacient
6. rhythm method
7. abstinence
8. spermicides
9. ECP

Exercise 5

1. increase
2. induce
3. tocolytics

Exercise 6

1. third trimester
2. low or missing amniotic fluid
3. umbilical cord wrapped around the neck of the neonate
4. across horizontally
5. abnormal condition of pregnancy marked by hypertension, edema, and proteinuria

Exercise 7

1. B   2. D   3. C   4. A

5. -itis (inflammation) omphal/o (umbilicus)
Term: omphalitis (of the newborn)
6. -osis (abnormal condition) erythr/o (red blood cell) blast/o (immature)
Term: erythroblastosis fetalis
7. -ia (condition, state of) macro- (large) som/o (body)
Term: macrosomia

Exercise 8

1. kernicterus
2. neonatal hypertension
3. hyaline membrane syndrome
4. ophthalmia neonatorum
5. neonatal craniotabes
6. hydrops fetalis
7. meconium staining
8. congenital hypotonia
9. hypothermia of newborn

Exercise 9

1. F   2. A   3. C   4. H   5. E   6. G
7. D   8. B

9. -y (process of) syn- (joined, together) dactyl/o (fingers, toes)
Term: syndactyly
10. -plasia (condition of formation) a- (no, not, without) chondr/o (cartilage)
Term: achondroplasia
11. -y (process of) poly- (many, much) dactyl/o (fingers, toes)
Term: polydactyly
12. gastr/o (stomach) + -schisis (split)
Def: split stomach (opening in abdomen)
13. omphal/o (umbilicus) + -cele (herniation, protrusion)
Def: umbilical herniation
14. ankyl/o (stiffening) gloss/o (tongue) -ia (condition)
Def: condition of stiffened tongue
15. -ia (condition) crypt- (hidden) orchid/o (testis)
Term: cryptorchidism
16. -ism (condition) an- (no, not, without) orch/o (testis)
Term: anorchism
17. epi- (above) -spadias (a rent or tear)
Term: epispadias
18. hypo- (below) -spadias (a rent or tear)
Term: hypospadias

Exercise 10

1. B   2. C   3. D   4. A   5. E   6. F

7. levo (left) + -cardia (heart condition)
Def: left side heart condition
8. dextr/o (right) + -cardia (heart condition)
Def: right side heart condition

9. trache/o (trachea) + -malacia (condition of softening)
   Def: condition of softening of the trachea
10. crani/o (skull) + rach/i (vertebra) + -schisis (split)
    Def: split of the skull and vertebra
11. an- (no, not, without) + encephal/o (brain) + -y (noun ending)
    Def: without brain
12. trache/o (trachea) -stenosis (narrowing)
    Term: tracheostenosis
13. hydr/o (water) -cephalus (head)
    Term: hydrocephalus
14. -ia (condition) macro- (large) ot/o (ear)
    Term: macrotia
15. -ia (condition) micro- (small) ot/o (ear)
    Term: microtia

Exercise 11
1. large for gestational age
2. abnormal
3. patent ductus arteriosus, patent foramen ovale
4. jaundice or hyperbilirunemia
5. transient tachypnea of newborn

Chapter 7 Review

Word Part Definitions-Pregnancy and the Perinatal Period:
1. primi-
2. neo-
3. -para, -tocia
4. -metry
5. multi-
6. nulli-
7. peri-
8. -rrhea
9. -para, -tocia
10. ante-
11. -amnios
12. post-
13. -gravida
14. blast/o
15. gravid/o
16. galact/o
17. cret/o
18. nat/o
19. cephal/o
20. prurit/o
21. amni/o
22. episi/o
23. troph/o
24. hydatid/i
25. olig/o
26. part/o
27. chori/o
28. pelv/i
29. omphal/o
30. placent/o
31. hydr/o

Wordshop-Pregnancy and the Perinatal Period:
1. trophoblast
2. diamniotic
3. ectopic
4. nulligravida
5. postnatal
6. primipara
7. cephalopelvic
8. chorioamnionitis
9. oligohydramnios
10. polyhydramnios
11. dystocia
12. agalactia
13. episiotomy
14. blastocyst
15. monochorionic

Term Sorting-Pregnancy and the Perinatal Period:
Anatomy and Physiology: allantois, amnion, blastocyst, chorion, EDD, embryo, gestation, gravida, hCG, LMP, morula, parturition, placenta, puerperium, zygote
Pathology: abruptio placentae, chorioamnionitis, choriocarcinoma, dystocia, erythroblastosis fetalis, HELLP syndrome, hydatidiform mole, hyperemesis gravidarum, hypogalactia, oligohydramnios, placenta accreta, placentitis, preeclampsia, PUPP, TTTS
Procedures: AFP, amniocentesis, cephalic version, cerclage, C-section, CST, CVS, episiotomy, pelvimetry, VBAC

Translations-Pregnancy and the Perinatal Period:
1. pelvimetry, cephalopelvic disproportion
2. amniocentesis
3. neonate, nuchal cord
4. hyperemesis gravidarum, gestational phlebitis
5. breech presentation, cephalic version
6. ectopic pregnancy
7. primigravida, cerclage
8. abruptio placentae, cesarean section (CS)
9. twin-to-twin transfusion syndrome (TTTS)
10. episiotomy
11. hypogalactia
12. dystocia, puerperal sepsis

Word Part Definitions-Congenital Conditions:
1. micro-
2. poly-

3. -cele
4. tetra-
5. syn-
6. -cardia
7. -malacia
8. crypt-
9. a-, an-
10. -schisis
11. -stenosis
12. -spadias
13. epi-
14. macro-
15. levo-
16. hypo-
17. crani/o
18. ankyl/o
19. dextr/o
20. trache/o
21. ot/o
22. gastr/o
23. chondr/o
24. cephal/o
25. omphal/o
26. encephal/o
27. orch/o
28. dactyl/o

Wordshop-Congenital Conditions:

1. levocardia
2. tracheomalacia
3. macrotia
4. gastroschisis
5. omphalocele
6. anencephaly
7. polydactyly
8. achondroplasia
9. ankyloglossia
10. hydrocephalus
11. tracheostenosis
12. anorchism
13. cryptorchidism
14. hypospadias
15. dextrocardia

Term Sorting-Congenital Conditions:
Digestive: ankyloglossia, esophageal atresia, gastroschisis, Hirschsprung's disease, levocardia, omphalocele, pyloric stenosis
Circulatory: coarctation of the aorta, dextrocardia, PDA, septal defect, tetralogy of Fallot
Musculoskeletal: achondroplasia, polydactyly, spinal bifida occulta, syndactyly, talipes, torticollis
Male Repro: anarchism, chordee, cryptorchidism, epispadias, hypospadias

Translations-Congenital Conditions:

1. polydactyly, syndactyly
2. spina bifida occulta
3. cleft palate, palatoplasty
4. orchiopexy, cryptorchidism
5. patent ductus arteriosus (PDA)
6. tetralogy of Fallot
7. spina bifida, meningocele or meningomyelocele
8. macrotia, otoplasty
9. pyloric stenosis, pyloromyotomy
10. hypospadias, balanoplasty
11. hydrocephalus, ventriculoperitoneostomy

Chapter 8

Exercise 1
A:

1. I	2. J	3. E	4. A	5. M	6. K
7. L	8. F	9. D	10. C	11. H	12. G
13. B	14. N				

B:

1. J	2. A	3. E	4. H	5. I	6. B
7. G	8. D	9. C	10. F		

11. poly- (many) + nucle/o (nucleus) + -ar (pertaining to)
    Def: pertaining to many nuclei
12. a- (without) + granul/o (little grain) + cyt/o (cell) + -ic (pertaining to)
    Def: pertaining to cells without little grains
13. lymphat/o (lymph) + -ic (pertaining to)
    Def: pertaining to lymph
14. a- (without) + nucle/o (nucleus) + -ar (pertaining to)
    Def: pertaining to without a nucleus
15. poly- (many) + morph/o (shape) + -ic (pertaining to)
    Def: pertaining to many shapes

Exercise 2
1. A, B, AB, O
2. antigens
3. A and AB
4. donor, recipient
5. Rh factor

Exercise 3
1. Nonspecific immunity is a general defense against pathogens. Specific immunity involves recognition of a given pathogen and a reaction against it.
2. mechanical: skin, mucus; physical: sneezing, coughing, vomiting, diarrhea; chemical: saliva, tears, perspiration

3. phagocytes via neutrophils and monocytes, inflammation, fever, protective proteins
4. active artificial
5. passive natural
6. passive artificial
7. active natural

8. B   9. F   10. D   11. E   12. C
13. A   14. G   15. H   16. I   17. J

Exercise 4
1. K   2. C   3. D   4. F   5. A   6. H
7. B   8. J   9. E   10. I   11. G

12. iron (sider/o) condition of deficiency (-penia)
   Term: sideropenia
13. blood (hem/o) protein (globin/o) disease process (-pathy)
   Term: hemoglobinopathy
14. red (erythr/o) embryonic, immature (blast/o) condition of deficiency (-penia)
   Term: erythroblastopenia
15. wasting (-phthisis) bone marrow (myel/o)
   Term: myelophthisis
16. all (pan-) cell (cyt/o) condition of deficiency (-penia)
   Term: pancytopenia

Exercise 5
1. A   2. D   3. E   4. H   5. N   6. K
7. I   8. G   9. J   10. M   11. F   12. B
13. L   14. C   15. O

16. thromb/o (clotting) + cyt/o (cell) + -penia (condition of deficiency
   Def: condition of deficiency of clotting cells
17. eosin/o (rosy-colored) + -philia (condition of attraction)
   Def: condition of attraction to pink
18. plasm/a (plasma) + -cytosis (condition of abnormal increase of cells)
   Def: condition of abnormal increase of plasma cells
19. a- (without, no) + splen/o (spleen) + -ia (condition)
   Def: condition of no spleen
20. septic/o (infection) + -emia (blood condition)
   Def: condition of infection in the blood

Exercise 6
1. E   2. A   3. F   4. B   5. C   6. D

Exercise 7
1. G   2. I   3. B   4. D   5. F   6. H
7. A   8. E   9. C   10. J

Exercise 8
1. I   2. H   3. G   4. A   5. B   6. J
7. K   8. D   9. A   10. D   11. C   12. E
13. F

Exercise 9
1. potassium (K) level = 3.7
2. sodium level = 142
3. BU or bun = 15

Exercise 10
1. E   2. D   3. C   4. A   5. F   6. B

7. cutting out (-ectomy) spleen (splen/o)
   Term: splenectomy
8. cutting out (-ectomy) pharyngeal tonsils (adenoid/o)
   Term: adenoidectomy
9. stopping (-stasis) blood (hem/o)
   Term: hemostasis
10. cutting out (-ectomy) lymph node (lymphaden/o)
   Term: lymphadenectomy

Exercise 11
1. J   2. C   3. E   4. I   5. B   6. A
7. H   8. G   9. F   10. D

Exercise 12
1. mildly pyrexic
2. pharyngeal inflammation
3. cervic/o (neck) + -al (pertaining to) lymphaden/o (lymph gland) + -pathy (disease)
   Def: lymph gland disease pertaining to the neck
4. splenomegaly
5. lymphocytosis

Exercise 13
1. Principal Diagnosis: Sickle Cell Crisis
2. No. His mother and father have sickle cell trait. Those who have the trait do not exhibit symptoms of sickle cell disease.
3. appendix

Chapter 8 Review

Word Part Definitions:
1. -cyte
2. -gen
3. -cytosis
4. -globin
5. -poiesis
6. -phthisis
7. -philia
8. -penia

9. -siderin
10. -emia
11. hem/o
12. eosin/o
13. phag/o
14. nucle/o
15. sider/o
16. myel/o
17. splen/o
18. pyr/o
19. erythr/o
20. thromb/o
21. fibrin/o
22. cyt/o
23. globin/o
24. immun/o
25. leuk/o
26. ser/o
27. granul/o
28. plasm/o
29. thym/o
30. lymph/o
31. morph/o
32. tonsill/o

Wordshop:
1. pancytopenia
2. leukocytosis
3. eosinophilia
4. thrombocytopenia
5. lymphadenectomy
6. erythrocytosis
7. asplenia
8. erythroblastopenia
9. agranulocyte
10. anemia
11. hemosiderin
12. sideropenia
13. polymorphonucleocyte
14. hemoglobinopathy
15. myelophthisis

Term Sorting:
Anatomy and Physiology: agglutinogen, antigen, cytokine, eosinophil, hematopoiesis, hemoglobin, homeostasis, interferon, interleukin, monokine, morphology, phagocytosis, plasma, prothrombin, thrombocyte
Pathology: CML, DIC, erythroblastopenia, G6PD, hemoglobinopathy, hemophilia, monocytosis, myelophthisis, purpura, sarcoidosis, septicemia, sickle cell trait, sideropenia, splenitis, thalassemia
Procedures: adenoidectomy, apheresis, autotransfusion, BMP, BMT, CBC, CMP, diff count, ELISA, Hct, lymphadenectomy, MCH, Schilling test, splenectomy

Translations:
1. splenitis, splenectomy
2. pancytopenia, aplastic anemia
3. leukocytosis, blood culture
4. graft-versus-host disease (GVHD)
5. bone marrow transplant (BMT), acute myelogenous leukemia (AML)
6. sickle cell crisis, hypersplenism
7. plateletpheresis, thrombocytopenia
8. acute posthemorrhagic anemia, blood transfusion
9. myelophthisis
10. hemophilia, partial thromboplastin time (PTT)

Chapter 9

Exercise 1
1. D, F   2. E   3. G   4. K   5. B   6. J
7. I   8. A, C, H

9. endo- (within) + vascul/o (vessel) + -ar (pertaining to)
   Def: pertaining to within the vessel
10. intra- (within) + ven/o (vein) + -ous (pertaining to)
    Def: pertaining to within a vein
11. peri- (surrounding) + cardi/o (heart) + -al (pertaining to)
    Def: pertaining to surrounding the heart

Exercise 2
A:
1. E	2. G	3. N	4. L	5. I	6. A
7. J	8. D	9. H	10. M	11. F	12. K
13. B	14. C	15. O	16. P	17. Q	18. R

B:
1. I	2. H	3. L	4. D	5. J	6. N
7. M	8. S	9. Q	10. T	11. R	12. P
13. E	14. B	15. G	16. K	17. C	18. O
19. A	20. F				

Exercise 3
A:
| 1. G | 2. H | 3. C | 4. D | 5. B | 6. F |
| 7. I | 8. A | 9. E | 10. J | | |

B:
| 1. J | 2. E | 3. B | 4. H | 5. I | 6. C |
| 7. D | 8. A | 9. F | 10. G | 11. K | |

Exercise 4
A:
| 1. G | 2. E | 3. D | 4. F | 5. I | 6. B |
| 7. H | 8. J | 9. A | 10. C | | |

B:
| 1. G | 2. C | 3. J | 4. F | 5. H | 6. E |
| 7. I | 8. D | 9. B | 10. A | 11. K | |

Exercise 5

A:

1. I	2. F	3. J	4. E	5. C	6. G
7. A	8. H	9. M	10. D	11. K	12. L
13. B	14. N				

B:

1. E	2. N	3. H	4. M	5. O	6. D
7. J	8. K	9. F	10. C	11. L	12. G
13. I	14. A	15. B			

Exercise 6

A:

1. D	2. H	3. K	4. F	5. J	6. C
7. E	8. B	9. I	10. A	11. L	12. G

B:

1. A	2. I	3. D	4. L	5. O	6. G
7. N	8. P	9. F	10. C	11. K	12. M
13. E	14. J	15. H	16. B		

Exercise 7

A:

1. J	2. H	3. L	4. O	5. G	6. C
7. A	8. D	9. M	10. N	11. B	12. E
13. F	14. P	15. K	16. I	17. R	18. Q

B:

1. I	2. F	3. L	4. D	5. N	6. J
7. K	8. O	9. C	10. E	11. Q	12. M
13. B	14. A	15. G	16. P	17. H	
18. R					

Exercise 8

1. during
2. neck, brain
3. within
4. narrowing

Exercise 9

1. A	2. I	3. E	4. F	5. C	6. H
7. J	8. D	9. G	10. B		

11. brady- (slow) + -cardia (heart condition)
    Def: condition of slow heart(beat)
12. orth/o (straight) + -pnea (breathing)
    Def: difficulty breathing unless straight (upright)
13. cardi/o (heart) + -algia (pain)
    Def: heart pain

Exercise 10

1. C	2. D	3. E	4. A	5. B

Exercise 11

1. dysrhythmia
2. fibrillation
3. flutter
4. block
5. sick sinus syndrome
6. premature ventricular contractions, premature ventricular depolarizations
7. ventricular tachycardia
8. acute cor pulmonale
9. mitral stenosis
10. mitral regurgitation
11. cardi/o (heart) + -megaly (enlargement)
    Def: enlargement of the heart
12. tachy- (rapid) + -cardia (heart condition)
    Def: condition of rapid heart (beat)
13. endocardi/o (endocardium) + -itis (inflammation)
    Def: inflammation of the endocardium
14. cardiomy/o (heart muscle) + -pathy (disease condition)
    Def: disease condition of the heart muscle
15. pericardi/o (pericardium) + -itis (inflammation)
    Def: inflammation of the pericardium
16. pulmon/o (lung) + -ary (pertaining to) hyper- (excessive) + -tension (pressure)
    Def: excessive pressure pertaining to the lungs

Exercise 12

1. C	2. K	3. A	4. J	5. D	6. H
7. B	8. L	9. F	10. I	11. E	12. G
13. N	14. O	15. M			

16. vascul/o (vessel) + -itis (inflammation)
    Def: inflammation of a vessel
17. arteri/o (artery) + -sclerosis (hardening)
    Def: hardening of the arteries
18. thromb/o (clot) + phleb/o (vein) + -itis (inflammation)
    Def: inflammation and clot in a vein
19. hypo- (below, deficient) + tens/o (stretching) + -ion (process of)
    Def: condition of below (normal) blood pressure
20. a- (without) + phas/o (speech) + -ia (condition)
    Def: condition of without speech
21. mono- (one) + -plegia (paralysis)
    Def: paralysis of one (body part)

Exercise 13

1. lymphaden/o (lymph gland) + -pathy (disease state)
    Def: disease state of a lymph gland
2. splen/o (spleen) + -megaly (enlargement)
    Def: enlargement of the spleen
3. lymphangi/o (lymph vessel) + -ectasis (dilation)
    Def: dilation of a lymph vessel
4. lymph/o (lymph fluid) + -edema (swelling)
    Def: swelling (due to) lymph fluid

5. lymphangi/o (lymph vessel) + -itis (inflammation)
   Def: inflammation of a lymph vessel
6. lymphaden/o (lymph gland) + -itis (inflammation)
   Def: inflammation of a lymph gland

Exercise 14
1. D   2. A   3. C   4. B

5. hemangioma
6. cardiac myxosarcoma
7. atrial myxoma
8. hemangiosarcoma

Exercise 15
1. coronary arteries
2. normal heart rhythm (beat)
3. arrhythmia
4. the upper chambers of the heart
5. enlarged

Exercise 16
1. J   2. A   3. F   4. I   5. E   6. D
7. B   8. H   9. G   10. C

11. spleen (splen/o) fixing (-pexy)
    Term: splenopexy
12. heart (cardi/o) turning (-version)
    Term: cardioversion
13. crushing (-tripsy) vein (ven/o)
    Term: venotripsy
14. lymph vessel (lymphangi/o) -graphy (recording)
    Term: lymphangiography
15. suturing (-rrhaphy) artery (arteri/o)
    Term: arteriorrhaphy
16. vessel (angi/o) surgically forming (-plasty)
    Term: angioplasty
17. sac surrounding the heart (pericardi/o) releasing (-lysis)
    Term: pericardiolysis
18. valve (valvul/o) surgically forming part or all (-plasty)
    Term: valvuloplasty

Exercise 17
1. C   2. A, C, D   3. A, E   4. A, D, E   5. A, D, E
6. A, E   7. B   8. F   9. G

Exercise 18
1. A. difficult or painful breathing
   B. profuse sweating
   C. high blood pressure
2. substernal—below the breastbone
3. extremities had no cyanosis or clubbing

4. echocardiography
5. coronary artery bypass graft, CABG
6. the lungs

Chapter 9 Review

Word Part Definitions:
1. -cardia
2. -ectasis
3. -pathy
4. brady-
5. -sclerosis
6. echo-
7. tachy-
8. -graphy
9. -um
10. -megaly
11. arteri/o
12. cardi/o or coron/o
13. pulmon/o
14. thromb/o
15. hem/o
16. endocardi/o
17. angi/o or vascul/o
18. mesenter/o
19. myocardi/o
20. phleb/o
21. lymphaden/o
22. aort/o
23. lymphangi/o
24. coron/o or cardi/o
25. ather/o
26. epicardi/o
27. lymph/o
28. atri/o
29. sept/o
30. vascul/o or angi/o
31. cyan//o
32. pericardi/o

Wordshop:
1. cardiomyopathy
2. thrombophlebitis
3. tachycardia
4. echocardiography
5. lymphangiectasis
6. angioplasty
7. dysrhythmia
8. endocarditis
9. cardialgia
10. pericardiocentesis
11. atrioventricular
12. phlebectomy
13. arteriosclerosis
14. endarterectomy
15. venotripsy

Term Sorting:

Anatomy and Physiology: annulus, aorta, atrium, bundle of His, capillary, diastole, endocardium, mesentery, Purkinje fibers, septum, spleen, systole, tricuspid valve, ventricle, venule

Pathology: angina pectoris, arrhythmia, arteriosclerosis, BBB, bradycardia, cardiomegaly, cyanosis, endocarditis, hemorrhoid, hypertension, ischemia, lymphadenitis, MVP, SOB, splenomegaly

Procedures: angiocardiography, angiotripsy, CABG, cardioplegia, cardioversion, ECG, electrocardiogram, endarterectomy, MIDCAB, pericardiocentesis, pericardiolysis, phlebography, phlebotomy, septoplasty, splenopexy

Translations:

1. myocardial infarction, coronary artery bypass graft
2. cerebral infarction, monoplegia
3. edema, heart failure (HF)
4. coronary artery atherosclerosis, cardiodynia
5. phlebography, phlebitis
6. diaphoresis, tachycardia
7. angina pectoris, ischemia
8. pericardiocentesis, cardiac tamponade
9. tricuspid stenosis (TS), valvuloplasty
10. cardiomyopathy, left ventricular assist device (LVAD)

Chapter 10

Exercise 1

1. R	2. L	3. Q	4. T	5. M	6. O
7. G	8. C	9. X	10. Y	11. E	12. F
13. P	14. D	15. S	16. B	17. V	18. BB
19. I	20. Z	21. W	22. J	23. AA	24. U
25. H	26. K	27. A	28. CC	29. EE	30. DD
31. N					

Exercise 2

1. K	2. J	3. O	4. D	5. A	6. F
7. T	8. E	9. G	10. S	11. M	12. I
13. B	14. H	15. N	16. C	17. P	18. R
19. L	20. Q				

21. condition (-ia) excessive (hyper-) carbon dioxide (capn/o)
    Term: hypercapnia
22. blood condition (-emia) deficient (hypo-) oxygen (ox/o)
    Term: hypoxemia
23. condition (-ia) without (a-) sound (phon/o)
    Term: aphonia

24. chest (thorac/o) pain (-dynia)
    Term: thoracodynia
25. fast (tachy-) breathing (-pnea)
    Term: tachypnea

Exercise 3

1. D	2. B	3. F	4. A	5. E	6. C

7. nas/o (nose) + laryng/o (larynx) + -itis (inflammation)
   Def: inflammation of the nose and larynx (voice box)
8. trache/o (trachea) + -itis (inflammation)
   Def: inflammation of the trachea
9. bronchiol/o (bronchiole) + -itis (inflammation)
   Def: inflammation of the bronchioles

Exercise 4

1. H	2. C	3. A	4. E	5. I	6. D
7. G	8. B	9. F			

10. spasm condition (-ismus) larynx (laryng/o)
    Term: laryngismus
11. abnormal condition (-osis) fungus (myc/o) nose (rhin/o)
    Term: rhinomycosis
12. dilation (-ectasis) bronchus (bronchi/o)
    Term: bronchiectasis
13. abnormal condition (-osis) lung (pneum/o) dust (coni/o)
    Term: pneumoconiosis

Exercise 5

1. I	2. B	3. D	4. A	5. F	6. H
7. G	8. E	9. C			

10. bronch/o (bronchus) + -spasm (sudden, involuntary contraction)
    Def: sudden involuntary contraction of the bronchus
11. a- (not) + tel/e (complete) + -ectasis (dilation)
    Def: incomplete dilation, or collapse (of a lung)
12. py/o (pus) + -thorax (chest, pleural cavity)
    Def: pus in the chest pleural cavity
13. hydr/o (water, fluid) + -thorax (chest, pleural cavity)
    Def: fluid in the pleural cavity

Exercise 6

1. papilloma
2. mesothelioma
3. oat cell carcinoma
4. adenocarcinoma

Exercise 7

1. clear to auscultation

2. no wheezes
3. no crackles
4. chest x-ray
5. atelectasis

Exercise 8

1. C   2. A   3. G   4. H   5. N   6. M
7. O   8. E   9. J   10. L   11. I   12. B
13. F   14. K   15. D

16. recording (-graphy) bronchi (bronch/o)
    Term: bronchography
17. cutting out (-ectomy) ethmoid bone
    (ethmoid/o)
    Term: ethmoidectomy
18. fixation (-desis) pleura (pleur/o)
    Term: pleurodesis
19. new opening (-stomy) trachea (trache/o)
    Term: tracheostomy
20. cutting out (-plasty) turbinate (turbin/o)
    Term: turbinectomy
21. surgically forming (-plasty) nose (rhin/o)
    Term: rhinoplasty
22. surgical puncture (-centesis) pleura (pleur/o)
    Term: pleurocentesis

Exercise 9

1. C   2. E   3. D   4. A   5. B

6. hand-held nebulizer, HHN
7. inhaler
8. ventilator

Exercise 10

1. lungs
2. breathing in
3. bronchoscopy
4. nose, pharynx, and lungs
5. nasopharyngitis with symptoms of
    pneumonia

Exercise 11

1. slight degree of excessive sweating; slight
    bluish discoloration of the nail beds
2. a pulse oximeter is clipped onto the earlobe or
    the finger
3. wheezes are whistling sounds on breathing;
    rhonchi are rumbling sounds heard on
    auscultation
4. a peak flow meter measures breathing capacity

Chapter 10 Review

Word Part Definitions:

1. tachy-
2. hyper-

3. hypo-
4. brady-
5. -pnea
6. -ptysis
7. -thorax
8. dys-
9. -ismus
10. -ectasis
11. capn/o
12. pneum/o
13. pector/o
14. spir/o
15. apic/o
16. pleur/o
17. nas/o or rhin/o
18. sept/o
19. coni/o
20. myc/o
21. pharyng/o
22. muc/o
23. ox/i
24. phren/o
25. trache/o
26. py/o
27. cost/o
28. sin/o
29. tonsill/o
30. salping/o
31. laryng/o
32. rhin/o or nas/o

Wordshop:

1. hypercapnia
2. rhinomycosis
3. pneumoconiosis
4. tracheoesophageal
5. exhalation
6. pleurodynia
7. rhinopharyngitis
8. septoplasty
9. pyothorax
10. tracheoitis
11. pleurodesis
12. intercostal
13. oximetry
14. bronchoscopy

Term Sorting:

Anatomy and Physiology: alveolus, diaphragm,
   epiglottis, eustachian tube, exhalation,
   mediastinum, mucus, olfaction, oropharynx,
   oxygen, oxyhemoglobin, phonation, pleura,
   sinus, trachea

Pathology: aphonia, apnea, ARDS, atelectasis,
   bronchiectasis, COPD, diphtheria, emphysema,
   epistaxis, hyperpnea, laryngismus, pneumonia,
   rhinomycosis, rhonchi, sinusitis

Procedures: bronchoscopy, CPAP, CXR, nebulizer, PEEP, pleurocentesis, pleurolysis, PSV, pulmonary resection, pulse oximetry, septoplasty, sinusotomy, tracheotomy, tracheostomy, ventilation

Translations:
1. dyspnea, shortness of breath (SOB)
2. dysphonia, laryngitis
3. stridor, epiglottitis
4. thoracodynia, pleural effusion
5. chest x-ray, pneumonia
6. pharyngitis, laryngitis
7. pulse oximetry, spirometry
8. deviated septum, septoplasty
9. pleurocentesis, hemothorax
10. bronchiectasis, chronic obstructive pulmonary disease (COPD)
11. laryngeal, tracheostomy

Chapter 11

Exercise 1
1. central nervous system (CNS), peripheral nervous system (PNS)
2. transmit, to
3. efferent, from
4. somatic, autonomic

Exercise 2
1. D   2. B   3. E   4. A   5. C

6. peri- (surrounding, around) + neur/o (nerve) + -al (pertaining to)
   Def: pertaining to surrounding a nerve
7. olig/o (scanty, few) + dendr/o (dendrite) + -itic (pertaining to)
   Def: pertaining to few dendrites
8. micro- (small) + -glia (glue) + -al (pertaining to)
   Def: pertaining to small glue (cells)

Exercise 3
A:
1. H   2. J   3. F   4. A   5. C   6. I
7. D   8. B   9. G   10. E
B:
1. H   2. B   3. A   4. D   5. C   6. F
7. I   8. E   9. G   10. J

11. intra- (within) + ventricul/o (ventricle) + -ar (pertaining to)
    Def: pertaining to within a ventricle
12. epi- (above) + dur/o (dura mater) + -al (pertaining to)
    Def: pertaining to above the dura mater

13. para- (near, beside) + spin/o (spine) + -al (pertaining to)
    Def: pertaining to near the spine
14. infra- (down, below) + cerebell/o (cerebellum) + -ar (pertaining to)
    Def: pertaining to below the cerebellum

Exercise 4
1. M   2. I   3. D   4. F   5. L   6. H
7. J   8. E   9. G   10. B   11. K   12. N
13. C   14. A

15. a- (without) + phas/o (speech) + -ia (condition)
    Def: condition of without speech
16. dys- (difficult) + phag/o (eat, swallow) + -ia (condition)
    Def: condition of difficult swallowing
17. hemat/o (blood) + -oma (tumor, mass)
    Def: mass of blood

Exercise 5
1. Parkinson's disease
2. Alzheimer's disease
3. migraine
4. epilepsy
5. transient ischemic attack (TIA)
6. multiple sclerosis (MS)
7. seizure (-lepsy) sleep (narc/o)
   Term: narcolepsy
8. difficult (dys-) sleep (somn/o) condition (-ia)
   Term: dyssomnia

Exercise 6
1. F   2. A   3. K   4. L   5. C   6. I
7. D   8. J   9. B   10. H   11. E   12. G

13. caus/o (burning) + -algia (pain)
    Def: burning pain
14. mer/o (thigh) + -algia (pain) par- (abnormal) + -esthetica (sensation)
    Def: abnormal sensation of thigh pain
15. poly- (many) + neur/o (nerve) + -pathy (disease process)
    Def: disease process of many nerves
16. hemi- (half) + -plegia (paralysis)
    Def: paralysis of half
17. di- (two) + -plegia (paralysis)
    Def: paralysis of two (sides)

Exercise 7
1. ganglia (gangli/o) nerve (neur/o) tumor (-oma)
   Term: ganglioneuroma
2. meninges (meningi/o) tumor (-oma)
   Term: meningioma
3. star (astr/o) cell (cyt/o) tumor (-oma)
   Term: astrocytoma

4. nerve (neur/o) fiber (fibr/o) tumor (-oma)
   Term: neurofibroma
5. medulla (medull/o) embryonic (blast/o) tumor
   (-oma)
   Term: medulloblastoma
6. nerve (neur/o) embryonic (blast/o) tumor (-oma)
   Term: neuroblastoma

Exercise 8
1. vertigo is dizziness; syncope means fainting
2. TIA is transient ischemic attack; a temporary
   lack of cerebral blood circulation due to an
   occlusion or a cerebral hemorrhage.
3. Aphasia is a condition of inability to speak.
4. Ataxia is a lack of muscular coordination.

Exercise 9
1. F   2. B   3. N   4. J   5. G   6. A
7. D   8. L   9. C   10. H   11. M   12. E
13. I   14. K

15. chem/o (chemical, drug) + thalam/o
    (thalamus) + -ectomy (cutting out)
    **Def: "cutting out" thalamus tissue using
    chemicals**
16. phren/o (phrenic nerve) + -emphraxis
    (crushing)
    Def: crushing the phrenic nerve
17. echo- (sound) + encephal/o (brain) + -graphy
    (recording)
    **Def: recording the brain using sound
    (waves)**
18. vag/o (vagus nerve) + -tomy (cutting)
    Def: cutting of the vagus nerve
19. neur/o (nerve) + -plasty (surgically forming)
    Def: surgically forming a nerve
20. ventricul/o (ventricle) + peritone/o
    (peritoneum) + -stomy (making a new opening)
    **Def: making a new opening between a
    ventricle and the peritoneum**

Exercise 10
1. H   2. G   3. E   4. C   5. B   6. D
7. F   8. A

Exercise 11
1. hemiparesis
2. dysarthria
3. parietal epidural hematoma
4. above

Chapter 11 Review

Word Part Definitions:
1. quadri-
2. -paresis

3. hemi-
4. poly-
5. mono-
6. -lepsy
7. -oma
8. para-
9. -emphraxis
10. -plegia
11. cortic/o
12. phag/o
13. tax/o
14. rhiz/o or radicul/o
15. cerebell/o
16. esthesi/o
17. blast/o
18. myel/o or cord/o
19. dur/o
20. phas/o
21. ventricul/o
22. encephal/o
23. cord/o or myel/o
24. dendr/o
25. narc/o or somn/o
26. neur/o
27. cerebr/o
28. astr/o
29. radicul/o or rhiz/o
30. somn/o or narc/o
31. pallid/o
32. mening/o

Wordshop:
1. polyneuropathy
2. encephalitis
3. quadriplegia
4. echoencephalography
5. neurotomy
6. aphasia
7. dysphagia
8. epilepsy
9. paresthesia
10. polysomnography
11. rhizotomy
12. neurexeresis
13. medulloblastoma
14. dyssomnia
15. hemiparesis

Term Sorting:
Anatomy and Physiology: BBB, cauda
   equina, cerebellum, CNS, CSF, dendrite,
   dura mater, ganglia, glia, meninges, neuron,
   neurotransmitter, synapse, thalamus, ventricle
Pathology: amnesia, aphasia, causalgia, diplegia,
   epilepsy, fasciculation, hematoma, meningioma,
   meningitis, MS, polyneuropathy, PPS, spasm,
   syncope, TIA

Procedures: chemothalamectomy, cordotomy, craniotomy, EEG, myelography, neurectomy, nerve block, neurexeresis, neuroplasty, phrenemphraxis, rhizotomy, sympathectomy, TENS, vagotomy, ventriculoperitoneostomy

Translations:
1. transient ischemic attack (TIA), contralateral
2. hemiparesis, aphasia
3. hematoma, amnesia
4. vertigo, syncope
5. migraine
6. hydrocephalus, ventriculocisternostomy
7. tremors, dysphagia
8. hemispherectomy, epilepsy
9. lumbar puncture, meningitis
10. polysomnography, dyssomnia

Chapter 12

Exercise 1
1. A   2. C   3. G   4. B   5. E   6. D
7. F

8. condition (-ia) without (an-) pleasure (hedon/o)
   Term: anhedonia
9. excessive (hyper-) movement (-kinesis)
   Term: hyperkinesis

Exercise 2
1. F   2. A   3. D   4. M   5. N   6. E
7. K   8. C   9. I   10. L   11. B   12. G
13. J   14. H   15. O   16. P

17. schiz/o (split) phren/o (mind) -ia (condition)
    Def: condition of split mind
18. para- (abnormal) -noia (condition of the mind)
    Def: abnormal condition of the mind
19. psych/o (mind) -osis (abnormal condition)
    Def: abnormal condition of the mind
20. cycl/o (recurring) -thymia (condition of the mind)
    Def: recurring condition of the mind
21. oneir/o (dream) -ism (state)
    Def: dream state

Exercise 3
1. L   2. G   3. A   4. P   5. Q   6. H
7. O   8. C   9. M   10. B   11. J   12. E
13. N   14. D   15. I   16. F   17. K

18. condition of fear (-phobia) marketplace (agora-)
    Term: agoraphobia
19. condition of fear (-phobia) female (gyn/e)
    Term: gynephobia

20. condition (-ia) without (in-) sleep (somn/o)
    Term: insomnia
21. condition of madness (-mania) woman (nymph/o)
    Term: nymphomania
22. condition of fear (-phobia) heights, extremes (acro-)
    Term: acrophobia
23. condition (-ism) walking (ambul/o) sleep (somn/o)
    Term: somnambulism

Exercise 4
A:
1. L   2. A   3. B   4. F   5. I   6. C
7. G   8. D   9. K   10. H   11. E   12. M
13. J   14. N
B:
1. C   2. E   3. A   4. F   5. B   6. G
7. D

8. pyr/o (fire) + -mania (condition of madness)
   Def: condition of madness concerning fires
9. trich/o (hair) + till/o (to pull) + -mania (condition of madness)
   Def: condition of pulling hair madness
10. necr/o (death) + phil/o (attraction) + -ia (condition)
    Def: condition of attraction to death or the dead

Exercise 5
1. full affect range
2. euthymic
3. no evidence of delusion
4. PTSD (post-traumatic stress disorder)

Exercise 6
1. D   2. B   3. F   4. C   5. G   6. A
7. E   8. H

Exercise 7
1. behavioral therapy
2. light therapy
3. ECT (electroconvulsive therapy)
4. psychoanalysis
5. cognitive therapy
6. narcosynthesis
7. adaptive behavioral therapy
8. biofeedback
9. treatment (-therapy) drugs (pharmac/o)
   Term: pharmacotherapy
10. process of (-ation) removal (de-) poison (toxic/o)
    Term: detoxification
11. pertaining to (-ic) power (dynam/o) mind (psych/o)
    Term: psychodynamic

12. state (-sis) sleep (hypn/o)
    Term: hypnosis

Exercise 8
1. G   2. C   3. E   4. H   5. D   6. B
7. A   8. F

Exercise 9
1. Panic disorder is an anxiety disorder characterized by recurrent severe panic attacks.
2. autistic disorder; manifested by abnormal development of social interaction, impaired communication, and repetitive behaviors
3. anxiety
4. sleepwalking

Chapter 12 Review

Word Part Definitions:
1. -lalia
2. -mania
3. an-
4. -phobia
5. -thymia
6. agora-
7. eu-
8. -oid
9. cata-
10. -ism
11. acro-
12. -kinesis
13. para-
14. hedon/o
15. cycl/o
16. orex/o
17. ment/o or psych/o or phren/o
18. somat/o
19. anthrop/o
20. nymph/o
21. oneir/o
22. pol/o
23. psych/o or ment/o or phren/o
24. klept/o
25. calcul/o
26. hypn/o or somn/o
27. somn/o or hypn/o
28. phren/o or psych/o or ment/o
29. phil/o
30. pyr/o
31. claustr/o
32. phor/o
33. ped/o

Wordshop:
1. anhedonia
2. dyscalculia
3. gynephobia
4. psychosis
5. pyromania
6. hyperkinesis
7. oneirism
8. acrophobia
9. hypnosis
10. somnambulism
11. trichotillomania
12. hypersomnia
13. cyclothymia
14. echolalia
15. schizophrenia

Translations:
1. blunted affect, panic disorder (PD)
2. anorexia nervosa, cyclothymia
3. hypersomnia, somnambulism
4. light therapy, anhedonia
5. dysphoria, euphoria, bipolar disorder (BD or BP)
6. anxiety, posttraumatic stress disorder (PTSD)
7. acrophobia, claustrophobia
8. obsessive-compulsive disorder (OCD)
9. psychosis, hallucinations
10. attention-deficit hyperactivity disorder (ADHD)

Chapter 13

Exercise 1
A:
1. B   2. F   3. H   4. C   5. D   6. I
7. A   8. E   9. G
B:
1. D   2. E   3. A   4. G   5. B   6. C
7. F   8. H   9. I

Exercise 2
A:
1. C   2. G   3. D   4. E   5. F   6. B
7. A
B:
1. H   2. I   3. O   4. L   5. A   6. M
7. B   8. D   9. J   10. C   11. G   12. F
13. K   14. E   15. N

Exercise 3
1. D   2. A   3. K   4. P   5. G   6. J
7. M   8. B   9. F   10. O   11. L   12. C
13. I   14. E   15. H   16. N

17. eyelid (blephar/o) drooping (-ptosis)
    Term: blepharoptosis
18. tear gland (dacryoaden/o) inflammation (-itis)
    Term: dacryoadenitis
19. cornea (kerat/o) softening (-malacia)

Term: keratomalacia
20. eyelid (blephar/o) slackening (-chalasis)
    Term: blepharochalasis

Exercise 4
1. K   2. A   3. J   4. B   5. I   6. C
7. F   8. E   9. H   10. D   11. G

12. no (a-) lens (phak/o) condition (-ia)
    Term: aphakia
13. optic disk (papill/o) swelling (-edema)
    Term: papilledema
14. all (pan-) eye (ophthalm/o) inflammation (-itis)
    Term: panophthalmitis

Exercise 5
1. B   2. A   3. D   4. I   5. J   6. C
7. L   8. K   9. N   10. F   11. M   12. H
13. G   14. E

15. visual condition (-opia) double (dipl/o)
    Term: diplopia
16. mass (-oma) darkness (scot/o)
    Term: scotoma
17. condition (-ia) not (an-) equal (is/o) pupil
    (cor/o)
    Term: anisocoria
18. state of (-iasis) dilation (mydr/o)
    Term: mydriasis
19. tumor (-oma) embryonic (blast/o) retina (retin/o)
    Term: retinoblastoma
20. vision condition (-opia) old age (presby-)
    Term: presbyopia

Exercise 6
1. E   2. G   3. B   4. H   5. F   6. C
7. D   8. A   9. I

Exercise 7
1. A   2. F   3. H   4. B   5. D   6. I
7. G   8. C   9. E

10. blephar/o (eyelid) + -plasty (surgically forming)
    Def: surgically forming the eyelid
11. irid/o (iris) + -ectomy (cutting out)
    Def: cutting out the iris
12. conjunctiv/o (conjunctiva) + -plasty (surgically
    forming)
    Def: surgically forming the conjunctiva
13. vitr/o (vitreous humor) + -ectomy (cutting out)
    Def: cutting out the vitreous humor

Exercise 8
1. C   2. E   3. B   4. A   5. D

Exercise 9
1. cataract

2. before the operation
3. broken down and removed
4. posterior lens implant
5. topical

Exercise 10
1. diplopia is double vision; cephalgia is headache
2. nearsighted due to malcurvature of the cornea
3. tonometry
4. near or around the limbus

Chapter 13 Review

Word Part Definition:
1. -ptosis
2. -metry
3. -scopy
4. extra-
5. -chalasia
6. pan-
7. -malacia
8. -opia or -opsia
9. -plasty
10. eso-
11. -opsia or -opia
12. ec-
13. lacrim/o or dacry/o
14. kerat/o
15. dacry/o or lacrim/o
16. ophthalm/o
17. dacryocyst/o
18. cycl/o
19. opt/o
20. scot/o
21. blephar/o or palpebr/o
22. irid/o
23. nyctal/o
24. retin/o
25. core/o
26. phot/o
27. canth/o
28. papill/o
29. palpebr/o or blephar/o
30. goni/o
31. dacryoaden/o
32. phac/o
33. scler/o

Wordshop:
1. aphakia
2. achromatopsia
3. dacryoadenitis
4. blepharoptosis
5. photophobia
6. presbyopia
7. esotropia

8. panophthalmitis
9. hypermetropia
10. anisocoria
11. cyclodiathermy
12. keratoplasty
13. canthorrhaphy
14. mydriasis
15. hemianopsia

Term Sorting:
Anatomy and Physiology: accommodation, annulus of Zinn, canthus, conjunctiva, cornea, iris, lacrimation, limbus, macula lutea, oculus sinistra, palpebration, pupil, Schlemm's canal, sclera, uvea
Pathology: aphakia, blepharitis, chalazion, dacryocystitis, exophthalmos, glaucoma, hyphema, keratomalacia, nyctalopia, optic papillitis, photophobia, pinguecula, retinoblastoma, scotoma, strabismus
Procedures: Amsler grid, canthorrhaphy, conjunctivoplasty, cyclodiathermy, diopters, enucleation of eyeball, fluorescein angiography, gonioscopy, iridoplasty, LASIK, radial keratotomy, slit lamp, tonometry, VA, vitrectomy

Translations:
1. photophobia, epiphora
2. miosis, synechia, iridocyclitis
3. anisocoria, hyphema
4. achromatopsia, myopia
5. papilledema
6. glaucoma, tonometry
7. blepharoplasty, blepharoptosis
8. scleral buckling, retinal detachment
9. strabismus
10. Amsler grid test, age-related macular degeneration (ARMD)
11. Schirmer tear test
12. nyctalopia, retinitis pigmentosa

Chapter 14

Exercise 1
1. E, I   2. B   3. K   4. A   5. H, J 6. F
7. N   8. D   9. C   10. L   11. M 12. G

13. eustachian tube
14. mastoid process
15. outer, middle, inner
16. pinna, auricle
17. vestibule, semicircular canals, cochlea
18. utricle, saccule

Exercise 2
1. A   2. H   3. E   4. B   5. G   6. C
7. D   8. F

9. tympan/o (tympanum, eardrum) + -sclerosis (abnormal condition of hardening)
   Def: abnormal condition of hardening of the eardrum
10. chol/e (bile) + steat/o (fat) + -oma (mass, tumor)
    Def: mass of fat and cholesterol
11. ot/o (ear) + -itis (inflammation) + medi/o (middle) + -a (noun ending)
    Def: inflammation of the middle ear

Exercise 3
1. E   2. H   3. A   4. B   5. G   6. C
7. F   8. D

9. excessive (hyper-) hearing (-acusis)
   Term: hyperacusis
10. inflammation (-itis) inner ear (labyrinth/o)
    Term: labyrinthitis
11. discharge (-rrhea) ear (ot/o)
    Term: otorrhea
12. pain (-algia) ear (ot/o)
    Term: otalgia
13. mass (-oma) earwax (cerumin/o)
    Term: ceruminoma

Exercise 4
1. A   2. G   3. C   4. J   5. D   6. I
7. H   8. F   9. B   10. E

11. tympan/o (eardrum) + -metry (measuring)
    Def: measuring the eardrum
12. -plasty (surgically forming) + ot/o (ear)
    Def: surgically forming the ear
13. -metry (measuring) + audi/o (hearing)
    Def: measuring hearing

Exercise 5
1. C   2. D   3. A   4. B

Exercise 6
1. no lymphadenopathy
2. no wheezing
3. tympanic membrane
4. oropharynx
5. otitis media

Chapter 14 Review

Word Part Definitions:
1. presby-
2. -acusis
3. -plasty
4. -oma
5. -peri
6. endo-

7. -metry
8. -sclerosis
9. staped/o
10. helic/o
11. cerumin/o
12. myring/o or tympan/o
13. audi/o or acous/o
14. auricul/o
15. chondr/o
16. acous/o or audi/o
17. ot/o
18. labyrinth/o
19. tympan/o or myring/o
20. salping/o

Wordshop:
1. otorrhea
2. presbycusis
3. tympanoplasty
4. otosclerosis
5. labyrinthitis
6. audiometry
7. perichondrium
8. pharyngotympanic
9. diplacusis
10. hyperacusis
11. stapedoplasty
12. myringotomy or tympanotomy
13. electrocochleography
14. cholesteatoma

Term Sorting:
Anatomy and Physiology: auricle, cerumen, cochlea, endolymph, eustachian tube, helix, labyrinth, organ of Corti, pinna, stapes, tympanic membrane, vestibule
Pathology: acoustic neuroma, ceruminoma, diplacusis, mastoiditis, Ménière's disease, myringitis, OM, otalgia, otitis externa, otorrhea, otosclerosis, presbycusis, tinnitus, tympanosclerosis
Procedures: audiometry, cochlear implant, ECOG, mastoidectomy, myringotomy, ossiculectomy, otoplasty, otoscopy, stapediolysis, tympanometry, UNHS

Translations:
1. otoscope, otitis media
2. audiometry, presbycusis
3. tinnitus, acoustic neuroma
4. otoplasty
5. otosclerosis
6. mastoiditis, mastoidectomy
7. ossiculectomy, ankylosis of ear ossicles
8. eustachian salpingitis, myringitis
9. tympanosclerosis
10. diplacusis

Chapter 15

Exercise 1
1. I   2. N   3. T   4. U   5. R   6. D
7. S   8. P   9. A   10. Q   11. J   12. G
13. F   14. M   15. L   16. H   17. K   18. B
19. E   20. O   21. C

Exercise 2
1. hypophysis
2. hypothalamus
3. adenohypophysis
4. metabolism, calcium
5. kidneys
6. medulla, cortex
7. glucagon, insulin
8. ketones
9. mediastinum, immune
10. pineal, melatonin, sleep

Exercise 3
1. D   2. E   3. H   4. F   5. G   6. A
7. C   8. B

9. hyper- (excessive) + glyc/o (sugar, glucose) + -emia (blood condition)
Def: Condition of excessive glucose in the blood
10. glycos/o (sugar, glucose) + -uria (urinary condition)
Def: Condition of sugar in the urine

Exercise 4
1. C   2. B   3. A   4. H   5. G   6. F
7. I   8. Q   9. P   10. O   11. D   12. L
13. N   14. E   15. K   16. M   17. J

18. excessive (hyper-) thyroid gland (thyroid/o) condition (-ism)
Term: hyperthyroidism
19. deficient (hypo-) glucose (glyc/o) blood condition (-emia)
Term: hypoglycemia
20. extremities (acro-) enlargement (-megaly)
Term: acromegaly
21. before (pro-) old age (ger/o) condition (-ia)
Term: progeria

Exercise 5
1. F   2. B   3. A   4. D   5. G   6. J
7. C   8. I   9. E   10. H   11. K

12. hyper- (excessive) + lipid/o (fat) + -emia (blood condition)
Def: blood condition of excessive fats

13. hypo- (deficient) + calc/o (calcium) + -emia (blood condition)
    Def: blood condition of deficient calcium
14. hyper- (excessive) + cholesterol/o (cholesterol) + -emia (blood condition)
    Def: blood condition of excessive cholesterol

Exercise 6
1. B   2. F   3. D   4. C   5. E   6. A

Exercise 7
1. Type 2 diabetes mellitus (non-insulin-dependent diabetes mellitus)
2. diabetic retinopathy
3. Body Mass Index (BMI)
4. hypothyroidism

Exercise 8
1. RIA
2. A1c
3. total calcium
4. urine glucose
5. TFTs

Exercise 9
1. cutting out (-ectomy) pancreas (pancreat/o) duodenum (duoden/o)
   Term: pancreatoduodenectomy
2. suturing (-rrhaphy) adrenal gland (adrenal/o)
   Term: adrenalorrhaphy
3. cutting out a stone (-lithotomy) pancreas (pancreat/o)
   Term: pancreatolithotomy
4. viewing (-scopy) thyroid gland (thyroid/o)
   Term: thyroidoscopy
5. cutting out (-ectomy) pituitary gland (pituit/o)
   Term: pituitectomy

Exercise 10
1. C   2. A   3. D   4. B

Exercise 11
1. parathyroid hormone
2. subtotal parathyroidectomy
3. calcium
4. intraoperative PTH monitoring
5. parathyroid hyperplasia

Chapter 15 Review

Word Part Definitions:
1. -graphy
2. -uria
3. endo-
4. hyper-
5. supra-
6. hypo-
7. -emia
8. exo-
9. -crine
10. acro-
11. poly-
12. -ectomy
13. kal/i
14. hypophys/o or pituitar/o
15. chrom/o
16. natr/o
17. gluc/o or glyc/o
18. gonad/o
19. parathyroid/o
20. trop/o
21. aden/o
22. thym/o
23. glyc/o or gluc/o
24. phe/o
25. crin/o
26. thyr/o
27. thalam/o
28. adren/o
29. calc/o
30. pancreat/o
31. cyt/o
32. pituitar/o or hypophys/o

Wordshop:
1. suprarenal
2. hyperglycemia
3. polydipsia
4. hypothyroidism
5. acromegaly
6. hypokalemia
7. ketoacidosis
8. pheochromocytoma
9. pancreatoduodenectomy
10. hyponatremia

Term Sorting:
Anatomy and Physiology: ADH, adrenal cortex, calcitonin, hypothalamus, insulin, islets of Langerhans, ketone, melatonin, metabolism, neurohypophysis, oxytocin, parathyroid, suprarenals, thymosin, TSH

Pathology: adiposity, Cushing's syndrome, cystic fibrosis, dehydration, DI, DM, GHD, glycosuria, hyperthyroidism, hypoglycemia, ketonuria, polydipsia, progeria, SIADH, thymoma

Procedures: A1c, adrenalectomy, ERP, FPG, OGTT, pancreatoduodenectomy, pinealotomy, RIA, TFTs

Translations:
1. polydipsia, polyuria
2. exophthalmos, hyperthyroidism
3. hypocalcemia, tetany, hypoparathyroidism
4. hyperglycemia, hypokalemia
5. hyperinsulinism, hypoglycemia
6. islet cell carcinoma, pancreatoduodenectomy
7. type 1 diabetes, oral glucose tolerance test (OGTT)
8. thyroidectomy, goiter
9. hyponatremia, syndrome of inappropriate antidiuretic hormone (SIADH)
10. fasting plasma glucose (FPG), type 2 diabetes
11. acromegaly, adenohypophysis

Index

Note: Page numbers followed by "f" indicate figures "t" indicate tables and "b" indicate boxes.

Root Operations That Have Common Suffixes

Root Operation	Suffixes	Definition
Alteration	-plasty surgically forming -ectomy cutting out	Modifying the natural anatomic structure of a body part without affecting the function of the body part.
Bypass	-stomy making a new opening	Altering the route of passage of the contents of a tubular body part.
Destruction	-emphraxis obstruting, crushing	Physical eradication of all or a portion of a body part by the direct use of energy, force, or a destructive agent.
Dilation	-plasty surgically forming	Expanding an orifice or the lumen of a tubular body part.
Division	clasis intentional breaking -tomy cutting	Cutting out or off, without replacement, a portion of a body part.
Drainage	-centesis surgical puncture -stomy making a new opening -tomy cutting	Taking or letting out fluids and/or gases from a body part.
Excision	-ectomy cutting out	Cutting out or off, without replacement, a portion of a body part.
Extirpation	-ectomy cutting out -lithotomy cutting out a stone	Taking or cutting out solid matter from a body part.
Extraction	-abrasion scraping of -exeresis tearing out	Pulling or Stripping out or off all or a portion of a body part.
Fragmentation	-tripsy crushing	Breaking solid matter in a body part into pieces.
Fusion	-desis binding	Joining together portions of an articular body part rendering the articular body part immobile.
Inspection	-scopy viewing	Visually and/or manually exploring a body part.
Occlusion	-tripsy crushing	Completely closing an orifice or lumen of a tubular body part.
Perfusion	-apheresis removal	Extracorporeal treatment by diffusion or therapeutic fluid.
Release	-lysis breaking down -tomy cutting	Freeing a body part from an abnormal physical constraint.
Removal		Taking out or off a device from a body part.
Repair	-pexy suspension -plasty surgically forming -rrhaphy suturing	Restoring, to the extent possible, a body part to its normal anatomic structure and function.
Replacement	-plasty surgically forming	Putting in or on biological or synthetic material that physically takes the place and/or function of all or a portion of a body part.
Reposition	-pexy suspension -plasty surgically forming	Moving to its normal location or other suitable location all or a portion of a body part
Resection	-ectomy cutting out	Cutting out or off, without replacement, all of a body part
Supplement	-plasty surgically forming -rrhaphy suturing	Putting in or on biological or synthetic material that physically reinforces and/or augments the function of a portion of a body part.